Eye Movements and Their Role in Visual and Cognitive Processes

Reviews of Oculomotor Research

ELSEVIER

AMSTERDAM · NEW YORK · OXFORD

Reviews of Oculomotor Research
Volume 4

Eye Movements and Their Role in Visual and Cognitive Processes

Edited by

Eileen Kowler

Department of Psychology
Rutgers University
New Brunswick, New Jersey
U.S.A.

1990

ELSEVIER

AMSTERDAM · NEW YORK · OXFORD

ISBN 0-444-81254-7 (volume)
ISSN 0168-8375 (series)

Published by:
Elsevier Science Publishers B.V.
(Biomedical Division)
P.O. Box 211
1000 AE Amsterdam
The Netherlands

Sole distributors for the U.S.A. and Canada:
Elsevier Science Publishing Company, Inc.
655 Avenue of the Americas
New York, NY 10010
U.S.A.

Library of Congress Cataloging in Publication data

Eye movements and their role in visual and cognitive processes /
edited by E. Kowler.
p. cm. -- (Reviews of oculomotor research, ISSN 0168-8375 ;
v. 4)
Includes bibliographical references.
Includes index.
ISBN 0-444-81254-7 (alk. paper)
1. Eye -- Movements. I. Kowler, E. II. Series.
[DNLM: 1. Cognition -- physiology. 2. Eye Movements -- physiology.
3. Neuropsychology. 4. Visual Perception -- physiology. W1 RE253JNM
v. 4 / WW 400 E975]
QP477.5.E94 1990
152.14 -- dc20
DNLM/DLC
for Library of Congress 90-3562
CIP

Printed on acid-free paper
Printed in The Netherlands

Preface

This is the first book to deal exclusively with oculomotor performance in a series that, up to this point, has been devoted largely to reviews of research on oculomotor anatomy and physiology. I take the significance of the publication of this book in the present series to be recognition that a genuine understanding of eye movement will not come about through studies of neurons alone. We need to know about the capacity to make different kinds of eye movement, and about how such oculomotor capacity is used to accomplish different sorts of visual and cognitive tasks. In other words, we need to know how the eye can move and why it moves in particular ways.

Most oculomotor researchers (and visual and cognitive scientists as well) share a general idea of what eye movements accomplish. We make saccades to bring selected, eccentric images to the fovea, and we make smooth eye movements to keep them there. These ideas are not controversial, but, by themselves, are far too vague to play an important role in theories of eye movement, vision, cognition, or neural organization. It is one thing, for example, to view the saccadic system as designed to rapidly direct the line of sight to a single, simple eccentric target, and then to develop one's behavioral and neural models accordingly. It is quite another to ask how human beings program brisk sequences of saccades to *selected* regions within detailed, patterned, visual environments with sufficient accuracy to perceive the relevant visual details. This is, of course, precisely what we do so effortlessly when we read. Similarly, we recognize that smooth eye movements keep images sufficiently stable to support clear vision, but unless we know how stable images are supposed to be (too little slip can be as harmful as too much), and the 'tricks' the visual system has evolved to cope with inevitable oculomotor imprecision, we will end up with distorted ideas about smooth oculomotor function and miss completely the important ways that visual, cognitive and oculomotor capacities evolved together for mutual compatibility. In short, considering eye movements separately from the visual and cognitive tasks they are designed to perform can give a misleading impression of how the system works. Considering eye movement, vision, and cognition together is a potentially powerful tool for understanding brain function. This book attempts to link these three areas.

Attemps to link theories of eye movement with theories of vision and cognition are not new. One of the oldest examples is Lotze's (1884) theory of 'local signs'.

'Local signs' were the location-codes attached to each retinal cell that allowed us to properly sense the spatial position of the stimulating light. According to Lotze, local signs could not be innate because the 'soul has no spatial extent'. Instead, Lotze proposed that local signs were learned as a result of reflexive eye movements evoked by the stimulation of eccentric retinal cells. The local signs were memory traces of the "magnitude of the achievement" necessary to bring the line of sight to eccentric retinal points.

Lotze's theory of local signs contained many of the elements found in modern theories that attempt to link visual, cognitive and oculomotor events. He recognized, for example, the inherent limitation of vision without eye movements, that is, he recognized the poor resolving capability of eccentric retinal locations. He also included an underlying model of oculomotor control. His was a simple, reflexive model in which stimulation of a receptor is sufficient to evoke the appropriate saccade automatically. Lest one be tempted to regard Lotze's proposal of retinal local signs merely as a quaint historical curiosity, consider that a current area of controversy among visual scientists is the question of how we 'know' the location of the receptors with sufficient accuracy to resolve the extremely fine lines of interference fringes imaged on the retina.

Memories of Lotze are also triggered by the classical problem of the way in which non-visual (sometimes called 'extraretinal') signals accompanying eye movements (either proprioceptive signals or an efferent copy of the issued oculomotor command) are involved in the ability to determine the location of an object with respect to ourselves. Discussion of this classical problem is the primary topic of two of the chapters in this volume. Skavenski discusses the contribution of non-visual signals to both perceptual and motor localization. He reviews long-standing controversies about the accuracy of non-visual signals and about the relative contribution of proprioceptive signals and the efferent copy to localization. Wallach evaluates the role of smooth pursuit eye movements in the perception of motion by showing how the perceptual system resolves experimentally-produced conflicts between object-relative cues and subject-relative cues to motion (the former consist of changes in the retinal position of objects relative to each other, the latter consist of either retinal image motion or non-visual signals accompanying smooth pursuit). Collewijn and Erkelens consider the contribution of non-visual signals accompanying vergence eye movements to the perception of depth when they review the role of eye movements in binocular vision. Sperling discusses both the visual and the non-visual events accompanying saccades when he considers how we perceive a clear image of a stationary world despite continual movements of the eye. Viviani reviews the evidence for the participation of non-visual signals in the control of saccades.

There is a surprising degree of consensus among these authors – surprising given the divergence of styles and approaches – that non-visual signals are important for motor localization, which is based on the *absolute* location of a target in space with respect to the viewer. Non-visual signals appear to be less important for judging the apparent position or motion of an object. Such perceptual judgments, expressed by a verbal report rather than a movement of the eye or limb, are often based on the *relative*, rather than absolute, location of an object with respect to other objects in the visual field.

The analysis of relative visual location may come into play very early in the processing of visual information, according to Steinman and Levinson's chapter. They discuss the remarkable tolerance of vision for fairly large amounts of image motion in their review of the significance of eye movements for the detection of contrast and spatial detail. Similarly, Collewijn and Erkelens show that percepts of motion-in-depth tolerate large amounts of binocular image motion, produced by changes in vergence eye movements, because the percepts depend on changes in relative, rather than absolute, binocular disparity. These chapters point out that the significance of the visual system's tolerance for large amounts of image motion was not appreciated until quite recently, when recordings of eye movements in freely-moving people showed retinal image velocities to be much higher than observed in traditional studies, in which the head is supported by a biteboard. The reliance of vision and perception on relative, rather than absolute, position or motion is clearly valuable to the organism. It means that perceptual judgments remain unchanged despite the retinal perturbations generated by eye movements.

Another major message emerging from various chapters in this volume is the rejection of the view, going back at least to Lotze, that eye movements are pure reflexes evoked by changes in the position of lights in the visual field. Eye movements are guided by visual information, but they also depend on such things as decisions about where one might want to look to find useful information, and on how quickly new information must be obtained. The importance of voluntary decisions to the programming of saccades, for example, has long inspired researchers to try to infer the nature of hidden cognitive processes from examination of the overt, readily observable, movements of the eyes. The chapters by Viviani and by Suppes critically examine such attempts as part of their general reviews of the role of saccades in visual search and visual problem-solving. Each concludes, for somewhat different reasons, that there is little hope of reading thoughts from saccadic scan patterns, at least not without the guidance of a well-developed theory of the underlying cognitive processes accompanying the scanning. O'Regan, in his chapter reviewing eye movements and reading, maintains that the link between saccadic eye movements and cognitive processes can be understood provided that both high-level (i.e., decisional) and low-level (i.e., visuo-motor) constraints on the eye movements are known.

The contribution of both low-level visuo-motor factors and high-level cognitive factors to the control of saccades and smooth eye movements is reviewed in my chapter. I argue that the contribution of selective attention, expectations and memory (high-level control) to the programming of eye movements is far more pervasive than has been conventionally assumed. Models neglecting high-level control do not capture the fundamental characteristics of human oculomotor performance. Pavel's chapter deals with one aspect of high-level control, namely, predictive eye movement. He discusses attempts to build mathematical models of predictive eye movements, and offers some new models based on theories of adaptive neural networks.

My reading of all these chapters leads me to the conclusion that while there may be important differences between the *sensory* information controlling eye movements and perception – signals of absolute position or motion controlling the former, and signals of relative position or motion controlling the latter – there is but *one* set of *cognitive* decisions participating in the joint control of movement and mentation. The challenge is to trace the pathway from thought to eye movement. Such attempts will be guided by ideas about the function of eye movements obtained from the study of vision and cognition while the eye is in motion. At the same time, theories of vision and cognition must take into account the constraints imposed by the need for eye movements in the acquisition of accurate visual information. It is my hope that this book has illustrated the benefits of considering eye movements, vision and cognition all in consort for the understanding of human thought and action.

A word about our approach to the assigned topics: I encouraged the authors to evaluate research on their respective topics critically. They were asked to try to lay out the fundamental problems researchers have been (or should be) trying to solve. They were encouraged to examine the assumptions made in prior research, and, in addition, to consider limitations imposed by currently popular methodology, by currently popular experimental paradigms, or by available instrumentation. This charge has led to a set of chapters in which authors were, to say the least, not shy about expressing their points of view. If readers find themselves persuaded by any of our arguments, or sufficiently disturbed to return to the source papers for detailed study, or to invent new experiments or new theories to deal with the many, important unsolved problems highlighted in this volume, then we will feel that we have accomplished a lot.

Preparation of this book was supported, in part, by the U.S. Air Force Office of Scientific Research, Life Sciences Directorate (grant number 88-0171). I thank several individuals who made important intellectual and technical contributions at various stages of this project: Vin Asarpota, Han Collewijn, Genevieve Haddad, Peiyuan He, Eli Krantz, Thomas V. Papathomas, Zygmunt Pizlo, 'Martin' Regan, Robert Steinman, Douglas Williams and Guo-Liang Zhu. I also thank Nello Spiteri, Tine Peereboom and Roger Borthwick of Elsevier for their help and patience. Finally, I joyfully dedicate this book to my daughters, Lea Kowler Steinman and Anna Kowler Steinman, who arrived on February 18, 1990, a scant few days ahead of the page proofs.

Eileen Kowler
New Brunswick, New Jersey
May, 1990

List of Authors

H. COLLEWIJN
Department of Physiology I, Faculty of Medicine, Erasmus University Rotterdam, P.O. Box 1738, 3000 DR Rotterdam, The Netherlands

C.J. ERKELENS
Department of Physiology I, Faculty of Medicine, Erasmus University Rotterdam, P.O. Box 1738, 3000 DR Rotterdam, The Netherlands

E. KOWLER
Department of Psychology, Rutgers University, New Brunswick, NJ 08903, U.S.A.

J.Z. LEVINSON
Department of Psychology, University of Maryland, College Park, MD 20742, U.S.A.

J.K. O'REGAN
Groupe Regard, CNRS, 28 rue Serpente, 75006 Paris, France

M. PAVEL
Department of Psychology, Stanford University, Stanford, CA 94305, U.S.A.

A.A. SKAVENSKI
Department of Psychology, Northeastern University, 360 Huntington Avenue, Boston, MA 02115, U.S.A.

G. SPERLING
HIP Laboratory, Department of Psychology and Center for Neural Science, New York University, 6 Washington Place, Room 980, New York, NY 10003, U.S.A.

R.M. STEINMAN
Department of Psychology, University of Maryland, College Park, MD 20742, U.S.A.

P. SUPPES
Institute for Mathematical Studies in the Social Sciences, Stanford University, Stanford, CA 94305, U.S.A.

P. VIVIANI
Faculty of Psychology and Educational Sciences, University of Geneva, 24 rue du Général Dufour, 1211 Geneva, Switzerland

H. WALLACH
Department of Psychology, Swarthmore College, Swarthmore, PA 19081, U.S.A.

Contents

Eye movements and their role in visual and cognitive processes
E. Kowler, Editor

CHAPTER 1

The role of visual and cognitive processes in the control of eye movement

Eileen Kowler

Department of Psychology, Rutgers University, New Brunswick, NJ 08903, U.S.A.

1. Introduction

1.1. Theme

The understanding of human eye movement has always seemed a natural prerequisite to the understanding of many visual, perceptual and cognitive processes. This is because eye movements determine the position and the velocity of the retinal image. An accurate interpretation of performance on any visual task requires that we either know what the eye is doing or make some reasonable assumptions based on known oculomotor characteristics. So, the better we understand the processes that determine human eye movement, the better will we be able to predict the state of the retinal image in a wide variety of circumstances.

This chapter examines some of the visual and cognitive processes that determine human eye movements. This is an ambitious goal considering that we lack a comprehensive explanation of human oculomotor performance. A major obstacle has been the difficulty of finding invariant relationships between characteristics of the visual stimulus, such as the position or the velocity of the retinal image, and the movements of the eye. Many different eye movement patterns can be observed with the same visual stimulus. Similarly, large changes in the visual stimulus often have no systematic effect on the eye movements. Obscuring these sought-for invariant stimulus-response relationships are the 'cognitive' factors – choice, effort, selective attention, expectations and memory.

To appreciate how serious a challenge cognitive factors present for the development of theories, consider what has happened in the study of visual perception. The most complete theories have been those which account for the relationships consistently observed between a psychophysical report (the detection of the bars of a grating, for example) and the characteristics of the stimulus (the contrast and the spatial frequency of the grating). But as soon as investigators begin to consider the aspects of perception more susceptible to cognitive activity, such as the role of selective attention or past experience in the recognition of an alphanumeric character, consensus about theories disappears. Moreover, the prospect of relating the psychophysical observations to currently available physiological data becomes remote.

Those who study human eye movements, like those who study visual recognition, are confronted with the problem of incorporating the influence of both stimulus variables and cognitive factors. Unfortunately, the solution to this problem that has been adopted too often in oculomotor research has been not to deny cognitive influences, but rather to ignore, minimize or postpone their consideration in an attempt to develop models of the supposedly simpler lower-level processes, namely, sensorimotor relationships and their underlying physiology. I will argue in this chapter that such approaches will not work. We will not succeed in understanding eye movements unless cognitive factors are incorporated from the outset. Selective attention, expectations and memory play essential and inescapable roles in the programming of eye movements. Their contribution will be shown to be pervasive and effortless, becoming more apparent the closer the laboratory situation approaches that of the natural world. No special procedures are needed to elicit cognitive contributions: indeed, if anything, special procedures are often devised in the hope of keeping them at bay. Even the types of eye movement that are insensitive to willful, deliberate control (smooth pursuit, for example) are nevertheless unavoidably tied to what we expect and to what we attend.

Pervasive, effortless, cognitive influences make trouble for the prevailing models, which typically envision eye movements as under the control of passive, mechanistic processes, producing automatic reactions to external events. The picture to be painted here is that of an active oculomotor system, which creates a purposeful pattern of action based on the internal states of the organism. The 'internal states' might include representations of selected portions of the immediate visual environment, as well as representations of relevant memories, plans and beliefs. The central thesis of the chapter is that we have to understand the role of cognitive processes in order to devise theories of oculomotor control that capture the essence of how eye movements work in the natural world.

1.2. Organization of the chapter

This chapter will describe some of the visual and cognitive processes which determine three kinds of eye movement: eye movements of maintained fixation, smooth eye movements, and saccades. Vergence is reviewed in the chapters by Collewijn and Erkelens, and certain phenomena related to vestibularly driven eye movements in the chapter by Steinman and Levinson. The chapters by O'Regan, Pavel, Skavenski and Viviani also contain material relevant to the programming of saccades and smooth eye movements. This chapter deals mainly with human oculomotor performance, and with attempts to relate the performance to the properties of the visual stimulus, and to what the subject perceives, knows, wants, expects, attends to and remembers. Performance of other species and neurophysiological results, with a few exceptions, will not be described.

I have tried in many places to take a somewhat historical perspective, in which the background, as well as the contemporary status, of various lines of research is presented. This was done in an attempt to portray present work in the context of how we got to where we are today, and to show that many contemporary ideas (including ideas about cognitive influences) are, in fact, revivals of themes developed by oculomotor pioneers – Dodge and Ter Braak, in particular – during the first half of the century.

There have been several recent discussions of the relative contributions of cognitive and stimulus factors to eye movement control. See Berthoz and Melvill Jones (1985) and Collewijn (1989) for discussions of vestibularly driven eye movements, Erkelens et al. (1989a,b) for discussion of vergence, and Robinson (1986), Steinman (1986a) and Steinman et al. (1990) for different views of the contribution of the 'systems' approach to oculomotor research. There are also classical treatments of the role of cognitive processes in motor activity in general, rather than eye movements in particular. Dodge (1931), Craik (1947) and Lashley (1951) are particularly interesting, thoughtful and influential treatments of motor control, all of which, for a variety of different reasons, reject mechanistic approaches in favor of central control and organization.

2. Maintaining stable gaze

This section discusses the eye movements made while we attempt to look steadily at a stationary target. This is often referred to in the oculomotor literature as 'maintained fixation'. I am starting out with a discussion of fixation for two reasons. First, it is useful to know the characteristics of these eye movements in order to specify the retinal image conditions that typically confront our visual and cognitive systems. Second, the studies of fixation offer a relatively simple situation in which to search for, and model, invariant relationships between the retinal stimulus and the oculomotor response. The lessons learned from the studies of fixation may prove quite valuable when we come to the task of understanding the eye movements used to look about or to follow moving targets. These tasks, however, demand attentional resources and sophisticated decisions, and so, clearly, performance becomes harder to interpret. So let us start with something which seems to be relatively simple, namely, the eye movements made to look at a single stationary target.

2.1. Maintained fixation of stationary targets is extremely stable when the head is firmly supported

Studies of the eye movements during maintained fixation of stationary targets, the first eye movement studies to employ highly accurate recording techniques, began in the early 1950s. These studies were inspired by a prediction of the 'dynamic theories' of visual acuity (e.g., Jones and Higgins, 1947; Marshall and Talbot, 1942). The dynamic theories proposed that high-frequency oscillations of the retinal image provide the basis for a neural sharpening process, which computes the average position of a single visual feature with a precision better than the width of a single cone. Before 1950 there were longstanding disagreements about the true characteristics of fixational eye movements, so no one knew whether the image actually moved around enough to provide the kind of rapidly changing visual input that the averaging process needed. (See Steinman and Levinson's chapter for further discussion of the dynamic theories; and Ratliff and Riggs (1950) for a review of the disagreements in the early studies of fixational eye movements.)

To resolve these disagreements a technique for making accurate measurements of eye movements was developed independently by Ratliff and Riggs (1950) and by Ditchburn and Ginsborg (1953) (see also Yarbus, 1967). They made cinematographic records of a small spot of light reflected from a plane mirror mounted on the surface of a custom-fitted scleral contact lens. This method, known as the 'contact lens optical lever', could detect eye rotations of well under a minute of arc. By virtue of the use of a plane mirror, the recordings were insensitive to translational movements. Insensitivity to translations is important and deserves brief discussion here. Contamination of recordings by translational movements, a property of corneal reflection or diffuse reflection monitors, limits the accuracy with which one can estimate the true motion of the retinal image from the eye recordings. This is because translations and rotations have different effects on the retinal image. For example, consider an extreme case: only eye rotations change the position of the retinal image of a very distant target; translations do not. The size of the eye rotation is equivalent to the angular motion of the retinal image when targets are very far away, and approximately equivalent (within 5%) when targets are as close as 0.1 m (see Ratliff and Riggs, 1950; Steinman et al., 1982; Ferman et al., 1987; and the footnote on p. 10 for discussion of the sources of error in estimating retinal image motion from measurements of eye rotation.) Accurate inferences about the motion of the retinal image from recordings of eye movements can be made when recordings show pure rotational movements, uncontaminated by translations. It might seem that one way to remove translations, regardless of the type of eye monitor used, is to hold the head firmly in place. This technique will be only partially successful because translations cannot be prevented completely, even with firm head support (see Skavenski and Steinman, 1970; Cornsweet, 1976, for further discussion). The contact lens optical lever method of recording eye movements offers a better solution because its output is insensitive to translations. Moreover, by using a distant target any translations that might occur will not change the position of the retinal image. Other eye movement monitors, developed more recently, have adopted different solutions to minimizing or eliminating translations from the measurements (see, for example, Cornsweet and Crane, 1973; Skavenski et al., 1979; Steinman and Collewijn, 1980; Ferman et al., 1987; and Steinman and Levinson's chapter).

The contact lens optical lever requires the head to be firmly supported in order to keep the eye within the very limited recording range of the instrument (± 5°). The consequences of head support for interpreting the visual significance of the stability of gaze did not become apparent until well after the pioneering studies of maintained fixation had been done, and will be discussed in section 2.3.

The studies of maintained fixation in the 1950s described a fairly stereotypical, and by now well-known, pattern of eye movements when subjects fixated small, stationary targets, such as points of light, or thin lines or cross-hairs. The eye movement pattern consisted of a high-frequency (30–80 Hz), small-amplitude (15 sec arc) tremor, which was superimposed on low-frequency (2–5 Hz) slow oscillations whose amplitude was about 1′–3′. Interrupting these movements at intervals ranging from 0.2 to several seconds were small (5′–10′) saccades (microsaccades). An example of this 'typical' fixation pattern is shown in Fig. 1a. The immediate significance of these findings was that the amplitude of the high-frequency tremor, less than the width of a single cone, was clearly too small to play any important role in visual acuity, in contrast with the proposals of the dynamic theorists.

The most striking characteristic of maintained fixation was its remarkable stability. Ratliff and Riggs (1950) estimated that the "total movement (of the eye) over a period of 3 to 4 seconds is 10 to 20 min of arc". A similar conclusion was reached by Ditchburn and Ginsborg (1953). To appreciate how small a region this is, realize that the 'bouquet of central cones', the central retinal area described by Polyak (1941) as containing the 'most delicate', slenderest cones, is 20′ in diameter.

These early estimates of fixation stability were extended in later work. Nachmias (1959), for example, studied the 2-dimensional properties of fixational eye movements. This required mounting the plane mirror so as to be normal to a stalk on the contact lens that was parallel to the line of sight. The earlier method of resting the plane mirror on (or embedding it into) the surface of the contact lens (Ratliff and Riggs, 1950; Ditchburn and Ginsborg, 1953) was fine for horizontal movements, but confounded vertical eye rotations with torsions. Nachmias (1959) described the 2-dimensional stability of the line of sight by means of a bivariate contour ellipse area, which represented the area in which the line of sight would be located 68% of the time. The bivariate contour ellipse areas, determined from random samples of eye position taken during 30-s fixation trials, was about 60–100 min of arc². This would be equivalent to standard deviations of 3′–4′ on either the horizontal or vertical meridian, assuming no correlation between the horizontal and vertical eye movements.

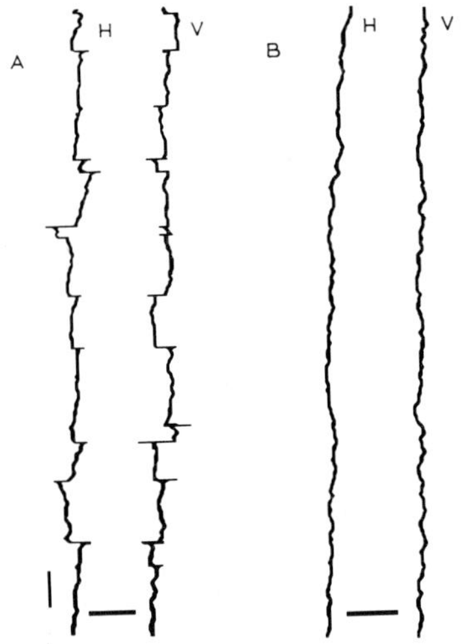

Fig. 1. (A) Horizontal (H) and vertical (V) eye movements of a subject fixating a point of light in darkness. Records were made with a contact lens–optical lever. The record begins at the top. The horizontal black bar at the bottom represents 15 min arc, the vertical bar a 1 s interval. The abrupt changes in eye position are saccades. (B) Same, except the subject has elected not to make saccades. (From Steinman et al., 1973)

There was also evidence that the stable fixation described above for relatively brief intervals (less than about 30 s) would also be maintained for far longer periods. Steinman (1965) found that the mean eye positions were almost the same across sets of trials (the standard error of the trial mean eye positions was only 2′–3′), leading him to conclude that the fixation target was consistently placed within the same 10′ retinal region.

The estimates of fixation stability, described above, were remarkably similar to those obtained by Barlow (1952), who used a recording technique that was, in principle, sensitive to translations. Barlow photographed a droplet of mercury placed on the limbus. Translations of the head were minimized by having subjects lie on a stone slab with their heads wedged tightly inside a rigid iron frame. Barlow asked the subjects to indicate when they believed that they were actually looking at the target. The standard deviation of eye positions at the beginning of such intervals, corrected for the estimated contribution of head movements, was only about 5′.

The fixational eye movement pattern discovered by the scientists working with highly accurate eye movement monitors in the 1950s and 1960s had several implications:

First, stable fixation was a boon to psychophysical research. It meant that reliable placement of the retinal image could be achieved simply by asking subjects to look at a suitable fixation target. Even the choice of a suitable target proved to be easy. Neither the stability of fixation nor the mean position of the eye depended in any important way on the color of the target or on its luminance (Steinman, 1965; Boyce, 1967b), provided that luminance remained above absolute foveal threshold (Steinman and Cunitz, 1968). The size of the target (Steinman, 1965; Rattle, 1969) and its shape (Murphy et al., 1974) did not have much effect either, at least for targets confined to the fovea. Stability suffered, but only modestly, with targets as large as 30 deg in diameter (see Fig. 2) (Sansbury et al., 1973). Fixational eye movements were as stable for naive, inexperienced subjects as they were for the experienced subjects (Winterson and Collewijn, 1976). So, for all practical purposes, concern that sloppy eye position control would send a visual stimulus far from a small, central retinal position could be safely dismissed.

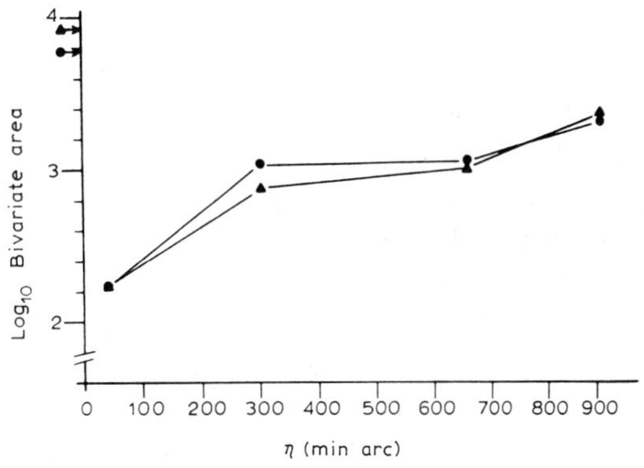

Fig. 2. Inverse fixation stability (log bivariate area) of two subjects who were instructed to maintain the line of sight in the center of target configurations of various sizes. Targets were either a single, homogeneous disc (1.3° diameter), or two of the same discs separated horizontally by 21.8°, or four of the same discs separated horizontally and vertically by 10, 21.8 and 29.5°. Data are plotted as a function of the distance between the target and the line of sight. The arrows on the ordinate show log bivariate area for each subject in complete darkness. (From Sansbury et al., 1972)

The second implication of the studies of fixational eye movements was that the eye, although quite stable, was obviously not completely stationary. The small amount of wandering of the image proved to have profound visual consequences. Abolishing all image motion, by moving the stimulus in the same spatiotemporal pattern as the eye, led to the fading of the stimulus within a few seconds (Ditchburn and Ginsborg, 1952; Ratliff et al., 1953). The fading of stablized images and more generally the role of retinal image motion in vision is discussed extensively in Steinman and Levinson's chapter.

The third implication of the studies of fixation in the 1950s was methodological. These studies introduced into eye movement research the highly accurate and precise recording techniques and the procedures for testing performance under the rigorous conditions that had been established in the visual psychophysical laboratory; that is, intensive investigation of a few committed observers trying to do the task as well as they could. The virtues of this approach became more apparent when the statistical properties of fixational eye movements were examined in attempts to discover how the eye remained so stable.

2.2. Stable fixation is accomplished by smooth eye movements, not by saccades

Cornsweet (1956) was probably the first to take a serious interest in the role of the saccades and smooth movements in the control of eye position during fixation. He recorded horizontal eye movements with the contact lens optical lever technique while subjects fixated a narrow vertical line. He found that neither the saccades nor the slow oscillations were correlated with the amount of fading of a retinally stabilized target, suggesting that neither type of movement functioned specifically for the purpose of providing the retinal motion needed to keep images visible. This led Cornsweet to investigate the role of saccades and slow movements in maintaining stable fixation. Cornsweet found that the further the eye was from its mean position, the more likely a saccade was to occur. Moreover, the saccades were corrective: they returned the eye to within 1′–2′ of its mean position. The velocities of the slow, intersaccadic drift movements, on the other hand, were not correlated with the distance of the eye from the mean position. Cornsweet suggested that the slow movements were oculomotor instabilities, which produced fixation errors. The errors then triggered the appropriate corrective saccades.

Cornsweet (1956) also made a suggestion that has since appeared frequently in the oculomotor literature (e.g., Becker and Jurgens, 1979), namely, that the size and direction of saccades are programmed independently. He made this suggestion based on analysis of the average saccade direction and average saccade size as a function of eye position before the start of saccades. Recall that he found that the direction and the size of saccades were both appropriate to return the eye approximately to its mean position. This implies that any saccades which might occur when the eye was already at its mean position should be very small and be equally likely to be directed to the right or to the left. But this turned out to be only partly true. The average size of the saccades was smallest (3′) when the eye was 1′ to the left of its mean position before the start of the saccade. Direction was a different story. The proportion of rightward and leftward saccades was equal when the eye was located 1.5′ to the right of its mean position before the start of the saccade. Cornsweet reconciled this discrepancy between size and direction by suggesting that there are separate 'size' and 'direction' mechanisms, which select different goal positions for the line of sight.

Cornsweet's (1956) model got things off to a good start. It proposed a clear, quantitative relationship between eye movement and retinal input signals. But as others began detailed analyses of fixation it soon became apparent that the 'drift away–saccade back' pattern that Cornsweet had described was by no means universal. Nachmias (1959), who recorded two-dimensional eye movements and analysed the components of eye movements along 8 meridians, was able to confirm Cornsweet's result for some meridians but found that the slow 'drift' movements could be corrective along others. He concluded that the compensatory 'drifts' were really smooth pursuit of a stationary target, much as the eye smoothly pursues moving targets (see section 3). Fiorentini and Ercoles (1966) and St. Cyr and Fender (1969a) also found that the drifts could be corrective. Others found that the velocity of drift increases in total darkness, supporting the idea that drifts were not 'instabilities' (Cornsweet, 1956) but were controlled by visual input (Ditchburn and Ginsborg, 1953; Nachmias, 1961; Proskuryakova and Shakhnovich, 1968; Matin et al., 1970; Skavenski and Steinman, 1970; Sansbury et al., 1973; Becker and Klein, 1973). Fig. 3 shows a comparison of fixational eye movements in the light and in the dark.

Saccades, like the drifts, did not follow the pattern expected from Cornsweet's data. Saccades were supposed to correct fixation errors, but several investigators reported that saccades would create fixation errors as well (Glezer, 1959; Proskuryakova and Shakhnovich, 1968; Barlow, 1952; Boyce, 1967a). An analysis of the movements of both eyes during fixation supports the same conclusion. Krauskopf et al. (1960) found no correlation between the drifts in the two eyes (determined from

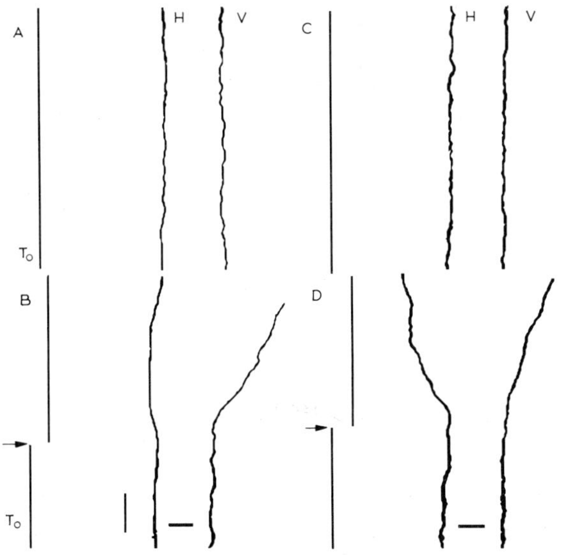

Fig. 3. (A) A two-dimensional record of the eye movement pattern during maintained fixation of a point located directly in front of the subject's right eye. The record begins at the bottom (T_O). (B) A record made under similar conditions except that the target was removed from view in the 2nd second at the time indicated by the black arrow. (The vertical black bar shows a 1 s interval.) Four seconds later the eye had drifted down (the vertical trace (V) went to the right) and had reached the recording limits of the apparatus. The size of the drift can be estimated from the black bar at the bottom of the record which shows 15 minutes of arc. (C) A record made under the same conditions as (A) except that the target was located about 30 degrees to the right of the subject. (D) A record made with the target in the same position shown in (C) except that the target was removed from view at the time indicated by the black arrow. The eye drifted toward the straight-ahead position when the target was removed (left in the horizontal trace (H)). It also drifted downward (to the right in the vertical (V) trace). (From Steinman et al., 1973)

eye positions taken from 2-s saccade-free drift samples), but a near perfect correlation of the occurrence, direction and size of saccades in each eye. The discrepant correlations implied that saccades were likely to be producing a fixation error in at least one of the two eyes.

There were other reasons to believe that saccades were not position-correcting fixation reflexes. Barlow (1952) found that saccades began to drop out of the fixation pattern the longer the subject kept looking at the target. He thought that saccades had more to do with the interest in the task than with basic mechanisms of oculomotor control. Barlow also speculated that saccade rates could be controlled voluntarily. His speculation was confirmed by Steinman et al. (1967). They found that the simple instruction to concentrate on keeping the eye still, rather than on 'fixating' the target, brought saccade rates down from about 1 to 2 each second, to 1 saccade every 2 or 3 seconds. The ability to reduce saccade rates in compliance with simple instructions has since been demonstrated often, including with naive, inexperienced eye movement subjects (Steinman et al., 1973; Winterson and Collewijn, 1976; Schor and Hallmark, 1978; Ciuffreda et al., 1979), and is consistent with the early reports of occasional long periods (many consecutive seconds) of saccade-free fixation (e.g., Barlow, 1952; Ditchburn and Ginsborg, 1953; Fiorentini and Ercoles, 1966; Proskuryakova and Shakhnovich, 1968; Ratliff and Riggs, 1950; Yarbus, 1967).

Steinman et al.'s (1967) demonstration that saccades could be easily suppressed at will made the saccades less like reflexes and more like voluntary behaviors, and, more importantly, showed that saccades were not necessary to achieve stable fixation. The slow movements, which had come to be called 'slow control' instead of drifts (Steinman et al., 1973), were sufficient to keep the eye in place. Figs. 1b and 3a,c show examples of slow control. Slow control has since been demonstrated in young children (Kowler and Martins, 1982), as well as in several species, such as cat (Winterson and Robinson, 1975), rabbit (Collewijn and Van der Mark, 1972), and monkey (Skavenski et al., 1975; Snodderly, 1987). So far, no useful function (either oculomotor or visual) for small saccades has been found, despite many attempts to unearth their role (Kowler and Steinman, 1977, 1979a, 1980; Winterson and Collewijn, 1976; Bridgeman and Palca, 1980). (See section 4.3 for further discussion of the characteristics and utility of small saccades.)

The rejection of Cornsweet's model, featuring noisy drifts and corrective saccades, simplified things because the number of different types of eye movement that had to be accounted for was reduced. There was no longer good reason to believe that the small saccades during fixation were different from the large, voluntary saccades we use to scan a visual scene (Cunitz and Steinman, 1969). To use Dodge's (1927) criteria for voluntary behavior, it had been established that small saccades could be 'voluntarily inhibited and arbitrarily initiated', the latter property demonstrated by Haddad and Steinman (1973), who showed that subjects could make 5′ saccades away from a single stationary target in specified directions.

The number of different types of smooth movement to be accounted for had also been reduced. The smooth eye movements during fixation of a stationary target could now be regarded as essentially the same as the smooth eye movements made to follow moving targets (Nachmias, 1961), as Dodge had assumed in 1903 (see also Walls, 1962). So, one implication of the discovery of slow control was that the smooth pursuit of intrinsically produced retinal image motion may not operate on principles fundamentally different from those involved in the smooth pursuit of targets that are truly in motion.

How did slow control work? Did it correct retinal position errors in order to maintain the image at some optimal place, or did it correct velocity errors in order to keep the image stable? This issue is still not clearly resolved, but at this point velocity correction seems more plausible. For one thing, the line of sight does not drift toward single targets at eccentricities greater (Whittaker et al., 1988) or less than 5° (Kowler et al., 1990a). Other reasons that position correction is unlikely are based on examining what happens when subjects fixate targets other than the small points or lines or cross-hairs used in most studies. Murphy et al. (1974) asked subjects to try to maintain a stable line of sight at some designated position, either along the boundary or inside outline drawings of small (<80′) simple forms. (Fig. 4 shows their stimuli.) They found that the stability of fixation was the same with the forms as with the traditional single point target. Fixation stability, as well as the mean position of the line of sight, was independent of the shape of the fixation target and independent of where, within the form or on the boundary, the subject was told to look. The same results were obtained regardless of whether subjects made small saccades while they fixated, or whether they refrained from making saccades, maintaining the line of sight exclusively with slow control.

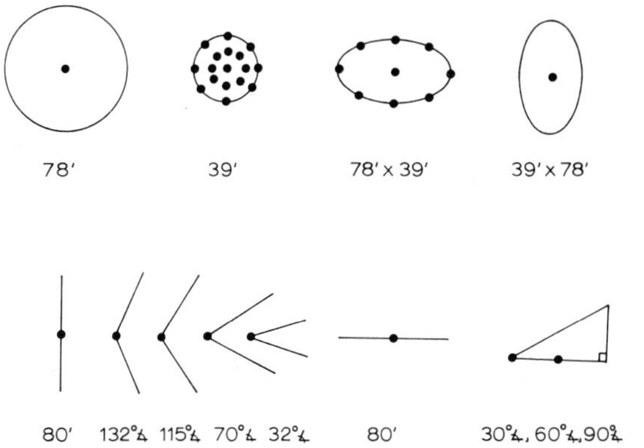

Fig. 4. The stimuli used in the Murphy et al. (1974) study of the effect of stimulus shape on fixation. The superimposed points show the different fixation positions studied. These points were not present during the experimental trials. Subjects were able to maintain a stable line of sight on any of the fixation positions. (From Murphy et al., 1974)

Murphy et al.'s (1974) experiment showed that there was no simple one-to-one relationship between position error signals and the slow control movements of the eye. In their experiment, position error signals of assorted sizes and directions were present when a location within a form was fixated. Yet the eye was never dragged over to a boundary. It would seem to be simpler to account for the stability Murphy et al. (1974) observed by a fixation system designed to keep images stationary rather than one designed to bring images to a particular location. This is because Murphy et al.'s results show that any position-correcting system would have to be under the subject's, rather than under stimulus control. To appreciate the greater complexity that would be introduced by a subject-controlled position system, consider the position-correcting system based on stimulus control described by Steinman (1965) in an attempt to explain how fixation stability and mean fixation position were about the same for small point targets and for 87′ discs. He proposed that position error signals are determined by averaging the location of each element on the target's boundary with respect to the location of the line of sight. The resulting error signal would be zero when fixation was maintained at one location inside the target (presumably, the center). This model was consistent with Steinman's (1965) data, but could not explain Murphy et al.'s finding of equally stable fixation at a variety of places on or inside the contour of a form. To explain Murphy et al.'s results with a position-correcting model, it would be necessary for the position-error signal to be defined with respect to an invisible reference position determined by the subject based on information in the contour of the target. Such a process cannot be ruled out based on current evidence, and if confirmed it would show a far greater control over fixational error signals by voluntary processes than has been envisioned in all prior work.

Murphy et al.'s (1974) results also led to a reinterpretation of Kaufman and Richards's (1969) and Richards and Kaufman's (1969) finding that subjects tended to fixate near the center of simple shapes. They had tried to relate the centering tendencies to Blum's (1973) theory of shape coding, in which a shape is represented according to its symmetric axis. Richards and Kaufman speculated that symmetric axis transformations might be occurring in the visual system to produce the effective stimulus for eye movements. But Murphy et al.'s demonstration of the independence of eye movements from the shape of the target, in an experiment in which subjects were told where to look, showed that Kaufman and Richards had actually measured their subject's preferences rather than inviolate oculomotor tendencies. (The role of centering tendencies will come up again in the discussion of saccadic eye movements to eccentric targets in section 4.7.1.)

The story of fixational eye movements told so far may be summarized by saying that the line of sight is maintained on a chosen target, or at a chosen location within a target, by means of slow eye movements which appear to be designed to keep images stable on the retina. The question of how stable images have to be in order to ensure clear vision is discussed in the next section, which will show that fixational characteristics change considerably when the head is not artificially supported.

2.3. Fixation stability diminishes when the head is free to move

The studies of fixation up through the 1970s employed accurate and precise eye movement monitors which, as noted earlier, required stable placement of the subject's head. It seemed reasonable to expect that the same excellent control of fixational eye movements described in the earlier sections would be found even when the head was not artificially supported. This is because both the vestibulo-ocular response and the visually activated slow control mechanism should be able to compensate for any additional retinal image motion caused by motions of the unsupported head.

Techniques to measure eye movements while the head is unsupported were developed in the 1970s. These methods employed a magnetic field sensor coil technique and will be briefly described here. (See Ferman et al., 1987, for a recent detailed treatment.) The magnetic field sensor coil method, developed initially by Robinson (1963), is based on the principle that the voltage induced in a coil of wire located inside an a.c. magnetic field is proportional to the sine of the angle between the coil and the field. In the sensor coil technique, eye movements are recorded while the subject sits inside a magnetic field generated by passing alternating current through Helmholtz coils. The sensor coil is attached to the eye by means of a contact lens, or, for better adherence of the coil to the eye, by means of a silicone annulus (Collewijn et al., 1975). Translations of the eye will have no effect on the eye recordings, provided that the eye remains confined to the small, homogeneous central region of the magnetic field. So, the extent to which head motions can be permitted without introducing contamination by translations depends on the size of this homogeneous region. In conventional sensor coil instruments, with magnetic fields generated by 60 or 90 cm diameter round Helmholtz field coils, the homogeneous region is too small to dispense with head supports.

Skavenski et al. (1979) built a sensor-coil monitor using a set of square Helmholtz field coils, 2 m on a side, which generated magnetic fields large enough to permit head translations of up to ± 1 cm without introduction of translational artifacts of more than 1 minute of arc into the recordings. They measured eye movements of subjects instructed to sit or stand as still as possible while looking at a single point target located at optical infinity. Asking subjects to sit or stand as still as possible should make only minimal demands on systems which compensate for head motions and provide an estimate of the best possible fixation stability achievable without the use of head support.

Skavenski et al. found that movements of the unsupported head were appreciable and were not compensated fully by eye rotations, even when subjects tried to hold the head as still as possible. Fig. 5 shows examples of the head and eye movements made while trying to sit or stand as still as possible. (Note that both the head and eye traces show movements with respect to earth-fixed coordinates, which means that the eye traces represent motion of the retinal image*.) The 2-dimensional dispersion of the line of sight (bivariate contour ellipse area) was about 1.5 – 3-times greater when the head was not artifically supported. Eye speed increased from about ¼°/s with artificial head support to about ½°/s when the head was free. Clearly, the compensation for head motion was incomplete.

If the stability of gaze suffers without artificial head support, even when subjects try to keep as still as possible, what would happen with the sorts of head motion we normally make when going about ordinary activities? This problem was investigated with new instrumentation developed by Collewijn and co-workers – the revolving magnetic field sensor coil monitor used with a cube-surface, rather than Helmholtz, field coil arrangement. This instrument allowed greater freedom of head movement without sacrificing the precision of measurement or introducing translational artifacts. It also provided linear indications of eye orientation and absolute calibration of rotations. Briefly, this instrument employed a rotating magnetic field so that the measure of eye position was based on the phase (not the amplitude) of the voltage induced in the sensor coil mounted on the eye or head. With suitably large, homogeneous regions of the field, eye movements of less than 1′ could be recorded accurately while the head was in motion. Head translations can be quite large (>60 cm) when large cube-surface coils are used without introducing artifacts into the recordings (see Erkelens et al., 1989a). (See Collewijn, 1977; Steinman and Collewijn, 1980; and Collewijn et al., 1983, for more detailed descriptions of this device, and Steinman, 1986b, for a history of the development of the instrumentation currently in use for measuring eye movements in subjects whose heads are free to move naturally.)

The studies of eye fixation using the revolving field monitor showed that the dispersion of eye position and the mean eye speed both increased when subjects attempted active head motion while looking at a small, distant target. Eye rotations compensated for about 95–98% of the head rotations. Although this sounds like very good compensation (indeed, it may be unrealistic to expect better performance of biological systems), it nevertheless led

* Eye rotation in space is not always exactly equivalent to retinal image motion. This is because: (1) the center of rotation of the eye is not coincident with the nodal point of the eye (see Ratliff and Riggs, 1950; Steinman et al., 1982; and Collewijn and Erkelens, this volume, for further discussion), (2) the center of rotation of the head is not coincident with the center of rotation of the eye, requiring the eye to rotate through a slightly greater angle than the head to fully compensate for head rotation, and (3) eye rotations made to compensate for translations of the head will not result in motion of the retinal image. It can be shown than none of these three factors is large enough to warrant consideration for targets at optical infinity, which were used in the experiments described in the text. Mis-estimates of retinal image motion will be well under 1% (Steinman et al., 1982). See Collewijn et al. (1990) and Kowler et al. (1990b) for studies in which retinal image motion was measured accurately for near targets.

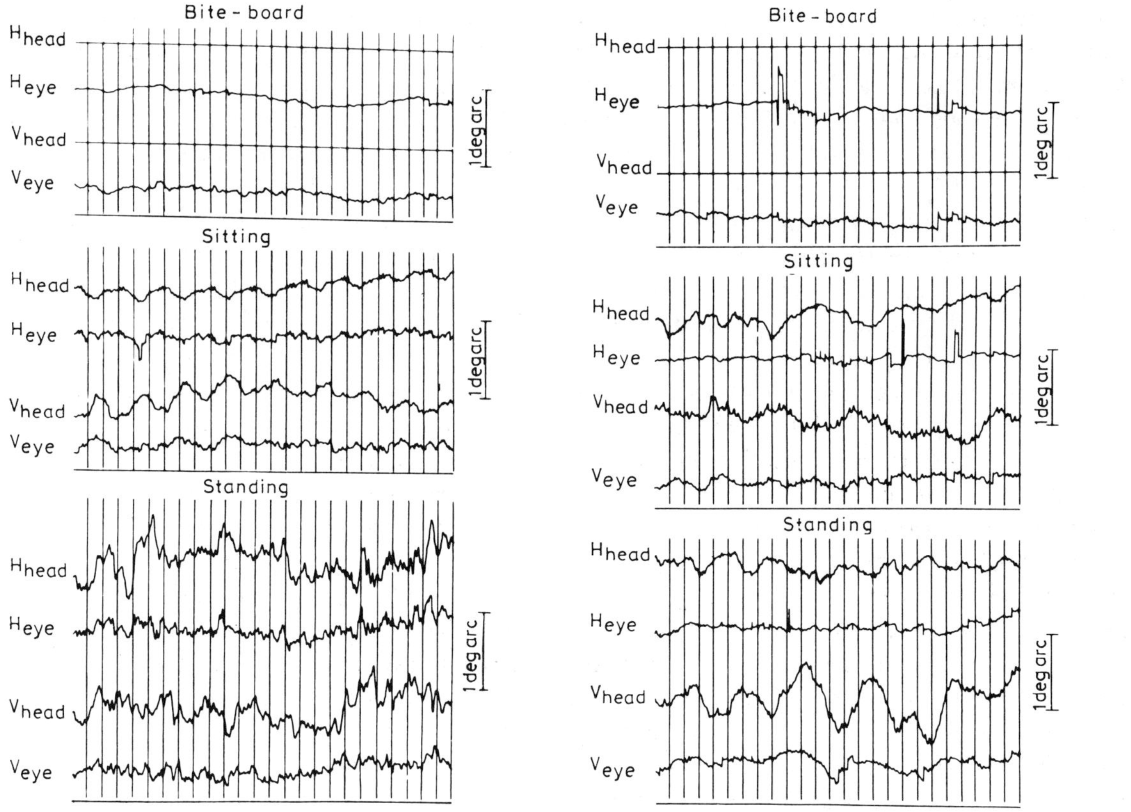

Fig. 5. Representative records of the horizontal (H) and vertical (V) positions of the head and eye in space of two subjects, AS (left) and RS (right), fixating a target at optical infinity, while their heads were supported by a bite-board or while sitting or standing as still as possible without artificial support. Time began on the right and repetitive vertical stripes indicate 1-s intervals. The length of the vertical bars on the right corresponds to a 1° arc rotation on either meridian. Upward changes in head and image traces signify rightward movements in (H) and upward movements in (V). (From Skavenski et al., 1979)

to residual retinal image speeds of about 1–2°/s for modest head rotations (frequency < 1 Hz, amplitude 10–15°). Image motion frequently exceeded 5°/s for more vigorous rotations. Fig. 6 shows several examples of eye movements during both modest and vigorous rotations of the head, and Fig. 7 shows distributions of 100-ms retinal image velocities. The sorts of head motion shown are typical of those we make in daily life, and the subjects in these experiments were under the impression, as we typically are, that the world appears stable and continues to be seen clearly. (Several chapters in this volume discuss different aspects of vision while the head is mobile. See Wallach's and Skavenski's chapters for discussion of perceptual stability, Steinman and Levinson's chapter for discussion of contrast detection and visual resolution, and Collewijn and Erkelens' chapter for discussion of stereovision during head motion.)

Ferman et al. (1987) recently confirmed and extended the initial measurements of fixational stability in subjects whose heads were not artificially supported. The important new feature of their study was the use of experimental and analytical techniques to eliminate possible sources of measurement artifacts that might have contributed in the prior work. Measurement artifacts might have come from misalignment of the annulus on the eye or from cross-coupling of the head movements. Ferman et al. replicated the results of the prior studies,

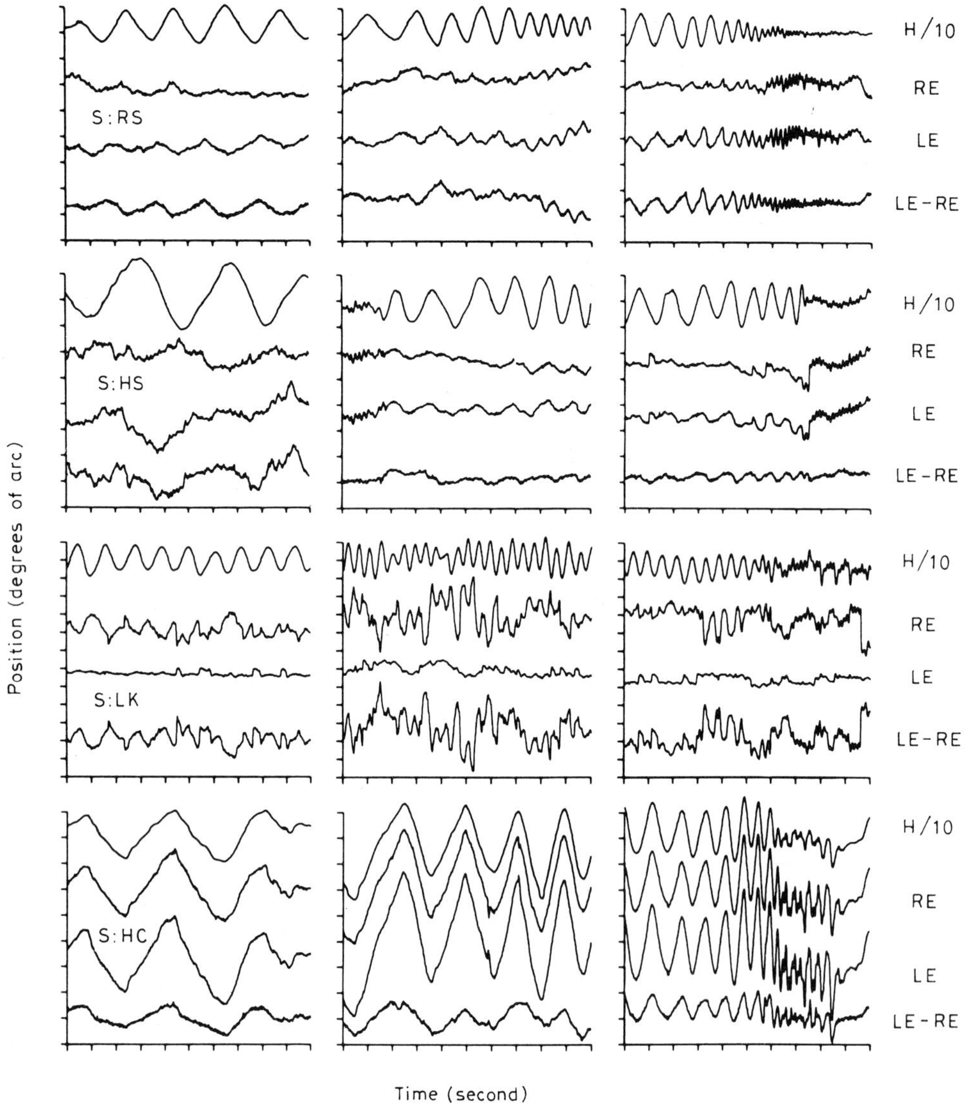

Fig. 6. Representative records of horizontal head and eye movements of four subjects (RS, HS, LK and HC) while they fixated a distant object as they moved their heads. Each record begins on the left. The time-scale marks signify 1-s intervals. The ordinate in each record shows the position of the head and eyes in space. The position scale-marks signify 1° distances. The head position trace (H/10) shows the position of the head scaled to 1/10 of its actual value. The position of the retinal image in the right eye (RE) is shown just below the head, the position of the retinal image in the left eye (LE) just below the right eye, and the vergence of the eyes (LE-RE) is shown at the bottom of each record. Position changes upwards in the head and eye records signify rightward movements. Upwards changes in the vergence trace signify convergence. (From Steinman and Collewijn, 1980)

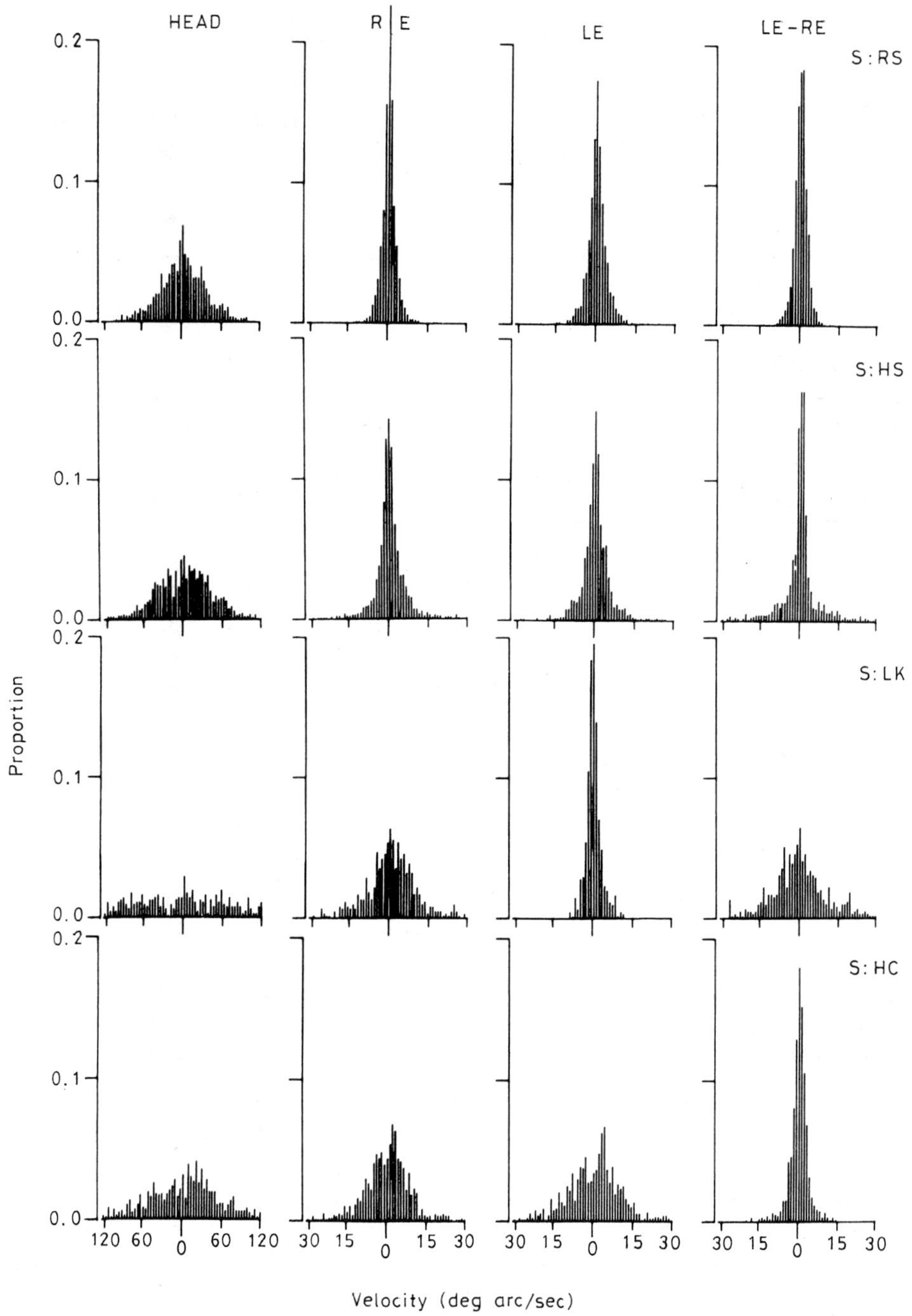

Fig. 7. Horizontal retinal image velocity histograms of four subjects (RS, HS, LK and HC) while they fixated a distant object as they moved their heads. The histograms plot proportions of velocities. Leftward velocities are plotted to the left of zero and rightward velocities to the right of zero. Head velocities (HEAD) are grouped in 4°/s bins. Right eye (RE), left eye (LE) and vergence (LE-RE) velocities are grouped in 1°/s bins. Vergence velocities to the right of zero signify convergence. Vergence velocities to the left of zero signify divergence. (From Steinman and Collewijn, 1980)

described above, and showed that any misalignment of the annulus or cross-coupling of the head motions was too small to be of significance.

The relatively large amounts of eye motion, when normal freedom of head movement is allowed, need not imply that visual or vestibular compensatory systems are too poor or imprecise to serve the needs of vision. Skavenski et al. (1979) suggested that the imperfect compensation may represent the operation of finely-tuned processes whose goal is not to abolish as much retinal image motion as possible, but to maintain the retinal image motion at a value that may be optimal for clear vision.

The suggestion that a briskly oscillating retinal image is useful for vision, made 30 years after the beginning of the modern studies of fixational eye movements, challenges the fundamental assumption that the goal of eye movements is to achieve the stable placement of the retinal image in a central retinal location whose size is but a few minutes of arc in diameter. A complete description of the pattern of retinal image motion that eye movements are trying to achieve cannot be made now because the appropriate concurrent oculomotor and visual experiments to address this fundamental question have yet to be done.

2.4. Overview

We have seen that stable gaze is accomplished by smooth eye movements, not by saccades. The stability most commonly observed in the oculomotor or psychophysical laboratory is indeed impressive, but is rarely achieved in natural environments where the head is not supported artificially. The velocity of the retinal image when the head is free to move ranges from about ½ to several degrees per second.

The oculomotor performance described in this section is presumably controlled by low-level sensorimotor circuitry, perhaps involving systems that sense retinal image motion and then program the appropriate compensatory eye movements. The next section deals with the smooth eye movements made to track moving targets, a task which makes greater demands on the attention, interest and knowledge of the observer.

3. Smooth tracking eye movements

3.1. Human beings cannot voluntarily initiate smooth tracking eye movements in the absence of a moving stimulus

Smooth tracking eye movements cannot be initiated at will in the absence of a smoothly moving stimulus. Efforts to voluntarily initiate smooth eye movements within a stationary visual field result in a sequence of saccades. This event has always seemed curious because it contradicts subjective impressions. Dodge (1931), for example, felt as if his eyes were gliding smoothly across the line of text as he was reading. He proved that his subjective impression of smooth eye motion was wrong by observing the successive jumps of an afterimage as he read a line of text. His subjective impression of smooth eye motion might have reflected the continuous acquisition of information from the text, and not the actual movements of the eye.

The inability to voluntarily initiate smooth tracking eye movements in the absence of a smoothly moving target, and the corresponding inability to completely suppress them in the absence of a stationary target (e.g., Murphy et al., 1975), has made it seem quite sensible to regard smooth eye movements as a sensorimotor reflex, operating under the control of the stimulus rather than free will*. I will begin the discussion of smooth tracking eye movements by reviewing reflexive approaches, which are

* Voluntary initiation of pursuit in some individuals has been noted, although this is rare (e.g. Westheimer and Conover, 1954; Heywood, 1972). The interpretation of these rare instances is not clear. For example, I know of individuals who can voluntarily initiate pursuit on the horizontal meridian, but not on the vertical. This argues that the rare instances of horizontal voluntary pursuit are idiosyncratic phenomena (perhaps related to vergence; Gertz, 1916, cited in Heywood, 1973) rather than a result of subjects' mastery of particular strategies or tricks that can be used by anyone to control smooth eye movement once they know how.

centered on attempts to discover and interpret invariant stimulus-response relationships. I will then describe several phenomena which are inconsistent with many of the basic tenets of these reflexive approaches. These phenomena demonstrate the crucial role of central and subjective factors, such as selective attention and expectations, in the programming of smooth eye movements.

Most of the research to be described will deal with the way in which alert and attentive subjects track small, smoothly moving targets. Some oculomotor researchers might take this to mean that I will be describing an active 'smooth pursuit' response rather than a more primitive 'optokinetic nystagmus' (OKN). OKN usually refers to the smooth eye movements evoked by the motion of a large pattern, typically a pattern of stripes painted on the inner surface of a moving cylinder that surrounds a stationary subject (cf. Collewijn, 1985). This large moving pattern is assumed to represent the image motion of the natural, stationary world as the subject rotates the head and the eyes (Ter Braak, 1936; Walls, 1962). In this sense the 'OKN' is assumed to represent the eye movements made to stabilize stationary environments, rather than to track smoothly moving objects. Recall that the stabilization of stationary environments was also supposed to be the function of the slow control movements, described in section 2. Slow control, however, is a smooth response to the retinal motion of a genuinely stationary environment produced by the observer's own eye movements, and it is studied in the laboratory just that way: with stationary targets viewed by observers whose heads are either stabilized or free to move, and who actively attend to the visual target. By contrast, the observer in an OKN experiment is often told to stare straight ahead at a large moving pattern and to let the eye be dragged along with the stimulus motion, rather than actively trying to track it (Ter Braak, 1936; Ter Braak and Buis, 1970). Sometimes investigators will also talk about 'OKN' when they study the smooth eye movements made while the observer is rotated within a stationary, patterned cylinder. 'Smooth pursuit', in contrast to 'OKN' or 'slow control', traditionally refers to the smooth tracking of fairly small, smoothly moving targets.

Oculomotorists continually talk about whether any of these distinctions, made on the basis of the type of stimulus used in the laboratory (large vs. small; stationary vs. moving), or on the basis of the presumed functions of eye movements, actually reflect the operation of distinct and independent smooth oculomotor subsystems. So far, the attempt to separate smooth subsystems has led to quite a muddle. A clear separation cannot be made based on the choice of stimulus – large moving pattern vs. small moving point – because the main characteristics of the smooth eye movements are essentially the same for both. For example, the differences between the pursuit of patterns and points are relatively modest (e.g., larger aftereffects following prolonged stimulation with large moving patterns than with moving points (Muratore and Zee, 1979), or higher maximal eye velocities with large moving patterns than with moving points (Van den Berg and Collewijn, 1986)), and could well be due to differences in the way a single, smooth subsystem responds to large and small stimuli. Certainly, resorting to separate mechanisms seems to be an option to be taken only after this simpler alternative has been eliminated (and so far it has not).

Anatomical distinctions between 'smooth pursuit' and 'OKN' are also obscure. In the late 1970s and early 1980s several investigators proposed that smooth pursuit is controlled by a special, fast 'direct' pathway that operates in parallel with a slower 'OKN' pathway (Cohen et al., 1977; Lisberger et al., 1981a; Robinson, 1981). The evidence offered to support such a proposal is the finding that lesions to this 'direct' pathway reduce the velocity of smooth pursuit of point targets in humans or in monkeys while producing little impairment of the steady-state velocity of the pursuit of large patterns (e.g., Zee et al., 1976, 1981; Westheimer and Blair, 1973). Such results might suggest parallel pathways, but there are several reasons why they do not distinguish 'OKN' from 'smooth pursuit'. One is that the smooth pursuit of small targets might be more vulnerable to the effects of lesions simply because the task is harder. For example, falling behind a point target leads to potentially harmful displacements of the target from the fovea and to subjective uncertainty about where the target actually is. On the other hand, there is no such thing as falling behind the large striped pattern because the stripes are everywhere. Complicating the comparison of points and patterns even further has been a tendency to use different kinds of motion pattern in studies of the two kinds of stimulus, i.e., points are often moved back and forth, and stripes in a single direction. Finally, it turns out that two parallel pathways, one fast and another slow, were proposed several years before the two pathways were proposed for primates, in order to explain the dynamic properties of the optokinetic response of the rabbit (Collewijn, 1972, 1981, 1985) – an animal which is often said to lack genuine 'smooth pursuit'. (The rabbit is discussed in section 3.3.)

The important point for the purposes of the present chapter is that the present evidence does not allow us to attribute some characteristics of smooth eye movements in human beings to a 'smooth pursuit subsystem' and others to an 'optokinetic subsystem' solely on the basis of the type of stimulus, waveform of the target motion, or the enthusiasm of the subject. I will not, therefore, presuppose the existence of two distinct smooth subsystems, but instead try to describe smooth oculomotor capacities of human beings who try to maintain the line of sight on a smoothly moving target. Active tracking seems to be more representative of how we use eye movements in natural viewing than letting the eye be dragged off by whatever motion happens to come along. (Indeed, we may never engage in the sort of passive following of full-field visual scenes described in the studies of OKN; passive following may be no more than a voluntary reduction in the velocity of smooth eye tracking (Steinman et al., 1969).) The existence or nature of any smooth oculomotor subdivisions remains to be worked out once we better understand the sensory, motor, attentional and predictive processes which are involved in the tracking of moving targets. It may turn out that smooth oculomotor performance in human beings is best viewed as under the control of a single subsystem whose input is selected by the observer from among the various stationary or moving patterns in the visual field at any given time.

3.2. Smooth eye movements may reduce, but do not abolish, the motion of a target on the retina

A relatively early and well-known attempt to find out how smooth eye movements are initiated and maintained was Rashbass's (1961) study of smooth pursuit of constant-velocity target motions. He found that smooth eye movements in the direction of the target motion began about 150 ms after the onset of the target motion. Rashbass (1961) wanted to find out whether the smooth response was evoked by the change in the target position or by the smooth motion itself. To distinguish between the effects of these two kinds of stimulus error signals – position error and velocity error – Rashbass measured pursuit with a target that jumped in one direction and immediately began to move smoothly in the opposite direction. If smooth pursuit eye movements were driven by position errors, then the eye should start off by drifting toward the eccentric target, opposite to the direction of smooth motion, but in the direction that would bring the line of sight closer to the position of the target. Rashbass found that the eye moved smoothly in the direction of the smooth target motion, just as if the jump had not occurred (see Fig. 8). Rashbass's observation confirmed the earlier suggestion by Dodge and Fox (1928) that smooth eye movements function to keep retinal images stable, not to bring them to a central retinal location. Recall that a case for the importance of velocity errors, rather than position errors, was made earlier in the discussion of slow control movements with stationary targets (section 2.2).

The question of whether smooth pursuit is sensitive to position error reappears periodically and requires brief discussion here. Smooth responses to abrupt target displacements (target 'steps' in the conventional jargon) are seen occasionally. For ex-

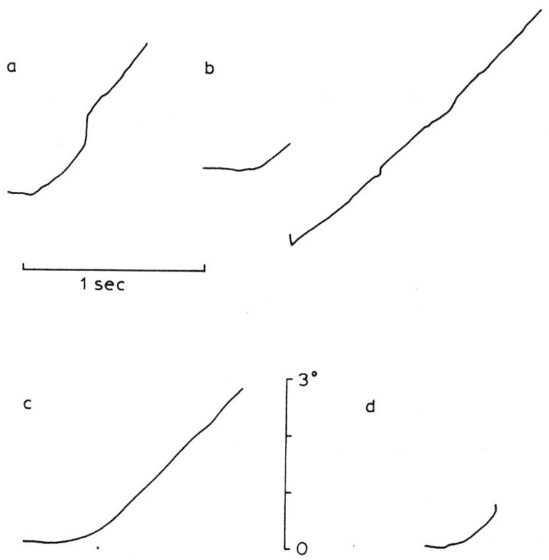

Fig. 8. Tracking responses to a target moving with uniform velocity preceded by a variety of displacements: (a) no displacement; (b) 3° displacement in a direction opposite to the velocity; (c) 1° displacement in a direction opposite to the velocity; (d) 1° displacement in the same direction as the velocity. (From Rashbass, 1961)

ample, Wyman and Steinman (1973a) found instances of smooth correction, but only for very small (7′) steps; larger steps had no effect on smooth eye movements. Carl and Gellman (1987) found smooth responses to 2° steps, but only when the steps were presented in the context of an experimental session containing mostly ramp motions. This result shows that the expectation of encountering smooth motion, or recent past experience tracking smooth motion, was needed to provoke the smooth response to the steps. Carl and Gellman also observed smooth responses to 2° steps imposed on ongoing smooth target motion while pursuit was under way. But the dominant response to the steps larger than 2° was a reduction in eye velocity, regardless of the direction of the steps. Reductions in eye velocity that are independent of step direction do not suggest sensitivity to position, because subjects are known to be able to reduce pursuit velocity voluntarily (Steinman et al., 1969) and might have chosen to do so in Carl and Gellman's experiment in response to the sudden, unexpected disappearance of the moving target from the central fovea. Wyatt and Pola (1981) claimed to find smooth responses to steps, but they used an unusual stimulus. They presented an eccentric target that jumped once, at the beginning of the trial. Subsequent jumps were triggered by saccades, that is, whenever a saccade occurred the size and direction of the jump was the same as the measured size and direction of the saccade. As a result, saccades should not have affected the target's retinal eccentricity, at least within the limits imposed by the speed, accuracy and precision of their image-stabilization system. They found no response to the initial target step, which occurred independently of the saccade. Smooth responses did occur to the subsequent target steps, which were triggered by the saccades. Results obtained with such 'open-loop' stimuli (called open-loop because the normal effects of eye movements on the position of the retinal image are prevented, i.e., retinal feedback signals are removed) do not necessarily support a role for position sensitivity. This is because open-loop stimuli can produce strong subjective impressions of smooth motion. Also, open-loop performance is characterized by a variety of oculomotor idiosyncrasies (described in sections 3.4 and 3.5), and therefore tends not to produce performance which can be directly related to the stimulus conditions, or to performance under normal, 'closed-loop', conditions. On balance, the best that might be said, in agreement with Carl and Gellman's (1987) conclusion, is that certain abrupt displacements of the target may provide adequate stimuli for smooth motion detectors (e.g., Burt and Sperling, 1976) and, in that way, allow smooth oculomotor responses. Unambiguous support for the sensitivity of smooth eye movements to pure position errors is still lacking (Kowler et al., 1990a).

Given the evidence that velocity errors appear to be more important than position errors, let us return to the consideration of the characteristics of pursuit of constant velocity motion. Rashbass (1961) reported that eye velocity reached target velocity by about 400 ms after the onset of target motion, at least for target velocities up to 10°/s. He claimed that any mismatch between the velocity of the eye and the velocity of the target was negligible, about the same magnitude as the typical oscillations of the eye observed during maintained fixation (see section 2.1). Rashbass suggested that the close match of eye and target velocity meant that continual motion of the retinal image is not needed to maintain pursuit. He suggested that pursuit is initiated by the initial sweep of the target across the retina, which causes the eye to accelerate in the direction of the smooth target motion until it reaches the velocity of the target. Pursuit is then maintained at target velocity because the eye is able to remember and continually re-program smooth movements at its current velocity. The re-programming of the same response continues until a change in the motion of the target initiates acceleration of the eye to a new maintained velocity.

Rashbass's model of pursuit was the same model that Craik had proposed some years earlier (1947) for smooth manual tracking in one of the earliest papers to apply Control Theory to human motor performance. Craik believed that an ongoing motor response would be maintained by means of a positive feedback signal, which he suggested might be produced by reverberating circuits, to allow the system to 'go on doing whatever it was doing at the moment' (p. 59) until a change in stimulation was detected. It was a predictive process of sorts, in which the standard prediction was that things would always stay as they are.

Things did not stay as they were. Rashbass's (1961) observation that eye velocity matched target velocity after 400 ms of pursuit was not confirmed by Puckett and Steinman (1969). They found that the eye always lagged behind the target. Eye velocity during the final half-second of target motion, when performance was expected to be at its best, was 70–90% of the velocity of the target. The finding that the eye lagged behind the target meant that retinal image motion would be available all the time to stimulate pursuit, and the automatic maintenance of eye velocity suggested in the Craik-Rashbass model would not be needed.

The disagreement over velocity-matching encouraged precise quantitative evaluation of eye velocity in subsequent work in order to detect even small mismatches. Subsequent studies confirmed that the eye lagged behind the target, on average (Murphy, 1978; Kowler and McKee, 1987; Collewijn and Tamminga, 1984, 1986; Van den Berg and Collewijn, 1986). These studies showed that the average ratio of eye velocity to target velocity (sometimes referred to as pursuit 'gain') tends to decrease as target velocity increases (see Fig. 9 (from Collewijn and Tamminga, 1984)). Sustained pursuit at target velocity was found only in special cases, namely after considerable practice tracking

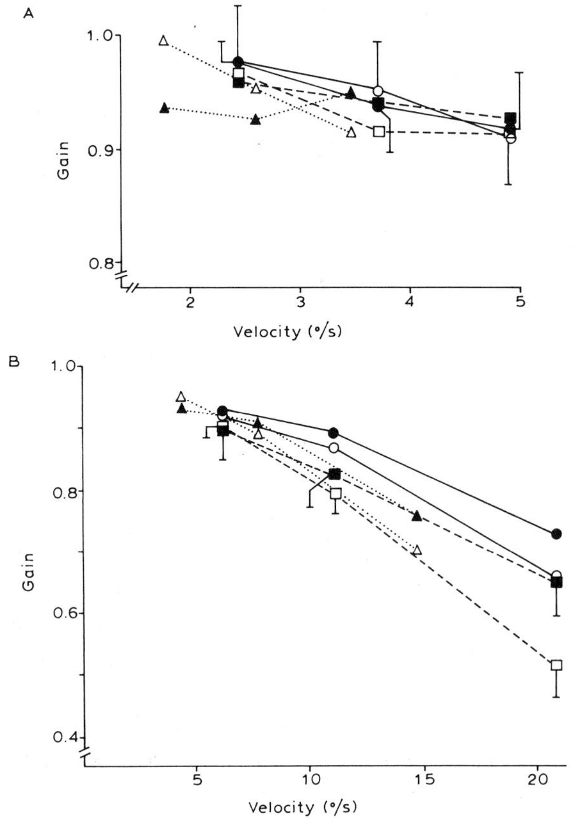

Fig. 9. Gain (eye velocity/target velocity) of horizontal (filled symbols) and vertical (open symbols) smooth eye movement responses to triangular-wave stimuli moving in one dimension with an amplitude of 10° (continuous lines), or in two dimensions simultaneously with an amplitude of 7.07° (dotted lines) or 10° (dashed lines). Means ± S.D. for five subjects for low (A) and high (B) target velocities. (From Collewijn and Tamminga, 1984)

low-velocity (2°/s) periodic target motions (Kowler et al., 1978).

These studies of pursuit implied that retinal image motion is necessary to maintain pursuit, unless extensive practice tracking simple, slow periodic motions was provided. The significance of retinal motion for models of smooth pursuit is described in the next section, where performance of the rabbit is described briefly.

3.3. Smooth eye movements of human beings are similar in several (but not all) respects to smooth eye movements of rabbits

Comparisons of smooth eye movements in the human with smooth eye movements in the rabbit have been popular since the classic work of Ter Braak (1936). The rabbit has provided us with the prototypical smooth-following system, whose basic principles appear to be fairly well understood, and despite many differences between the smooth eye movements of humans and rabbits, which I will discuss later, the models developed for the rabbit (discussed below) form the core of many of the models developed to account for performance of primates. It is, therefore, instructive to consider the rabbit at this point in the chapter to understand the sort of basic smooth sensorimotor tracking mechanism one might hope to find in humans, and to provide a context for the discussion, in later sections, of the contributions of central and subjective factors to human performance.

Rabbits readily pursue high-contrast textured patterns that occupy the large central 'visual streak' of their retina (the region where the density of ganglion cells is highest) (Dubois and Collewijn, 1979a). Rabbits will also pursue small targets, but will not pursue targets moving against stationary, structured visual backgrounds (Collewijn, 1981). (This result demonstrates that the rabbit lacks selective capacity (see section 3.6), not that it lacks a 'smooth pursuit' subsystem.) Like the human being, the rabbit tracks constant velocity motion with an average eye velocity that is less than target velocity, and the ratio of eye velocity to target velocity falls off as target velocity increases (Collewijn, 1969).

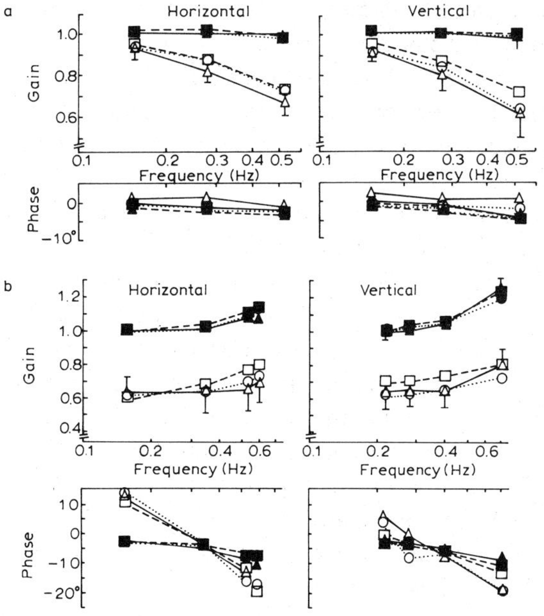

Fig. 10. (a) Gain and phase of the tracking of one-dimensional sinusoidal motion with an amplitude of 10° (continuous lines), or a two-dimensional stimulus with an amplitude of 7.07° (dashed lines) or 10° (dotted lines). Filled symbols show performance including saccades, open symbols show the pure smooth component after the contribution of saccades was removed from the eye traces. Means ± S.D. for five subjects. (b) Same, for pseudo-random target motion (sums of sinusoids). (From Collewijn and Tamminga, 1984)

Performance in human and rabbit is also similar in that the gain of pursuit of sinusoidal target motion (expressed as eye amplitude/target amplitude) decreases as either the frequency or the amplitude of the motion increases (Fig. 10a shows this relation for human smooth eye movement). Collewijn (1969, for rabbit) and Collewijn and Tamminga (1984, for human) argued that effects of both frequency and amplitude on the pursuit of sinusoidal motion represents the dependence of pursuit on the peak velocity of the target. This conclusion may hold for target frequencies below 0.5 Hz. Higher-frequency target motions, however, are harder for humans to track even when a reduction in amplitude makes the peak velocity slow enough so that near perfect pursuit would be expected (Martins et al., 1985). High target frequencies are detrimental for rabbit as well (Collewijn, 1981).

The gain of the rabbits' pursuit of sinusoidal motions and the gain and time course of pursuit of constant velocity motions were predicted by a linear systems model in which retinal slip signals (the difference between eye velocity and target velocity) were integrated by two parallel pathways to produce the smooth oculomotor command (Collewijn, 1972). One pathway had a short time constant and low gain and simulated the initial increase in eye velocity that occurred 100 ms after the onset of constant-velocity stimulus motion. The other pathway contained a 'leaky' integrator, was characterized by high gain and a long time constant, and simulated the more gradual rise in eye velocity to its maximal value. This model predicted the rabbit's response more accurately than alternatives, such as a single pathway with one or two integrators placed in series.

Additional information about the sensory input to smooth eye movement in rabbit was obtained by means of open-loop experiments. Recall that in such experiments special techniques are used so that the motion of the retinal image remains unaffected by the eye movements. This effectively opens the feedback loop containing the eye-motion signal, which normally combines with the target motion to produce the retinal slip. Open-loop measurements make it possible to discover the response to experimentally controlled amounts of retinal image motion.

Open-loop conditions were established in Collewijn's (1969) experiments by allowing the rabbit to view the moving stimulus through an immobilized eye, while movements of the other, occluded eye were recorded. An interesting aspect of the open-loop results was that the pattern of variation in eye velocity as a function of target velocity turned out to be remarkably close to the pattern of variation in the firing rate of retinal ganglion cells as a function of target velocity (Oyster et al., 1972). This similarity pointed to the ganglion cells as the likely source of the image motion signals used to drive the smooth eye movement. It also suggested that the eye velocity command is computed in a relatively simple way, namely, by summation of the firing rates of the active neurons. More elaborate schemes, such as those based on relationships between the outputs of different types of velocity-sensitive cell, did not appear to be necessary. A temporal-coding scheme comparable to that proposed for rabbit has also been suggested for the monkey, except that the relevant velocity-sensitive cells were assumed to be located in extrastriate cortical regions (Lisberger et al., 1987).

Later work caused some of the confidence in the simple temporal-coding scheme for rabbit to be lost. The shape of the velocity-tuning curves for neurons in the rabbit's central motion pathways was different from the shape of the velocity-tuning curves of the ganglion cells, and, therefore, different from the shape of the function relating eye velocity to stimulus velocity (Collewijn, 1975, 1981). Another complication was the surprising dependence of open-loop gain on the method used to control the retinal motion of the target. Gain fell off less steeply with increasing stimulus velocity when the movements of the viewing eye were compensated electronically, by feeding back the recorded eye motion into the stimulus motion, than when the movements of the viewing eye were prevented by immobilization of the eye (Dubois and Collewijn, 1979a). This result suggested that non-visual signals (proprioception or efferent copy), available when the viewing eye was free to move, had contributed to the pursuit. So, there are clearly unsolved problems even with the rabbit – the animal that has been introduced here as providing a well-understood, prototypical smooth tracking machine.

Despite these complications, there has clearly been a good deal of significant progress in developing models of smooth eye tracking in the rabbit, and in relating performance to the underlying physiology. So, to the extent that the stimulus-response relationships in primate and rabbit are similar, we may be able to gain useful insight into the primate by using what we know about the rabbit to guide the research. For example, we have already seen attempts to draw parallels between the primate and the rabbit in the previous discussions of the role of retinal slip in maintaining pursuit (section 3.2), the interpretation of the velocity-tuning curves in monkey extrastriate cortex (this section, see above), and the proposed contribution of separate fast and slow pathways to smooth eye movement (section 3.1).

The strategy of taking advantage of what has been learned about a simpler animal to tackle problems of human performance has worked exceedingly well in the study of motion perception. Reichardt's (1961) models of motion detection, developed originally to account for the optomotor response of the beetle, embodies general principles of motion detection which can also account for some aspects of motion perception in humans (Van Santen and Sperling, 1984, 1985). (In his influential book, Marr (1982) assumed that Reichardt's model of the fly's optomotor response would also apply to human smooth pursuit. This view, we shall soon see, is not correct.)

Will the same good fortune that has befallen investigators of motion perception, who learned something about humans from studies of insects, also fall on the oculomotorists hoping to understand human eye movement from observations of a simpler species? Not necessarily. The models of motion-processing developed for insects are most useful in accounting for phenomena at relatively early levels of processing, such as the detection of motion, or the discrimination of its direction. Incorporation of higher-level perceptual phenomena, such as perceptual illusions derived from the relative motion of different objects in the visual field, can legitimately be delayed until more basic processes are better understood. Those who study eye movements, in contrast with those who study motion perception, do not necessarily have the luxury of studying more primitive (rabbit-like?) aspects of the response in isolation from higher-level processes, such as selective attention, learning, memory and expectations. In studies of motion perception, investigators will attempt to control the contribution of these higher-level processes by making the stimulus and task fairly simple (i.e., detection or discrimination) and by relying on well-established psychophysical techniques to make sure that the contribution of expectations, decision criteria and other sorts of response bias are distinguished in the experimental design and analyses from the contribution of the lower-level sensory processes. But eye movement research is at a much more primitive stage. We are still in the midst of finding out what the higher-level factors are, whether they can be removed, or whether their effects can somehow be taken into account, or even whether trying to bypass higher-level processes is a good research strategy. After all, in perceptual research, the internal experience is the main issue, and extraneous factors which affect the report of the experience can legitimately be regarded as nuisances, to be circumvented as cleanly as possible. But in eye movement research, the responses themselves are the issue, and in trying to side-step what are assumed to be nuisances one can end up distorting the very processes under study.

The next several sections will discuss a variety of influences on smooth tracking eye movements, and evaluate the attempts to isolate the supposedly more primitive sensorimotor mechanisms from the contribution of cognitive processes. I will attempt to show that a complete understanding of smooth eye tracking requires incorporating cognitive factors into models, rather than delaying their appearance in the hope that more primitive and low-level processes will be understood first.

I begin by reviewing the research on human eye movements measured under open-loop conditions, a situation which has proven to be invaluable for understanding stimulus-response relationships in the rabbit, but has so far proven intractable for the human.

3.4. When the normal relationship between eye movements and retinal image motion is disrupted, smooth eye movements are no longer related to the pattern of stimulus motion in a systematic way

3.4.1. The role of orbital signals

Measurement of open-loop performance permits the testing of a straightforward hypothesis. If retinal-slip velocity signals are the main effective input for maintenance of smooth eye movements, as has been proposed for human (Puckett and Steinman, 1969) and rabbit (Collewijn, 1969), then removing slip by stabilizing the image on the retina should make the smooth eye movement mechanism blind to the target. The eye should drift, just as it does in darkness. This is in fact what happens in rabbit: stability is lost and the eye drifts about its mean position, resembling the drifts the rabbit makes in the dark (Collewijn and Van der Mark, 1972).

In human the story is different. Performance with a retinally stabilized visual stimulus (an afterimage, for example) does not resemble smooth eye movements in the dark. Recall that in the dark the eye tends to drift in idiosyncratic directions (Fig. 3) (Skavenski and Steinman, 1970; Matin et al., 1970; Hansen and Skavenski, 1977). But with an afterimage a variety of different types of smooth eye movement pattern have been observed. For example, some subjects can voluntarily initiate certain patterns of directed smooth eye motions (Heywood and Churcher, 1971; Heywood, 1972; Steinbach and Pearce, 1972; Cushman et al., 1984; Kommerell and Klein, 1971; Mach and Bachant, 1969). This is a surprising result, because voluntary initiation of smooth eye movements is normally not possible in darkness, or in a visual field containing nothing but stationary targets (see footnote on p. 14). Subjects can voluntarily reduce eye velocity to specified fractions of target velocity (Steinman et al., 1969). They cannot voluntarily track faster than the target (Steinman et al., 1969) or voluntarily change direction (Kowler and Steinman, 1979b).

The observation that smooth eye movements observed with afterimages are different from the smooth eye movements observed in total darkness means that some signal, other than retinal slip, must be contributing to the smooth oculomotor command. A complete model of pursuit would have to specify this signal. One well-known response to this challenge has been a revival of the Craik-Rashbass model. In the revival, eye velocity was once again said to be maintained in the absence of retinal slip. Maintenance of eye velocity was accomplished by adding a positive feedback signal, representing the velocity of the eye in the orbit, to the usual retinal slip (Young, 1971; Robinson, 1971; Yasui and Young, 1975; Lisberger et al., 1981b). This combination represents the velocity of the target in orbital coordinates, which then becomes the effective stimulus for pursuit. The revival of the Craik-Rashbass model differed from the original in that the pathway carrying the copy of the eye velocity was given a gain of less than 1 to prevent instabilities (Yasui and Young, 1975). As a result, the new version of the Craik-Rashbass model, unlike Rashbass's (1961) version, did not predict that the eye would match the velocity of the target.

Yasui and Young (1975) argued that their model would account for the pursuit of an afterimage in the following way. The sum of retinal velocity and eye velocity was said to represent the 'perceived' velocity of the target, which is the signal they believed drives the smooth pursuit. In the case of the afterimage, for which the retinal velocity is zero, the 'perceived' velocity would be equal to (or slightly less than, given the reduced gain of the positive feedback) the velocity of the smooth motion of the eye. Once pursuit of the afterimage gets going, the 'perceived' velocity signal would continue to generate new pursuit movements. To support this model, Yasui and Young (1975) noticed that the eye movements compensating for sinusoidal rotation of the head in darkness could be enhanced by providing the subject with an afterimage. They argued that the perceived motion of the afterimage was the stimulus responsible for the enhanced smooth eye movements. Note that it was not necessary to call the combination of retinal velocity and eye velocity the 'perceived velocity' of the target. 'Orbital velocity' would have been more appropriate, as will be shown in the next section.

The suggestion that a positive feedback signal carrying a copy of eye velocity contributes to smooth pursuit has appeared frequently and has been justified on a variety of grounds. For example, the positive feedback signal has been proposed in order to better account for dynamic properties of pursuit (Robinson et al., 1986), to account for similarities between the precision of pursuit and velocity perception (Kowler and McKee, 1987) and to account for the firing patterns of neurons in the cerebellum (Miles and Fuller, 1975). There has also been a suggestion that the signal contributes to smooth tracking in rabbit (Collewijn, 1985). The observations that pursuit occasionally 'runs on' for a brief period following the removal of the moving target (Whittaker and Eaholtz, 1982; Van den Berg, 1988; for human; Eckmiller and Mackeben, 1978, for monkey; Collewijn, 1985, for rabbit), or following a brief period of retinal stabilization of a moving target (Van den Berg, 1988), have also been attributed to the contribution of a positive feedback signal representing eye velocity. (A timely and accurate copy of the eye *position* signal also plays a role in perceptual and in motor (arm) localization, an idea that goes back to Helmholtz and that undoubtedly contributed to the attraction of using such a signal to control smooth eye tracking; see Skavenski's chapter.) Yet the one thing that the positive feedback signal does not adequately explain is the pattern of smooth eye movements observed with retinally stabilized targets, the mystery which had prompted its appearance in smooth pursuit models in the first place. Smooth eye movements with retinally stabilized targets are described in greater detail in the next section.

3.4.2. Performance idiosyncrasies

Inclusion of a positive feedback signal predicts that smooth eye movement with a retinally stabilized target should be different from smooth eye movements in darkness. But the positive feedback signal, by itself, does not explain the characteristics of the smooth eye movements with stabilized targets. For example, as already noted, one unexplained phenomenon is the emergence of some voluntary control over eye speed or direction. More disturbing, however, the positive feedback signal does not explain the observation, described below, that pursuit of stabilized targets is subject to large individual differences.

Individual differences were demonstrated by Cushman et al. (1984), who asked subjects to try to smoothly pursue an afterimage so as to mimic a variety of simple constant-velocity or periodic target motions. They found a remarkable range of variation in the performance. Some subjects could initiate smooth eye movements in only one direction. Others could make smooth eye movements in either direction but could not control the speed. Fig. 11 illustrates the limited voluntary control over smooth eye movements with stabilized targets. Performance is shown for the two subjects who, of the four tested, had the most voluntary control. The figure shows that each could smoothly pursue a target moving under normal, closed-loop conditions (top graphs in Fig. 11a and b) but that neither could accurately mimic the same patterns of motion with either an electronically stabilized target (middle graphs) or an afterimage (bottom graphs).

Individual differences in smooth eye movements with eccentric afterimages were also prominent. Previous workers had reported that the eye drifts in the direction of eccentric afterimages (e.g., Steinbach and Pearce, 1972). But Cushman et al. (1984) found that the eye would drift toward eccentric afterimages only in some of their subjects. Other subjects could just as easily drift away from as towards the afterimage, and others could not drift at all. The individual differences seen with afterimages, which were the same with electronically stabilized targets, disappeared when very small amounts of image slip were permitted (i.e., compensation for 94%, rather than 100%, of eye motion; Cushman et al., 1980). This last result has an important methodological implication. It shows that highly precise stabilization is essential in order to draw correct conclusions about performance un-

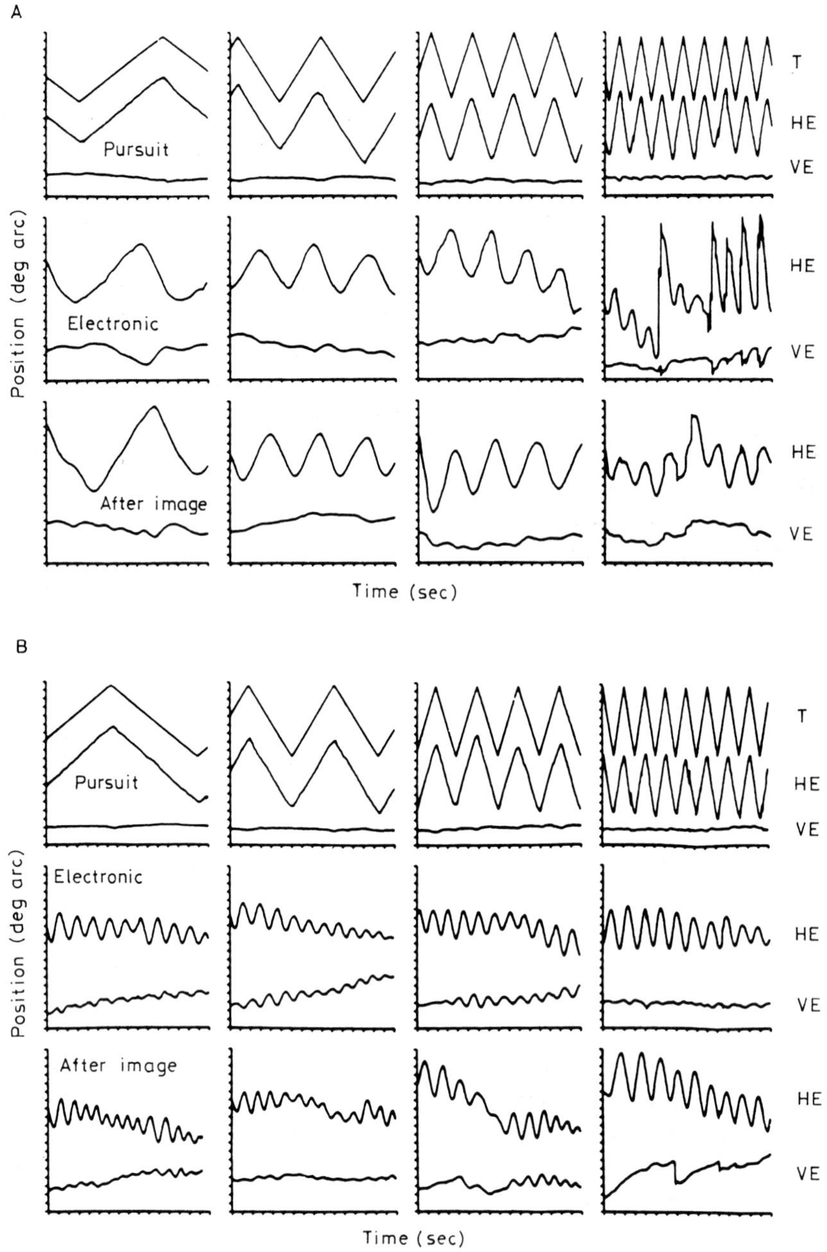

Fig. 11. Best-case analog records of subject JT (A) and subject WC (B) pursuing a triangular target motion (top four graphs in (A) and (B)), attempting to make the same eye movement pattern with an electronically stabilized target (middle four graphs in (A) and (B)) and with an afterimage (bottom four graphs in (A) and (B)). Target velocities were 1, 2, 4 and 8°/s. Traces are reproduced for the target (T), the horizontal position of the eye (HE) and the vertical position of the eye (VE). The time scale shows 1-s intervals. The position scale shows 1° distances. Upward displacements of the traces signify eye movements to the right or upward. (From Cushman et al., 1984)

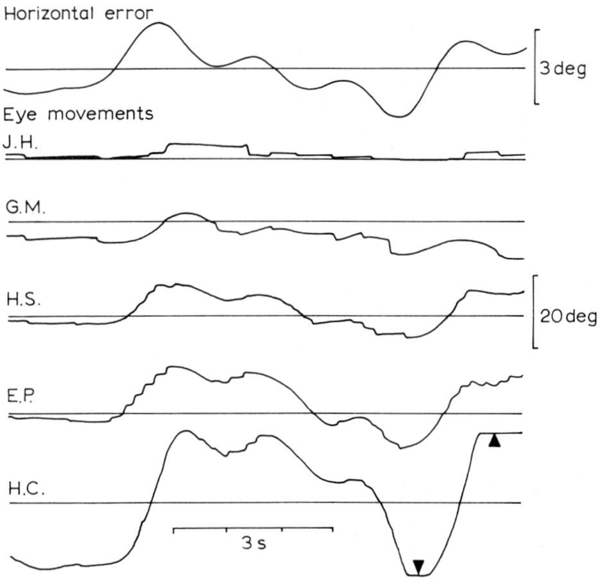

Fig. 12. Horizontal eye movements of five subjects who were asked to smoothly pursue stabilized targets with the same pattern of pseudo-random motion superimposed. The upper calibration bar applies to the retinal stimulus position; the lower one applies to the eye movements. The arrows in the lower trace mark saturations of the recording range. (From Collewijn and Tamminga, 1986)

der open-loop conditions.

Individual differences, comparable to those observed with stabilized targets, are equally striking when experimentally controlled patterns of retinal image motion are imposed on the stabilized target. Pursuit of controlled patterns of retinal image motion has been studied as part of attempts to discover the human 'open-loop' response. Dubois and Collewijn (1979b) found that some subjects vigorously pursued imposed retinal image motion in certain directions, while other directions were not pursued at all. The preferred directions differed among the subjects. (The idiosyncrasies were observed only for large (15 deg) stimuli centered on the fovea; eccentric stimuli were always tracked faster when they moved away from, rather than toward, the fovea.) Large individual differences in both the speed and the direction of pursuit have also been found under 'open-loop' conditions when pseudo-random image motions (sums of sinusoids) were imposed on stabilized targets (see Fig. 12) (Collewijn and Tamminga, 1986).

This section has shown two things so far. First, there are good reasons to believe that the effective stimulus for pursuit includes a positive feedback signal, representing eye velocity. This means that the effective stimulus for pursuit is defined in an orbital, rather than in a retinal, frame of reference. Second, the inclusion of such a signal will not explain pursuit under open-loop conditions. The large individual differences observed under open-loop conditions show that the open-loop technique is useless for discovering invariant, lawful relationships between retinal motion and eye motion in human smooth pursuit, thus depriving investigators of a potentially valuable analytic tool. Open-loop conditions open the way for all kinds of processes, their nature still unknown, to influence and control human smooth eye movements.

3.4.3. An alternative proposal for measuring 'open-loop' performance: the initial pursuit response

We have just seen how difficult it is to interpret smooth tracking under conventional open-loop conditions, in which controlled patterns of image motion are imposed on stabilized targets. An alternative method which has been tried is the study of the initial portion of pursuit. The initial portion of pursuit is taken to be a good estimate of the open-loop performance because, given that the eye is relatively stationary before the target starts to move, the pattern of the target motion in space should be about the same as the pattern of motion on the retina. So, measurements of the initial pursuit should allow the relationship between retinal motion and eye motion to be determined without the need for special techniques to experimentally control the retinal motion. (Actually, the eye does drift before the onset of target motion. These anticipatory smooth movements will be ignored for the present, and discussed later in section 3.7.2.)

Reasonably strong claims about the significance of initial pursuit have been made. For example, the initial response has been said to be a "direct reflection of visual processing in the input pathways of pursuit" (Tychsen and Lisberger, 1986, p. 956). The question of whether such a strong claim is justified will be discussed later in this section after a few properties of initial pursuit have been described.

Tychsen and Lisberger (1986) studied the dependence of the initial pursuit response on several stimulus variables, in particular the velocity, intensity and retinal eccentricity of the moving target. They found that the average acceleration of the initial pursuit, measured over the first 100 ms following the onset of the pursuit response, was highest for targets that moved horizontally toward the fovea, starting from an eccentricity of about 3 deg. Eye acceleration fell off steadily as the starting position was shifted to locations farther from, or closer to, the approximate position of the line of sight. Vertical pursuit showed a different pattern. Eye acceleration was higher for targets located in the lower portion of the visual field than for targets located in the upper portion, regardless of whether the motion was toward or away from the fovea. Reducing the intensity of the target from about 2.8 to 0.8 log units above a psychophysically determined detection threshold caused eye acceleration to decrease, but only for targets moving 45°/s or faster. Pursuit of lower target velocities was unaffected by intensity. Thus, it seems that the initial pursuit response, at least on the horizontal meridian, is fastest when the target's initial motion crosses the fovea. In addition, fast-moving, dim targets do not produce a brisk initial response.

Do any or all of these effects of stimulus variables on initial pursuit derive exclusively from the status of signals in the afferent pathways to pursuit, as has been claimed? Perhaps. For example, afferent signals from the fovea may be stronger (e.g., more contributing neurons) than extrafoveal signals, thus accounting for the faster pursuit of foveal targets. By the same token, signals from dim, fast-moving targets may be relatively weak. These proposed relationships between neural signals and smooth pursuit must be viewed carefully, however, because they do not imply that the status of afferent signals is the only, or even the principal, determinant of pursuit velocity, nor that the straightforward transformation of sensory signals to the oculomotor command, described for the rabbit (section 3.3), necessarily applies to human beings. Smooth eye tracking is a complex phenomenon, and the tight links between stimulus variables and responses which characterize smooth eye movements in the rabbit are hard to nail down in human beings. For example, in human beings, pursuit velocity declines when the subject's focus of attention does not correspond to the position of the moving target (see section 3.6), in much the same way that the initial reponse velocity was found to decline with increasing eccentricity or decreasing stimulus intensity. This implies that attentional, not sensory, factors can account for, or at least contribute to, the decline in pursuit velocity with increasing eccentricity or decreasing intensity. The velocity of initial pursuit is also sensitive to the past history of stimulus motions, and to the length of time the target is expected to remain in motion (section 3.7). These effects often outweigh those of sensory variables. It seems, then, that we are far from being able to distill the precise contribution of afferent signals to pursuit, and, more importantly, far from a theory of *how* afferent (and other) signals determine the pursuit response. Achieving these goals will require a better appreciation of the way in which central and subjective factors determine pursuit. Consideration of these factors begins next with a discussion of the relationship between perceived motion and pursuit. Following this, the role of selective attention and expectations will be reviewed*.

---

* In a recent paper Van den Berg (1988) took advantage of the influence of past history on pursuit in an attempt to characterize the open-loop response. He stabilized the image briefly (1.5 s) during ongoing pursuit of either sinusoidal or pseudo-random motions. He found that individual differences between the five subjects he tested were small, at least during the first 0.7 s of stabilization, and that pursuit characteristics were determined largely by the pattern of prior target motion, much as if subjects were trying to continue to mimic the motion they had been tracking (see section 3.7 on predictive eye movements). The extent to which this technique of brief image stabilization during ongoing pursuit proves to be successful in untangling the role of sensory processes, learning and expectations on smooth eye movement remains to be determined in future applications.

3.5. We pursue a highly organized motion signal, but we do not 'pursue what we perceive'

Section 3.4.1 introduced the suggestion that perceived motion is the effective stimulus for pursuit (Yasui and Young, 1975) but pointed out that, given the available evidence, it is not necessary to label the stimulus for pursuit 'perceived velocity'. 'Orbital velocity' (retinal velocity + eye velocity with respect to the head) is the better choice, as becomes clear by considering what happens when orbital motion is in conflict with perceived motion. The conflict will occur whenever the distance between the target and the observer is changed. Changes in the distance of the moving target will, of course, change the orbital velocity, but will not affect perceived velocity, at least within the limits of velocity constancy (cf. Mack, 1986). Smooth eye movements, unlike percepts of motion, must ignore distance cues, and other cues that promote velocity constancy, and try to match the orbital velocity, at least if accurate tracking is to be maintained. (For additional discussion of the implication of taking distance cues into account in the evaluation of oculomotor theories, see Steinman, 1986b.)

The dissociation between 'perceived' and 'orbital' motion allows us to quickly move from the question of whether perceived motion drives pursuit to the more precise question of the extent to which perceived motion and pursuit depend on the same motion analysers.

One reason to believe that pursuit and perception share motion analysers, at least at some level of processing, comes from studies of the smooth pursuit of targets moving in a sequence of small jumps (Westheimer, 1954), a stimulus that produces the percept of 'optimal' apparent motion (Wertheimer, 1912). This was studied in a clever experiment by Morgan and Turnbull (1978), who measured both perceived motion and smooth pursuit in an attempt to discover whether both varied in the same way as a function of the spatiotemporal pattern of the jumps. Their stimulus display consisted of a row of points, with each point illuminated briefly in succession. The trick to their measurement of the apparent smoothness of the motion was that each point was presented to one eye slightly before the other. As a result, the observer perceived the target as moving smoothly in depth whenever the intervals between the presentation of the adjacent points was sufficiently short. Morgan and Turnbull (1978) used the proportion of correct judgments of depth (i.e., whether the motion was towards or away from the observer) to represent the perceived smoothness of the motion. They found that depth judgments became increasingly less accurate as the interval between the successive flashes of adjacent points increased, with the judgments falling to chance levels for interflash intervals of 150 ms or longer (Fig. 13a). Coincidentally, the effectiveness of smooth pursuit, assessed by the standard deviation of eye position around a trajectory representing perfect tracking, deteriorated markedly when the interflash interval exceeded 150 ms (Fig. 13b). Their results argue that the same motion analysers serve perception and pursuit.

A different sort of demonstration linking pursuit eye movements to apparent motion is the finding that intermittently illuminated (10–100 Hz) arrays of stationary points can be pursued, provided that both the smooth eye movements and the percepts of smooth motion are initiated by a continuously moving target; e.g., Heywood (1973); also Behrens and Grusser (1979), who called this phenomenon 'sigma OKN'. The perceived motion with the 'sigma OKN' stimulus depends on taking eye velocity signals into account, and it is in this sense comparable to the perceived motion of afterimages. The perceived motion of 'sigma OKN' is, to stay within the terminology used in this chapter, apparent motion in orbital coordinates.

Another argument for perception and pursuit sharing motion analysers comes from a study by Kowler and McKee (1987). They compared the ability of smooth eye movements and perception to discriminate differences in target velocity. (This is different from most of the measures encountered so far in this chapter, where the emphasis was placed on how fast the eye traveled relative to the speed of the target.) Kowler and McKee measured

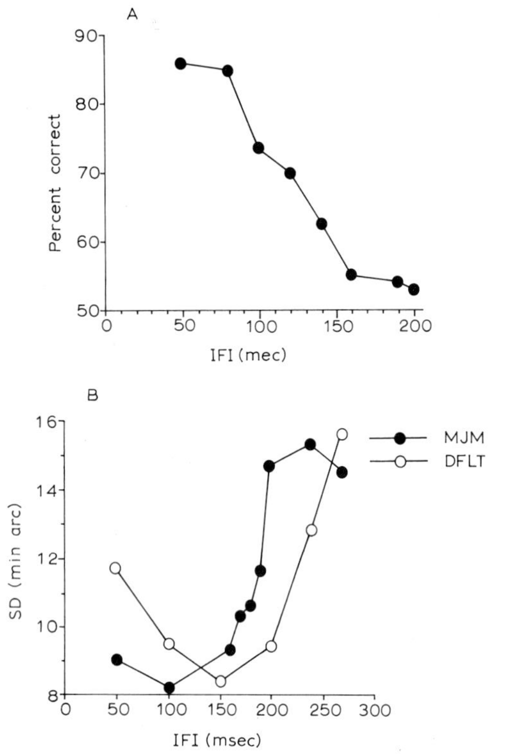

Fig. 13. (A) Percent correct judgments of depth as a function of the time between successive flashes of a target (IFI), which was perceived as moving in depth because each flash was presented to one eye slightly before the other. Data are the means over three observers. (B) The smoothness of the tracking of the same target motion. The graph shows the standard deviations of eye position around the best-fit regression of eye position over time. Data are from two observers. (Based on Morgan and Turnbull, 1978)

'oculomotor velocity discrimination' by having subjects pursue a different constant-velocity motion on each trial, with velocity selected at random from a set of five closely spaced values. Examples of velocity time-course functions, obtained from four different sets of target velocity, are shown in Fig. 14. Distributions of eye velocities in each velocity set were analysed to determine the proportion of each falling above a criterion value (the criterion was set to the mean eye velocity for the mean target velocity of the set). These proportions, plotted as a function of target velocity, constituted what they called the 'oculometric function', analogous to the conventional psychometric function. These functions, which were determined separately for each velocity set, were then used to find the 'oculomotor difference threshold', the smallest difference in target velocity that was needed to produce statistically distinguishable eye velocities. Kowler and McKee found that the oculomotor discrimination of velocity was very poor during the first few hundred milliseconds following the onset of target motion. The oculomotor difference threshold decreased steadily over time after the onset of target motion, reaching the lowest (hence, best) levels by about 600–700 ms after the target had begun to move (Fig. 15a). This shows that the initial velocity signal is imprecise, despite the fact that the eye could quickly achieve a velocity near the mean of the set of stimuli. (One reason that the pursuit response can be fast, yet imprecise, for several hundred milliseconds involves the consideration of predictive aspects of pursuit and will be taken up in section 3.7.3.) Kowler and McKee also found that oculomotor velocity discrimination depended on the velocity of the target. Once oculomotor velocity discrimination had reached its best levels (about 600–700 ms after the onset of target motion), both oculomotor and perceptual velocity discrimination varied in the same way with the velocity of the target (Fig. 15b), suggesting that both perception and smooth eye movement might be served by common motion analysers. The similarity between perception and smooth eye movements has limits, however. Principally, the similarity does not apply to the initial portion of pursuit. Oculomotor velocity discrimination is poor during the first few hundred milliseconds following the onset of target motion, as it is for very brief (200 ms) target motions. On the other hand, perceptual velocity discrimination with only 200 ms of exposure to the target motion is quite good and does not benefit much from increasing the stimulus duration. Perceptual velocity discrimination with only 200 ms exposures is as good as oculomotor velocity discrimination becomes much later in pursuit (Fig. 15b). This discrepancy between characteristics of motion perception and characteristics of the initial

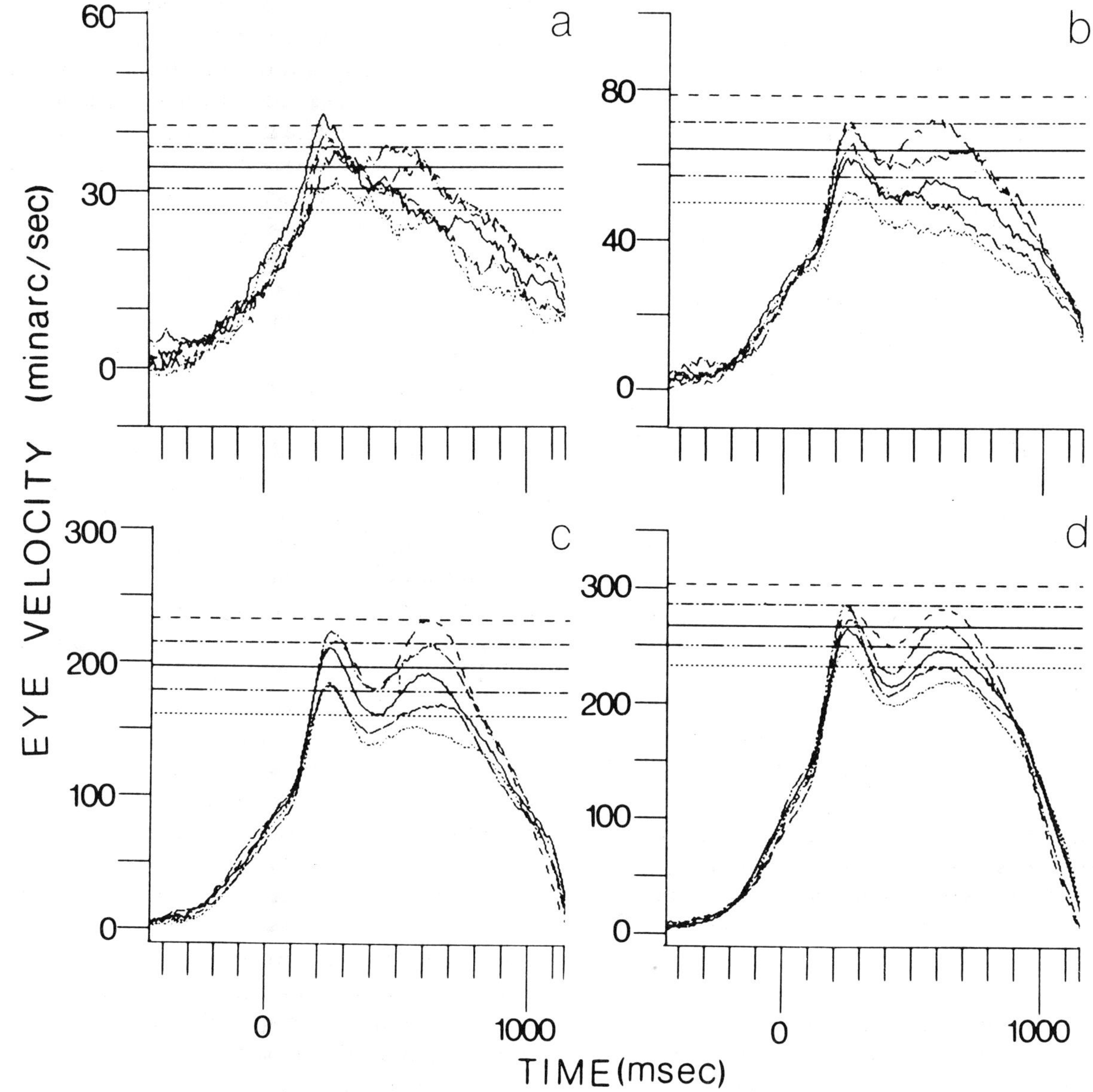

Fig. 14. Mean 100-ms eye velocity for subject EK pursuing leftward target motions in four different sets of constant-velocity target motions. Eye velocity is shown as a function of the midpoint of successive 100-ms intervals whose onsets are separated by 10 ms. Target motion began at 0 ms on the abscissa and ended at 1000 ms. Velocities less than 0′/s indicate rightward eye motion. The horizontal lines indicate the velocities of the targets. (From Kowler and McKee, 1987)

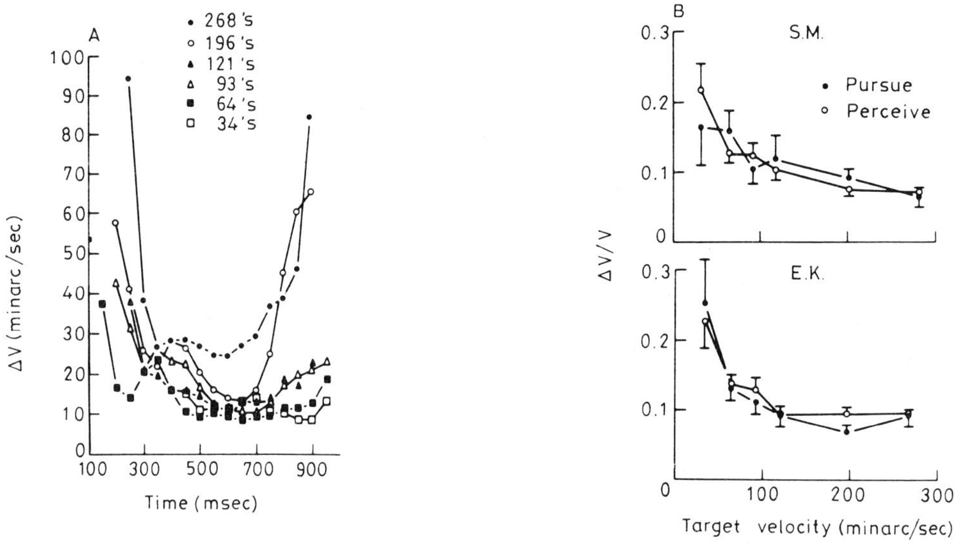

Fig. 15. (A) Oculomotor difference threshold (Δ *V*) as a function of time relative to the onset of target motion. Data are for subject EK. Difference thresholds were computed based on distributions of 100-ms eye velocities and are plotted as a function of the midpoint of the velocity sample. Each function shows the difference threshold for a different velocity set; the mean velocity of each set is listed on the figure. Difference thresholds decreased over time, reaching lowest values about 600–700 ms after the onset of target motion. The subsequent increases in the difference thresholds occurred when the eye began to slow down in anticipation that the target was going to stop moving. (B) Weber fractions (Δ *V*/*V*) (the ratio of the difference threshold to the mean velocity of the set) as a function of the mean velocity of the set for subjects SM and EK. Filled symbols are Weber fractions based on the lowest difference threshold obtained for each velocity set. Open symbols are Weber fractions representing perceived differences of the same target velocities. (From Kowler and McKee, 1987)

portion of pursuit provides yet another reason to be cautious about concluding that initial pursuit reflects the information in neural motion-processing centers (see also section 3.4.3).

Links between pursuit and perception have also been demonstrated by reports of pursuit of centrally generated moving stimuli, which, clearly, require higher levels of motion processing than would be needed for velocity discrimination. For example, moving stereoscopic contours (Fox et al., 1978) and segments of dynamic visual noise (Ward and Morgan, 1978) can be pursued. Some individuals can pursue the movements of their own hand or finger in darkness (e.g., Steinbach, 1969; Gauthier and Hofferer, 1976). This response is weak and intermittent, however, and may be improved by allowing periodic, brief glimpses of the moving hand (Steinbach, 1969, 1976; Jordan, 1970) (see Fig. 16).

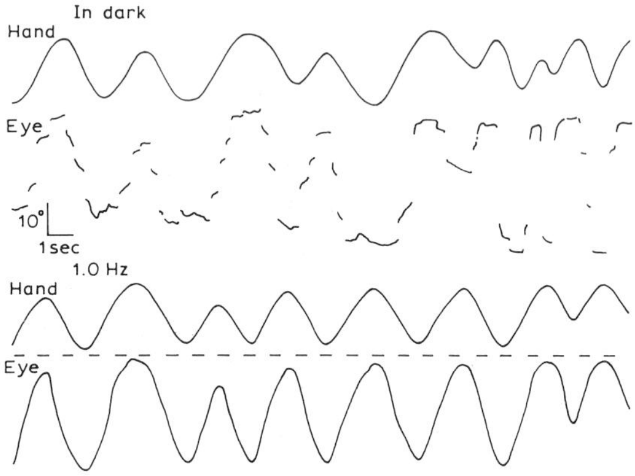

Fig. 16. The top pair of traces shows subject's attempt to track her own hand in complete darkness. There are some short episodes of pursuit, but tracking is mostly saccadic. The bottom pair of traces shows the marked improvement in pursuit that occurs when the hand is strobe-illuminated (microsecond pulses) at 1 Hz. (From Steinbach, 1976)

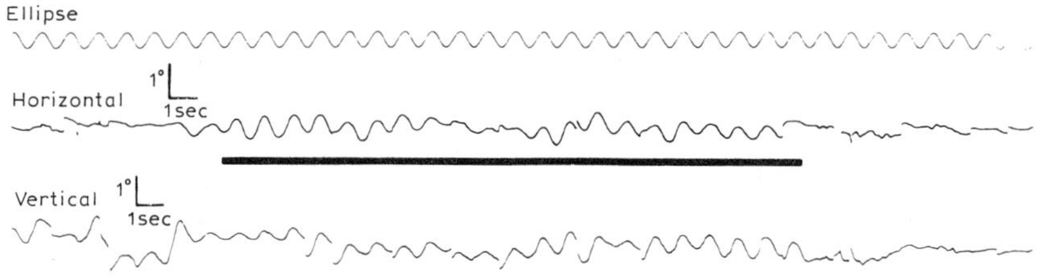

Fig. 17. Horizontal and vertical component of eye movements made while the subject tracked an ellipse (tilted at 45°) moving horizontally behind a narrow slit. Driving function for the ellipse is on the top trace. The heavy black line shows when the subject perceived the stimulus as an ellipse moving behind a slit, rather than two spots of light moving vertically in counterphase. The occurrence of horizontal pursuit is correlated with the percept of an 'object' seen moving behind the narrow slit. (From Steinbach, 1976)

Illusions of motion can be pursued. Steinbach (1976) reported that subjects were able to pursue the perceived, horizontal motion of a moving ellipse seen through a narrow vertical slit (Fig. 17). In this well-known illusion, often called 'anorthoscopic perception' (cf. Anstis and Atkinson, 1967), the only retinal motion was the vertical oscillation of the edges of the ellipse as it passed behind the slit. Steinbach's result confirmed an earlier suggestion of Anstis and Atkinson (1967), who used a subjective measure of eye motion (the perceived location of afterimages) to infer the pursuit of the anorthoscopic stimuli. Pursuit of anorthoscopic motion was also observed by Morgan (1981) and by Mack et al. (1982).

There have also been attempts to demonstrate that the same cortical regions serve both motion perception and smooth eye movements. These studies consisted of demonstrations that lesions to extrastriate areas implicated in motion perception (e.g., the middle temporal area; Newsome and Paré, 1988) decrease the velocity of smooth pursuit (Newsome et al., 1985, 1988; Dursteler et al., 1987; Dursteler and Wurtz, 1988). Electrical stimulation can produce a small, brief increase in pursuit velocity, or a relatively larger and longer-lasting decrease, depending upon which location is stimulated (Komatsu and Wurtz, 1989). Decreases in eye velocity are hard to interpret because, as noted earlier, subjects can voluntarily decrease pursuit velocity (Steinman et al., 1969) and may do so if distracted from the task or stimulus. So it is possible that some or all of the effects of lesions and stimulation on pursuit might represent the animal's behavioral reaction to an alteration in the appearance of the moving target, rather than distortion of the motion signals necessary to generate smooth pursuit. More elaborate behavioral testing will be needed to sort out the various alternative interpretations of the animal's performance.

The studies reviewed in this section illustrate various ways in which smooth pursuit and motion perception appear to share common motion analysers. Despite these demonstrations, it has nevertheless become clear that oculomotorists will go astray if they choose to simply borrow ideas about the central processing of pursuit stimuli from researchers in motion perception. This is because stimuli producing vivid percepts of motion are not often able to stimulate pursuit. For example, Mack et al. (1979, 1982) found that neither motion aftereffects nor induced motion (perceived motion of a stationary target inside a moving surround) were pursued. These results were also obtained with retinally stabilized targets so that, in principle, the position and velocity errors which would have discouraged the continued pursuit of illusions would be absent. Collewijn and Tamminga (1986) also found that the induced motion of a stationary target was not pursued when the target was either unstabilized or retinally stabilized and was superimposed on a large moving background. (The story for stabilized images became a bit more complicated, as might be expected from the research described in section 3.4, when Van den Berg and Collewijn, 1987, demonstrated that subjects could choose to pursue a superimposed, stabilized target either in or opposite to the direction of the moving background.)

Mack et al. (1982) attempted to reconcile the various instances in which perceived motion did and did not influence pursuit by suggesting that percepts are influential only when the stimulus perceived as moving has no competing 'retinal counterpart'. Stimuli with no retinal counterpart can be pursued, they argued, because "there is no retinal feedback which can constrain or inhibit pursuit" (p. 86). The anorthoscopic stimulus does not have a retinal counterpart because the entire ellipse is never present on the retina, but is instead generated centrally. Although it is not completely clear why the portion of the ellipse seen through the slit, or the portion of the ellipse painted on the retina as the eye pursues the percept, should not qualify as 'retinal counterparts', the hypothesis of Mack et al. (1982) is interesting because it reminds us that there are different ways of coding motion. Some kinds of codes, such as the motion of a target with respect to the observer (including even centrally generated targets, such as the stereoscopic contours or the moving ellipse), may influence both pursuit and perception. Other codes, such as the relative motion of two regions of the retinal image, may influence only the percepts. Why should one type of motion – motion relative to the observer – be able to influence smooth eye movement, while another, which is so important for perception – motion relative to other objects in the field – apparently does not? Perhaps the decision rules about which types of motion will and will not be influential are hardwired into the perceptual or the oculomotor machinery. Alternatively, the smooth oculomotor system may contribute to the formation or selection of its own moving stimulus by evaluating the effectiveness of the tracking eye movements. For example, pursuit of a target undergoing induced motion will not bring the line of sight closer to the target, and so may not be maintained. The capacity of smooth eye movements to make internal adjustments depending on the effectiveness of prior responses is discussed in more detail in the section on predictive eye movements (3.7.4) and is also discussed in Pavel's chapter. See also Collewijn and Erkelens' chapter for a related discussion of the relationship between binocular eye movements and the perception of depth.

This section has shown that central representations of motion serve as stimuli for smooth pursuit. This is *not* the same as saying that perceived motion drives pursuit because the stimuli for perception and pursuit are different: pursuit depends on motion relative to the observer, while percepts often depend on the relative motion of different objects in the visual field. The emphasis on central representations of motion as stimuli for pursuit moves us away from the view that the pursuit stimulus is simply an internal replica of retinal velocity, with perhaps a signal representing the motion of the eye added in at some stage. The description of the central representation of stimulus motion will be extended in the next section, which deals with the role of selective attention in determining the target for smooth eye movement.

3.6. Selective attention determines which one of many possible retinal signals serves as the input to the smooth oculomotor system

3.6.1. Visual fields containing more than one pattern of motion

At the beginning of the section on smooth eye movement we saw that there are profound limits to the voluntary control over smooth eye movement. For example, we cannot voluntarily initiate smooth eye movements without a smoothly moving target, or voluntarily suppress them without a stationary target. This section describes what happens when a variety of targets, both stationary and moving, are present at the same time.

A straightforward way for smooth eye movements to respond to more than one target at the same time is to respond to the pooled contribution of all of the targets. Adding more targets would simply change the available input, and would not invoke any new oculomotor processes. The main problem that would face researchers who want to understand the response to multiple targets would be the need to discover how the various retinal velocity signals combine mathematically, and how stimulus attributes, such as intensity or retinal location, affect the relative contribution of each velocity signal to the pool.

This straightforward scheme is wrong. When the visual field contains a variety of targets, moving at different velocities, the observer selects which target is to be tracked. The ability to select the target for smooth eye movements was suggested as early as 1906 by Ernst Mach, who realized that selective capacity is essential to explain how we are able to keep looking at the goal ahead of us as we walk about, without the eye being dragged off by the retinal motion of the world streaming by. The ability to select the target for smooth eye movements means that velocity signals must be sorted out so that only the selected signals will reach the smooth oculomotor subsystem. The hard problem is to understand how this sorting and selectivity is achieved. I will review a few suggested solutions. These range from those proposed in some early studies, which stressed the importance of retinal location, to later work, which showed that voluntary selective attention is more important. I will then argue that the way in which selectivity is achieved has general implications for characterizing the stimulus for smooth eye movements.

3.6.2. Retinal position vs. voluntary selection

Much of the early work on selection of the target for smooth eye movements emphasized not so much the voluntary selective capacities, but rather the apparent advantage accorded to stimuli that fall on the fovea relative to stimuli falling on more eccentric retinal locations. Investigators were surprised to find that the smooth pursuit of a large, moving striped pattern (the classic 'OKN' stimulus; see section 3.1) could be inhibited easily by fixation of a mere stationary point superimposed on the stripes (Dodge and Fox, 1928; Fisher and Kornmuller, 1930; Stark, 1971).

Later studies described the effects of retinal location more systematically and precisely. For example, Murphy et al. (1975) found that fixation of a superimposed stationary point or a small (30′ diameter) annulus was able to eliminate almost all traces of pursuit of a moving background grating. Extrafoveal annuli (147′ diameter) were much less effective. Similarly, Collewijn and Tamminga (1984) found that a moving point could be smoothly tracked across a stationary grating about as well as it could be tracked across a dark background, provided that the subjects looked directly at the moving point. [Note: There were small effects of the background on pursuit, just as there were small effects of a moving background on fixation of a superimposed stationary point (Collewijn and Tamminga, 1986). These effects were found in only some of the subjects, who may have allowed themselves to be distracted a bit by the background.] In contrast with the accurate tracking of a foveal point across a patterned background, Collewijn and Tamminga (1986) found that it was hard to pursue a point which was kept at an eccentricity of 5 deg as it moved across the stationary background, a situation in which the fovea was filled with the image of the moving visual pattern. In interpreting this result keep in mind that retinal eccentricities of a few degrees have little or no effect on smooth pursuit of targets moving across dark or homogeneous backgrounds (Winterson and Steinman, 1978; Collewijn and Tamminga, 1986). Eccentricities of a few degrees become important only when a competing pattern of motion is in the fovea. In such instances, the stimulus in the fovea has an advantage.

There is more to smooth oculomotor selectivity, however, than the advantageous placement of the chosen image on the fovea. For example, investigators who studied selectivity by superimposing a stabilized scotoma on a large moving pattern (Cheng and Outerbridge, 1975; Dubois and Collewijn, 1979b) noticed that the scotoma tended to inhibit the pursuit of the background, with the pursuit becoming slower as the scotoma became larger. Nevertheless, retinal location was not the whole story because special effort – what we would refer to

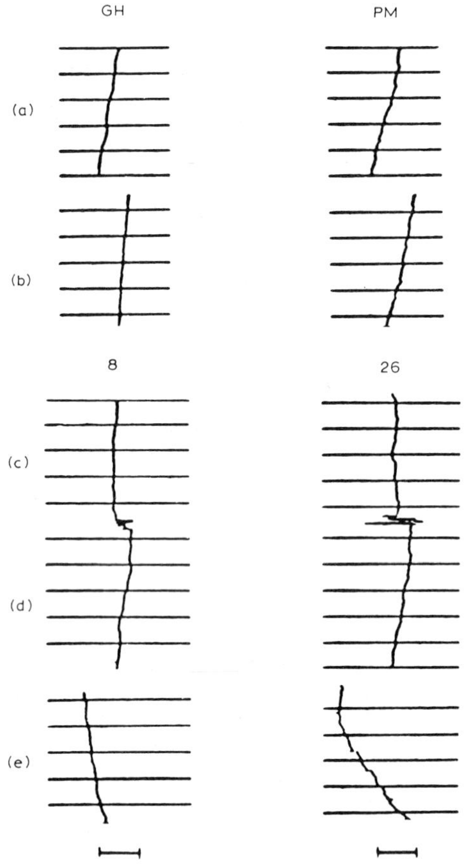

Fig. 18. (a) Representative records of horizontal eye movements of two subjects (GH and PM) who drift to the right when they use slow control to maintain the line of sight on a stationary point superimposed on a 4° diameter stationary grating. (b) Same as (a) except that the point was removed, leaving only the stationary grating. (c) The point was removed and the grating moved to the left at 8′/s for GH and at 26′/s for PM. Note that the grating's motion, in the absence of the superimposed point, nullified the rightward drifts. (d) The superimposed stationary point was restored to the display and subjects tried to fixate the point. Their usual rightward drift returned, despite the leftward motion of the grating. (e) Subjects successfully tried to track the leftward motion of the grating. Records are read from bottom to top. Horizontal lines are 1-s time-markers. The bar below each subject's records represents 1° arc rotation. (From Murphy et al., 1975)

colloquially as paying 'attention' to the background – could increase the velocity of pursuit (Dubois and Collewijn, 1979b). The contribution of 'effort' or 'attention' shows that the selection process is not simply a matter of positioning the desired target on the fovea. Selectivity is a matter of decisions made by the subject about which target to attend to. (I will discuss evidence linking oculomotor and perceptual attention in section 3.6.4.)

An unusual illustration of the power of selectivity to determine the target for smooth eye movements is shown in Fig. 18, taken from Murphy et al. (1975). Murphy et al. studied two subjects who had natural tendencies to drift horizontally when fixating a stationary target (Fig. 18a,b). The unusual aspect of the performance was that these subjects showed the same drifts when they tried to fixate a point superimposed on a grating which moved opposite to the direction of their natural drift (Fig. 18d). This meant that the smooth eye movements continued to be determined by the selected target (the stationary point) even as the line of sight was drifting away from the stationary point, across the moving grating.

3.6.3. Selection with stimuli occupying the same retinal location: implications for the central organization of the pursuit stimulus

The demonstrations summarized in the previous section, showing that the advantage for foveal over extrafoveal stimuli is not absolute, but instead depends on attention, suggest that an unambiguous estimate of the capacity to select the target for smooth eye movements requires targets whose retinal locations overlap completely. This situation was studied originally by Ter Braak (1957) and Ter Braak and Buis (1970). They used what they called 'ambivalent optokinetic stimulation'. This consisted of a drum painted with interleaved sets of stripes on its outer surface. The stripes were painted so that one set appeared to be moving to the right and the other to the left when the drum was rotated. Subjects were able to smoothly track either set of stripes, and they were able to switch from one set to the other at will. This shows that foveal placement of a stimulus does not ensure that it will serve as the target for smooth pursuit, because, with the 'ambivalent' stimuli, the images of both sets of stripes fell on the fovea, but it was up to the subject to decide which set to track.

Ter Braak (1957) and Ter Braak and Buis (1970) did not report eye velocities and, therefore, did not know whether the set of stripes moving in the background interfered with pursuit of the selected set of stripes. Kowler et al. (1984b) measured eye velocities with overlapping stimuli similar to those used by Ter Braak. Kowler et al.'s stimuli consisted of two, identical, superimposed, full-field patterns of randomly positioned dots, one stationary and the other moving to the left. The velocity of the moving pattern was deliberately set to a low value (1 deg/s) so that either field would be seen clearly regardless of which field the subject was tracking (Westheimer and McKee, 1975; Murphy, 1978). They found that subjects could keep the line of sight on either the stationary or the moving pattern with virtually no influence (<4%) of the background (Fig. 19). This result demonstrated that selectivity can be almost perfect when there were no differences in the retinal locations, indeed no differences of any sort, between the target and the background. Kowler et al. (1984b) also emphasized that subjects had tried their best to pay full attention to the target field. This kind of effort is important when drawing conclusions about selective capacity, because effects of backgrounds on smooth eye movements could easily result from instances of the subject not fully attending to the target, but allowing attention to wander to the background as well.

Kowler et al.'s (1984b) results had implications for the way in which the selectivity was achieved. A plausible view, consistent with the observations that had been made before their study, would be that selectivity is a matter of choosing velocity signals from one or another location in the display. This view is attractive because it is easy to envision neural motion detectors 'tagged' according to the location of their receptive fields. But selection of location could not explain how the subjects were able to pursue one dot pattern and eliminate influence of the other, superimposed pattern, because the stimulus fields were so dense that dots from one pattern were continually passing across dots of the

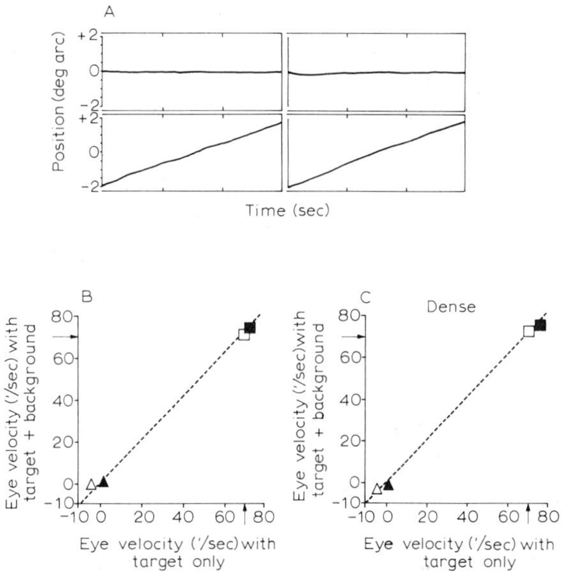

Fig. 19. (A) Representative records of horizontal eye movements for subject RS under instructions to maintain the line of sight on the stationary (top two graphs) or moving (bottom two graphs) field of random dots. In the lefthand graphs, only one field was present; in the right both were presented superimposed. Tick marks on the x-axis separate 1-s intervals. Upward deflections of the eye trace indicate movements to the left. (B) Mean 21-ms eye velocities for subjects HC (open symbols) and RS (solid symbols) under the instruction to maintain the line of sight on the random dot field presented either alone (abscissa) or with the superimposed background field (ordinate). Triangles show eye velocity when the stationary field was the target, squares when the moving field was the target. The density of the dots was 1 dot/deg^2. Standard errors were smaller than the plotting symbols. Negative values on the axes indicate rightward velocities. The arrow indicates the velocity of the moving field. Velocities falling on the dotted diagonal line indicate no effect of the background. Velocities falling above the line, when the stationary field was the target, indicate smooth eye movements in the direction of the moving background. Velocities below the line, when the moving field was the target, indicate smooth eye movements slowed by the stationary background. (C) Same as (B) except that the density of the dots was increased to 8 dots/deg^2. (From Kowler et al., 1984b)

other. So, selection based on location would not distinguish the target field from the background field. Selection of one or the other stimulus velocity (or, simply, direction of motion) could be ruled out as well because the vivid, compelling percept of induced motion of the stationary field was never reflected in the smooth eye movements (another example of not pursuing what we perceive; see section 3.5).

The elimination of both location and velocity as the basis for selection shows that selection was achieved by choosing a particular distinct perceptual configuration – a group of dots in the target field that was perceptually isolated from the dots in the background. This outcome means that the superimposed velocity signals must first be organized into distinct, segregated patterns before they reach the smooth oculomotor circuitry. This result, like the demonstrations of the pursuit of illusory motion, described in the previous section, provides another example of the significant central processing needed before motion signals are available for smooth eye movement control. Explaining the selectivity in Kowler et al.'s experiment requires the motion of the two superimposed fields to be segregated and the signals representing the velocity of each to remain 'tagged' according to the appropriate pattern of origin so that only the selected signals will be sent to the smooth oculomotor subsystem. How central motion analysers accomplish this is not known.

Kowler et al.'s (1984b) results also show that voluntary selective attention determines the target for smooth eye movement, but it does not determine smooth eye velocity directly. Had voluntary selection determined the eye velocity, the eye would have pursued the perceived induced motion. Instead, the eye velocity was determined by the retinal (or by the orbital) velocity of the selected field. This means that the voluntary selective processes are limited to telling the smooth oculomotor subsystem *what* to track. Information about the velocity of the chosen target, which is then used to compute the oculomotor commands, is carried separately by mechanisms that are not amenable to voluntary control and, unlike our percepts, blind to relative motion. (This 2-stage process, selection of input followed by computation of the motor command, will prove to be useful in accounting for some properties of saccadic eye movements, to be described in section 4.7.)

3.6.4. Perceptual and oculomotor selective attention

Is selecting the target for smooth eye movements equivalent to paying perceptual attention to the target? Or, do we have access to distinct selective processes, one serving the needs of perceptual judgments and the other of motor performance?

To answer this question Khurana and Kowler (1987) studied perceptual and oculomotor selection concurrently. Their experiment required subjects to pursue a target (a pair of rows of moving characters), while at the same time searching for a numeral located in the target rows and a numeral located in nearby, untracked background rows (Fig. 20). Subjects were better able to identify and locate the numeral in the tracked, target rows than in the untracked, background rows. Moreover, the superior performance for the target was due to attention – effects of retinal speed or retinal position were carefully ruled out. The results show that a single selective attentional decision determines the target for pursuit and for perception.

It is an ideal arrangement: we can control smooth eye movements by doing nothing other than paying attention to what we find of interest, regardless of the visual backgrounds streaming by. (And even this might not be too demanding. Khurana and Kowler (1987) found that shifting a bit of attention to the background improved its perceptibility slightly, while barely perturbing the ongoing pursuit.) Once we pay sufficient attention to our chosen target, the relevant velocity signals (whatever they may be) will determine the smooth eye movement command with no extra effort on our part.

This section on selective attention showed that central representations of the motion of selected (attended) targets provide the effective stimulus for pursuit. The next extends the description of the central representation of motion by showing that the effective stimulus consists of what we know about a target's future motion, as well as what we sense about its present motion.

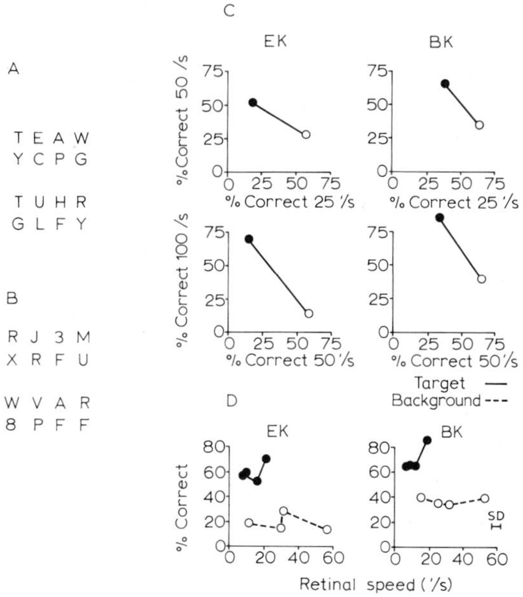

Fig. 20. (A) The stimulus used in an experiment which measured smooth eye movements and selective perceptual attention at the same time. An array of 16 characters began moving horizontally at the beginning of a trial. The velocity of characters in row 1 (top row) was the same as the velocity of row 3. Similarly, the velocity of row 2 matched that of row 4. (Velocities were as follows: when one pair of rows moved at 25′/s, the other moved at 50′/s; when one pair moved at 50′/s, the other moved at 100′/s.) The subject kept the line of sight in the vertical gap between rows 2 and 3 and tried to match horizontal eye velocity to one of the row-pairs (called the 'target' pair). When the line of sight reached the approximate center of the display, the characters were replaced briefly (200 ms) by an array such as that shown in (B). Note that one numeral is present in each pair of rows. In this example, a '3' is in row 1 and an '8' is in row 4. Subjects had to identify both numerals and report the row in which they were located. (C) Visual search performance. Percent correct reports for the slower pair of rows is shown on the abscissa, for the faster pair on the ordinate. The filled symbol shows performance when the slower pair was the target, the open symbol when the faster pair was the target. Performance was always better for the target rows. (D) The same data points as in (C) plotted as a function of measured retinal speed. Performance was always better for the target rows and retinal speed was largely irrelevant. (From Khurana and Kowler, 1987.)

3.7. Smooth eye movements depend on expectations about the future path of target motion

The discussion of smooth eye movements up to this point has described sensory, perceptual and attentional contributions to pursuit. This section will show that smooth eye movements can be initiated and maintained by internal signals, representing expectations of future target motion, which are not derived from any immediate sensory or perceptual cues. One of the major themes of this section is that the processes which operate to produce anticipatory pursuit will contribute regardless of whether the target motion is 'predictable' or 'random'.

3.7.1. Anticipatory reversals

The effect of expectations on smooth eye movement was observed in some of the earliest studies of smooth pursuit. Dodge (1931) and Dodge et al. (1930) discovered that the eye would often turn around before the target during pursuit of periodic target motion – a phenomenon they named 'anticipatory reversal'. They also noticed 'preliminary drifts' (Dodge et al., 1930, p. 29) (drifts before the start of target motion) and said that the origin of this sort of eye movement was 'not yet clearly understood'. (There will be more discussion of the 'preliminary drift' in section 3.7.2.)

Westheimer (1954) also encountered the 'anticipatory reversals' in the first study to suggest the application of control theory to the study of eye movement. Westheimer, like Dodge before him and several others to follow, believed that anticipatory reversals were due to learning. The idea was that a stereotypical smooth oculomotor response would be learned after repeated cycles of tracking the same periodic, oscillating motion. Pursuit of random target motions, unlike the pursuit of periodic motions, was assumed to be immune to learning and anticipation, and dependent only on the underlying sensorimotor relationships (what Westheimer called 'psycho-optic reflexes').

Interest in anticipatory reversals reappeared in the 1960s when several investigators, in attempts to apply linear systems analysis to smooth pursuit, tried to predict the pursuit of a complex pattern of motion from the pursuit of its sinusoidal components. This proved to be impossible, as might be expected from the earlier work of Dodge and Westheimer, because of the influence of anticipation on the pursuit of sinusoidal motions. Pursuit of sinusoidal motion showed higher gain and shorter phase lags than did pursuit of aperiodic, random motions (i.e., sums of sinusoids or bandwidth-limited Gaussian noise) (Stark et al., 1962; Dallos and Jones, 1963; Michael and Melvill Jones, 1966; St. Cyr and Fender, 1969b; Collewijn and Tamminga, 1984). Phase leads were often observed. The difference between the pursuit of the two types of motion can be seen in Fig. 10, which shows the average gain and phase of pursuit of sinusoidal motions (Fig. 10a) and random motions (Fig. 10b). Pursuit of random motions also depends on the bandwidth of the stimulus; the higher the bandwidth, the poorer the pursuit (Michael and Melvill Jones, 1966; Collewijn and Tamminga, 1984). In general, pursuit of random motions is quite poor and may not reduce retinal velocity sufficiently to support clear vision.

Modelers have tried to deal with the differences between the pursuit of sinusoidal and random target motions by assuming that a special, predictive element contributes only when the target motion is sinusoidal. For example, Dallos and Jones (1963) began their model with this assumption: "Probably the most straightforward way to think about these differences [between pursuit of sinusoidal and random stimulus motions] is to assume that all elements that are operating during the tracking of a randomly moving target will also be in the control loop during the following of a predictable input. The difference in system behavior for those two cases then must be sought in the presence of some compensating element during the tracking of periodic stimuli. This compensating element will be referred to as a predictor or learning operator" (p. 225).

Dallos and Jones provided a mathematical description of their 'predictor' by assuming that it was responsible for the observed differences between the response to sinusoidal and to random stimuli. The 'predictor' would have to 'know' when to participate, and Dallos and Jones suggested that it would be activated after the periodicity of the si-

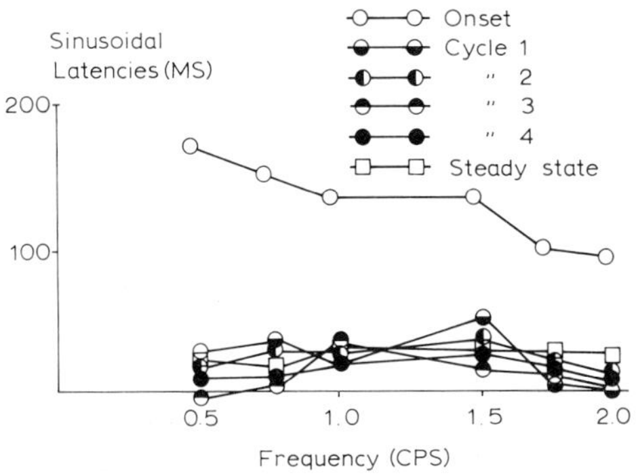

Fig. 21. Average latencies of one subject for the first few cycles of sinusoidal tracking. Steady-state latency is also shown. Note that latency reaches steady-state levels during the first cycle of tracking. (From Dallos and Jones, 1963)

nusoidal target motion had been detected. They assumed that the predictor was able to learn the repetitive pattern of motion and use what had been learned to pre-program the appropriate smooth oculomotor commands. But they found that phase lags dropped to asymptotic levels during the first cycle of pursuit (see Fig. 21), raising a major problem for the model because it seems unlikely that the 'predictor' would be able to learn the pattern of motion so quickly. Perhaps learning was not involved after all.

There were also problems with the assumption that anticipation was restricted to the tracking of sinusoidal motion. Studies showed that the gain of pursuit of random motions was low (as expected) but, surprisingly, tended to *increase* with increasing target frequency, at least for target frequencies below 1 Hz. This was noticed by St. Cyr and Fender (1969b) and later by Collewijn and Tamminga (1984), whose analysis eliminated saccades from the measurements and left the pure smooth response (Fig. 10b). Collewijn and Tamminga (1984) also found pronounced phase leads for the smooth pursuit of the lower-frequency components of the random motions (Fig. 10b) – hardly what would be expected of pure sensorimotor processes.

If anticipatory influences were not due to the learning of a response to a stereotyped pattern of target motion, then what was going on? Consideration of this question continues in the next section, which discusses modern studies of Dodge's 'preliminary drift'.

3.7.2. Anticipatory smooth eye movements before the onset of expected target motion

Recall that the 'preliminary drift' described by Dodge was a smooth eye movement that began before the start of target motion. This type of movement, which I will call 'anticipatory pursuit', does not conform to what investigators have come to expect of smooth eye movement, that is, anticipatory pursuits are not provoked by an immediately available sensory or perceptual signal because they occur while the target is still stationary. Also, anticipatory pursuits create, rather than correct, position and velocity errors because they take the eye away from the stationary target. Examples of anticipatory pursuit are shown in Fig. 22. An example of a particularly fast anticipatory pursuit (about 50 deg/s), is shown in Fig. 23.

Anticipatory pursuit has been observed often and has been studied in detail (e.g., Kowler and Steinman, 1979b,c, 1981; Kowler et al., 1984a; Becker and Fuchs, 1985; Boman and Hotson, 1988). These movements are about 10–25% of the velocity of the expected constant velocity motion. They are fastest when the direction of future target motion is known in advance, but they occur before motion in unpredictable directions as well (Kowler and Steinman, 1981). When the direction of target motion is unpredictable, the eye drifts in the direction the subject guesses the target will move (see Fig. 24). Anticipatory pursuits also occur before target motions at unpredictable times (Kowler and Steinman, 1979c) and at unpredictable velocities (Kowler and McKee, 1987). When the velocity of the target is unpredictable, the velocity of the anticipatory pursuit increases as the average velocity of the stimulus set increases (Kowler and McKee, 1987). These results show that randomization of stimulus parameters, by itself, does not prevent anticipatory pursuit. Instead, randomization affects the speed, direction or time of onset of the anticipatory pursuit so that these characteristics are best suited to the stimulus that is most likely to be presented.

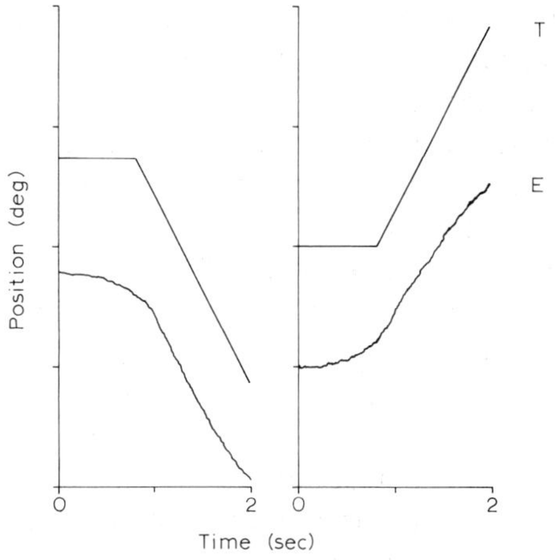

Fig. 22. Horizontal eye position (bottom traces) as a function of time during smooth pursuit of constant-velocity target motion (top traces) to the left (left-hand graph) and to the right (right-hand graph) for a naive subject. Note the start of pursuit about 300 ms before the target started to move. (From Kowler, 1989)

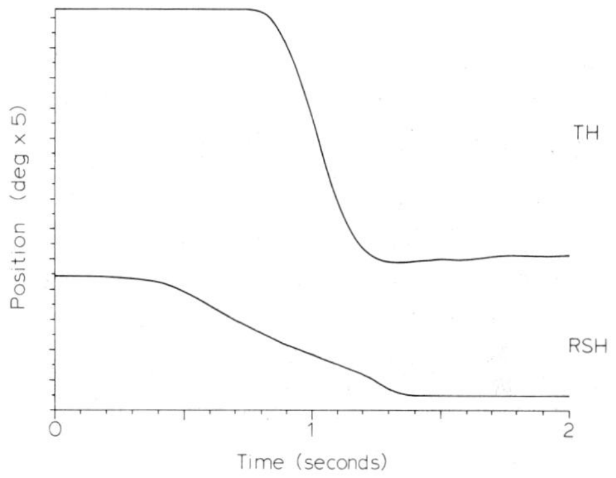

Fig. 23. Movements of the right eye (RSH) of a subject tracking a single point target (TH) moved by an experimenter across the subject's visual field. The subject knew the direction of target motion but did not know when the target was to begin moving relative to the onset of the trial. (Based on Collewijn et al., 1985)

The significance of finding anticipatory smooth eye movements before the onset of random target motions was stated clearly by Dodge (1931, p. 87):

"Some of our records show an important variant of the general picture of the first phase of pursuit. Possibly due to some more or less clear anticipation

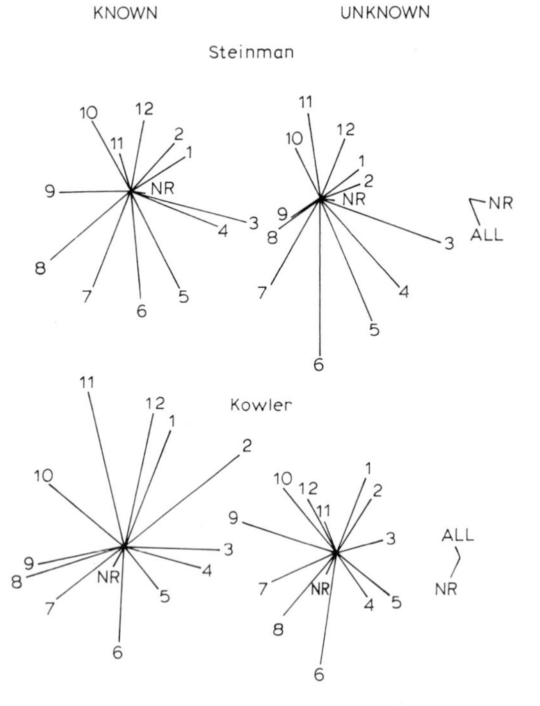

Fig. 24. The mean velocity of an anticipatory smooth pursuit eye movement before the onset of expected ramp motion away from center in the direction of the hours of the clockface. The numbers on the vectors denote the direction of ramp motion when ramp direction was *known* to the subject; the numbers when ramp direction was *unknown* denote the expected direction, which was reported before each trial. Mean eye velocity averaged over all directions (All) and in trials when no ramp motion was expected (NR) are also shown. (From Kowler and Steinman, 1981)

or set of which the record is the only indicator, the eye record may show a preliminary slow glide before the first saccadic refixation. In one record the preliminary glide is almost simultaneous with the beginning of objective motion in the other direction. It is obviously an anticipatory false reaction . . . *The unique feature of this record is the false anticipatory glide. If the start has been made in the right direction, this initial glide might have been read by the uninitiated as a true reaction with an extraordinarily short latency.* Such records should make us very conservative in measuring latencies from initial glides." (Italics mine.)

Dodge realized that anticipatory phenomena may easily escape notice, with significant consequences for the interpretation of the results. This is illustrated in the next section, which describes how expectations about future target motions continue to influence the pursuit response even after the target starts to move.

3.7.3. Effects of expectations on ongoing pursuit

As Dodge (1931) realized, anticipation is easy to detect when it produces something bizarre, such as a drift opposite to the direction of ongoing target motion (e.g., Kowler and Steinman, 1979c; Lisberger et al., 1981b). Anticipation is hard to detect when it produces something that, in principal, could have been accomplished by a reflexive sensorimotor process, such as an increase or a decrease in the speed of the eye relative to the speed of the target. Nevertheless, a role for anticipation during ongoing pursuit can be inferred because the pursuit response, even with randomly chosen stimuli, is modified according to the set of stimuli presented during an experimental session.

The effect of stimulus context is shown in Fig. 25. Each graph in the figure compares the response to the same constant-velocity target motion when it was tracked as part of a set of faster targets or a set of slower targets. The graphs show that the pursuit was faster when the target was tracked as part of the faster set.

The influence of the velocity-context is particularly clear during the first few hundred milliseconds of pursuit. Velocity-context acts to fashion a response that is suitable for the entire set of stimuli, rather than a response based exclusively on the current stimulus. As a result distinctions between responses to different stimuli are diminished. This is shown in Fig. 14, which contains eye velocity time-course functions taken from Kowler and McKee's (1987) study of oculomotor velocity discrimination (section 3.5). Each graph shows the response to the five target velocities tested during an experimental session. The particular target velocity was unknown to the subject and was selected at random before each trial. Each graph shows that the eye quickly accelerated to about the same value (near the mid-

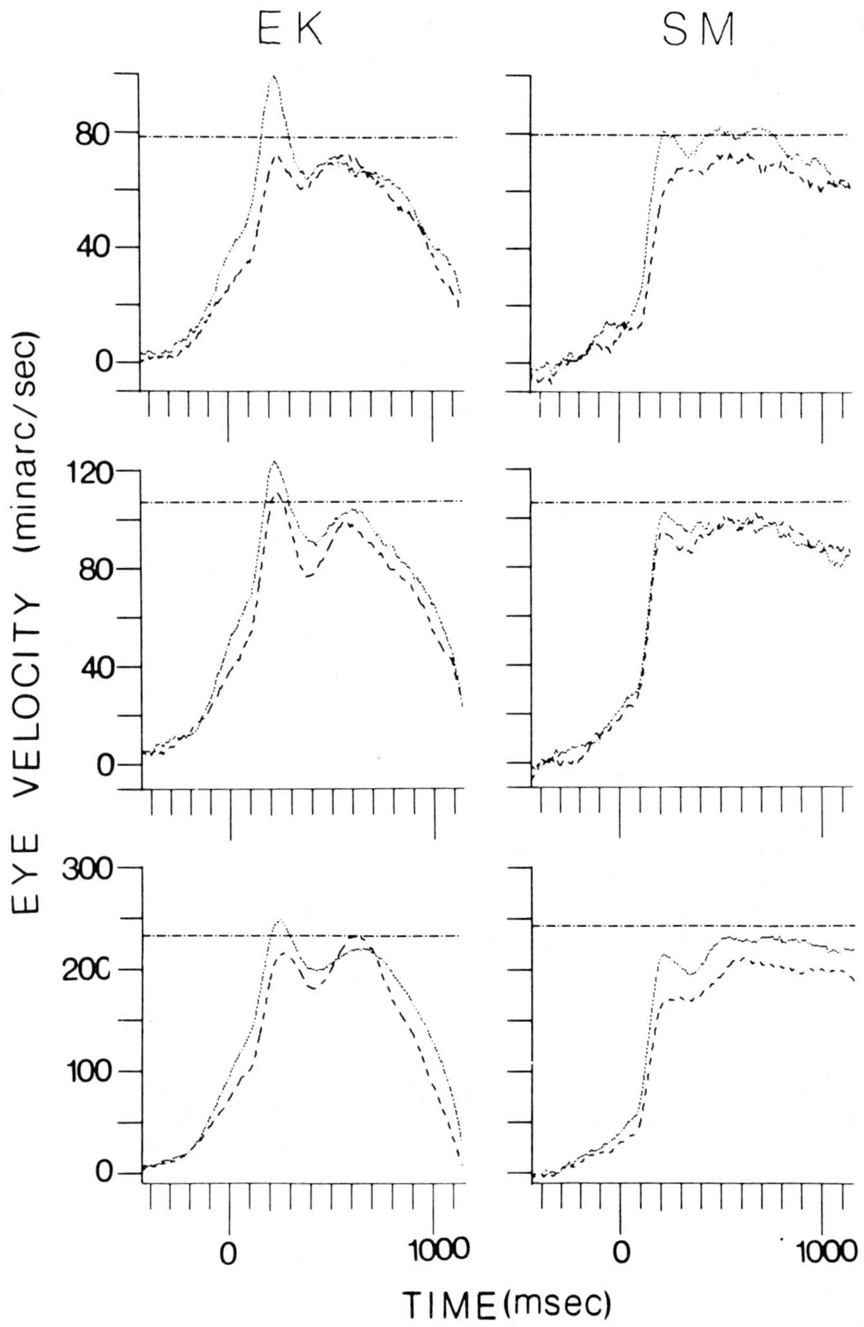

Fig. 25. Mean 100-ms eye velocity for subject EK (left) and SM (right) pursuing leftward target motion (target velocities given by the horizontal line in each graph). The dashed line shows eye velocity when the target was the fastest in a set of lower velocities, the dotted line when it was the slowest in a set of higher velocities. Eye velocity is shown as a function of the midpoint of successive 100-ms intervals whose onsets are separated by 10 ms. Target motion began at the interval labelled 0 on the absicissa and ended at 1000 ms for EK and at 1800 ms for SM. Velocities less than 0°/s indicate rightward motion. (From Kowler and McKee, 1987)

dle velocity of the set) for each of the five target velocities tested during an experimental session. The eye velocity functions did not fully sort themselves out until more than 0.5 s after the target had started to move – despite the fact that independent measurements of perceptual velocity discrimination showed that precise information about target velocity was available with 100–200-ms exposures. Evidently, smooth eye movements do not use such precise signals early in pursuit.

A similar tendency of context to obscure differences between responses to different targets was observed by Carl and Gellman (1987), whose data are shown in Fig. 26. One subject (Fig. 26c) tracked all the targets poorly. The other two (Fig. 26a,b) showed effects of context in that the slower targets in the set (5 and 10 deg/s) were tracked too fast and the faster targets (20 and 40 deg/s) too slowly. These effects of velocity-context are similar to the 'acceleration saturation' reported for smooth pursuit (e.g., Robinson et al., 1986) in that eye acceleration early in pursuit is slower than expected for the faster targets of a set, and faster than expected for the slower targets. It is tempting to attribute the 'acceleration saturation' to low-level sensory or sensorimotor phenomena, but the dependence of the initial acceleration on context suggests that higher-order processes are involved. These processes act before a target is presented to help generate a smooth response that is suitable for the likely, upcoming stimulus motion.

The dependence of the initial portion of pursuit on velocity-context shows that pursuit is launched based as much or more on the target motions of the immediate past, and the target motions expected in the near future, as on the current retinal signal. In this sense initial pursuit becomes an extension of the earlier, purely anticipatory portion. Becker and Fuchs (1985) also concluded that initial pursuit is an extension of the earlier anticipatory response based on their study of the pursuit of periodic, trapezoidal target motions. They found brisk initial pursuit during randomly selected episodes in which the visual target was removed from view just as the smooth target motion was expected to begin.

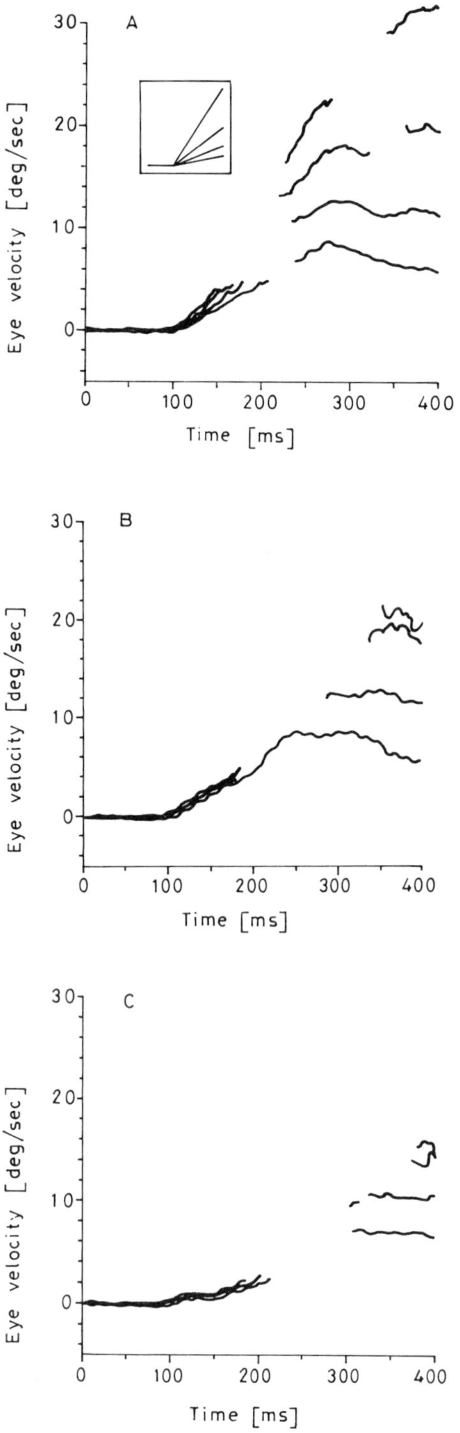

Fig. 26. Mean responses of three subjects to ramps of 5, 10, 20 and 40°/s. Each panel shows the responses of a different subject. (From Carl and Gellman, 1987)

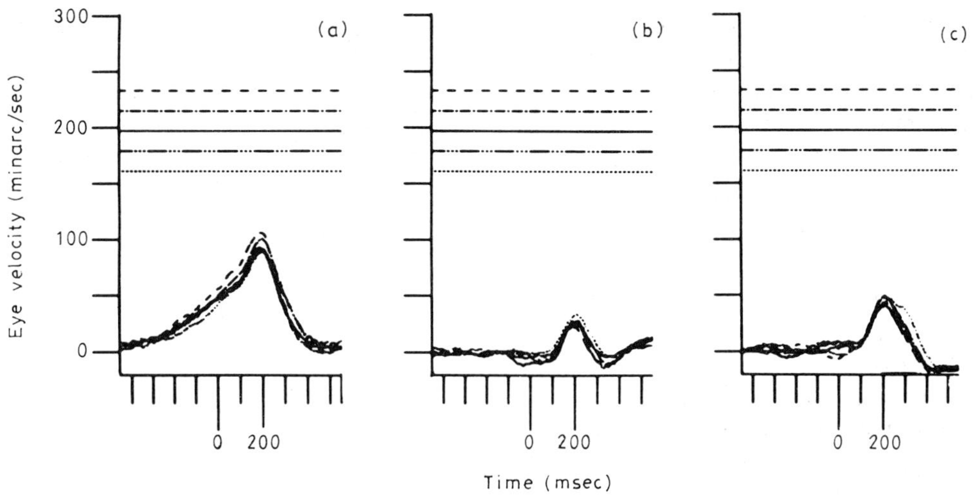

Fig. 27. Mean 100-ms eye velocity for subject EK pursuing briefly presented, constant-velocity target motion. (a) Leftward target motion when direction was known before the trial; (b) leftward and (c) rightward target motion when direction was selected at random. Eye velocity is shown as a function of the midpoint of 100-ms intervals whose onsets were separated by 10 ms. Target motion began at the interval labelled 0 on the abscissa and ended at the interval labelled 200. Velocities less than 0′/s indicate rightward eye motion in (a) and (b), and leftward motion in (c). The horizontal lines indicate the velocities of the targets. (From Kowler and McKee, 1987)

The dependence of the initial portion of pursuit on past history and expectations is shown vividly by the effects of expected duration. If the initial acceleration of the eye were to be evoked exclusively by the initial sweep of the target across the retina, then removing the target from view after the eye has had time to reach target velocity (usually within 200 ms of the onset of the target motion) should make no difference. But removing the target turns out to drastically inhibit the pursuit. When the duration of target motion is reduced to 200 ms, the eye hardly gets off the ground (see Fig. 27). Apparently, there is no brisk initial pursuit unless the target motion is expected to continue. Of course, it is possible to produce a faster response to the short-duration motions by mixing in some long trials. But this outcome does not mean that randomization lets the sensorimotor processes be revealed. It is another example of expectations intervening. When the duration of the target motion is randomized, the resulting pursuit response is a compromise: brief targets are tracked faster, and the longer-duration motions more slowly than when the duration of target motion is the same from trial to trial (see Fig. 28).

The evidence described in this section shows that the initial pursuit response is quite sensitive to the past history of stimulus motions and to expectations about future motion. In particular, past history and expectations reduce the sensitivity to stimulus differences in favor of the preparation of a response suited to the entire stimulus set. The contributions of past history and expectations make the initial response a poor indicator of the contents of the immediate sensory signals because these signals act on a system that is already predisposed to respond in a particular way. Indeed, the initial response may be the last place to look for fine-grain properties of the afferent signals, and one of the best to study past history and expectations.

3.7.4. Cognitive expectations vs. habits

The anticipatory phenomena described so far could have come from two sorts of process. One is the genuine cognitive expectation about the nature of the impending target motion. The second is more automatic and involuntary, for example, a trial-by-

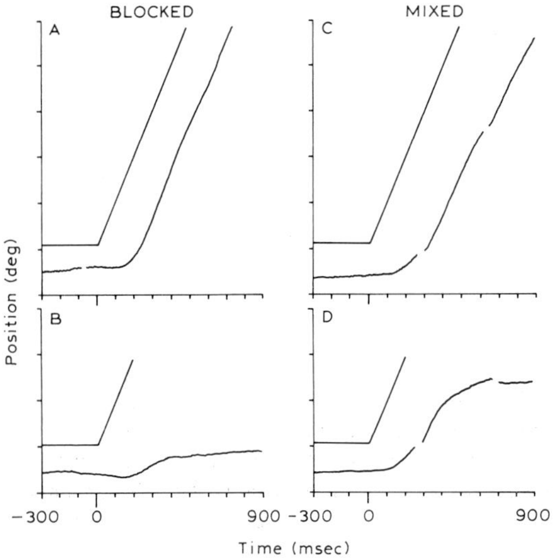

Fig. 28. Representative eye movement records showing smooth pursuit of 9.5°/s target motion, On the left (Blocked) the duration was set to a constant value of either 1 s (top graph) or 200 ms (bottom graph). On the right (Mixed), duration was selected randomly to be either 1 s or 200 ms on each trial. Note the brisk initial pursuit of the longer duration and the poor initial pursuit of the shorter duration motion in the Blocked condition. The initial response took on a value roughly in between these two extremes when durations were randomly mixed. The gaps in the eye traces indicate when saccades occurred. The eye traces were shifted by amounts roughly equal to the size of these saccades.

trial adaptive modification of some as yet unspecified aspect of pursuit whose goal is to promote the repetition of successful responses and discourage repetition of unsuccessful ones. Either of these processes could account for the findings summarized so far in this section, because in all cases the expectations about the future target motion were based on the past history of target motions.

Cognitive expectations and past history were separated in the following experiment (Kowler, 1989). Subjects pursued a target that moved downward inside an outline drawing of an inverted Y-shaped tube (see Fig. 29). At the junction of the right- and left-hand branches of the Y, the target would take either path with equal probability. The novel feature of this experiment was that in some sessions the path was disclosed before the trial by either an auditory cue (a synthesized voice saying 'right' or 'left') or by a visual cue (a barrier blocking access to the untravelled path).

In the sessions that did not contain cues, the velocity of anticipatory pursuit, measured before the target entered either oblique branch of the tube, was determined by the past history of target motions (Fig. 30a). The eye drifted rightward when prior stimulus motions were to the right and leftward when prior motions were to the left. The dependence on prior stimulus motions needs a bit more elaboration, because these 'sequential dependencies' illustrate the contribution of anticipatory processes when the subject does not know which motion will be presented. Kowler et al. (1984a) found the same pattern of sequential dependencies for anticipatory smooth eye movements before target steps in randomly chosen directions. Falmagne et al. (1975) had found an analogous pattern for two-choice manual reaction time in a button-pressing task. The sequential dependencies in both studies could be predicted by Falmagne et al.'s finite-state Markov model, in which the subject was assumed to prepare for one of the two possible stimuli before each trial. The model represents an adaptive process in that the preparatory state tends to be preserved following effective (accurate) responses and to change following ineffective (or inaccurate) responses (see Pavel's chapter for further discussion of adaptive models).

Adaptive processes, based solely on the effectiveness of prior responses, cannot, however, be the whole story. In the presence of the cues, which told the subject which stimulus would be presented, the anticipatory pursuits were determined by the direction in which the subject expected the target to move (Fig. 30b,c). Effects of the past were small, and clearly overridden by the cognitive expectations about future events.

This experiment shows that internal signals, representing expected target motion, and based on the processing of symbolic cues in the environment, can serve as stimuli for pursuit, just as if they were signals representing actual target motion. High-level, symbolic information, contained in the visual array, is being represented in a form that provides

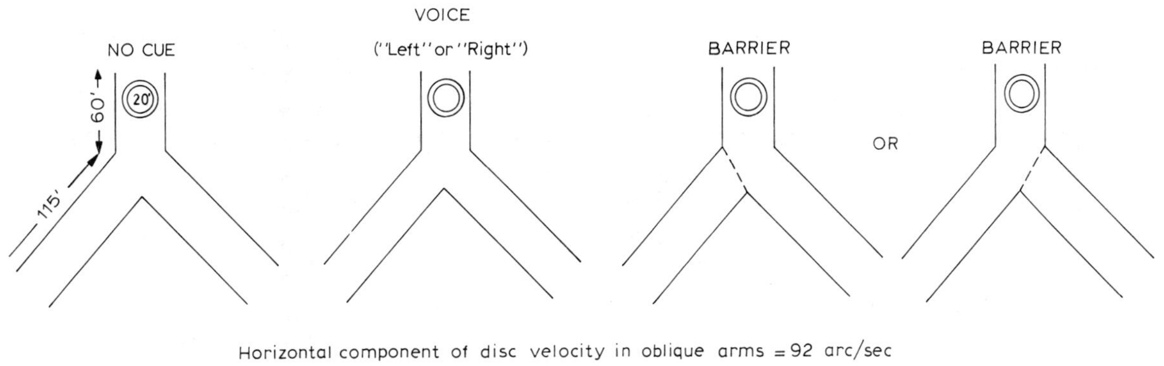

Fig. 29. The stimulus display in the experiment comparing habits to cognitive expectations. It consisted of a stationary inverted-Y-shaped tube and an annulus which served as the moving target. The velocity of the target was 130′/s. The target moved down the tube and continued at the same velocity down either the right-hand or left-hand oblique branch of the Y (horizontal component of velocity when the target was in either branch of the Y was 92′/s). The target was equally likely to travel down either branch. The branch in which the target moved was either undisclosed before each trial (*No Cue*), disclosed by a *Voice* cue, or disclosed by a visible *Barrier* cue blocking access to either the left-hand or right-hand branch. (From Kowler, 1989)

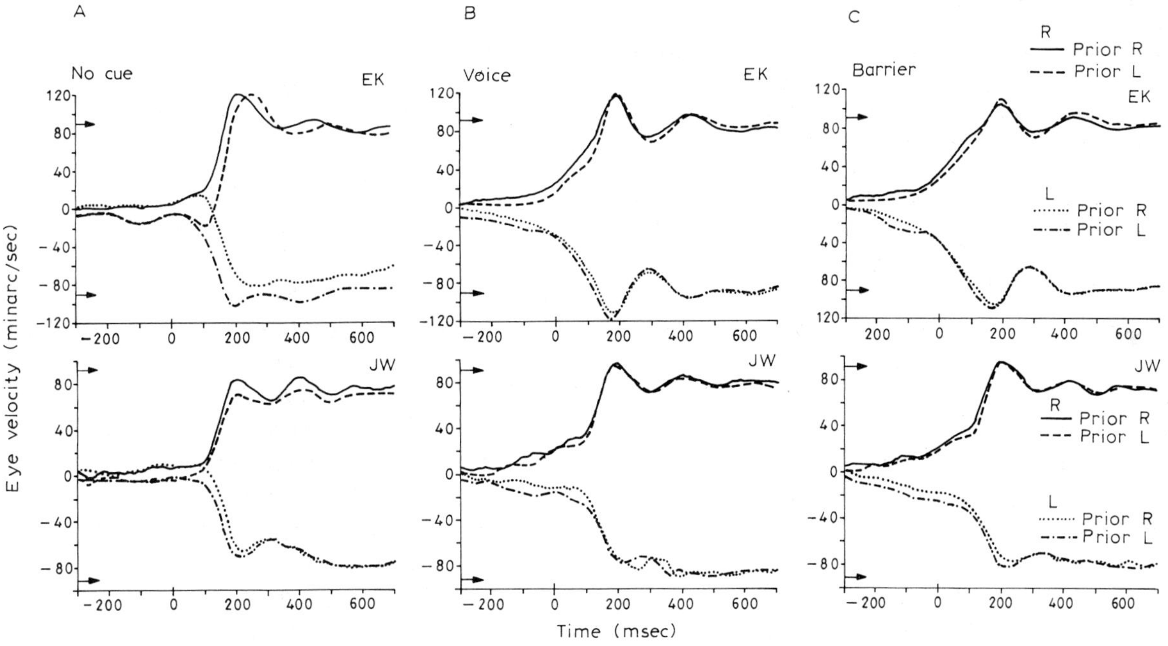

Fig. 30. Mean horizontal eye velocity during successive 100-ms intervals (onsets 10 ms apart) as a function of the midpoint of the interval when either (A) *No Cue,* (B) a *Voice* cue or (C) a *Barrier* cue about the direction of future horizontal target motion was given. Top graphs, EK; bottom, naive subject JW. Time 0 is the start of horizontal target motion (the first entry of the moving target into the oblique branch of the Y-shaped tube). Arrows on the ordinate show horizontal target velocity; negative values denote leftward motion. The top pair of functions in each graph show eye velocity when the eye moved down the left-hand branch. One function in each pair shows eye velocity when the target motion in the preceding trial was to the right; the other when the target motion in the preceding trial was to the left. Each mean is based on 80–100 observations. Standard errors were 1–2′/s and as high as 3′/s (5′/s with *No Cue*) only during the interval (0–200 ms) of most rapid eye acceleration. (From Kowler, 1989)

an effective, compelling signal to drive what is historically taken to be a low-level reflexive response.

3.7.5. Implications for the study of random target motions

The studies of anticipatory pursuit have implications for the interpretation of pursuit in the typical laboratory situation, in which stimuli are selected at random, often from large and diverse stimulus sets. This procedure has been defended on the grounds that randomization will eliminate or minimize the contribution of expectations, leaving the response solely in the hands of low-level sensorimotor processes. We have already seen that randomization, with no cues provided about the direction of future motion, does not eliminate the effects of stimulus set on pursuit (section 3.7.3) and does not eliminate anticipatory pursuit (Fig. 30a). Randomization is not eliminating expectations – it will not prevent guessing (Kowler and Steinman, 1979c, 1981) or sequential dependencies (Kowler et al., 1984a). Randomization is determining a particular preparatory state adopted before each experimental trial. An important consequence of this fact for models is that the stimulus-response relationships observed in one particular experimental context might not hold up in others. This limitation could be addressed by extensive investigation of various experimental contexts, or, preferably, by developing models which explictly incorporate *both* expectations and sensorimotor constraints, rather than models which assume that expectations can be ignored. It seems that incorporating expectations would be particularly useful because in most studies the random stimuli tested actually share many features (such as the duration or the meridian of the target motion), which would allow expectations to improve pursuit in ways that would not be readily noticeable in the data.

A different, and potentially more serious, problem with drawing conclusions based exclusively on studies with random motions is that such studies might not reveal the fundamental principles determining how smooth eye movements work. Realize that smooth pursuit is not particularly effective when randomization is sufficient to preclude accurate anticipatory movements. For example, pursuit of complex, random patterns is poor (3.7.1) and pursuit of randomly selected constant-velocity motions takes several hundred milliseconds to settle down (3.7.3). This suggests that, left to themselves, the low-level sensorimotor reflexes might not be able to guarantee pursuit which is accurate enough to support clear vision. And perhaps it is just as well. Random stimuli are unnatural. In natural environments, cues about the future direction and speed of target motion are plentiful. We have already seen that such cues can be used by observers for the programming of accurate anticipatory pursuits. Perhaps the best way to understand smooth eye movements, in the long run, will require studies of pursuit of cued patterns of motion, so that the stimulus to the lower-level sensorimotor circuits, consisting of the present target motion along with the expectations, will always be known.

3.8. Overview of smooth eye movement

This section on smooth eye movement has challenged the conventional assumptions, described in sections 3.1 and 3.2, that sensory signals operate in some automatic fashion to determine smooth oculomotor commands. This assumption may work very well for animals such as the rabbit (3.3), but for human beings the assumption was called into question because of the prominent role of central and subjective factors. We have seen, for example, that centrally organized motion signals can drive pursuit (3.5). We have also seen that velocity signals are organized into patterns before the selected signals reach the smooth oculomotor circuitry (3.6). And we have seen that the effective stimulus for pursuit includes a signal representing the stimulus motion hundreds of milliseconds into the future (3.7).

Cognitive and subjective factors are not, of course, the whole story. In the absence of normal visual feedback, idiosyncrasies are rampant (3.4). Moreover, the sequential dependencies show that the results of pursuit are closely monitored to keep the response within acceptable limits (3.7). At this point, we are very much in the dark because basic questions have not been addressed. What, for example, defines an acceptable pursuit response? Achievement of some optimal retinal velocity, or, perhaps, some indication that the target is seen clearly?

The theme of this section has been that answers to such questions, and a more complete understanding of pursuit, may be better obtained if we acknowledge the role of central and subjective factors from the outset and try to formulate as complete a description as possible of the complex input signals which are sent to the lower-level oculomotor circuitry. In the meantime, we might enjoy the cleverness of nature in linking the involuntary oculomotor pursuit to an active and busy consciousness. Why, after all, should one go to the trouble of designing a visual algorithm for selecting a target or computing its velocity purely from momentary sensory cues when the human being has already decided which target is of interest and already knows something about when and where it will begin to move?

The following section considers saccades. These are voluntary motor responses, in the sense that they can be initiated in whichever direction one wishes, regardless of the presence or the nature of the visual array. As a result no special demonstrations will be needed to show that central and subjective factors must be included in order to correctly interpret the performance.

4. Saccades

4.1. Saccades, unlike smooth eye movements, may be, and probably always are, initiated voluntarily

Voluntary control of saccades may be demonstrated simply by noticing that it is possible to look around all sorts of visual environment whenever or wherever you choose.

The wide appreciation of volitional control has encouraged the use of saccades as overt indicators of otherwise hidden cognitive processes. (For comprehensive reviews and evaluations, see the chapters by Suppes, Viviani and O'Regan.) Reading thoughts from saccades is a dangerous business if it is assumed that where one looks, or how long one looks in a given place, is completely a function of choice or interest, independent of the constraints imposed by the saccadic programming apparatus itself. On the other hand, equally troublesome would be a search for invariant relationships between the visual stimulus and saccades under the assumption that performance is completely a function of the stimulus configuration, ignoring the contributions of voluntary choice, selective attention and expectations. The following sections will summarize research on saccadic capacities with the goal of elucidating the constraints imposed by sensorimotor processes and by central and subjective factors.

4.2. The endpoint of saccades relative to a target stimulus may be controlled by the subject

A conventional way of studying saccades has been to ask a subject to move the eye to a small target that appears suddenly in eccentric vision. The reaction time, the size and the direction of the saccade are measured. The target usually disappears from its central location just as the new eccentric target appears; thus, the target is actually moving from one location to another and is appropriately called a 'target step'.

Observers often make saccades that are inaccurate ('undershooting' or 'overshooting') (e.g., Becker and Fuchs, 1969; Frost and Poppel, 1976; Wyman and Steinman, 1973a), sometimes with reliable errors of offset position of up to 30–50% of the size of the step (Timberlake et al., 1972). Such errors are not compulsory. Saccades to continuously visible targets can be far more accurate (Collewijn et al., 1988a,b; Lemij and Collewijn, 1989). Also, subjects can control the endpoint of the saccades. They can decide to make a saccade that either falls short of, or exceeds, the position of the target (Steinman et al., 1973), or is in a direction opposite to the direction of the target step (e.g., Hallett's (1978) 'anti-saccades'), or lands in a selected location within a simple outline drawing of a form (He et al., 1988). Some of the deliberate mislocalizations, such as the 'anti-saccades', occur at the cost of increased latency or decreased spatial precision. Nevertheless, the capacity to adjust saccade size shows that the endpoint can be chosen by the individual using visual information as a guide.

How precisely the chosen saccadic endpoint can be reached will depend on limitations imposed by sensorimotor processes. Examples of such limitations will be described in the next section.

4.3. The eccentricity of the visual target affects the spatial precision and the latency of saccades

The effect of the retinal eccentricity of the target on the spatial precision of saccades is shown by the increase in the variability of the size of the saccade as the size of the target step increases (Timberlake et al., 1972). Fig. 31, based on Timberlake et al.'s data, shows the effect of target eccentricity on the *relative* precision of saccades. Relative precision is described by the ratio of the standard deviation of saccade size to the size of the target step. (This measure is analogous to Fitts' (1954) 'index of difficulty' for manual responses and to the Weber fraction for perceptual reports.) Fig. 31 shows that the ratio of the standard deviation of saccade size to the size of the target step decreases as the size of the step increases, reaching an asymptotic value of about 0.1 at a step size of 2 deg. An interesting property of this curve is the discontinuity at 40′, near the edge of the foveal floor (Polyak, 1941), which represents a transition to a less precise localization mechanism. A discontinuity occurs at the same place in standard tests of visual acuity (e.g., Millodot, 1966), suggesting that the precision of visual mechanisms which code the spatial location of the target sets a limit on the spatial precision of saccades.

Limitations other than those imposed by visual mechanisms are probably needed to explain the reduction in the relative precision of saccades for target steps smaller than 30 minutes of arc, shown in Fig. 31. Nonvisual sources are involved because the relative precision of perceptual judgments of spatial distance is quite good for distances smaller than 30 minutes of arc. For example, observers can reliably discriminate differences of about 8% in the size of small target steps; perceptual discrimination improves to about 2% when the task is to discriminate the distance between two stationary references (Westheimer, 1979). Clearly, we can estimate small distances more precisely than we can track small displacements of a target.

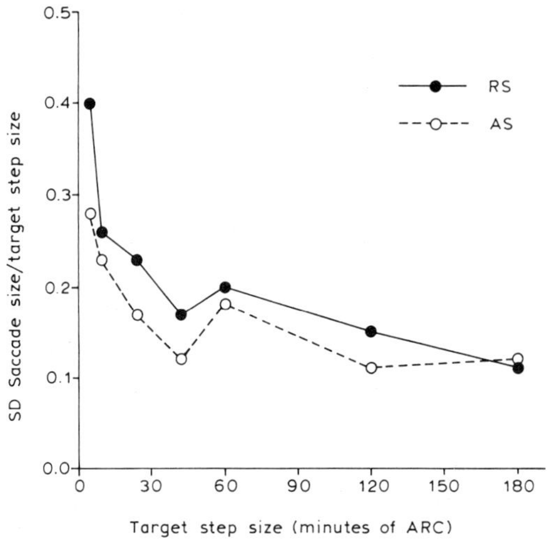

Fig. 31. The ratio of the standard deviation of saccade size to the size of the target step as a function of the size of the target step for subjects RS and AS. (Based on Timberlake et al., 1972)

The spatial imprecision of small saccades is not limited to the tracking of target steps. Haddad and Steinman (1973) asked subjects to make the smallest saccade they could away from a stationary point target. They found that the average size of the saccade was about 5.5′, with a standard deviation of 2.5′. The ratio of the standard deviation to the size of the saccade is about 0.45, about the same ratio observed for the saccades made to track 5′ target steps (see Fig. 31).

The large SD/step-size ratios for small target steps, described above, show that precise control of small saccades is difficult to achieve. The difficulty is further demonstrated by the long latency of the saccades made to track small target steps. Average saccadic latency in target step-tracking tasks increases only slightly (about 20 ms) as step size increases from 30′ to 40 deg (Bartz, 1962; White et al., 1962; Heywood and Churcher, 1980; Frost and Poppel, 1976), but latency increases sharply (by more than 100 ms) as step size decreases from 30′ to 3.5′ (see Fig. 32) (Wyman and Steinman, 1973b; Kowler and Anton, 1987). The long latency of the saccades made to track small target steps shows that the increase in the SD/step-size ratio for small saccades (Fig. 31) was not due to a decision to sacrifice the spatial precision of saccades in order to shorten the latency, and suggests that small saccades are relatively difficult to program.

The difficulty subjects have in exercising precise control over the spatial and the temporal properties of small saccades may account for previous beliefs in a ¼to ½deg saccadic 'dead zone'. The saccadic 'dead zone' was proposed by Rashbass (1961), who found that target steps this small were not tracked. Yet subjects will track target steps as small as 3′ if they are explicitly asked to do so (Wyman and Steinman, 1973a), showing that the 'dead zone' is not a hard-wired limit, and may represent no more than the understandable reluctance to try to do a hard task.

Fortunately, the difficulty subjects have controlling small saccades, and any consequent reluctance to use them, should not cause any visual difficulties. Psychophysical studies have so far turned up no useful role for saccades smaller than about 15′. For example, subjects choose to avoid making any saccades when they perform finely guided visuomotor tasks (such as threading a needle) which force attention to be paid to small, circumscribed areas (Winterson and Collewijn, 1976; also, Bridgeman and Palca, 1980, for the same result using a video version of a needle-threading task, which did not involve any movements of the arm or fingers.) Also, using saccades to count the items haphazardly arranged in a 30′ diameter field does not improve counting accuracy beyond what can be achieved with a stationary eye, even though larger saccades (about 20–30′) are helpful when items are contained in a 2° diameter field (Kowler and Steinman, 1977, 1979a). The retinal transients accompanying

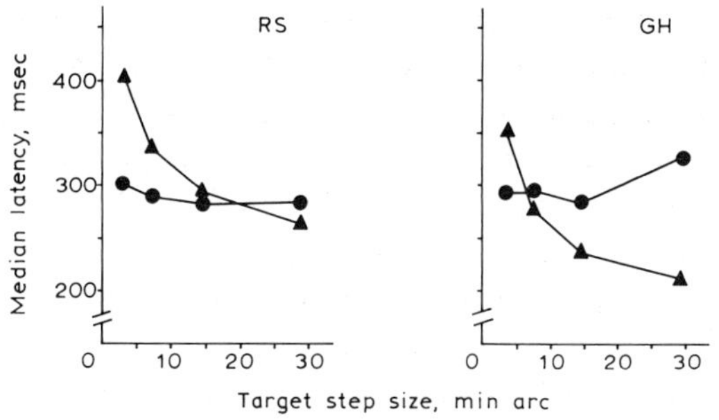

Fig. 32. Median latencies of the first saccade in the direction of the target step for target steps of different magnitudes when the subject was instructed to track the target step (triangles). The circles show latency when the target step served as a signal to go to a continuously visible second target located 14′ below the target that stepped (circles). Saccades to the continuously visible target were unaffected by step-size, showing that the long latency of the saccades used to track small steps (triangles) was due to factors connected with saccadic programming, rather than with stimulus detection. The left graph shows the data for subjects RS; the right graph for subject GH. (From Wyman and Steinman, 1973b)

saccades are not particularly helpful for vision (cf. Kowler and Steinman, 1980), or for visual information processing (Kowler and Sperling, 1980; 1983). Smooth movements of the eye are optimal for visibility (see Steinman and Levinson's chapter) and, if anything, saccades will produce retinal smears and rapid retinal image motion, which can impair various sorts of perceptual judgment (Volkmann, 1986; also, Sperling's chapter, this volume).

It is unlikely that any useful role for the small saccades will ever emerge. The studies of latency and spatial precision, described above, have shown that saccades are hardest to use just where we need them the least: in the central ½deg of the retina where visual discrimination is most acute. This makes previous ideas that small saccades control the position of the eye during maintained fixation (Cornsweet, 1956; Krauskopf et al., 1960), or constitute a controlled, miniature search pattern of small regions (Steinman et al., 1973), or reduce visual thresholds (Ditchburn, 1980), or contribute to the perception of forms (Gaarder, 1960), seem implausible. Small saccades are simply not up to any of these jobs, and they are not needed for them.

The precision of visual capacities in the central retina is much better than the precision of the saccades that can be made to inspect this region.

The spatial imprecision of small saccades, in contrast with the highly precise visual judgments in the central fovea, also implies that saccades do not have access to the same precise information about target position that is available for visual judgments, or else that saccades receive precise information about target position, which is then obscured by other sources of variability, such as limitations inherent in the oculomotor output machinery.

The material in this section summarizes some of the relationships between saccades and the spatial properties of the stimulus. The next section explores some of the relationships between saccades and the temporal properties of the stimulus. This discussion will bring back the issue of anticipation, which was considered in the section on smooth eye movements (see 3.7). For example, anticipation is needed to explain why saccades can be used to track 'predictable' target steps (square-wave target motion) with little or no latency (Stark et al., 1962; Dallos and Jones, 1963). Further discussion of the role of anticipation in saccadic performance begins in the next section.

4.4. Saccadic commands can be prepared, in whole or in part, before the appearance of the eccentric target

When a subject is asked to make some sort of manual response, a button press, for example, to indicate which of many possible stimuli were presented, the reaction time of the response is found to depend on the number of possible stimulus alternatives (see Luce, 1986, for a review and analysis of this phenomenon). The demonstration that the reaction time to a stimulus depends on the number of alternatives is a classic indication that the response is not evoked reflexively by a stimulus, but depends, in part, on preparations that occur before the stimulus appears.

Oculomotorists have not been able to agree about whether there is a comparable dependence of saccadic reaction time on the number of alternative stimuli, a disagreement which has led to some confusion about whether to treat saccades as voluntary motor responses, or as reflexes elicited by eccentric stimuli. Hackman (1940) found that saccadic latency decreased when subjects knew which one of 8 possible stimulus locations would contain the target. But Saslow (1967b), who criticized Hackman's experiment because an audible click accompanied each stimulus, found that reaction time remained the same (about 200 ms) as the number of possible target locations increased from 2 to 8, regardless of whether the locations were on the same or opposite sides of the fixation target. Saslow's (1967b) results were later confirmed by Heywood and Churcher (1980), who found no effect on saccadic latency of increasing the number of alternative target locations from 2 to 16, but not by Michard et al. (1974), who found that latency increased as the number of alternatives increased from 2 to 4. Interpretation of the relationship between reaction time and the number of possible stimulus alternatives is complicated because many unambiguously voluntary responses, such as speaking, do not show this dependence either (Luce, 1986).

The number of alternative stimuli did prove to be influential when the task was harder than the tracking of a single, stepping target. For example, Viviani and Swensson's (1982) subjects were told to look at a target form which was embedded in a field of many different background forms. They found that the latency of saccades was reduced by decreasing the number of alternative locations that might contain the target form.

There is less disagreement that saccades are affected by changing the relative probability of finding a target in a given location. Norcia et al. (1979) and Kowler et al. (1984a) found that the latency of saccades was shorter for targets in more probable locations. (Kowler et al. (1984a) also found sequential dependencies analogous to those observed for anticipatory pursuits (see section 3.7.4), i.e., shorter latency and improved accuracy for saccades to steps preceded by steps in the same direction.) He and Kowler (1989) found effects of location probability on saccadic accuracy when the task was to look as quickly as possible at a target presented in the company of a nontarget stimulus. Saccades were accurate, and location probability was not influential, in an easier task in which the target was presented alone, without a nontarget. (See section 4.7.1 for further discussion of this experiment.)

The studies summarized above show that location probability is most influential when the task is fairly difficult, and when subjects are encouraged to respond quickly, even if responding quickly diminishes the accuracy of the saccade. This is not too surprising. There have been several reports that subjects can trade-off saccadic latency for accuracy (e.g., Steinman et al., 1973; Findlay, 1981; Viviani and Swensson, 1982; Ottes et al., 1985; Coëffé and O'Regan, 1987). The need to respond quickly in a difficult task would encourage the preparation of saccadic programs before target localization was completed. Such programs would be expected to incorporate information about the likely location of targets, rather than be based exclusively on information acquired from the immediate visual display.

The studies of the effects of probability on saccades show that saccadic performance results from the combined influence of newly acquired visual information, along with the past experience and expectations of the subject. The same point was made about smooth eye movements in section 3. The discussion of how past experience, expectations and lower-level sensorimotor factors determine saccadic programming continues in the next section, which considers what happens when various sorts of stimulus appear (or disappear) in the field of view at about the time that the visual target appears.

4.5. Saccadic latency is affected by the abrupt appearance or disappearance of stimuli

4.5.1. Signals that facilitate or delay saccadic programming

A classic characteristic of manual responses is that a warning about the impending appearance of the stimulus reduces the reaction time (cf. Luce, 1986). Saccades show the conventional effects of warnings in that the latency is reduced when the warning stimulus precedes the appearance of the target (Saslow, 1967a; Ross and Ross, 1980).

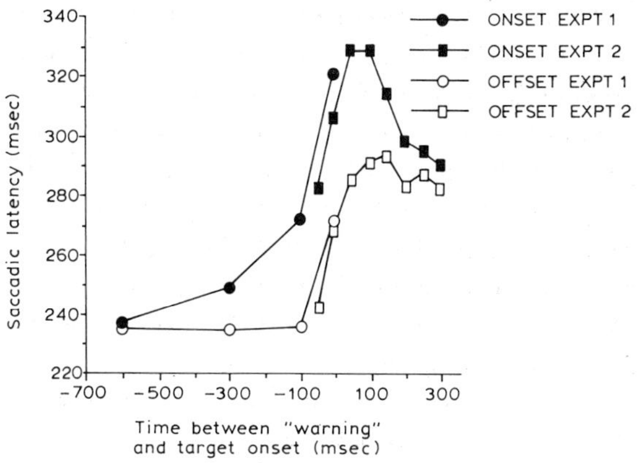

Fig. 33. Mean saccadic latency as a function of time between a warning signal and the appearance of an eccentric target. Filled symbols show latency when the warning was conveyed by the onset of a central stimulus, open symbols by the offset. Negative values on the abscissa indicate that the warning preceded the appearance of the target. Data are taken from experiments 1 (circles) and 2 (squares) of Ross and Ross (1980).

An example of the effects of warning signals on saccadic reaction time appears in Fig. 33, based on Ross and Ross (1980). They found that saccadic latency was shortened by warning signals which preceded the appearance of the target. Things were a bit more complicated, however, because warnings conveyed by the offset of a central stimulus (that is, the offset of a stimulus located near the initial fixation point) were more effective than warnings conveyed by the onset of a central stimulus. Moreover, central onsets that occurred while programming was in progress, i.e., during the 200 ms interval following the appearance of the visual target, were harmful, increasing saccadic latency by about 40 ms. Central offsets during this period had no effect. Mackeben and Nakayama (1988) demonstrated a comparable dissociation between the effects of central onsets and central offsets in a psychophysical task requiring a shift of attention to an eccentric target while the eye remained stationary.

These studies, describing what happens when central stimuli abruptly appear or disappear, have shown that saccades are clearly subject to conventional 'warning' effects. In addition, the abrupt appearance of a central stimulus can delay saccadic programming, and the abrupt disappearance of a central stimulus might facilitate programming, for reasons which appear to be unrelated to the preparatory processes usually invoked to explain the effects of warning signals.

4.5.2. 'Express' saccades

The effects of the onsets and offsets of central stimuli on saccades, described in the previous section, should not be confused with the so-called 'express' saccades (Fischer and Boch, 1983; Fischer et al., 1984; Boch et al., 1984; Boch and Fischer, 1986; Schiller et al., 1987, in monkey; Fischer and Ramsperger, 1984, 1986; Mayfrank et al., 1986; Fischer and Breitmeyer, 1987, in human beings). 'Express' saccades are said to have unusually short latencies (about 100 ms) and are observed when the sudden disappearance of a central fixation stimulus is followed after a temporal 'gap' of 200 ms by the onset of the eccentric target. ('Express' saccades are extremely rare when the fixation point remains visible; Mayfrank et al., 1986; Becker, 1989.) 'Express' saccades have been referred to at various times as 'reflex-like eye movements' governed by a distinct mechanism (Schiller et al., 1987; Fischer and Breitmeyer, 1987) or as a distinct 'population' of saccades attributed to a special 'internal state' of the visual or oculomotor system (Mayfrank et al., 1987).

Not all saccades are 'express', according to the references cited above. The latency distributions are said to be bimodal, with the second peak occurring at a latency of about 150 ms. Mayfrank et al. (1986) and Fischer and Breitmeyer (1987) have attributed the 'express' saccades to what they have called a 'disengagement of attention' from the central visual target. But the experiments are open to a simpler interpretation, namely, that the instances of extremely short latencies were due to conventional warning effects. In the experiments cited above, the offset was a completely reliable warning about the time of appearance of the target because the time between the offset and the appearance of the target (the 'gap') was always 200 ms. In one experiment in which 'gap' duration was randomized, the range of tested 'gaps' was small (200 vs. 220 ms) and the location of the eccentric target was always the same (Fischer and Ramsperger, 1984; Fig. 2c). Even in cases in which target position was randomly varied (4° right vs. 4° left) and the fixation point remained visible (a situation producing relatively few 'express' saccades) the target, nevertheless, appeared at a known time (2 s after the onset of the fixation point). So, the experimental arrangements that produce 'express' saccades offered considerable advance information about when or where the target would appear and, therefore, allowed the subjects to save time by preparing at least a portion of the saccadic program in advance.

The advanced preparation of saccadic programs would seem not to have played a role in Schiller et al.'s (1987) studies of 'express' saccades in monkey, because both the location of the target and the duration of the 'gap' were randomly chosen from among a few possibilities (fewer than 6 target locations and 7 gap durations). The distribution of saccadic latencies was bimodal, with the earlier saccades (latency 100 ms) representing the 'express' variety, and the rest representing ordinary saccades (latency about 150 ms). Distributions of saccadic endpoints were not provided, but for the purposes of the present discussion possible latency-accuracy relationships (see section 4.4) will be ignored and the distributions of the endpoints of the short- and long-latency saccades will be assumed to be the same. Could the advance preparation of saccades have accounted for Schiller et al.'s results?

An 'all-or-none' advanced preparation of saccades would not. By 'all-or-none' I mean that the subject prepares an unmodifiable saccadic program before the stimulus appears. This kind of advance preparation would be expected to lead to many errors, or to saccades occurring before the appearance of the target. It was the absence of either of these phenomena in Schiller et al.'s (1987) experiment (monkeys were not rewarded either for early or for erroneous saccades) that led the authors to discount advanced preparation. Nevertheless, there are other ways for advanced preparation to influence saccades which would not necessarily produce either errors or early saccades. These include: (1) the advanced preparation of a selected aspect of a future saccade, such as the preparation of the saccade size without specification of its direction until the stimulus appears (see Rosenbaum et al., 1984, who demonstrated the advanced preparation of selected aspects of finger movements); (2) the storage of prepared motor programs in a memory buffer, which is scanned for the appropriate program after the reaction signal is given to begin responding (Sternberg et al., 1978a,b; Zingale and Kowler, 1987); or (3) the establishment of overlearned, habitual motor sequences, which can be executed at unusually high speeds (Craik, 1947; Lashley, 1951; Levy-Schoen, 1981; Steinman et al., 1973). The kinds of preparatory process described above could have played a role in Schiller et al.'s (1987) experiments without producing either erroneous or early saccades. For example, consider the experiment which tested four gap durations (0, 50, 100, 200 ms) and four possible target locations. Suppose that the monkey begins to prepare motor programs for the four saccadic commands in sequence as soon as the warning stimulus occurs and stores the programs in short-term memory. (Properties of this memory, such as its capacity and the length of time its contents can be maintained without decay, would have to be determined experimentally.) The preparation continues until the eccentric target appears, when the monkey begins to search the set of prepared, stored programs for the one he needs. If the appropriate program had already been prepared, and was still present in the memory buffer, then saccadic latency would be quite short because all the monkey would need to do is retrieve the program from memory and begin execution. If, however, the appropriate program had not been prepared, then preparation would have to begin from scratch and, as a result, saccadic latency would be increased. This model predicts that the proportion of accurate 'express' saccades would increase with increasing 'gap' duration because the probability that the appropriate saccade was pre-programmed would increase the more time the monkey had to complete the preparation. In fact, the proportion of 'express' saccades did increase (from 32% to 94%, in the example given in Fig. 2 of Schiller et al.) as the 'gap' duration increased from 0 to 200 ms. Attributing the short-latency saccades made by Schiller et al.'s monkeys to a preparatory process, such as the simple one I have described, rather than to a special 'express' saccade generator, seems reasonable in the light of the fact that the animals were highly trained (Schiller et al. report that the animals performed 1000 to 2000 trials per day). Training would be expected to facilitate saccadic programming processes based on learning and memory, and would not be expected to influence low-level reflexes.

The research summarized in this section shows that, while the offset of a central stimulus can be a more effective 'warning' signal than the onset (Ross and Ross, 1980), central offsets (or 'disengagements of attention') do not evoke the so-called 'express' saccades. Evidence does not warrant attributing a subset of saccades with very short latencies to a special class of eye movements. Short-latency saccades can result from conventional 'warning' effects, or from a variety of potentially interesting phenomena involving the advanced preparation of saccades. The suggestion of bimodality in a response latency distribution is insufficient reason to posit separate classes of saccades.

To make this point more clearly, it is instructive to consider that the suggestion of bimodality in a distribution of latencies of finger movements is insufficient reason to posit a separate class of finger movements. There are other approaches to the analysis of latency distributions which do not propose different classes of responses. Studies of manual reaction time have long focused on the analysis of latency distributions and the development of analytic techniques to predict the parameters of the distributions based on the probabilities of the subject's being in one or another preparatory state. For example, in a model proposed by Falmagne et al. (1975) (mentioned briefly in section 3.7.4) to account for sequential dependencies in a two-choice manual reaction time task, subjects are assumed to be preparing for either one of the two possible stimuli before each trial. If the stimulus presented in a trial is the one the subject had anticipated, then reaction time is drawn from one distribution; if the other stimulus appeared, reaction time is drawn from a different distribution with a higher mean value. The resulting distribution of reaction times to the presentation of each stimulus is thus a weighted mixture of the two underlying distributions, one for the trials in which the subject had been prepared for the stimulus, and the other for trials in which he had not been prepared*. In other words, short latency responses aren't special reflexes; they are responses to those stimuli which happen to have been correctly anticipated by the subject. The important point is that the same preparatory process needed to explain distributions of manual reaction times may explain distributions of saccadic reaction times as well without proposing separate short and long-latency saccadic mechanisms. Development of saccadic models based on ideas about preparatory processes, and investigation of the different internal operations that constitute 'preparation', may in the long run lead to more satisfactory models of saccades than speculations about special saccadic mechanisms.

* Falmagne et al. (1975) described the preparatory process in terms of memory search. They proposed that the subject identifies the stimulus (consisting of one of two simple forms) presented on each trial by comparing it, in sequence, with memory representations of each of the two possible stimuli. So, preparation for stimulus 'A' meant that the actual stimulus presented on the trial was compared first to the memory representation of stimulus 'A' and then to the memory representation of stimulus 'B'. Although Falmagne et al. chose to describe preparation in terms of memory search, a variety of other internal preparatory processes would also be consistent with the formal properties of their model.

I will next consider inferences drawn about saccadic programming from what would appear to be simple variants on the typical single target-step experiment described so far. These are: (1) saccades to two consecutive target steps, which led to inferences about the integration of target-location information over time, and (2) saccades to a target among visual backgrounds, which led to inferences about the integration of target-location information across space.

4.6. Saccades to two consecutive target steps suggest an ability to adjust saccadic programs quickly on the basis of newly acquired stimulus information

Interest in studying the saccades made to track two consecutive target steps began with Westheimer (1954), who presented a target step away from center followed 40–240 ms later by a step back. He found that the subjects always tracked both target steps in sequence, even for the shortest interstep interval, when the target had already returned to the center before the first saccade was made. Westheimer's (1954) subjects obviously took the instruction to track the motion quite literally.

Subjects adopted a more lenient interpretation of the two-step tracking task in the 1960s and 1970s. Wheeless et al. (1967) found that 93% of saccades neglected the first target step and headed directly for the target's final position when the inter-step interval was as short as 50 ms; 77% went to the final position when the interval was 100 ms and 32% when it was 200 ms. What intrigued Wheeless et al. about their result was that so many of the saccades with the longest (200 ms) inter-step interval headed directly for the final target position. This seemed odd because the latency of saccades to the presentation of a single target step was only about 280 ms. This meant that as early as 80 ms before a saccade to the first step would have occurred, the saccade was cancelled and replaced by a new saccade to the final target position. One strong assumption contained in this interpretation is that the neglect of the first step was due exclusively to cancellation and re-programming, rather than to the programming of a single saccade to the final target position based on the expectation that a second step might occur. Wheeless et al., aware of this problem, tried to dissuade subjects from expecting double steps by testing mostly single-step trials. Nevertheless, the expectation of a double step probably played some role, because they noted that the latency to single steps was 25 ms longer in experimental sessions containing both single- and double-step trials than in sessions containing single-step trials exclusively.

Subsequent studies of the tracking of two consecutive target steps explored effects of the spatial properties of the stimulus. For example, saccades were more often directed to the final target position when the second step brought the target closer to, rather than further from, the starting fixation point (Levy-Schoen and Blanc-Garin, 1974). Also, the average latency of saccades made to the final target position was shorter if both targets were on the same side (rather than opposite sides) of the starting fixation point (Komoda et al., 1973). The effects of the spatial properties of the stimulus suggested to these authors that the 'cancellation' of a saccade, described by Wheeless et al. (1967), was not complete, but was more a matter of revising certain programmed saccadic parameters based on newly acquired visual information.

A case for the revision of parameters was also made by Becker and Jurgens (1979), who found that subjects often tracked a sequence of two consecutive target steps (both on the same side of the fixation point) with a single saccade that landed between the endpoints of the two steps. The 'averaging' of the two target endpoints suggested to Becker and Jurgens (1979) that saccadic amplitude is computed after saccadic direction, and that the amplitude computation pools all the positional information that is available within a certain temporal window. The generality of this pooling process would have to be limited, however, because Becker and Jurgens (1979) found that 'averaging' occurred more often, and required less time, when the second step brought the target closer to, rather than further from, the fixation point. This implied that it is

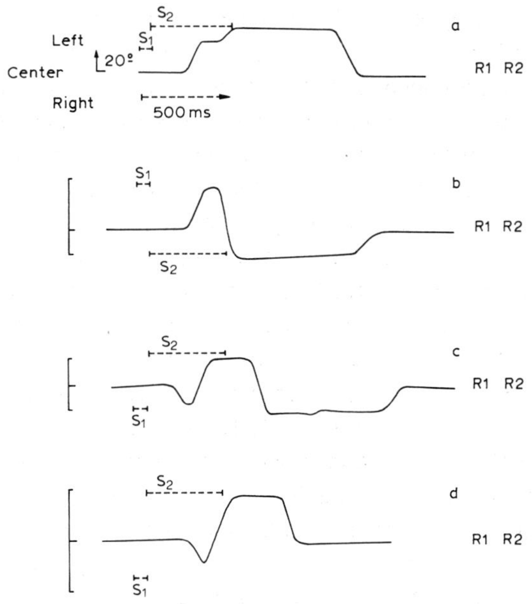

Fig. 34. Records c and d show examples of exceptionally brief pauses between saccades. (From Levy-Schoen and Blanc-Garin, 1974)

easier to decrease the size of saccades than increase it. Ottes et al. (1984) found that the proportion of 'averaging' saccades depended on the distance between the first and second locations of the target, with 'averaging' occurring only rarely when the distance between the endpoints of the two consecutive target steps exceeded 15 deg.

There were also suggestions that the programming of two saccades could occur at the same time, provided that the programming of each saccade was at a different stage. This conclusion was based on the timing pattern of the two consecutive saccades made to track two consecutive target steps. The latency of the second saccade was found to be independent of both the interval between the two target steps and the interval between the two saccades (Becker and Jurgens, 1979). The programming of one saccade was not completely independent of the programming of the other, however, because there was usually a minimum pause of about 100–150 ms between the saccades. One of the rare exceptions to this minimum pause is shown in Fig. 34, taken from Levy-Schoen and Blanc-Garin (1974), which shows instances of unusually brief pauses between successive saccades.

The studies of saccades made to track two consecutive target steps suggest that we have the capacity to modify saccadic programs shortly before their execution, based on newly acquired visual information. Alternatively, instead of modifying programs, we might instead delay specification of saccadic parameters as long as possible (see Rosenbaum et al., 1984, who advocate such a model for the control of finger movements). Either of these two schemes might prove to be valuable in natural situations, where the retinal image is always moving about due to incomplete compensation for head movements (section 2.3). Delaying the final, irrevocable specification of the saccadic program as long as possible is one way of making it more likely that perturbations of the retinal location of the target will be taken into account in the final saccadic program. (See Collewijn et al., 1990, for discussion of the current status of saccadic control with the head unrestrained.)

There is, however, one caveat before we leap from the laboratory to natural scanning, or before we claim to understand how the saccadic parameters are specified. As was pointed out earlier in the discussion of Wheeless' et al.'s (1967) experiment, it was always clear to the subject that on some portion of the trials the target would be taking a second step. The expectation that modification of an initial saccadic program might be required could make it easier to carry out the modification. This could occur in a variety of different ways. For example, the expectation that modification might be required could encourage preparation of more than one saccadic program, or could affect the way in which new visual information is sampled while programming is in progress. Of course, any such processes which make it easier to modify saccadic programs would be expected to operate in natural situations, as well as the laboratory, because in natural situations we expect the retinal location of the target to be perturbed by our own eye or head movements. The important point for the present discussion is that until we understand the role of the subject's expectations, it may not be correct to assume that the specification of saccadic parameters necessarily operates in a purely automatic fashion. The relative contribution of expectations and lower-level processes to the rapid modification of saccadic parameters has yet to be determined.

The relative contribution of expectations and lower-level, sensorimotor processes to saccadic programming is also considered in the next section, which deals with the spatial analog of the 2-step experiments. Here, the target appears in the company of other, nontarget stimuli.

4.7. Is the endpoint of a saccade influenced by the presence of a visual background?

4.7.1. 'Center-of-gravity' tendencies

When we scan natural visual scenes, we try to look at chosen targets, which appear not in isolation, as they do in the laboratory, but in the midst of patterned visual backgrounds. The problem facing us is to bring the line of sight to the chosen location without it being drawn to features in the background. In section 3.6 we saw that we can smoothly track targets moving across visual backgrounds with little or no influence of the background on the eye movements. Does the same selective capacity hold for saccades, that is, how well can we bring the line of sight to a stationary visual target which is presented along with visual background stimuli?

Surprisingly, and in apparent contrast to the successful elimination of background influence on smooth eye tracking, there have been several reports that background stimuli do influence the endpoint of saccades (e.g. Findlay, 1982; Ottes et al., 1984, 1985; Coëffé and O'Regan, 1987). These studies reported that saccades often land in the center of the entire stimulus configuration, consisting of the target stimulus, along with neighboring visual background stimuli. For example, Ottes et al. (1985) asked subjects to look at a green target spot which was presented along with a red, nontarget spot. One spot was above and to the right, and the other below and to the right, of the central fixation target. The subject did not know which of the two locations would contain the target until the stimuli

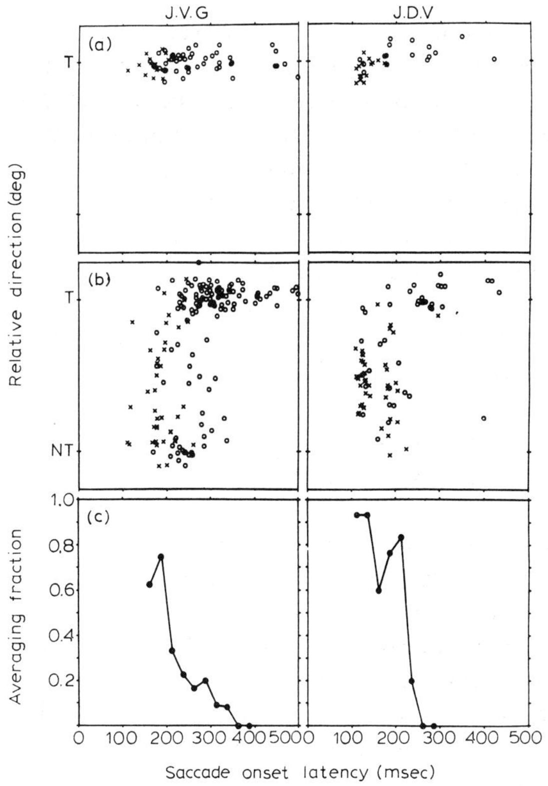

Fig. 35. Direction of first saccade to a single spot (row a) and a double-spot stimulus (row b) (directional separation = 30 deg) plotted as a function of saccadic latency. The vertical axis scaling is relative to the first saccade directions of responses to single spots at each of the double-spot positions. The data from the stimuli with a target direction of +15 deg have been pooled with those with a target direction of −15 deg after direction reversal of the latter responses. Two instructions were used: saccade as fast as possible (crosses) or as accurately as possible (circles). In row (c) the fraction of 'averaging' responses to the double spots, within each 25-ms latency bin containing at least 5 saccades, is plotted against mean latency of the same saccades. Data in (c) are pooled across instruction. A saccade is defined as 'averaging' if its direction is in between the two 95% ranges of the single-spot response. Left-hand column of panels contains the data of subject JVG, right-hand of subject JDV. (From Ottes et al., 1985)

appeared. Ottes et al. found that saccades with shorter latencies (less than about 300 ms) landed in between the two spots, provided that the directional separation of the spots was 30 deg or less. This is shown in Fig. 35, which shows the endpoints of the saccades as a function of their latency. More widely separated stimuli led to errors of a different sort in which the saccades were often directed either to the target or to the nontarget, and less frequently in between the two. Saccades with latencies longer than 300 ms were accurate, regardless of the directional separation. Ottes et al. (1985) attributed the centering tendency of the short-latency saccades to poor spatial resolution of the sensory stimulus, and proposed two hypotheses to explain why spatial resolution was poor. One was that centering saccades are produced by a separate, fast, saccadic subsystem with poor spatial resolution. This subsystem was said to program saccades 'automatically' based on stimulus 'energy content and relative timing'. The second hypothesis was that there was a single saccadic subsystem whose input became more precise over time. Short-latency saccades were assumed to be drawn toward the center of this poorly resolved spatial input, rather than to a selected location within it.

Coëffé and O'Regan (1987) later showed that short-latency saccades did not necessarily have to be drawn to the center of the stimulus array. They found that if the target location was known in advance, centering tendencies would be reduced and saccadic accuracy improved. They proposed that the improvement in saccadic accuracy came from the contribution of an independent 'target extraction' process. This process was assumed to operate concurrently with a tendency of saccades to land in what they called a 'gaze attraction position', which was said to depend on the 'summed influence of all the elements in the whole stimulus configuration'.

He and Kowler (1989) obtained results leading them to question whether two subsystems, or two independent processes, one directing saccades to the center and the other directing saccades to the true target location, were needed to explain performance. They presented a target stimulus ('+') and a nontarget stimulus ('x') at the same time, with one of the stimuli above and to the right and the other above and to the left of the central fixation point. The new feature of the study was that the probability that the target would appear in the right-hand location was varied (see section 4.4 for discussions

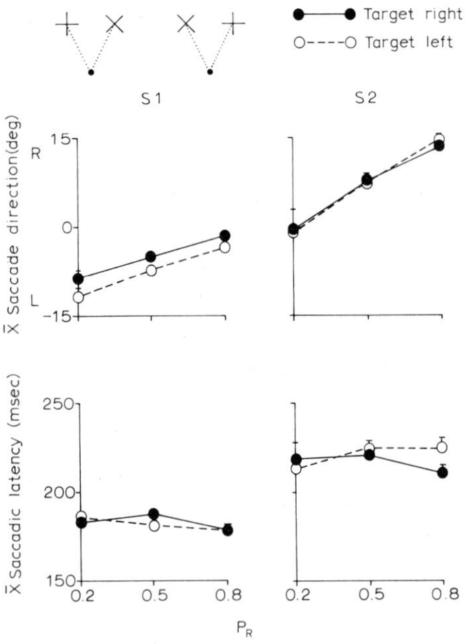

Fig. 36. Mean saccadic direction (top) and latency (bottom) as a function of the probability (P_R) of the target's appearing on the right for two naive subjects (S1 and S2). The target was either on the right (solid lines) or on the left (dotted lines). The directional separation of the target and nontarget was 30 deg. Standard errors were smaller than the plotting symbols except where noted by vertical bars. (From He and Kowler, 1989)

of effects of probability on saccades). They found that the saccadic endpoints were biased toward the more probable location, as is shown in Fig. 36, which plots the mean saccadic endpoint as a function of location probability. (Note that the mean latency, in contrast to the mean endpoint, was unaffected by probability.) Fig. 36 also shows that the actual location of the target did not matter too much – saccadic endpoints were about the same regardless of whether the target had appeared on the right or on the left. This suggests that the bias to direct saccades toward the more probable location did not require a special saccadic mechanism with information about the actual location of the target. The bias was due to the influence of the memory for the past history of target locations. Given that biases can draw the line of sight away from the center of the array, it is reasonable to suppose that biases could have been responsible for drawing saccades toward the center of the array in the first place. If this is true, then 'centering' tendencies need not be automatic, or require special saccadic subsystems, or imply poorly resolved spatial inputs. 'Centering' saccades might be no more than an efficient visual search strategy employed when one is asked to make a saccade before the target has been located. Genuine 'centering' tendencies, if they exist at all, would be best described as tendencies to look to the center of *selected* regions of the display, with the selection process under high-level control (He and Kowler, 1989; He et al., 1988).

These studies of saccadic 'centering' illustrate how complicated it is to correctly interpret the performance of subjects who are asked to make saccades before they have distinguished a target from its background. Such situations may encourage the reliance on memory for prior target locations and expectations about future locations. Interestingly, this is *not* the experimental strategy that was successful in demonstrating that smooth eye movements can be made to track selected targets, independently of visual stimuli in the background (section 3.6). In such experiments subjects were not confused about which stimulus was target and which was background. Indeed, to have encouraged such confusion would be an inappropriate test of selective capacity because the failure to eliminate the influence of the background on the eye movement would have represented a failure to pay full attention to the target, and not an automatic integration of the visual information in the target and the background. The same point can be made about saccades: if we want to describe the capacity to look at a selected target in the presence of backgrounds, it is necessary to be certain that the saccade is being programmed when the visual target can be clearly distinguished from the background. Otherwise, we risk confusing perceptual or attentional limitations with lower-level oculomotor events.

We still do not understand the extent to which saccadic programs are influenced by background stimuli when subjects have fully distinguished the target from its background. It is possible that backgrounds will make no difference, provided that the subject is paying sufficient attention to the target. This would imply that saccadic programs are determined by a two-stage process, similar to that proposed for smooth eye movement (section 3.6), in which a target is selected by paying attention to it and a saccadic program is then computed based on the position signals contained in the selected target.

There is some suggestive evidence in support of a two-stage model (target selection followed by computation of the saccadic response) (He and Kowler, 1989; He et al., 1988), but this support is only tentative, because a firm link between selective attention and saccades has yet to be established. This issue is discussed in the next section.

4.7.2. Saccades and selective attention

Despite the plausibility of a link between selective attention and saccades, it is still not clear that such a link exists. Selective attention can be moved about without saccades (Reeves and Sperling, 1986), but this shows that shifts of attention do not require saccades, and leaves open the question of whether saccades require corresponding attentional shifts. Klein (1980) did conclude that saccades could be made without shifts in attention based on experiments in which saccades were programmed while, in the same block of trials, subjects were also preparing to press a button in response to the appearance of a light. The light and the target for the saccade were either on the same, or on the opposite, side of the fixation point. Klein found that the reaction time of the button press was the same regardless of the location of the light, and he concluded that the programming of saccades did not compel a shift of attention to the saccadic target. Klein's interpretation can be questioned, however, because the saccadic and the button-pressing tasks were not performed concurrently. Instead, subjects were told which task to do before each trial. So, it is possible that the reaction time of the button press was not affected by saccadic programming because subjects did not program saccades in the button-press trials.

At this point the question of whether saccades require corresponding shifts of attention, or whether saccades and attention shifts can be carried out independently (e.g., in different directions), has not been resolved.

4.8. Saccades are planned as patterned sequences

Much of the research on saccades up to this point has dealt with the performance of subjects who were uncertain about the location of the target or the time of its appearance. This section will describe characteristics of saccades when uncertainty about the spatial or temporal properties of the stimulus was reduced, and subjects had to look from one stationary target to the next. These studies show that high-level plans for the entire sequences of saccades place constraints on their spatio-temporal pattern.

The rationale for studying sequences of movements is given quite clearly in Lashley's famous (1951) paper, 'The Problem of Serial Order in Behavior'. Lashley's eloquent description and insightful analysis of voluntary motor action is as timely today for the study of saccades as it was several decades ago for the study of voluntary movements.

Lashley argued that motor responses are organized into structured sequences whose main feature was the spatial and temporal integration of distinct elements into an effective, purposeful pattern of activity:

"Certainly language presents in a most striking form the integrative functions that are characteristic of the cerebral cortex and that reach their highest development in human thought processes. Temporal integration is not found exclusively in language; the coordination of leg movements in insects, the song of birds, the control of trotting and pacing in a gaited horse, the rat running the maze, the architect designing a house, and the carpenter sawing a board present a problem of sequences of action which cannot be explained in terms of successions of external stimuli" (p. 113).

Lashley looked for what he called "a syntax of movement", or, "an habitual order or mode of relating the expressive elements... which may be imposed upon a wide range and a wide variety of specific acts" (p. 122). For example, different motor activities were not triggered by independent sensory inputs, but were made with reference to a central "system of space coordinates", which defined the location of an object in external space and also with reference to the position of the organism as a whole. This, argued Lashley, would not only account for the spatial integration of distinct movements, but would also explain the remarkable capacities of animals to adjust quickly to gross distortions or deprivations of sensory information: the system of space coordinates was a product of all sorts of signals, including memories, and so could survive the loss of some of the signals without disruption of its essential character.

Movements were temporally organized as well. This is shown most clearly by the pervasiveness of rhythmic patterns of movements, found in speech, in walking, and even in breathing. The rhythmic action not only provides for temporal coordination of a single motor activity, but also suggests the existence of an internal clock, which ensures the temporal coordination of different movements carried out at the same time.

Lashley's arguments have been very influential in modern research on voluntary motor control. Studies have sought to discover the nature of the spatial and temporal coordination of specific motor activities and, in so doing, lead to a better understanding of the neural processes underlying the control of coordinated movements. For example: (1) Viviani and Terzuolo (1980) studied the consistent spatial and temporal patterns of handwriting, which survived changes in the overall speed of writing or the size of the written characters; (2) Sternberg et al. (1978a,b) studied the temporal pattern of sequences of typed keystrokes or spoken syllables. They found that both the latency for the initiation of a sequence and the time between successive movements depended on the length of the sequence as a whole. This led them to propose that all the motor programs for a sequence of responses are stored in a special memory buffer, which is scanned for the appropriate program before the execution of each response; (3) Rosenbaum at al. (1983) concluded that motor programs are stored in a hierarchically structured memory, and that programs may be elaborated to specify particular parameters of the movement right before the execution of a sequence begins (Rosenbaum et al., 1984).

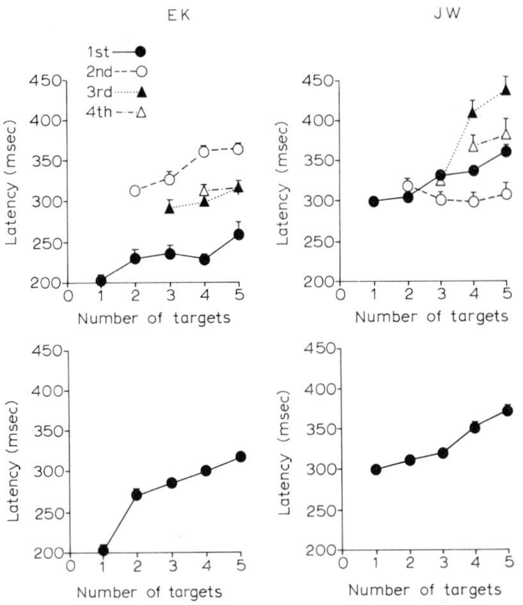

Fig. 37. The mean latency of the 1st–4th saccades of a sequence (top) and averaged overall saccades (bottom). as a function of the number of targets in the sequence for subject EK and naive subject JW. Vertical bars represent 1 SE. (From Zingale and Kowler, 1987)

It is not obvious that the spatial or temporal patterning of movements, described above for voluntary motor responses, must also apply to saccades. Unlike movements of the fingers, or spoken syllables, which can be initiated without a specific sensory cue, saccades are usually directed toward eccentric, selected, visual targets. In principle, the visual target can provide all the information needed to program the size or direction of the movement, so that remembered motor commands, or patterned sequences of motor responses, would not appear to be needed.

Zingale and Kowler (1987) demonstrated that both remembered motor commands and patterned sequences of responses do apply to saccades, much as they apply to finger movements or to speech. Their experiment was modeled after Sternberg et al.'s (1978a,b) experiment, in that the subjects ex-

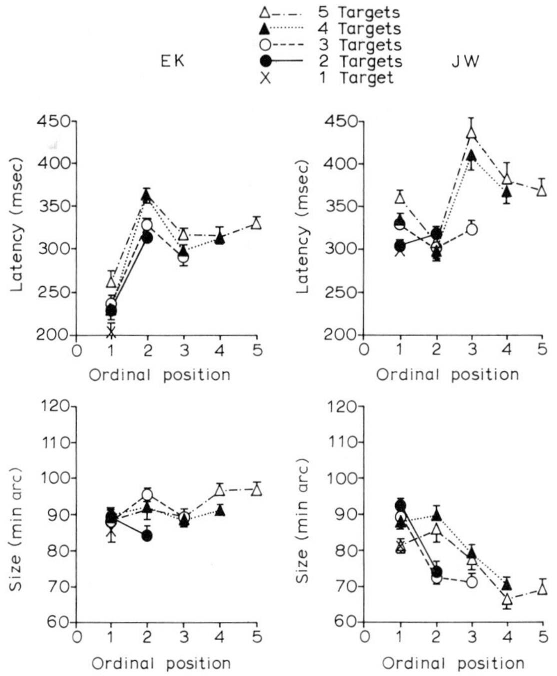

Fig. 38. Mean latency (top graphs) and mean saccade vector size (bottom graphs) as a function of the ordinal position of the saccade in the sequence for each of five sequence lengths. (From Zingale and Kowler, 1987)

ecuted saccadic sequences of different lengths. Specifically, subjects scanned a sequence of from 1 to 5 points, arranged in a simple 2-dimensional pattern. Zingale and Kowler (1987) (also Kowler, 1982; Inhoff, 1986) found that the latency of the first saccade, and the time between successive saccades, increased with the number of points that had to be scanned (Fig. 37). This suggests that the kind of memory-scanning process that Sternberg et al. (1978a) proposed for typing and speech may apply to saccades as well.

The dependence of the properties of a single saccade on the properties of the sequence in which it occurs, shown by the increase in latency with increasing sequence length, is also illustrated by the variation of intersaccadic interval as a function of the serial position of the saccade in the sequence (Fig. 38). The variation in intersaccadic interval as a function of serial position was quite similar to the pattern of inter-response times that characterizes sequences of spoken syllables (Sternberg et al., 1978b). The temporal pattern of the saccades made to look at the visual targets was also remarkably similar to the pattern of saccades observed when the targets were removed right before the execution of the sequence was to begin, and subjects had to direct saccades to remembered target locations. The visual targets were not completely irrelevant, however: saccades to remembered locations were about 20% too large, showing that the retrieved programs could be modified 'on-line' by the visual information.

What is the benefit of programming sequences of saccades? The answer to this may lie in remembering Lashley's insights about the importance of successfully integrating distinct motor response elements into coordinated patterns of activity. Saccades are only one kind of response element, and are rarely made in isolation. In natural situations, saccades are part of general searching or scanning patterns, which include movements of the head, limbs and fingers, as well as movements of the eyes. Perhaps the programming of saccadic sequences reflects not a process unique to saccades, but the operation of a single central motor controller, which uses the rhythm of the sequence to link the disparate motor elements into an effective pattern of activity.

4.9. Overview

The section on saccades described ways in which performance is limited by both low-level, sensorimotor constraints, and higher-level, central and subjective, factors. For example, the spatial precision of saccades is limited by mechanisms that code the location of the image (section 4.3). The precision of saccades smaller than 30′ is limited by other factors, however, because we can estimate the distance between two points far more precisely than we can make saccades from one to the next. In general, small saccades are hard to use and visually useless. The goal of saccades may not be to bring the target of interest to a central 'king' cone, but rather to a larger region, perhaps as large as 30′ – a region only slightly larger than the foveal bouquet which might contain the 'chamber of deputies' most concerned with the limits of visual resolution (Le Grand, 1967).

There is ample evidence that saccadic programs can be prepared, at least in part, before the location of targets is fully discerned. For example, 'warning' signals reduce latency (4.5), and advanced information about the probable locations of targets influences both saccadic latency and accuracy (4.4 and 4.7.1). Any programs prepared in advance are by no means immune to the influence of new, visual signals. For example the abrupt disappearance of a central stimulus can facilitate programming and the abrupt appearance of a central stimulus can delay the initiation of a saccade (4.5.1). There is, however, no convincing evidence that the facilitation acts by invoking a special class of reflexive 'express' saccades (4.5.2). The effects of the abrupt appearance or disappearance of central stimuli may be one of the many threads linking saccades to spatially selective attention, a link which is still not well understood (4.7.2).

Abrupt changes in target location that occur while saccadic programming is in progress can also influence the endpoint of the saccade (4.6). This suggests a remarkable ability to incorporate new visual information into programs on rather short notice. On the other hand, the abrupt changes produced experimentally were never a complete surprise to the subjects, so that some of the groundwork for the expected modifications might have been incorporated into the preparation of the initial response.

The problem of how saccades are programmed in patterned visual environments is still unsolved (4.7). Automatic 'center-of-gravity' tendencies have been described, but these seem to work in opposition to voluntary process, which would presumably take the line of sight to a chosen location in the visual array. The conflict between these two is discomfiting. The resolution may lie in a 'centering' mechanism that receives only the spatial information selected (attended to) by the subject. This general description, however, succeeds only in better defining, rather than resolving, the issue, namely, that separate constraints may be imposed from two different sources, (1) our ability to focus attention on one stimulus to the exclusion of others, and (2) the way in which a lower-level mechanism goes about computing a single saccadic endpoint from a spatially extended input. Solving the problem of saccadic programming in patterned environments requires more studies of saccades made to inspect stationary environments in which subjects are more certain about where they are trying to look, rather than more studies in which randomly chosen stimuli are used to try to elicit automatic responses. Randomization makes it more difficult to distinguish the operation of the always-present high-level selection processes from the lower-level computations of the oculomotor command.

Studies of other voluntary motor responses – finger movements or speech, for example – have made a great deal of progress of late by rejecting randomization and seeing how well subjects can execute specified sequences of movements. The temporal patterns of these responses are remarkably similar to those found when subjects use saccades to scan sequences of visible points (4.8). This suggests that saccades, like other voluntary movements, are planned as patterned sequences, not one at a time. Planning of saccadic sequences may be essential for the proper temporal coordination of saccades with the movements of the head, limbs and fingers, which usually accompany eye movements in natural viewing.

5. Future directions

This chapter has summarized some of the evidence showing that human eye movement is a product of both visual and cognitive influences, both of which need to be taken into account if theories are to truly represent the way in which eye movements operate in the natural world. We saw that eye movements depend on attentional decisions, expectations, memories and plans and, at the same time, are constrained by the structure of the visual array. Cognitive processes (in particular, expectations and memory for the past history of stimuli and responses) were shown to play a role even when the experimental stimuli were chosen at random. The role of selective attention and the capacity to plan patterned sequences of movements were discovered by testing more complicated stimuli than the conventional point of light moving in darkness; for example, studies of eye movements in the presence of background stimuli, and studies of saccades made to track sequences of target points.

We are still a long way from understanding how visual and cognitive influences combine to determine the effective eye movement patterns we rely on to see the world clearly. I suspect that if we are to succeed in developing new models and approaches, two things will have to happen.

The first is to ask anew the most basic question about eye movements: what are they good for? 'Producing the retinal conditions that are adequate for vision' was an acceptable answer for Raymond Dodge's time, when we knew what adequate conditions meant. But we can no longer be confident that achieving stationary images, every millisecond, is the goal. A little (or a lot) of motion may be harmful, helpful, or ignored. It may depend on what you are trying to see or do while the eye is moving. Concurrent study of visual, cognitive and oculomotor performance is needed. The directions for this research are suggested in many of the remaining chapters in this book, which deal explicitly with the role of eye movements in the performance of visual and cognitive tasks.

The second task for the future is to begin to seriously consider 'natural' oculomotor demands. We oculomotorists play fast and loose with the term 'natural'. Uncover an eye to do binocular recording, include a visual background stimulus, leave the room lights on, or unbolt the head and all of a sudden, we're 'natural'. Let me not discourage this development, but instead argue that there is a long way to go. The most important of the natural demands may be the coordination of different concurrent activities (again, Lashley was right). Small retinal errors are harmless. But sending an arm in one direction and eyes and head in another might be a disaster. Equally disastrous would be to make the task of coordinating the separate activities an active, deliberate process rather than something that the motor systems are naturally and automatically predisposed to do. This I believe to be the central message of the last few years of the research: that oculomotor performance, voluntary or involuntary, smooth or saccadic, is automatically and effortlessly coordinated because the motor commands are derived from one set of decisions, plans and ideas that we have about perceived objects in the world. Verification of this idea and the development of new oculomotor models which emphasize the central coordination of eye movements with the other sensorimotor and cognitive activities seems to be an appropriate goal for future oculomotor research. Achieving this goal will require new research techniques which let us simultaneously explore eye movements along with the many other activities that naturally occur at the same time.

Acknowledgement

Supported by grant 88-0171 from the Air Force Office of Scientific Research, Life Science Directorate. I thank V. Asarpota, P. He, E. Krantz, D. Pepper and G.L. Zhu for assistance.

References

Anstis, S.M. and Atkinson, J. (1967) Distortions in moving figures viewed through a stationary slit. Am. J. Psychol. 80, 572–587.

Bahill, A.T. and McDonald, J.D. (1983) Model emulates human smooth pursuit system in producing zero-latency target tracking. Biol. Cybern. 48, 213–222.

Barlow, H.B. (1952) Eye movements during fixation. J. Physiol. 116, 290–306.

Bartz, A.E. (1962) Eye-movement latency, duration, and response time as a function of angular displacement. J. Exp. Psychol. 64, 318–324.

Becker, W. (1989) Metrics. In: R.H. Wurtz and M.E. Goldberg (Eds.), The Neurobiology of Saccadic Eye Movements, Elsevier, Amsterdam, pp. 13–67.

Becker, W. and Fuchs, A.F. (1969) Further properties of the human saccadic system: eye movements and correction saccades with and without visual fixation points. Vision Res. 9, 1247–1258.

Becker, W. and Fuchs, A.F. (1985) Prediction in the oculomotor system: smooth pursuit during transient disappearance of a visual target. Exp. Brain Res. 57, 562–575.

Becker, W. and Jurgens, R. (1979) An analysis of the saccadic system by means of double step stimuli. Vision Res. 19, 967–983.

Becker, W. and Klein, H.M. (1973) Accuracy of saccadic eye movements and maintenance of eccentric eye positions in the dark. Vision Res. 13, 1021–1034.

Behrens, F. and Grusser, O.J. (1979) Smooth pursuit eye movements and optokinetic nystagmus elicited by intermittently illuminated stationary patterns. Exp. Brain Res. 37, 317–336.

Blum, H. (1973) Biological shape and visual science (Part I). J. Theor. Biol. 38, 205–287.

Boch, R. and Fischer, B. (1986) Further observations on the occurrence of express-saccades in the monkey. Exp. Brain Res. 63, 487–494.

Boch, R., Fischer, B. and Ramsperger, E. (1984) Express-saccades of the monkey: reaction times versus intensity, size, duration, and eccentricity of their targets. Exp. Brain Res. 55, 223–231.

Boman, D.K. and Hotson, J.R. (1988) Stimulus conditions that enhance anticipatory slow eye movements. Vision Res. 28, 1157–1165.

Boyce, P.R. (1967a) Monocular fixation in human eye movements. Proc. R. Soc. Lond. B167, 293–315.

Boyce, P.R. (1967b) The effect of change of target field luminance and colour on fixation eye movements. Optica Acta 14, 213–217.

Bridgeman, B. and Palca, J. (1980) The role of microsaccades in high acuity observation tasks. Vision Res. 20, 813–817.

Burt, P. and Sperling, G. (1980) Time, distance and feature trade-offs in visual apparent motion. Psychol. Rev. 88, 171–195.

Carl, J.R. and Gellman, R.S. (1987) Human smooth pursuit: stimulus-dependent responses. J. Neurophysiol. 57, 1446–1463.

Cheng, M. and Outerbridge, J.S. (1975) Optokinetic nystagmus during selective retinal stimulation. Exp. Brain Res. 23, 129–139.

Ciuffreda, K.J., Kenyon, R.V. and Stark, L. (1979) Suppression of fixational saccades in strabismic and anisometropic amblyopia. Ophthal. Res. 11, 31–39.

Coëffé, C. and O'Regan, J.K. (1987) Reducing the influence of non-target stimuli on saccade accuracy: predictability and latency effects. Vision Res. 27, 227–240.

Cohen, B., Matsuo, V. and Raphan, T. (1977) Quantitative analysis of the velocity characteristics of optokinetic nystagmus and optokinetic after-nystagmus. J. Physiol. 270, 321–344.

Collewijn, H. (1969) Optokinetic eye movements in the rabbit. Input output relations. Vision Res. 9, 117–132.

Collewijn, H. (1972) An analog model of the rabbit's optokinetic system. Brain Res. 36, 71–88.

Collewijn, H. (1975) Direction-selective units in the rabbit's nucleus of the optic tract. Brain Res. 100, 489–508.

Collewijn, H. (1977) Eye and head movements in freely moving rabbits. J. Physiol. 266, 471–498.

Collewijn, H. (1981) The oculomotor system of the rabbit and its plasticity. In: V. Braitenberg (Ed.), Studies of Brain Function, Vol. 5, Springer-Verlag, Berlin.

Collewijn, H. (1985) Integration of adaptive changes of the optokinetic reflex, pursuit and the vestibulo-ocular reflex. In: A. Berthoz and G. Melvill Jones (Eds.) Adaptive Mechanisms in Gaze Control, Elsevier, Amsterdam, pp. 51–69.

Collewijn, H. (1989) The vestibulo-ocular reflex: an outdated concept? In: J.H.S. Allum and M. Hulling (Eds.), Afferent Control of Posture and Locomotion; Progress in Brain Research, Vol. 80, Elsevier, Amsterdam, pp. 197–209.

Collewijn, H. and Tamminga, E.P. (1984) Human smooth and saccadic eye movements during voluntary pursuit of different target motions on different backgrounds. J. Physiol. 351, 217–250.

Collewijn, H. and Tamminga, E.P. (1986) Human fixation and pursuit in normal and open-loop conditions: effects of central and peripheral retinal targets. J. Physiol. 379, 109–129.

Collewijn, H. and van der Mark, F. (1972) Ocular stability in variable feedback conditions in the rabbit. Brain Res. 36, 47–57.

Collewijn, H., van der Mark, F. and Jansen, T.C. (1975) Precise recording of human eye movements. Vision Res. 15, 447–450.

Collewijn, H., Curio, G. and Grusser, O.J. (1982) Spatially selective visual attention and generation of eye pursuit movements. Human Neurobiol. 1, 129–139.

Collewijn, H., Martins, A.J. and Steinman, R.M. (1983) Compensatory eye movements during active and passive head movements: fast adaptation to changes in visual magnification. J. Physiol. 340, 259–286.

Collewijn, H., Steinman, R.M. and van der Steen, H. (1985) The performance of the smooth pursuit eye movement system during passive and self-generated stimulus motion. J. Physiol. 366, 19P.

Collewijn, H., Erkelens, C.J. and Steinman, R.M. (1988a) Binocular coordination of horizontal saccadic eye movements. J. Physiol. 404, 157–182.

Collewijn, H., Erkelens, C.J. and Steinman, R.M. (1988b) Binocular coordination of human vertical saccadic eye movements. J. Physiol. 404, 183–197.

Collewijn, H., Steinman, R.M., Erkelens, C.J., Pizlo, Z., and Van der Stein, J. (1990) The effect of freeing the head on eye movement characteristics during 3-D shifts of gaze and tracking. In: A. Berthoz, W. Graf and P.P. Vidal (Eds.), The Head-Neck Sensory Motor System, Oxford University Press, New York, in press.

Cornsweet, T.N. (1956) Determination of the stimuli for involuntary drifts and saccadic eye movements. J. Opt. Soc. Am. 46, 987–993.

Cornsweet, T.N. (1976) The Purkinje image method of recording eye position. In: R.A. Monty and J.W. Senders (Eds.), Eye Movements and Psychological Processes, Erlbaum, Hillsdale, NJ, pp. 161–165.

Cornsweet, T.N. and Crane, H.D. (1973) An accurate eye tracker using first and fourth Purkinje images. J. Opt. Soc. Am. 63, 921–928.

Craik, K. (1947) Theory of the human operator in control systems. Br. J. Psychol. 38, 56–61.

Crane, H.D. and Steele, C.S. (1978) Accurate three-dimensional eye tracker. Appl. Opt. 17, 691–705.

Cunitz, R.J. and Steinman, R.M. (1969) Comparison of saccadic eye movements during fixation and reading. Vision Res. 9, 683–693.

Cushman, W.B., Tangney, J.F., Steinman, R.M. and Ferguson, J.L. (1980) Characteristics of smooth eye movements under open loop conditions. Recent Advances in Vision Workshop, WB6.

Cushman, W.B., Tangney, J.F., Steinman, R.M. and Ferguson, J.L. (1984) Characteristics of smooth eye movements with stabilized targets. Vision Res. 24, 1003–1009.

Dallos, P.J. and Jones, R.W. (1963) Learning behaviour of the eye fixation control system. IEEE Trans. Autom. Control AC8, 218–227.

Ditchburn, R.W. (1980) The function of small saccades. Vision Res. 20, 271–272.

Ditchburn, R.W. and Ginsborg, B.L. (1952) Vision with a stabilized retinal image. Nature 170, 36–37.

Ditchburn, R.W. and Ginsborg, B.L. (1953) Involuntary eye movements during fixation. J. Physiol. 119, 1–17.

Dodge, R. (1903) Five types of eye movements in the horizontal meridian plane of the field of regard. Am. J. Physiol. 8, 307–327.

Dodge, R. (1927) Elementary Conditions of Human Variability, Columbia University Press, New York.

Dodge, R. (1931) Conditions and Consequences of Human Variability, Yale University Press, New Haven.

Dodge, R. and Fox, J.C. (1928) Optic nystagmus. Arch. Neurol. Psychiat. 20, 812–823.

Dodge, R., Travis, R.C. and Fox, J.C. (1930) Optic nystagmus III. Characteristics of the slow phase. Arch. Neurol. Psychiat. 24, 21–34.

Dubois, M.F.W. and Collewijn, H. (1979a) The optokinetic reactions of the rabbit: relation to the visual streak. Vision Res. 19, 9–17.

Dubois, M.F.W. and Collewijn, H. (1979b) Optokinetic reactions in man elicited by localized retinal motion stimuli. Vision Res. 19, 1105–1115.

Dursteler, M.B. and Wurtz R.H. (1988) Pursuit and optokinetic deficits following chemicals lesions of cortical areas MT and MST. J. Neurophysiol. 940–965.

Dursteler, M.B., Wurtz, R.H. and Newsome, W.T. (1987) Directional pursuit deficits following lesions of the foveal representation within the superior temporal sulcus of the macaque monkey. J. Neurophysiol. 1262–1287.

Eckmiller, R. (1987) The neural control of pursuit eye movements. Physiol. Rev. 67, 797–857.

Eckmiller, R. and Mackeben, M. (1978) Pursuit eye movement and neural control in the monkey. Pflugers Arch. 377, 15–23.

Erkelens, C.J., Steinman, R.M. and Collewijn, H. (1989a) Ocular vergence under natural conditions I. Continuous changes of target distance along the median plane. Proc. R. Soc. Lond. B, 236, 417–440.

Erkelens, C.J., Steinman, R.M. and Collewijn, H. (1989b) Ocular vergence under natural conditions II. Gaze shifts between real targets differing in distance and direction. Proc. R. Soc. Lond. B, 236, 441–465.

Falmagne, J.C., Cohen, S.P. and Dwivedi, A. (1975) Two-choice reactions as an ordered memory scanning process. In: P. Rabbitt and S. Dormic (Eds.), Attention and Performance V, Academic Press, New York.

Fender, D.H. and Nye, P.W. (1961) An investigation of the mechanisms of eye movement control. Kybernetik 1, 81–88.

Ferman, L., Collewijn, H., Jansen, T.C. and van den Berg, A.V. (1987) Human gaze stability in the horizontal, vertical and torsional direction during voluntary head movements evaluated with a three-dimensional scleral induction coil technique. Vision Res. 27, 811–828.

Findlay, J.M. (1981) Spatial and temporal factors in the predictive generation of saccadic eye movements. Vision Res. 21, 347–354.

Findlay, J.M. (1982) Global visual processing for saccadic eye movements. Vision Res. 22, 1033–1046.

Fiorentini, A. and Ercoles, A.H. (1966) Involuntary eye movements during attempted monocular fixation. Atti Fond. Giorgio Ronchi 21, 199–217.

Fischer, B. and Boch, R. (1983) Saccadic eye movements after extremely short reaction times in the monkey. Brain Res. 260, 21–26.

Fischer, B. and Breitmeyer, B. (1987) Mechanisms of visual attention revealed by saccadic eye movements. Neuropsychologia 25, 78–83.

Fischer, B. and Ramsperger, E. (1984) Human express saccades: extremely short reaction times of goal directed eye movements. Exp. Brain Res. 57, 191–195.

Fischer, B. and Ramsperger, E. (1986) Human express saccades: effects of randomization and daily practice. Exp. Brain Res. 64, 569–578.

Fischer, B., Boch, R. and Ramsperger, E. (1984) Express-saccades of the monkey: effect of daily training on probability of occurrence and reaction time. Exp. Brain Res. 55, 232–242.

Fischer, M.H. and Kornmuller, A.E. (1930) Optokinetische ausgeloste. Bewegungswahrnehmungen und optokinetischer nystagmus. J. Psychol. Neurol. 41, 273–308.

Fitts, P.M. (1954) The information capacity of the human motor system in controlling the amplitude of movement. J. Exp. Psychol. 47, 381–391.

Fox, R., Lehmkuhle, S. and Leguire, L.E. (1978) Stereoscopic contours induce optokinetic nystagmus. Vision Res. 18,

1189–1192.

Frost, D. and Poppel, E. (1976) Different programming modes of human saccadic eye movements as a function of stimulus eccentricity: Indications of a functional subdivision of the visual field. Biol. Cybern. 23, 39–48.

Gaarder, K.R. (1975) Eye Movements, Vision and Behavior: A Hierarchical Visual Information Processing Model, Hemisphere, New York.

Gauthier, G.M. and Hofferer, J.M. (1976) Eye tracking of self-moved targets in the absence of vision. Exp. Brain Res. 26, 121–139.

Glezer, V.D. (1959) The eye as a scanning system. Fiziol. Zh. SSSR 453, 271–279.

Hackman, R.B. (1940) An experimental study of variability in ocular latency. J. Exp. Psychol. 27, 546–558.

Haddad, G.M. and Steinman, R.M. (1973) The smallest voluntary saccade: implications for fixation. Vision Res. 13, 1075–1086.

Haegerstrom-Portnoy, G. and Brown, B. (1979) Contrast effects on smooth-pursuit eye movement velocity. Vision Res. 19, 169–174.

Hallett, P.E. (1978) Primary and secondary saccades to goals defined by instructions. Vision Res. 18, 1279–1296.

Hansen, R.M. (1979) Spatial localization during pursuit eye movements. Vision Res. 19, 1213–1221.

Hansen, R.M. and Skavenski, A.A. (1977) Accuracy of eye position information for motor control. Vision Res. 17, 919–926.

Hansen, R.M. and Skavenski, A.A. (1985) Accuracy of spatial localizations near the time of saccadic eye movements. Vision Res. 25, 1077–1082.

He, P. and Kowler, E. (1989) The role of location probability in the programming of saccades: implications for 'center-of-gravity' tendencies. Vision Res. 29, 1165–1181.

He, P., Kowler, E. and Leyton, M. (1988) Saccadic eye movements to simple forms. Invest. Ophthalmol. Vis. Sci. Suppl. 29, 135.

Hening, W., Vicario, D. and Ghez, C. (1988) Trajectory control in targeted force impulses. Exp. Brain Res. 71, 103–115.

Heywood, S. (1972) Voluntary control of smooth eye movements and their velocity. Nature 238, 408–410.

Heywood, S. (1973) Pursuing stationary dots: smooth eye movements and apparent movement. Perception 2, 181–195.

Heywood, S. and Churcher, J. (1971) Eye movements and the afterimage, I. Tracking the afterimage. Vision Res. 11, 1163–1168.

Heywood, S. and Churcher, J. (1980) Structure of the visual array and saccadic latency: implications for oculomotor control. Q. J. Exp. Psychol. 32, 335–341.

Inhoff, A.W. (1986) Preparing sequences of saccades under choice reaction conditions: effects of sequence length and context. Acta Psychol. 61, 211–228.

Jones, L. and Higgins, G. (1947) Photographic granularity and graininess. III. Some characteristics of the visual system of some importance in the evaluation of graininess and granularity. J. Opt. Soc. Am. 37, 217–263.

Jordan, S. (1970) Ocular pursuit movement as a function of visual and proprioceptive stimulation. Vision Res. 10, 775–780.

Kaufman, L. and Richards, W. (1969) Spontaneous fixation tendencies for visual forms. Percept. Psychophys. 5, 85–88.

Khurana, B. and Kowler, E. (1987) Shared attentional control of smooth eye movement and perception. Vision Res. 27, 1603–1618.

Klein, R. (1980) Does oculomotor readiness mediate cognitive control of visual attention? In: R.S. Nickerson (Ed.), Attention and Performance VIII, Erlbaum, Hillsdale, NJ, pp. 259–276.

Komatsu, H. and Wurtz, R.H. (1988a) Relation of cortical areas MT and MST to pursuit eye movements. I. Localization and visual properties of neurons. J. Neurophysiol. 60, 580–603.

Komatsu, H. and Wurtz, R.H. (1988b) Relation of cortical areas MT and MST to pursuit eye movements. III. Interaction with full-field visual stimulation. J. Neurophysiol. 60, 621–644.

Komatsu, H. and Wurtz, R.H. (1989) Modulation of pursuit eye movements by stimulation of cortical areas MT and MST. J. Neurophysiol, 62, 31–47.

Kommerell, G. and Klein, U. (1971) Über die visuelle regelung der okulomotorik: Die optomotorische wirkung exzentrischer nachbilder. Vision Res. 11, 905–920.

Komoda, M.K., Festinger, L., Phillips, L.J., Duckman, R.H. and Young, R.A. (1973) Some observations concerning saccadic eye movements. Vision Res. 13, 1009–1020.

Kowler, E. (1982) Characteristics and visual consequences of saccades used to inspect visual displays. AFOSR Technical Review Meeting, Sarasota, FL.

Kowler, E. (1989) Cognitive expectations, not habits, control anticipatory smooth oculomotor pursuit. Vision Res. 29, 1049–1057.

Kowler, E. and Anton, S. (1987) Reading twisted text: implications for the role of saccades. Vision Res. 27, 45–60.

Kowler, E. and McKee, S.P. (1984) The precision of smooth pursuit. Invest. Ophthalmol.. Vis. Sci. Suppl. 25, 262.

Kowler, E. and McKee, S.P. (1987) Sensitivity of smooth eye movement to small differences in target velocity. Vision Res. 27, 993–1015.

Kowler, E. and Martins, A.J. (1982) Eye movements of preschool children. Science 215, 997–999.

Kowler, E. and Sperling, G. (1980) Transient stimulation does not aid visual search: implications for the role of saccades. Percept. Psychophys. 27, 1–10.

Kowler, E. and Sperling, G. (1983) Abrupt onsets do not aid visual search. Percept. Psychophys. 34, 307–313.

Kowler, E. and Steinman, R.M. (1977) The role of small saccades in counting. Vision Res. 17, 141–146.

Kowler, E. and Steinman, R.M. (1979a) Miniature saccades: eye movements that do not count. Vision Res. 19, 105–108.

Kowler, E. and Steinman, R.M. (1979b) The effect of expecta-

tions on slow oculomotor control. I. Periodic target steps. Vision Res. 19, 619–632.
Kowler, E. and Steinman, R.M. (1979c) The effect of expectations on slow oculomotor control. II. Single target displacements. Vision Res. 19, 633–646.
Kowler, E. and Steinman, R.M. (1980) Small saccades serve no useful purpose. Vision Res. 20, 273–276.
Kowler, E. and Steinman, R.M. (1981) The effect of expectations on slow oculomotor control. III. Guessing unpredictable target displacements. Vision Res. 21, 191–203.
Kowler, E., Murphy, B.J. and Steinman, R.M. (1978) Velocity matching during smooth pursuit of different targets on different backgrounds. Vision Res. 18, 603–605.
Kowler, E., Martins, A.J. and Pavel, M. (1984a) The effect of expectations on slow oculomotor control. IV. Anticipatory smooth eye movements depend on prior target motions. Vision Res. 24, 197–210.
Kowler, E., van der Steen, J., Tamminga, E.P. and Collewijn, H. (1984b) Voluntary selection of the target for smooth eye movement in the presence of superimposed, full-field stationary and moving stimuli. Vision Res. 24, 1789–1798.
Kowlwe, E., Pizlo, Z., Epelboim, J., and Steinman, R.M. (1990a) Slow control is driven by velocity, not position, signals. Invest. Ophthal. Vis. Sci. Suppl., 31, 532.
Kowler, E., Pizlo, Z., Zhu, G.L., Erkelens, C.J., Steinman, R.M., and Collewijn, H. (1990b) Coordination of head and eye during the performance of natural (and unnatural) visual tasks. In: A. Berthoz, W. Graf, and P.P. Vidal (Eds.) The Head-Neck Sensory Motor System. Oxford University Press, New York, in press.
Krauskopf, J., Cornsweet, T.N. and Riggs, L.A. (1960) Analysis of eye movements during monocular and binocular fixation. J. Opt. Soc. Am. 50, 572–578.
Lashley, K.S. (1951) The problem of serial order in behavior. In: W.A. Jeffress (Ed.), Cerebral Mechanisms in Behavior: The Hixon Symposium, Wiley, New York, pp. 112–136.
Le Grand, Y. (1968) Light, Color and Vision, Chapman and Hall, London.
Lemij, H.G. and Collewijn, H. (1989) Differences in accuracy of human saccades between stationary and jumping targets. Vision Res. 29, 1737–1748.
Levy-Schoen, A. (1981) Flexible and/or rigid control of oculomotor scanning behavior. In: D.F. Fisher, R.A. Monty and J.W. Senders (Eds.), Eye Movements: Cognitive and Visual Perception, Erlbaum, New York.
Levy-Schoen, A. and Blanc-Garin, J. (1974) On oculomotor programming and perception. Brain Res. 71, 443–450.
Lisberger, S.G., Miles, F.A., Optican, L.M. and Eighmy, B.B. (1981a) Optokinetic response in monkey: underlying mechanisms and their sensitivity to long-term adaptive changes in vestibuloocular reflex. J. Neurophysiol. 45, 869–890.
Lisberger, S.G., Evinger, C., Johanson, G.W. and Fuchs, A.F. (1981b) Relationship between eye acceleration and retinal image velocity during foveal smooth pursuit in man and monkey. J. Neurophysiol. 46, 229–249.
Lisberger, S.G., Morris, E.J. and Tychsen, L. (1987) Visual motion processing and sensory-motor integration for smooth pursuit eye movements. Annu. Rev. Neurosci. 10, 97–129.
Luce, R.D. (1986) Response Times: Their Role in Inferring Elementary Mental Organization, Oxford University Press, New York.
Mach, E. (1906/1959) Analysis of Sensations, Dover, New York.
Mack, A. (1986) Perceptual aspects of motion in the frontal plane. In: K.R. Boff, L. Kaufman, and J.P. Thomas (Eds.) Handbook of Perception and Human Performance, Vol. I, Wiley, New York.
Mack, A. and Bachant, J. (1969) Perceived movement of the afterimage during smooth eye movement. Percept. Psychophys. 6, 379–384.
Mack, A., Fendrich, R. and Pleune, J. (1979) Smooth pursuit eye movements: is perceived motion necessary? Science 203, 1361–1363.
Mack, A., Fendrich, R. and Wong, E. (1982) Is perceived motion a stimulus for smooth pursuit? Vision Res. 22, 77–88.
Mackeben, M. and Nakayama K. (1988) Fixation release facilitates rapid attentional shifts. Invest. Ophthalmol. Vis. Sci. Suppl. 29, 22.
Marr, D. (1982) Vision, W.H. Freeman, San Francisco.
Marshall, W.H. and Talbot, S.A. (1942) Recent evidence for neural mechanisms in vision leading to a general theory of sensory acuity. Biol. Symp. 7, 117–164.
Martins, A.J., Kowler, E. and Palmer, C. (1985) Smooth pursuit of small-amplitude sinusoidal motion. J. Opt. Soc. Am. 2, 234–242.
Matin, L., Matin, E. and Pearce, D.G. (1970) Eye movements in the dark during the attempt to maintain a prior fixation position. Vision Res. 10, 837–857.
Mayfrank, L., Kimmig, H. and Fischer, B. (1987) The role of attention in the preparation of visually guided saccadic eye movements in man. In: J.K. O'Regan and A. Levy-Schoen (Eds.), Eye Movements: From Physiology to Cognition, Elsevier, Amsterdam, pp. 37–45.
Mayfrank, L., Mobashery, M., Kimmig, H. and Fischer, B. (1986) The role of fixation and visual attention in the occurrence of express saccades in man. Eur. Arch. Psychiatr. Neurol. Sci. 235, 269–275.
Megaw, E.D. and Armstrong, W. (1973) Individual and simultaneous tracking of a step input by the horizontal saccadic eye movement and manual control systems. J. Exp. Psychol. 100, 18–28.
Melvill Jones, G. and Berthoz, A. (1985) Mental control of the adaptive process. In: A. Berthoz and G. Melvill Jones (Eds.), Adaptive Mechanisms of Gaze Control, Elsevier, Amsterdam, pp. 203–208.
Michael, J. and Melvill Jones, G. (1966) Dependence of visual tracking capability upon stimulus predictability. Vision Res. 6, 707–716.

Michard, A., Tetard, C. and Levy-Schoen, A. (1974) Attente au signal et temps de réaction oculomoteur. Année Psychol. 74, 378–402.

Miles, F.A. and Fuller, J.H. (1975) Visual tracking and the primate flocculus. Science 189, 1000–1002.

Millodot, M. (1966) Foveal and extrafoveal acuity with and without stabilized retinal images. Br. J. Psysiol. Opt. 23, 75–106.

Morgan, M.J. (1981) How pursuit eye movements can convert temporal to spatial information. In: D.F. Fisher, R.A. Monty and J.W. Senders (Eds.), Eye Movements: Cognition and Visual Perception, Erlbaum, Hillsdale, NJ, pp. 111–133.

Morgan, M.J. and Turnbull, D.F. (1978) Smooth eye tracking and the perception of motion in the absence of real movement. Vision Res. 18, 1053–1059.

Muratore, R. and Zee, D.S. (1979) Pursuit after-nystagmus. Vision Res. 19, 1057–1059.

Murphy, B.J. (1978) Pattern thresholds for moving and stationary gratings during smooth eye movement. Vision Res. 18, 521–530.

Murphy, B.J., Haddad, G.M. and Steinman, R.M. (1974) Simple forms and fluctuations of the line of sight: implications for motor theories of form processing. Percept. Psychophys. 16(3), 557–563.

Murphy, B.J., Kowler, E. and Steinman, R.M. (1975) Slow oculomotor control in the presence of moving backgrounds. Vision Res. 15, 1263–1268.

Nachmias, J. (1959) Two-dimensional motion of the retinal during monocular fixation. J. Opt. Soc. Am. 49, 901–908.

Nachmias, J. (1961) Determiners of the drift of the eye during monocular fixation. J. Opt. Soc. Am. 51, 761–766.

Newsome, W.T. and Paré, E.B. (1988) A selective impairment of motion. Perception following lesions of the middle temporal visual area (MT). J. Neurosci. 2201–2211.

Newsome, W.T., Wurtz, R.H., Dursteler, M.R. and Mikami, A. (1985) Deficits in visual motion processing following ibotenic acid lesions of the middle temporal visual area of the macaque monkey. J. Neurosci. 5, 825–840.

Newsome, W.T., Wurtz, R.H. and Komatsu, H. (1988) Relation of cortical areas MT and MST to pursuit eye movements. II. Differentiation of retinal from extraretinal inputs. J. Neurophysiol. 604–620.

Norcia, A.M., Yonas, A. and Warren, W.H. (1979) Saccadic eye movement latencies as a function of target directional uncertainty. Invest. Ophthalmol. Vis. Sci. Suppl. 19, 147–148.

Ottes, F.P., Van Gisberger, J.A.M. and Eggermont, J.J. (1984) Metrics of saccade responses to visual double stimuli: two different modes. Vision Res. 24, 1169–1179.

Ottes, F.P., Van Gisbergen, J.A.M. and Eggermont, J.J. (1985) Latency dependence of colour-based target vs. nontarget discrimination by the saccade system. Vision Res. 25, 849–862.

Oyster, C.W., Takahashi, E. and Collewijn, H. (1972) Direction selective ganglion cells and control of optokinetic nystagmus in the rabbit. Vision Res. 12, 183–193.

Polyak, S.L. (1941) The Retina, University of Chicago Press, Chicago.

Proskuryakova, N.G. and Shakhnovich, A.R. (1968) Quantitative characteristics of fixation micromovements of the eye. Biofizika 13, 133–143.

Puckett, J. de W. and Steinman, R.M. (1969) Tracking eye movements with and without saccadic correction. Vision Res. 9, 695–703.

Rashbass, C. (1961) The relationship between saccadic and smooth tracking eye movements. J. Physiol. 159, 326–338.

Ratliff, F. and Riggs, L.A. (1950) Involuntary motions of the eye during monocular fixation. J. Exp. Psychol. 40, 687–701.

Rattle, J.D. (1969) Effect of target size on monocular fixation. Optica Acta 16, 183–192.

Reeves, A. and Sperling, G. (1986) Attention gating in short-term visual memory. Psychol. Rev. 93, 180–206.

Reichardt, W. (1961) Autocorrelation: a principle for the evaluation of sensory information by the central nervous system. In: W.A. Rosenblith (Ed.), Sensory Communication, Wiley, New York, pp. 303–317.

Richards, W. and Kaufman, L. (1969) Center-of-gravity tendencies for fixations and flow patterns. Percept. Psychophys. 5, 81–84.

Riggs, L.A., Ratliff, F., Cornsweet, J.C. and Cornsweet, T.N. (1953) The disappearance of steadily fixated test objects. J. Opt. Soc. Am. 43, 495–501.

Robinson, D.A. (1963) A method of measuring eye movements using a scleral search coil in a magnetic field. IEEE Trans. Bio-Med. Eng. 10, 137–145.

Robinson, D.A. (1965) The mechanics of human smooth pursuit eye movement. J. Physiol. 180, 569–591.

Robinson, D.A. (1971) Models of Oculomotor Neural Organization. In: P. Bach-y-Rita, C.C. Collins and J.E. Hyde (Eds.), The Control of Eye Movements, Academic Press, New York–London, pp. 519–538.

Robinson, D.A. (1981) Control of eye movements. In V.B. Brooks (Ed.), Handbook of Physiology, Vol. II, Part 2, The Nervous System, Williams & Wilkins, Baltimore, pp. 1275–1320.

Robinson, D.A. (1986) The systems approach in the oculomotor system. Vision Res. 26, 91–99.

Robinson, D.A., Gordon, J.L. and Gordon, S.E. (1986) A model of the smooth pursuit eye movement system. Biol. Cybern. 55, 43–57.

Rosenbaum, D.A., Kenny, S.B. and Derr, M.A. (1983) Hierarchical control of rapid movement sequences. J. Exp. Psychol. Hum. Percept. Perform. 9, 86–102.

Rosenbaum, D.A., Inhoff, A.W. and Gordon, A.M. (1984) Choosing between movement sequences: a hierarchical editor model. J. Exp. Psychol. Gen. 113, 372–393.

Ross, L.E. and Ross, S.M. (1980) Saccade latency and warning signals: stimulus onset, offset, and change as warning events. Percept. Psychophys. 27, 251–257.

Sansbury, R.V., Skavenski, A.A., Haddad, G.M. and Steinman,

R.M. (1973) Normal fixation of eccentric targets. J. Opt. Soc. Am. 63, 612–614.

Saslow, M.G. (1967a) Effects of components of displacement-step stimuli upon latency for saccadic eye movement. J. Opt. Soc. Am. 57, 1024–1033.

Saslow, M.G. (1967b) Latency for saccadic eye movement. J. Opt. Soc. Am. 57, 1030–1033.

Schiller, P.H., Sandell, J.H. and Maunsell, J.H.R. (1987) The effect of frontal eye field and superior colliculus lesions on saccadic latencies in the rhesus monkey. J. Neurophysiol. 57, 1033–1049.

Schor, C. and Hallmark, W. (1978) Slow control of eye position in strabismic amblyopia. Invest. Ophthalmol. 17, 577–581.

Skavenski, A.A. and Steinman, R.M. (1970) Control of eye position in the dark. Vision Res. 10, 193–203.

Skavenski, A.A., Robinson, D.A., Steinman, R.M. and Timberlake, G.T. (1975) Miniature eye movements of fixation in rhesus monkey. Vision Res. 15, 1269–1273.

Skavenski, A.A., Hansen, R.H., Steinman, R.M. and Winterson, B.J. (1979) Quality of retinal image stabilization during small natural and artificial body rotations in man. Vision Res. 19, 675–683.

Snodderly, D.M. (1987) Effect of light and dark environments on macaque and human fixational eye movements. Vision Res. 27, 401–415.

Snodderly, D.M. and Kurtz, D. (1985) Eye position during fixation tasks: comparison of macaque and human. Vision Res. 25, 83–98.

Stark, L. (1971) The control system for versional eye movements. In: P. Bach-y-Rita, C. Collins and J.E. Hyde (Eds.), The Control of Eye Movements, Academic Press, New York, pp. 363–428.

Stark, L., Vossius, G. and Young, L.R. (1962) Predictive control of eye tracking movements. IRE Trans. Hum. Factors Electron. HFE-3, 52–57.

St. Cyr, G.J. and Fender, D.H. (1969a) The interplay of drifts and flicks in binocular fixation. J. Opt. Soc. Am. 55, 1158–1165.

St. Cyr, G.J. and Fender, D.H. (1969b) Nonlinearities of the human oculomotor system: gain. Vision Res. 9, 1235–1246.

St. Cyr, G.J. and Fender, D.H. (1969c) Nonlinearities of the human oculomotor system: time delays. Vision Res. 9, 1491–1503.

Steinbach, M.J. (1969) Eye tracking of self-moved targets: the role of efference. J. Exp. Psychol. 82, 366–376.

Steinbach, M.J. (1976) Pursuing the perceptual rather than the retinal stimulus. Vision Res. 16, 1371–1376.

Steinbach, M.J. and Pearce, D.G. (1972) Release of pursuit eye movements using after-images. Vision Res. 12, 1307–1311.

Steinman, R.M. (1965) Effect of target size, luminance, and color on monocular fixation. J. Opt. Soc. Am. 55, 1158–1165.

Steinman, R.M. (1986a) The need for an eclectic, rather than systems, approach to the study of the primate oculomotor system. Vision Res. 26, 101–112.

Steinman, R.M. (1986b) Eye movement. Vision Res. 26, 1389–1400.

Steinman, R.M. and Collewijn, H. (1980) Binocular retinal image motion during active head rotation. Vision Res. 20, 415–429.

Steinman, R.M. and Cunitz, R.J. (1968) Fixation of targets near the absolute foveal threshold. Vision Res. 8, 277–286.

Steinman, R.M., Cunitz, R.J., Timberlake, G.T. and Herman, M. (1967) Voluntary control of microsaccades during maintained monocular fixation. Science 155, 1577–1579.

Steinman, R.M., Skavenski, A.A. and Sansbury, R.V. (1969) Voluntary control of smooth pursuit velocity. Vision Res. 9, 1167–1171.

Steinman, R.M., Haddad, G.M. Skavenski, A.A. and Wyman, D. (1973) Miniature eye movement. Science 181, 810–819.

Steinman, R.M., Cushman, W.B. and Martins, A.J. (1982) The precision of gaze. Human Neurobiol. 1, 97–109.

Steinman, R.M., Kowler, E. and Collewijn, H. (1990) New directions for oculomotor research. Vision Res., in press.

Sternberg, S., Monsell, S., Knoll, R. and Wright, C. (1978a) The latency and duration of rapid movement sequences: comparisons of speech and typewriting. In: G.E. Stelmach (Ed.), Information Processing in Motor Control and Learning, Academic Press, New York, pp. 117–152.

Sternberg, S., Wright, C., Knoll, R. and Monsell, S. (1978b) Motor programs in rapid speech: additional evidence. In: R.A. Cole (Ed.), The Perception and Production of Fluent Speech, Erlbaum, Hillsdale, NJ, pp. 507–534.

Ter Braak, J.W.G. (1936) Untersuchungen über optokinetischen Nystagmus. Arch. Neerl. Physiol. 21, 309–376.

Ter Braak, J.W.G. (1957) 'Ambivalent' optokinetic stimulation. Fol. Psychiat. Neurol. Neurochir. Neerl. 60, 131–135.

Ter Braak, J.W.G. and Buis, C. (1970) Optokinetic nystagmus and attention. Int. J. Neurol. 8, 34–42.

Timberlake, G.T., Wyman, D., Skavenski, A.A. and Steinman, R.M. (1972) The oculomotor error signal in the fovea. Vision Res. 12, 1059–1064.

Tychsen, L. and Lisberger, S.G. (1986) Visual motion processing for the initiation of smooth-pursuit eye movements in humans. J. Neurophysiol. 56, 953–968.

Van den Berg, A.V. (1988) Human smooth pursuit during transient perturbations of predictable and unpredictable target motions. Exp. Brain Res. 72, 95–108.

Van den Berg, A.V. and Collewijn, H. (1986) Human smooth pursuit: effects of stimulus extent and of spatial and temporal constraints of the pursuit trajectory. Vision Res. 26, 1209–1222.

Van den Berg, A.V. and Collewijn, H. (1987) Voluntary smooth eye movements with foveally-stabilized targets. Exp. Brain Res. 68, 194–204.

Van Santen, J.P.H. and Sperling, G. (1984) Temporal covariance model of human motion perception. J. Opt. Soc. Am. A 1, 451–473.

Van Santen, J.P.H. and Sperling, G. (1985) Elaborated Reichardt detectors. J. Opt. Soc. Am. 2, 300–321.

Viviani, P. and Swensson, R. (1982) Saccadic eye movements to peripherally discriminated visual targets. J. Exp. Psychol. Hum. Percept. Perform. 8, 113–126.

Viviani, P. and Terzuolo, C. (1980) Space-time invariance in learned motor skills. In: G.E. Stelmach and J. Requin (Eds.), Tutorials in Motor Behavior, North-Holland, Amsterdam, pp. 525–533.

Walls, G.L. (1962) The evolutionary history of eye movements. Vision Res. 2, 69–80.

Ward, R. and Morgan, M.J. (1978) Perceptual effect of pursuit eye movements in the absence of a target. Nature 274, 158–159.

Wertheimer, M. (1912) Experimentalle studien uber das Sehen von Bewegung. Zeitschrift fur Psychologie 61, 247–250 (Translation in: R.J. Herrnstein and E.G. Boring (Eds.), A Sourcebook in the History of Psychology, Harvard University Press, Cambridge, MA, pp. 259–261).

Westheimer, G. (1954) Eye movement response to a horizontally moving visual stimulus. Arch. Ophthalmol. 52, 932–941.

Westheimer, G. (1979) The spatial sense of the eye. Proctor lecture. Invest. Ophthalmol. Vis. Sci. 18, 893–912.

Westheimer, G. and Conover, D.W. (1954) Smooth eye movements in the absence of a moving visual stimulus. J. Exp. Psychol. 47, 283–284.

Westheimer, G. and McKee, S.P. (1975) Visual acuity in the presence of retinal image motion. J. Opt. Soc. Am. 65, 847–850.

Wheeless, L.L., Jr., Boynton, R.M. and Cohen, G.H. (1966) Eye-movement responses to step and pulse-step stimuli. J. Opt. Soc. Am. 56, 956–960.

Whittaker, S.G. and Eaholtz, G. (1982) Learning patterns of eye motion for foveal pursuit. Vision Sci. 23, 393–397.

Whittaker, S.G., Budd, J. and Cummings, R.W. (1988) Eccentric fixation with macular scotoma. Invest. Ophthalmol. Vis. Sci. 29, 268–278.

White, C.T., Eason, R.G. and Bartlett, N.R. (1962) Latency and duration of eye movements in the horizontal plane. J. Opt. Soc. Am. 52, 210–213.

Winterson, B.J. and Collewijn, H. (1976) Microsaccades during finely guided visuomotor tasks. Vision Res. 16, 1387–1390.

Winterson, B.J. and Robinson, D.A. (1975) Fixation by the alert but solitary cat. Vision Res. 15, 1349–1352.

Winterson, B.J. and Steinman, R.M. (1978) The effect of luminance on human smooth pursuit of perifoveal and foveal targets. Vision Res. 18, 1165–1172.

Woodworth, R.S. and Schlosberg, H. (1954) Experimental Psychology, Holt, Rinehart and Winston, New York.

Wyatt, H.J. and Pola, J. (1981) Slow eye movements to eccentric targets. Invest. Ophthalmol. Vis. Sci. 21, 477–483.

Wyman, D. and Steinman, R.M. (1973a) Small step tracking: implications for the oculomotor 'dead zone'. Vision Res. 13, 2165–2172.

Wyman, D. and Steinman, R.M. (1973b) Latency characteristics of small saccades. Vision Res. 13, 2173–2175.

Yarbus, A.L. (1967) Eye Movements and Vision, Plenum Press, New York.

Yasui, S. and Young, L.R. (1975) Perceived visual motion as effective stimulus to pursuit eye movement system. Science 190, 906–908.

Young, L.R. (1971) Pursuit eye tracking movements. In: P. Bach-y-Rita, C.C. Collins and J.E. Hyde (Eds.), The Control of Eye Movements, Academic Press, New York–London, pp. 429–443.

Zee, D.S., Yee, R.D. and Robinson, D.A. (1976) Optokinetic responses in labyrinthine-defective human beings. Brain Res. 113, 423–428.

Zee, D.S., Yamazaki, A., Butler, P.H. and Guger, G. (1981) Effects of ablation of flocculus and paraflocculus on eye movements in primate. J. Neurophysiol. 46, 878–889.

Zingale, C.M. and Kowler, E. (1987) Planning sequences of saccades. Vision Res. 27, 1327–1341.

Eye movements and their role in visual and cognitive processes
E. Kowler, Editor

CHAPTER 2

Predictive control of eye movement

M. Pavel

Department of Psychology, Stanford University, Stanford, CA 94305, U.S.A.

1. Introduction

Some of the earliest eye movement researchers noticed that stimuli moving in regular, periodic patterns are tracked more accurately than stimuli moving in aperiodic patterns (e.g. Dodge et al., 1930). The fact that periodic or 'predictable' motions are tracked more accurately than aperiodic or 'unpredictable' motions is indicative of the ability to estimate the future movements of a target and use these estimates to guide eye movements.

This chapter is primarily concerned with models of anticipatory oculomotor behavior and the relationship to the observed eye-movement data. Understanding prediction and anticipatory behavior is important for characterizing many aspects of oculomotor performance, because any data concerning the speed or accuracy of oculomotor responses (either smooth pursuit or saccades) will be interpreted differently if the responses are known to be the result of prediction.

Two types of predictive behavior will be considered in this chapter. In the first type the prediction of the future motion of a target is based on an extrapolation of its prior trajectory. In the second type, the prediction is based on decision-making processes. By this I mean that the motion of a target is predicted from contextual cues in the environment and the observers' common sense knowledge of the world. For example, the knowledge that a falling ball is likely to change its direction of motion upon contact with the floor may be reflected in the trajectory of the eye movements used to track the ball. In a laboratory experiment, the observer's context-based anticipation might be based on perceived regularities of prior target motions, or on cues about future target motion, or on pure guesses on the part of the subject. Both of these types of predictive behavior, trajectory extrapolation and decision-making, should be included in the oculomotor models for meaningful interpretation of the data.

I would like to emphasize that predictive behavior should never be ignored, because many organisms, including human observers, expect regularities and predictability even if there is none. Thus, even if the experimental paradigm is designed to discourage prediction by randomizing stimuli, observers acting on subjective probabilities will exhibit anticipatory behaviors. This means that data from any oculomotor (or more generally, behavioral) experiment may be the result of a combination of anticipatory and reflexive behaviors.

Predictive behavior has been addressed in oculomotor research. Early attempts to explain the difference between tracking of periodic and aperiodic (unpredictable) target motions in terms of linear time-invariant systems met with only marginal success. In this chapter I will argue that the reason for the limited success so far is that such models can only account for the extrapolation type of prediction and not for the nonlinear, decision-making type of prediction. In particular, the success of models in describing just about any oculomotor behavior will depend on their ability to include nonlinear decision-making processes, and in particular the information provided by contextual cues.

How can contextual inputs be included? One possibility is to use current methods in modern control systems theory, the so-called 'optimal control theory' (e.g., Bryson and Ho, 1968). These methods include algorithms capable of using complex information about the control problem. This chapter will summarize a few of these approaches and shows how optimal control theory can be applied to predictive oculomotor behavior. In addition, a different class of models, called decision-making models, developed to characterize anticipatory behaviors in cognitive experiments, will be described. Finally, I will suggest new approaches based on models of pattern recognition. The goal of these approaches is to combine aspects of models based on optimal control theory with aspects of models based on decision theory.

This chapter contains three parts. The first part will be concerned with the models of the extrapolation of target trajectory. I will first review some previous, well-known attempts to model predictive eye movements based on a classical linear control systems approach. Then, I will describe some more sophisticated signal estimation and prediction techniques based on modern optimal control theory which might be used to model more complex types of trajectory extrapolation. In the second part of this chapter I will describe decision-making models which incorporate expectation effects of voluntary choices made by an observer. This discussion includes a brief description of models which have been proposed to account for anticipatory phenomena in cognitive psychology and their application to oculomotor research. The third part of this chapter suggests a general approach to model the complex anticipatory behaviors based on more recent developments in pattern recognition techniques.

2. Trajectory extrapolation

Much of the classical work on predictive oculomotor behavior has been concerned with how a mechanical (mostly linear) system can use information in prior trajectories to predict the future paths. For the purpose of describing these models I assume that the fixed mechanical aspects of the eye movement system can be represented by a *black* box illustrated in Fig. 1a. The models I will describe were developed mainly (but not exclusively) to account for smooth eye movements. Keeping with convention, the input is the position $x(t)$ of a target and the output that of the eye, $u(t)$. The function x over time is the spatial *trajectory* of the target. I use 'position' despite the fact that in most current models of the smooth oculomotor system it is assumed that the critical inputs and outputs are velocities. In consideration of prediction, however, it is more conservative to operate on the target and eye positions as the more fundamental quantity because velocity can always be computed from position. Also, throughout this chapter I will be considering the role of prediction in either smooth eye movements or saccades, the latter assumed to be sensitive to position and not to velocity signals.

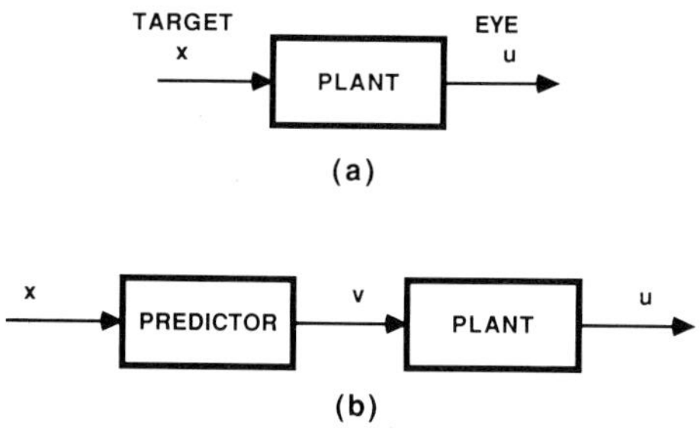

Fig. 1. Black box definition of (a) oculomotor 'plant' and (b) the 'plant' with a predictor.

The general paradigm for modeling anticipation can be described as defining a predictor which is interposed between the target position signal and the input to the oculomotor system. The output of the predictor $v(t)$ is then the actual input to the mechanically fixed oculomotor system. The goal of the modeling is to specify the characteristics of the predictor that will account for the observed anticipatory phenomena.

2.1. Classical linear systems approach

The models in this section are based on classical control theory (e.g., Kuo, 1982), and assume that the oculomotor system can be approximated by a linear system. The critical assumption is that the oculomotor system is 'designed', i.e., has evolved, to minimize the output error (to be defined below) under the constraint that the control system is composed of linear time-invariant components. In this section I first describe the oculomotor system as a linear system, and then several attempts to apply the classical control-theoretic approach to modeling predictive oculomotor behaviors.

2.1.1. The oculomotor system as a linear system

Although the oculomotor system is known to be nonlinear (St.-Cyr and Fender, 1969a; Collewijn and Tamminga, 1984), it is frequently represented by linear time-invariant components. Some of the system's nonlinearities are then represented by memory-less, threshold-like elements that limit the acceleration and velocity of the eye (e.g., Robinson et al., 1986). Many nonlinear systems of this type behave as if they were linear when confronted with small signals; that is, they obey superposition and homogeneity. Treating such systems as if they were linear is, therefore, a common practice in engineering. In keeping with this practice, the model in Fig. 2, used here for illustration of the principles of anticipation, is assumed to be essentially a linear system.

The behavior of the system is governed by its dynamics, its initial state, the input signal and the nonlinear limits. The dynamics of the system, together with the nonlinear limits, constrain how fast the system can change its state. In particular, in this example it is assumed that, at least for small signals, the system can be represented by a second-order linear system (Westheimer, 1954b). This particular system was chosen in order to illustrate various aspects of prediction, rather than as the best model of the eye movement system.

The behavior of a dynamical system can be described in either the frequency or the time domain.

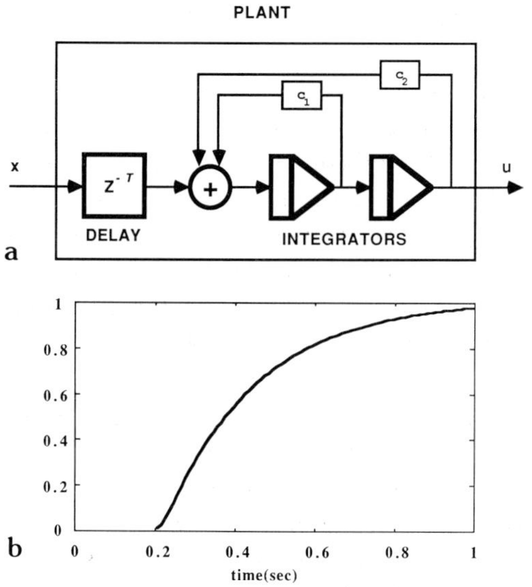

Fig. 2. (a) Linear second-order model of the eye movement dynamical system, or the 'plant'. A graphical representation of state variables and the linear operations. (b) Step response of the system in (a).

The frequency domain description is based on the property that if the input is a sinusoid of a given frequency, the output is a possibly delayed sinusoid of the same frequency. The ratio of the output to input amplitudes as a function of frequency characterizes the 'gain' of the linear system. The gain, together with the phase response as a function of frequency, comprise the frequency response of the system. More formally, a linear system can be characterized by its transfer function, i.e., the ratio of the Laplace transform of the output, $U(s)$, to the input $X(s)$ as a function of the complex frequency s. The use of complex numbers allows one to characterize the entire frequency response (i.e., gain and phase) by a single ratio, $U(s)/X(s)$. The Laplace transform can be thought of as a generalization of Fourier transform with $s = \alpha + i\omega$, and thereby a generalization of the frequency response. Thus, multiplication and division by s correspond to differentiation and integration, respectively. The transform of an exponential function $e^{-\alpha t}$ is $\frac{1}{s+\alpha}$.
In this example, the transfer function is given by:

$$H(s) = \frac{U(s)}{X(s)} = \frac{e^{-s\tau}}{(as+1)(bs+1)} \quad (1)$$

The constant τ, whose value is usually between 100 and 200 ms, represents a pure delay, and a and b are two time constants. If this dynamical system is thought of as the oculomotor 'plant' then the time constants a and b can be given values estimated by Keller (1973) to be 224 and 13 ms, respectively, for the monkey. (Robinson et al. (1986) used the same values in a study of human smooth pursuit.)

An alternative way to describe the behavior of a dynamical system involves an analysis of the *state* of the system in the time domain. The state of the system at any instant of time is characterized by a set of *state variables* whose values represent a complete summary of its history. That is, the response of a system to any future inputs can be determined if the state is known. For example, the state of a moving object is completely specified by its position and velocity. Knowledge of the position and velocity at a given time allows the computation of future positions and velocities by considering only current and future forces. The actual future behavior is determined by a solution of a set of differential equations (involving state variables) that describe the system's dynamics.* For example, a continuous time representation for the 'plant' in Fig. 2(b) is given by

$$\frac{d}{dt} u(t) = q(t)$$

$$k_2 \frac{d}{dt} q(t) + k_1 q(t) + u(t) = x(t-\tau) \quad (2)$$

where q and u are the state variables representing the state of the system at time t, and $k_1 = a+b, k_2 = ab$ are real constants. The set of differential equations can be solved to determine the response of the system to different inputs x. This *state-space* formulation of dynamical systems is a foundation for optimal control theoretic approaches to be discussed in later sections. At this point, the frequency domain description is more convenient.

Suppose that the purpose of this system is to smoothly pursue a moving target, that is, to minimize the difference between the input (target position) and output (eye position). This difference, $e(t) = x(t) - u(t)$, is called the 'tracking error'. When the error is represented in terms of velocities as $\dot{e}(t) = \frac{d}{dt} e(t)$ it is called 'retinal slip' or velocity error. If the target position is known only for the past $\tau \leq t$, the best the system can do in response to a step input is shown in Fig. 2(b). The large error is due to the response delay of the system and the fact that such a system cannot respond before it sees the stimulus. Systems that cannot respond before they see the stimulus are called *causal*.

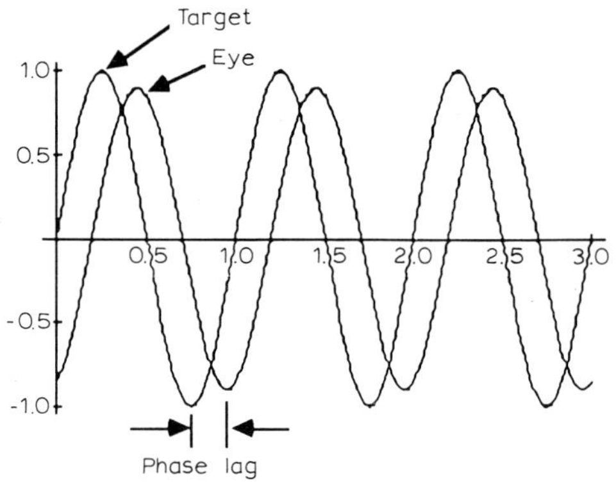

Fig. 3. The response of a linear system to sinusoidal target motion is sinusoidal eye motion with a possibly different amplitude and phase. The difference in phase is called a phase lag.

The response characteristics of this dynamical system are constrained by its physical limits. The response of such a system would be the same with periodic as with novel, unpredictable stimuli. For sinusoidal stimuli the response delay of a causal system is exhibited as a phase lag, as shown in Fig. 3. Sinusoidal and periodic stimuli in general have been used extensively because the phase lag, together with the amplitude response, as a function of frequency, completely characterizes a linear time-invariant system. Therefore, such a system with fixed characteristics (time-invariant) would not im-

* Differential equations are used for continuous-time system representations. For discrete-time representations, difference equations are used.

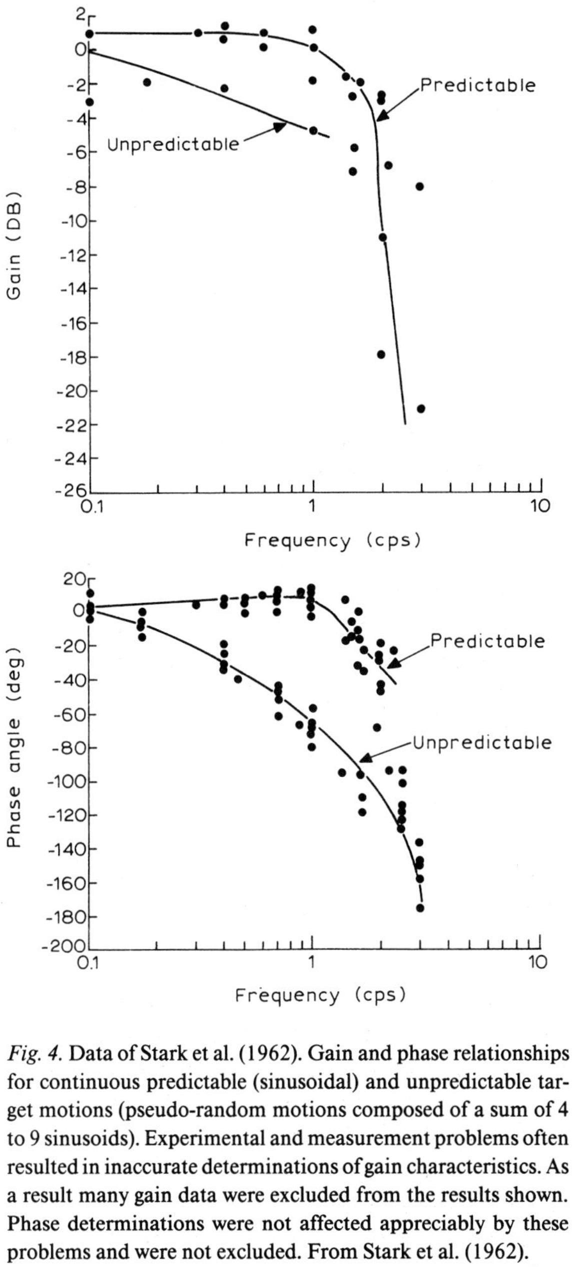

Fig. 4. Data of Stark et al. (1962). Gain and phase relationships for continuous predictable (sinusoidal) and unpredictable target motions (pseudo-random motions composed of a sum of 4 to 9 sinusoids). Experimental and measurement problems often resulted in inaccurate determinations of gain characteristics. As a result many gain data were excluded from the results shown. Phase determinations were not affected appreciably by these problems and were not excluded. From Stark et al. (1962).

prove its response (e.g. reduce its phase lag) over time.

The human oculomotor system is more flexible. In particular, smooth pursuit eye movements are more accurate for periodic, predictable stimuli than for aperiodic (random) stimuli. Fig. 4, taken from Stark et al. (1962), illustrates data of this sort obtained from the tracking of sinusoidal stimulus motions. A number of investigators have noticed a reduction in the phase lag for sinusoidal, in comparison with unpredictable stimuli (Westheimer, 1954b; Fender and Nye, 1961; Stark et al., 1962; Dallos and Jones, 1963).

There have been attempts to characterize the difference between tracking predictable and unpredictable inputs by methods commonly used for describing linear systems. For example, Stark et al. (1962), recognizing the need to study eye movements with both *predictable* and *unpredictable* stimuli, compared the amplitude and phase of the response as a function of frequency. They found an improved response for predictable motion for tracking both smooth and step target motions. An aspect of their study, which complicates interpretation of the results, is the way they constructed their unpredictable stimuli. Stark et al. (1962) composed their stimuli by summing a number of periodic stimuli. Such signals are more complex than simple sinusoids, but otherwise completely predictable. That is, given a sufficiently long sample of the waveform, the future target position is completely predictable. Since predictability of motion is not an all-or-none phenomenon, any predictability in the signal may have been used by the oculomotor system to improve its performance. So, the response obtained with the unpredictable stimuli might not accurately capture the oculomotor response to truly random inputs. The important point is that lack of periodicity, which can be attained by combining sinusoids with periods that are not related by rational numbers, does not necessarily imply unpredictability. Notions of the predictability of aperiodic signals will be discussed again in section 2.2.7.

Strictly speaking, the finding that human beings appear to learn over time to respond more accurately to predictable inputs would be inconsistent with hard-wired, time-invariant linear system models. In addition, the two essential properties of linear systems, superposition and homogeneity, were also found to fail for smooth eye movements (St.-Cyr and Fender, 1969a; Collewijn and Tamminga,

1984). Given such evidence, it may not seem wise to develop and evaluate models based on linear systems theory. But linear systems theory has many very attractive features, including simplicity, analytical tractability and robustness, so that it can be used to approximate some nonlinear systems. For example, for a limited range of signals it is possible to characterize a nonlinear system by computing the 'gain' as a function of frequency and signal amplitude. The technical term for the amplitude-dependent frequency response is the *describing function.* Because of these advantages it is useful to examine how well a linear system model can describe the instantaneous behavior of the oculomotor system after it has learned to anticipate the signal. Let me next discuss a few earlier attempts to model anticipatory behavior in the context of classical control theory with linear system components.

2.1.2. Classical control theory

Engineering application of classical, linear, automatic control theory consists of finding the best realizable linear system composed of discrete linear elements that would perform the desired control function. The control system would be designed with various negative and positive feedback loops to compensate for the undesirable characteristics of the system to be controlled. The main tools used in the description of systems in the frequency domain are based on Fourier or Laplace transforms. The major concern for the engineer was to produce the most sensitive controller while maintaining system stability. A successful control design would have small errors and small phase lags.

Researchers in eye movement systems reasoned that the classical control theory could, in principle, be used to explain some aspect of the predictive behavior of the oculomotor system. For example, Dallos and Jones (1963) studied the 'gain' and phase lag of pursuit as a function of the frequency of predictable and random target motions. They represented the observed anticipatory behavior of the oculomotor system by interposing a fixed, mechanical *predictor* in the signal path. In their model the predictor gets the original position error input and

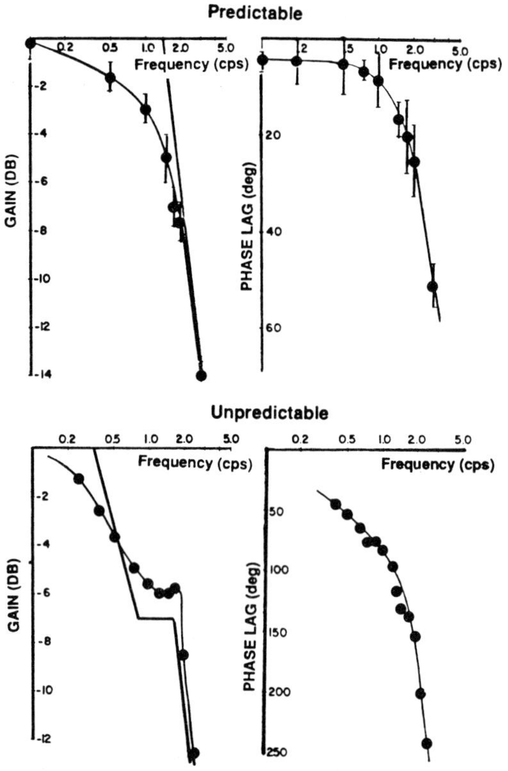

Fig. 5. Data of Dallos and Jones (1963). Average gain and phase as a function of frequency for predictable (sinusoidal) and unpredictable (Gaussian random noise) target motions. From Dallos and Jones (1963).

then generates an output signal that serves as the input into the 'plant' model of the oculomotor system. While this formulation is not necessarily the only way to represent the predictive behavior by a linear time-invariant system, it is sufficiently general to encompass a large class of theories. To characterize the predictor they compared the tracking of sinusoidal target motions with the tracking of motions generated by a low-pass (1.25 Hz) Gaussian random process (see their results in Fig. 5).

To characterize the predictor in mathematical form, they expressed the predictive effect as the ratio of gains obtained with predictable sinusoidal stimuli to the gain estimated for the unpredictable low-pass Gaussian stimuli. They assumed that the predictor was ineffective for the Gaussian stimuli, and computed the phase characteristics of the predictor by subtracting the phase for the Gaussian from that for the sinusoidal signals. The resulting predictor, obtained by fitting a fifth-order odd polynomial, had the following form:

$$K(i\omega) = \frac{28.1}{3.14+i\omega}\, e^{i(31.4\omega-6.7\omega^2+0.7\omega^3)} \tag{3}$$

This predictor has a high d.c. gain (approx. 10) and phase characteristics that are not physically realizable with conventional components. Dallos and Jones then proposed to approximate the predictor by a causal, physically realizable system with a rational transfer function. That approximation was equivalent to a concatenation of 11 second-order components.

A realizable linear predictive component has a transfer function of the form ($s\tau+1$). It is an approximation to a differentiator and can be realized in a circuit by a capacitor and a resistor. As such it is a causal system and the resulting phase lead is observed only for steady-state signals. There is no way that a system built of such components will produce a signal prior to getting its own input. This property will become important in evaluating the applicability of such predictors to 'non-causal' anticipatory responses.

Dallos and Jones incorporated their predictor into a complete oculomotor model, shown in Fig. 6. The model included a decision apparatus which chooses to include or exclude the predictor based on memory for prior events.

In addition to the steady-state smooth-pursuit data, Dallos and Jones also reported the improvement of tracking as a function of time for the sinusoidal target motions, as well as for square-wave motions tracked with saccades. They observed that the smooth tracking improved at a faster rate than the saccadic tracking of the square wave (see Fig. 7). For sinusoidal motion, the observers essentially eliminated the phase lag after only a single cycle. Depending on the repetition rate, it took more than three cycles for the square waves.

The work of Dallos and Jones represented an important step toward understanding the limitations of the linear time-invariant systems as models of predictive tracking. The basic limitation was that the resulting filter was not 'physically realizable', suggesting that additional mechanisms would be required to explain anticipatory responses. Although the notion of a physically realizable system has more specific meaning in engineering, one can think of it as a system composed of causal components such as differentiators, integrators, gain and summing elements. Also, while the linear model appeared to provide a reasonable account for their steady-state smooth-pursuit data, it failed to characterize the saccadic oculomotor response to square waves.

In addition to these limitations, there are some

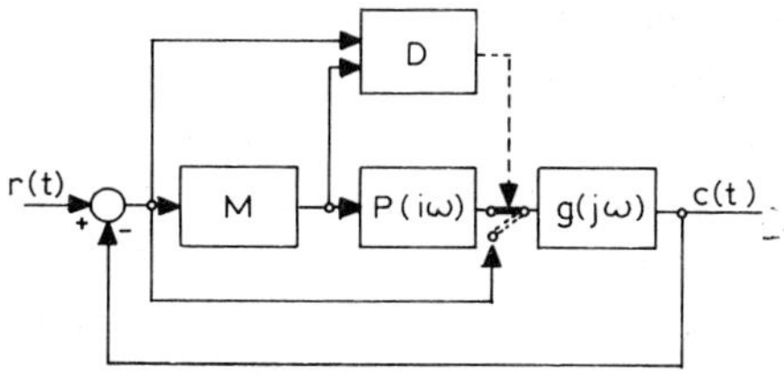

Fig. 6. The model of Dallos and Jones (1963). The memory system (M) generates an expected signal which is compared (D) to the actual signal. If they match the predictor with the transfer function $P(i\omega)$ is inserted into the loop. The plant is represented by its transfer function $g(j\omega)$, the input by r(t) and the eye motion by c(t). From Dallos and Jones (1963).

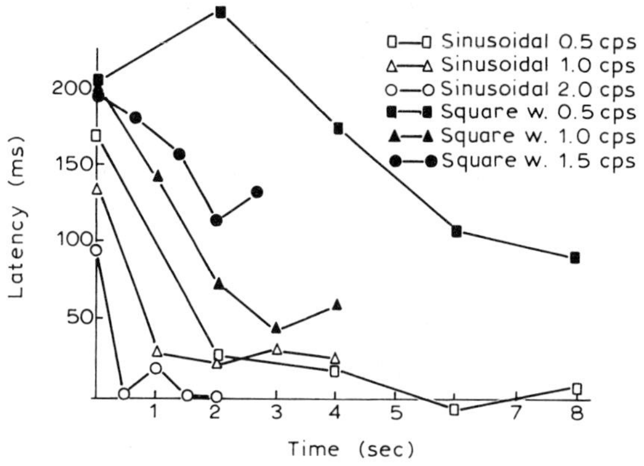

Fig. 7. Average latency as a function of time during trials tracking sinusoidal and square-wave target motions. From Dallos and Jones (1963).

other troublesome conclusions. First, they assumed that the predictor would be completely ineffective for a Gaussian (i.e., unpredictable) signal. The Gaussian signal they used, however, was filtered by a low-pass filter with a half-power point at 1.25 Hz. Even though such a signal has a random component, it is to some degree predictable (i.e., the signal cannot change its value arbitrarily in a very short time). The extent to which this signal is predictable is characterized by its autocorrelation function. Therefore, Dallos and Jones may have underestimated the actual contribution of the predictor to performance with the Gaussian stimulus.

Second, their analysis of pursuit did not eliminate the contribution of saccades. Therefore, the resulting frequency response was due, at least in part, to saccades. Finally, Dallos and Jones observed large trial-to-trial differences in tracking eye movements and concluded that averaging was necessary to "bring out the prevailing pattern". These large differences may be indicative of the fact that the prediction might arise, in whole or part, from observer strategies. Perhaps, for example, observers may *choose* a different strategy on each trial. There were indications that this may be so. For the more difficult (high-frequency) square-wave stimuli, the observers were not able to track for more than a few seconds at a time. Dallos and Jones interpreted this fact in terms of loss of the memory trace in their predictor, but a loss of sustained effort or attention might be an equally acceptable explanation.

On the theoretical level, the fixed linear predictor of Dallos and Jones can compensate for the phase lag in the steady-state response, but it has two serious shortcomings. First, it could not account for some anticipatory responses of the oculomotor system (Dodge et al., 1930), even those observed by these authors in their own square-wave tracking data. The second problem was identified by Michael and Melvill Jones (1966), who manipulated the degree of unpredictability of movement by varying the bandwidth and center frequency of their Gaussian random signals. They found that the ratio of predictable and unpredictable gains, which Dallos and Jones (1963) defined to be the contribution of the predictor, depended on the bandwidth of the random target motion. A single fixed predictor cannot explain the reduction in phase lag as a function of bandwidth.

St.-Cyr and Fender (1969b) criticized the Dallos and Jones model because of the many clearly nonlinear aspects of the oculomotor system. St.-Cyr and Fender (1969b) attempted to explain the dependence of phase lag on predictability by assuming that the lag is determined by a simple delay. The delay was attributed to signal processing and was assumed to be inversely proportional to the amount of information transmitted by the oculomotor system.

More specifically the processing delay T was given by:

$$T = T_i + \frac{H}{R} \tag{4}$$

where T_i is the dead time (approximately 65 milliseconds), H is the amount of information in the signal, and R is the amount of information transmitted between the stimulus and the eye movement. In particular the rate of transmission of information between x and y is given by:

$$R = \frac{1}{2} \log_2 \int \frac{S_x(\omega)S_y(\omega)}{|S_x(\omega)S_y(\omega) - S_{xy}(\omega)|^2} d\omega$$

in bits/second. The rate of transmission R was computed from the power spectra of the target trajectory and the eye movement, as well as their crosscorrelation. The value of H was computed from the slope of a linear regression of the estimated delay T on $1/R$; the estimate of H was 0.162 bits for one subject and 0.211 for the other. St.-Cyr and Fender (1969b) concluded that these linear regressions, shown in Fig. 8, provided a reasonable account for the data. Their model would be much more compelling if the information content of the stimulus H could have been determined independently of the eye movement data.

The basic premise of St.-Cyr and Fender's (1969b) model was that the delay T should vary as a function of the complexity of the target motion. This may be reasonable, but it does not explain

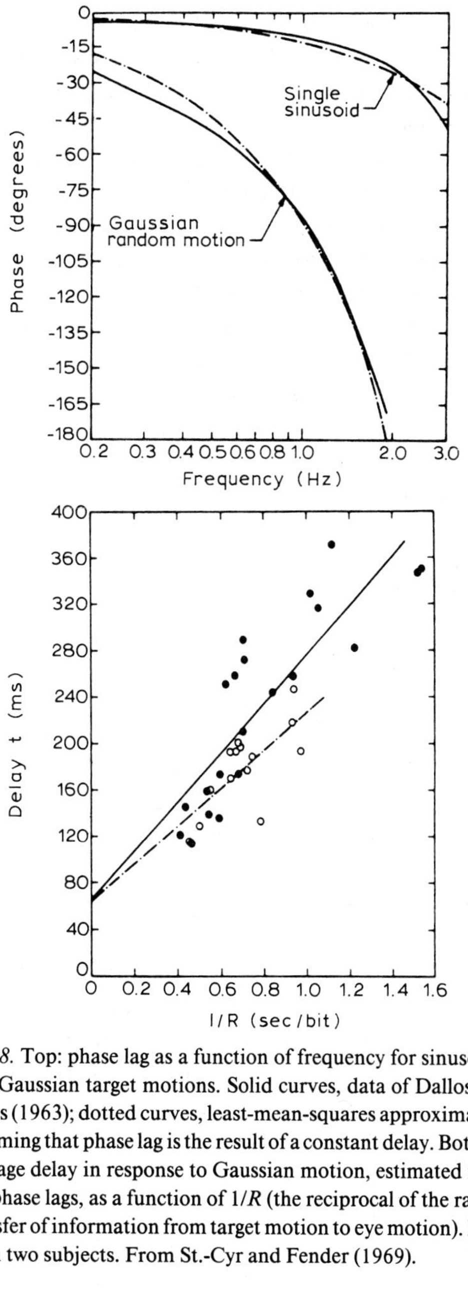

Fig. 8. Top: phase lag as a function of frequency for sinusoidal and Gaussian target motions. Solid curves, data of Dallos and Jones (1963); dotted curves, least-mean-squares approximation assuming that phase lag is the result of a constant delay. Bottom: average delay in response to Gaussian motion, estimated from the phase lags, as a function of $1/R$ (the reciprocal of the rate of transfer of information from target motion to eye motion). Data from two subjects. From St.-Cyr and Fender (1969).

anticipation. The authors did not worry about this because they believed that "... the direction of gaze never anticipates the target, but always lags behind it". Consequently, their model did not explain anticipatory effects where the eye movement occurs before the target. Also, note that, in spite of their rejection of linearity, they characterized the system's behavior by the frequency responses at a given amplitude. If the nonlinearity of the oculomotor system were taken seriously, the system would require a different description for each signal amplitude.

A further problem with most of the models described thus far is the fact that saccadic and smooth components of eye tracking were not distinguished. Because saccades are discrete events generated in response to continuous inputs, they should not be treated as a direct output of a linear system. Yasui and Young (1984) developed a model of anticipation in which they separated the saccadic components from the smooth pursuit components. They assumed that eye movements can be characterized by an *additive* combination of the output of the pursuit $u_p(t)$ and saccadic $u_s(t)$ subsystems, $u(t) = u_p(t)+u_s(t)$. The smooth-pursuit component was estimated by 'removing' saccadic jumps using a method described by Allum et al. (1975). Both the smooth-pursuit component and the composite eye movement confirmed previous results in that the more unpredictable target movements yielded longer phase lags and showed lower gains.

To analyse the saccadic system Yasui and Young computed the corresponding saccadic component by $u_s(t) = u(t)-u_p(t)$. They further argued that the effective ($x_{\text{eff}}(t)$) input to the saccadic system is the positional error after the smooth pursuit component has been removed, i.e.,

$$x_{\text{eff}}(t) = x(t)-u_p(t) \tag{5}$$

According to their model, the saccadic system does not see the actual target position nor does it see the error signal seen by the smooth pursuit. It has access only to the difference between where the eye is and where it would have been if the eye depended on the smooth pursuit movement alone. With these assumptions Yasui and Young then derived the hypothetical 'gain' of the saccadic system. Using the sampled data model of Young and Stark (1963) as a starting point, they introduced prediction as a compensating element with a transfer function:

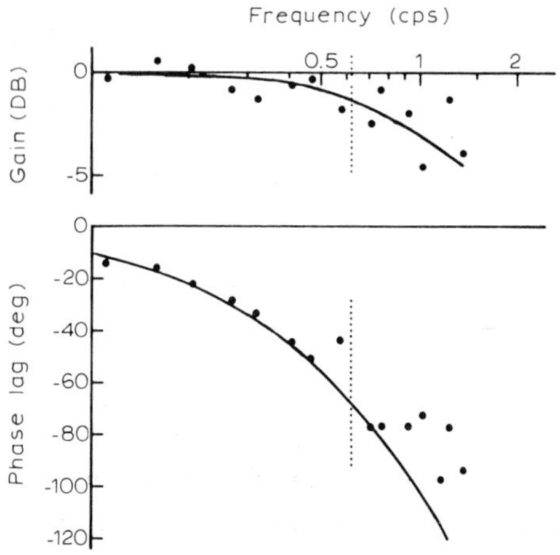

Fig. 9. Data of Yasui and Young (1984). Gain and phase of the saccadic response to pseudo-random target motions. The solid lines represent predictions from their control-theoretic model. The limits of the model validity (<0.62 Hz) are indicated by the vertical dotted line. From Yasui and Young (1984).

$$Q(s) = 1+i\omega T_{\mathrm{d}} \tag{6}$$

where T_d = 200ms is a delay reported by Westheimer (1954b). The resulting frequency response of the saccadic system is shown in Fig. 9.

This model uses a linear, time-invariant compensator and a periodic sampling of the input. The data analyses performed by Yasui and Young do not permit a complete evaluation of their hypotheses. In particular, their definition of the 'gain' of the saccadic subsystem depends on the performance of the smooth-pursuit system (which they did not model). Similarly, the validity of their assumption that the sampling mechanism is independent of the retinal position error needs to be demonstrated.

As these examples indicate, the models based on the classical control theory might account for some aspects of the difference in phase lag between responses to simple sinusoidal and more complex signals. These models were generally addressing selected steady-state input/output relationships. There were no mechanisms for explaining what information the oculomotor system might use to 'learn' to predict and how it might 'build' the predictor.*

The realistic scope of anticipatory behaviors is much greater than the reduction in phase lag. In particular, people can make anticipatory responses that precede the input events. The general idea is that the oculomotor system can make a response to a hypothetical internal signal, much in the same manner as an alert driver at night anticipates a left curve after he has seen the corresponding road sign. The models discussed so far cannot generate such anticipatory behaviors. An approach that comes closer to this goal is based on modern optimal control theory, which will be briefly described in the next section.

2.2. Optimal estimation and control theory

The previous section illustrated the scope and the limitations of the application of a traditional control-theoretic approach to oculomotor models. The most important limitation was the assumption that the oculomotor system is made up of linear time-invariant systems which act to minimize the output error. To overcome this inherent limitation of the classical approach, control engineers developed a less constrained approach called optimal control theory (Bryson and Ho, 1968). In this section I will first illustrate some of the basic principles of optimal control theory and its application to prediction in deterministic situations. I will then consider a framework for stochastic estimation and control, followed by a description of two examples of recursive algorithms. My approach will consist largely of a discussion of those aspects of optimal control methods which relate to eye movements and their predictive behaviors. There have been a few attempts to apply these notions to the oculomotor

---

* In a more recent attempt, Van den Berg (1988) proposed a model of smooth pursuit with a linear, adaptive compensator that adjusts its parameters by monitoring zero crossings of a moving target. While a step in the right direction (in that it is adaptive), this model, like other models based on classical control theory, is limited in that it is only capable of adjusting phase lags. It cannot explain how a predictable pattern of target motion is learned, nor account for the anticipatory responses, which occur prior to any signal change.

system, which I will summarize.

2.2.1. Definition of a control problem

In its most general sense, an optimal control approach consists of describing the system to be controlled, and finding appropriate control signals so that the system behaves in a desired manner. Unlike in the classical approach, the solutions need not necessarily be constrained by the availability or realizability of the analog, hard-wired systems. Because the control signal in optimal control theory is generated by computation, such systems can have the potential to learn to respond to new situations.

Application of the optimal control approach to eye movements is intended to describe mathematical input/output relationships without specific reference to the underlying neural processes. Nevertheless, optimal control models of human eye movements are physiologically plausible because the neural circuitry is not limited to the simple linear processes described in the previous section. The scope of this chapter does not permit an adequate treatment of modern control theory. I will limit myself to the description of some of the important engineering concepts and indicate their relevance to eye movements, and how they might remedy some of the limitations of the classical control-theoretic models of predictive behavior.

In optimal control theory the engineering control problem is characterized by specifying three things: (1) the dynamics of the system, (2) an objective function to be optimized, and (3) additional constraints. These specifications can be directly applied to the oculomotor system. For example:

1. The dynamics of the system is determined by the mechanical properties of the 'plant', for example Equation 2, and the linear and nonlinear properties of the controlling neural circuitry.
2. The objective function, which may depend on the task to be performed, involves the position or velocity of the eye. For example, the objective function may measure the extent to which the motion of the eye approximates the motion of a selected target, at least closely enough to allow clear vision. One such measure of quality of tracking performance is average squared difference between the target and eye positions.
3. Additional constraints may include various physiological limitations, such as limits on forces that can be delivered by orbital muscles or constraints on the effort necessary to achieve desired control. A typical objective function for discrete systems consists of the sum of squared error and the sum of squared signals.

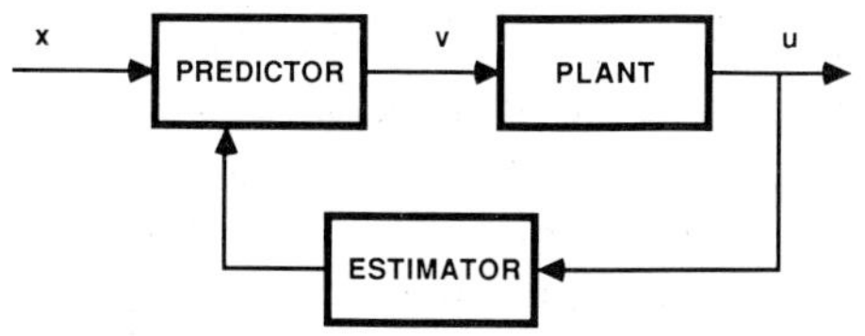

Fig. 10. Block diagram of an optimal control system. The estimator estimates the state of the plant and the predictor/controller generates the optimal signal with respect to a given objective.

The general paradigm for optimal control is illustrated in Fig. 10. The purpose of the controller is to generate a 'control signal' $v(t)$, i.e., a new input signal, which would produce optimal outputs with respect to the objective function while satisfying all the constraints. Such control can be achieved if the system has an estimate of the instantaneous and possibly future states of the plant. An estimate of the state of the plant is, therefore, determined by the estimator in Fig. 10.

If the properties of the system, the constraints on the systems and the desired output are all known exactly then one can construct a deterministic controller which would generate optimal oculomotor performance. I will use a deterministic approach to illustrate the critical role of prediction for optimal control, even though such a situation is not realistic for building biological models. I will then turn to the more biologically plausible stochastic models.

2.2.2. Deterministic systems

Suppose that the desired eye position (i.e., equal to target position) and the response dynamics of the oculomotor system are known exactly, and that there are no other constraints. Is it possible, in this simple case, to generate an input signal which will cause the eye to execute the desired trajectory? Such a signal would have to compensate for any of the characteristics of the oculomotor system which would normally cause the eye to track the target inaccurately. To the extent that such a signal can be generated, the tracking error can be completely eliminated.

To illustrate this unconstrained optimization I will compute the required input, or 'control' signal, required for perfect tracking by the 'plant' shown in Fig. 1. Such a signal is generated by a feed-forward controller. Because the only input to the controller is the desired trajectory x the control is said to be open-loop. The controller will be designed to generate the input signal v for the 'plant' so that the objective function $J = \int [x(t) - u(t)]^2 dt$ is minimized.

A general solution of this type of optimization problem usually requires quite sophisticated techniques based on calculus of variations applied to state-space representation of the dynamic system and the controller. In the case of a simple, linear, time-invariant, deterministic system, however, one can try to compute the control signal by computing the reciprocal transfer function $K(s) = \frac{1}{H(s)}$. The resulting transfer function of the controller K, which is itself a linear system, is

$$K(s) = \frac{1}{H(s)} = e^{s\tau}(as+1)(bs+1) = e^{s\tau}[1 + k_1 s + k_2 s^2] \quad (7)$$

where $k_1 = a+b$ and $k_2 = ab$. The resulting control signal in the time domain is

$$v(t) = x(t+\tau) + k_1 \frac{d}{dt} x(t+\tau) + k_2 \frac{d^2}{dt^2} x(t+\tau) \quad (8)$$

This equation illustrates that the ideal feed-forward controller does two things to counteract the distortions introduced by the response characteristics of the oculomotor plant. First, it requires the knowledge of the input τ seconds into the future. Second, it needs exact derivatives of the target motion. It is because of the shift into the future that this ideal controller must, in fact, be a predictor.

If such a predictor could be built, the error for many desired output signals could be reduced to zero. Consider the following examples of the behavior of such a predictor for sinusoidal, step and ramp stimuli. To compute the output of the controller for a sinusoidal signal we let the target motion be a sinusoid, $x(t) = \sin(\omega t)$. Then, substituting for x in Equation 8 we can find the new input control signal to be:

$$v(t) = (1 - k_2\omega^2)\sin[\omega(t+\tau)] + k_1\omega\cos[\omega(t+\tau)] \quad (9)$$

The controller, or predictor output (i.e., new oculomotor input), is a sinusoid of the same frequency with a different phase. Thus, for steady-state sinusoidal signals, this predictor behaves in a similar manner to the phase lead predictors of the classical control theory (Dallos and Jones, 1963; Yasui and Young, 1984).

Now consider the input to be a unit step function, which I denote $p_0(t)$. Unit step function is defined as zero for all $t \leq 0$ and equal to one everywhere else.

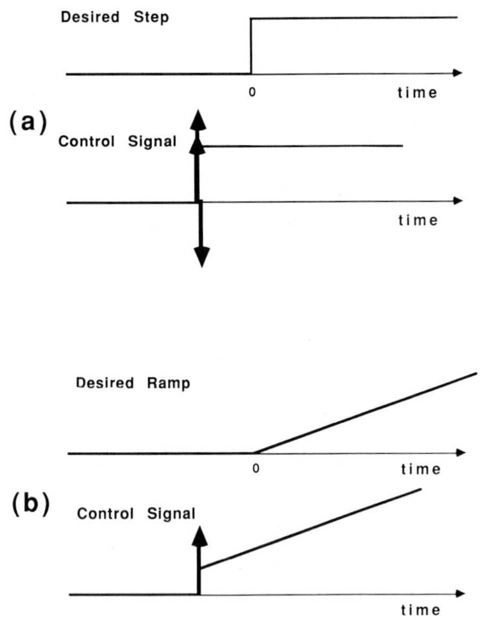

Fig. 11. Graphical representation of the desired eye position outputs and required control signals for (a) step and (b) ramp response. The output in each case is exactly equal to the desired input signal. The vertical arrows represent the impulse functions (functionals) delta.

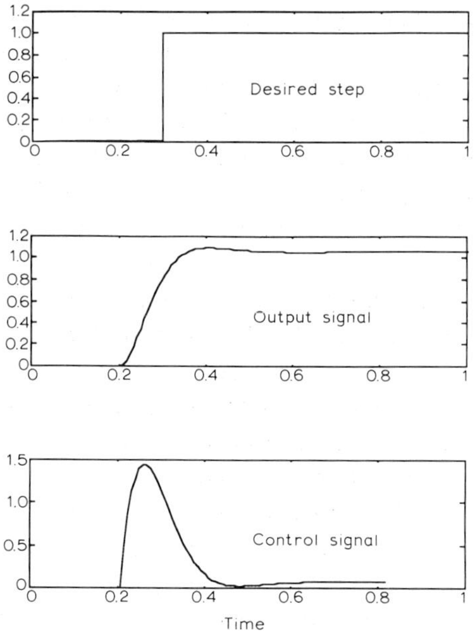

Fig. 12. A response of the plant (middle) to a step input (top) assuming full-state feedback control with perfect knowledge of the desired signal, and positive control signal. The predictor shifts the control signals (bottom) in time so that the control process starts before the actual input signal.

The step function corresponds to an instantaneous displacement of an otherwise stationary target. A graphical representation of the desired step function and the required control signal is shown in Fig. 11a. In order to compute the desired output of the controller it is necessary to differentiate the input. The first derivative of a step is an impulse $\delta(t)$ and the second derivative is a double impulse $\delta'(t)$. The impulse δ can be thought of as an infinitesimally short but very high amplitude pulse (burst). The resulting control signal for $x = p_0(t)$ is then given by

$$v(t) = p_0(t+\tau) + k_1\delta(t+\tau) + k_2\delta'(t+\tau) \tag{10}$$

Finally, consider an application to a constant-velocity (ramp) target motion. The desired output is a ramp which can be written mathematically as $r(t) = mtp_0(t)$ where m is the slope of the ramp and $p_0(t)$ is the unit step. If the target trajectory is a ramp $x(t) = r(t)$ then the predictor output is a combination of a ramp shifted in time, its derivative which is a pulse, and its second derivative consisting of two impulses. The predictor output is shown in Fig. 11b. Formally, the predictor output is given by

$$v(t) = r(t+\tau) + k_1 mp_0(t+\tau) + k_2 m\delta(t+\tau) \tag{11}$$

The reader can check that this v used as the input will produce the original ramp at the output.

If the deterministic, feed-forward, optimal controller described above can guarantee accurate tracking why is it not a desirable model of the eye movement system? There are several reasons. As illustrated on the previous examples, the deterministic approach requires very accurate spatial and temporal representation of the target trajectory and of the system characteristics. This is because the optimal controller essentially computes the inverse transfer function of the plant to be controlled. Such inverse transfer functions are very sensitive to noise and uncertainty and changes in the system parameters, and are not necessarily stable. The second difficulty arises because the control signals were computed without constraints on the magnitude of any forces and accelerations. The resulting signals, which required the impulse functions δ with infinite amplitudes, are not realizable in physical or biological systems. The third difficulty is that these systems are non-causal, i.e., their output at $t=t_0$ depends on values of the input for $t>t_0$. Such systems are not physically realizable.

Of course, it is possible to make the deterministic controller physically realizable. In a more realistic deterministic case, the control performance should be insensitive to small changes in the system dynamics and constrained by the maximum possible magnitude of torques and, possibly, the amount of energy (i.e., work) used for the control of eye movements. Fortunately, this is a typical set of constraints used by engineers to design optimal control systems. Applying these standard engineering approaches to the unit step input discussed above results in the oculomotor responses depicted in Fig. 12. While the tracking performance for the step and ramp is not perfect, it benefits from the knowledge of future target trajectory. An estimator of the future target trajectory is, therefore, critical in this deterministic control system.

But the control system described above, which was intended to be realistic, falls short of this goal for two reasons. First, almost all behaviors of biological systems exhibit some degree of randomness. This inherent randomness is characteristic of visual perception, memory and motor control. Human and animal subjects are likely to respond differently in identical situations and are unable to maintain absolute calibration. The inherent variability, therefore, must be included in the consideration of the optimal control problem. The second shortcoming of the deterministic system described above is that it lacks any mechanism to learn, and therefore does not explain a fundamental aspect of predictive behavior. Both of these characteristics will be considered in the following sections. I will first examine how to incorporate randomness by considering the stochastic systems approach.

2.2.3. Stochastic systems

If the target motion, the eye position and the system dynamics all have random components (noise), and are not known precisely in advance, the approach to modeling must be based on stochastic systems analysis. In the following few paragraphs I will describe a framework for characterizing noisy signals and systems, and an approach to estimation and control.

In real life most signals are contaminated by noise. Such signals, called stochastic signals or random processes, can be represented by lists or collections of random variables, one for each instant of time. These random variables will be denoted by upper case letters, e.g. $X(t)$. So, a stochastic trajectory is an ordered collection of periodic samples from a continuous trajectory represented by a list of random variables $\{X(t)\}$ indexed by the time parameter t. The complete knowledge about the random process is given by the joint probability distribution function:

$$Pr\{X(1)=x_1, X(2)=x_2, \ldots, X(t)=x_t\} = P(x_1, x_2, \ldots, x_t),$$

where P is a function of t arguments (discrete time samples). Frequently, stochastic signals are characterized only by their low-order moments, e.g., means and autocorrelation functions.

An important aspect of the deterministic optimal controller, as described in the previous section, was the ability to predict the input signal (target trajectory) τ seconds into the future. The same is true in the stochastic situation, and consequently the ability to control the eye movement is, in part, limited by the ability to predict the future target movement. While it is not possible to know the future target position exactly, it is often possible to find good estimates, $\hat{X}_{t+\tau}$, which will minimize the average (expected) squared error between the predicted and actual target position $X(t+\tau)$:

$$e(t+\tau) = E\,\{[\hat{X}(t+\tau) - X(t+\tau)]^2\} \tag{12}$$

Assuming no other source of information but the past, the best estimator can be shown to be the conditional expected value of the $X(t+\tau)$, given all the points on the trajectory that have been seen by the observer up to the time t. That is

$$\hat{X}(t+\tau) = E\,\{X(t+\tau) \mid X(\xi), 0 \leq \xi \leq t\} \tag{13}$$

This estimate, which minimizes the expected quadratic difference between the predicted and observed positions, is 'best' in the sense that it is unbiased and of minimum variance.

The objective of minimizing the errors defined as the difference between the desired and the actual outputs is somewhat arbitrary, but very widely used. The notion of prediction as minimizing errors can be traced to Galileo Galilei (1632, references cited in Wilson, 1972) and, in particular, the minimization of squared errors to Gauss (1795) (see Wilson, 1972). The chief advantages of the expected squared error measure are its mathematical properties, which frequently allow analytic solutions to difficult problems. Consequently, many control-theoretic problems use objective functions that have been based on the minimization of the squared error.

The input signal is not the only random variable. The output and the system dynamics may have random components as well. In a stochastic oculomotor system, for example, random components of neural firing may introduce uncertainties even if the input is known exactly. An important effect of randomness is that, even if the input is known, the error between the desired and the actual position can be minimized only in a statistical sense.

If all the statistical information were available, the oculomotor system could, theoretically, compute the optimal controlling signal by evaluating the expected value of its output (conditional on all the observations). Such calculations are, from a control-engineering perspective, usually computationally intractable. Moreover, the effectiveness of the method relies on the assumption that the information at the time of the calculation will remain correct over long periods of time. For these reasons, control engineers often resort to using simplifying assumptions about the system, and to using adaptive control schemes.

A typical approach to simplification is based on the assumption of linearity. In particular, the foundation of stochastic prediction theory, proposed by Kolmogorov (1941) and Wiener (1942; see Wiener, 1949), was based on the idea of finding the linear filter that minimizes the mean squared error between the predicted and the observed data. The prediction is computed, in discrete form

$$\hat{X}(t+\tau) = \sum_{\zeta=0}^{t} w(t,\zeta)X(t-\zeta) \tag{14}$$

where w are real weights that may depend on time t and the time interval τ. Note that for fixed t and τ the weights w can be interpreted as the impulse response of a linear time-invariant filter with finite impulse response. In that respect, this predictor is similar to those used in the classical approach described in the previous section. The important difference is that the weights can continuously change, depending on the previous experience with similar trajectories and on the prior part of the current trajectory. The critical question is, how might the system compute the weights of the predictor?

The problem of finding the set of weights that minimizes the error led to the formulation of the well known Wiener-Hopf (matrix) equation relating the crosscorrelation between the predicted position and the observed trajectory to the autocorrelation of the trajectory. This equation was extensively investigated several decades ago (e.g. Kolmogorov, 1941; Wiener, 1949). If the statistical properties (e.g., the autocorrelation) of the target trajectory are known a priori (e.g., from previous experience with similar trajectories) then the parameters of the filter can be computed using standard Fourier transform methods or, in the discrete case, a matrix inversion. But in other cases the computation of weights is more complicated. This occurs when the information about the trajectory is derived from the observations of the trajectory up to the point when the prediction is to be made. Then the Wiener-Hopf equation has to be solved by more sophisticated methods, for example, the spectral factorization method (Wiener, 1949).

The weights of the simplified linear predictor described above are not readily determined, particularly when the statistical properties of the trajectory are estimated only from the data observed prior to the point at which the estimate is to be made, $(X(\zeta), \zeta \leq t)$. The problem is that the solutions of the Wiener-Hopf equation require accurate estimates of the appropriate correlation matrices. To use this approach as a basis of a model of the oculomotor system would require a model which specifies how the oculomotor system can accurately compute, store and recall these crosscorrelation matrices. This may be particularly difficult if the trajectory is generated by an unknown and changing system.

The same difficulties were encountered by control engineers confronted with dynamical systems whose characteristics were changing in time. Attempts to solve these problems resulted in the development of adaptive techniques that gradually extract information from prior observations and continuously upgrade the predictions. These *recursive* techniques, to be described in the next section, appear quite promising for modeling the oculomotor system, because such models could explicitly learn from observed trajectories and use that information to generate predictions and thereby control signals.

2.2.4. *Recursive prediction models*

In this section I will describe two recursive techniques used in prediction and stochastic control. The two techniques differ in the assumptions made about the stochastic process to be predicted. The first method, called Kalman-Bucy, or simply the Kalman filter, is based on the assumption that the signal to be predicted is generated by a linear system (Kalman and Bucy, 1961). The other approach, closer in form to the Kolmogorov-Wiener theory, employs a linear discrete filter whose impulse response is continuously adjusted. With the oculomotor system in mind, my main focus is on techniques with incremental and recursive learning. In these processes new information is acquired in small steps and at each stage it is 'added' to what is already known.

2.2.5. *Kalman filter*

In many real-life situations, the observer is familiar with the system that generates the target trajectory. For example, for the relative motion of objects generated by self-locomotion through the environment, or for the motion of an object moving under the action of simple forces, it is possible for an observer to have an accurate, internal model of the process that generates the trajectory. In this section I will discuss a model of a prediction mechanism which is optimal if the target generating mechanism is linear and known. The type of predictor that recursively updates its predictions by estimating the state of the moving target is known as a Kalman filter.

An important aspect of modern control theory is that the control signal is obtained from the complete knowledge of the state of the controlled system. The advantage of Kalman filtering is that it can estimate the state of the system from available partial information. For example, the state of an object in motion is specified by its position, velocity and acceleration. If only instantaneous position is available to an observer, the Kalman filter can be used to estimate the remaining state variables, and thereby supply information for the optimal control of eye movements.

A simple example illustrating an application of the Kalman filter is the tracking of the motion of an object in a viscous environment, such as a ship moving in water. Let us suppose that the motion of the ship is governed by linear physical laws subject to observation noise and random currents. Any instantaneous observed position of the ship alone is not sufficient to predict its future positions. For example, estimates of velocity are also required to completely describe the current state of the ship and generate good predictions. The main purpose of the Kalman filter is to provide good estimates of the current state.

The Kalman filter is based on two assumptions. (1) The system that generates the target trajectory is well approximated by a linear system and the parameters of the system are known. For example, the target trajectory may be specified by linear physical laws governing the motion of the object. (2) Both the observation noise and the noise in the system are white (uncorrelated). In the case of the ship, random errors in the observed position and in the instantaneous velocity are uncorrelated from one observation to the next. The same must be true of the random deviations in the forces acting on the ship.

Under these conditions the Kalman filter can generate predictions in a recursive manner. By recursive I mean a process in which the prediction at time $t+1$ is a refinement of previous predictions. In particular, a good predictor like a Kalman filter can be implemented by computing a linear combination of two quantities: the earlier predictions and the observed prior positions

$$\hat{x}(t+1) = \alpha(t)\hat{x}(t) + \beta(t)y(t) \tag{15}$$

where $\hat{x}(t)$ is the estimate of the state of the ship at time t and $y(t)$ is the observed position of the ship at time t. The coefficients α and β determine the relative contribution of the two quantities so as to minimize the error in prediction. Note that both quantities y and $\hat{x}$ are potentially contaminated by noise: the position $y(t)$ by observation noise, and the current estimate $\hat{x}$ by errors in prediction. If the variance of the observations is greater than that of the calculated predictions, α should be large and β should be small. In the reverse case, when the observation is reliable, then β should be large and α should be small. In general these coefficients are calculated at each instant of time from the parameters describing the linear system which generates the trajectory and from the statistics of the random variables. The recursive process is started by guessing the initial state of the moving object and then updated after each independent observation.

The Kalman filter technique has been successfully applied as a component of a model of the human operator (e.g. Gai and Curry, 1976a). Despite its virtues there are several disadvantages in using a Kalman filter as a model of oculomotor predictive ability. First the target trajectory to be tracked must be generated by a system that is either linear, or well approximated by a linear system. This should not pose much of a problem, because many nonlinear systems are well approximated by linear systems.

A more serious objection to developing models based on the Kalman filter is that the organism must somehow acquire the exact parameters of the linear system which generates the trajectory (g in the above example), and must also estimate the statistics of the random variables. There is a question of whether it is feasible to assume that the oculomotor system can identify, compute and remember the parameters of the trajectory-generating system. In any case, the added complexity of this computation performed by the observer may make evaluation of the model very difficult. Therefore, we consider an alternative approach.

2.2.6. *Linear adaptive prediction*

When the target trajectory is generated by an unknown linear or nonlinear system, Kalman filtering may not be appropriate. It is customary to use a somewhat simpler but more robust strategy. One particularly convenient strategy, called linear adaptive prediction, is based on a class of linear models, as in the Kolmogorov-Wiener theory, whose parameters are recursively adapted to asymptotically minimize the mean squared error (Widrow and Stearns, 1985).

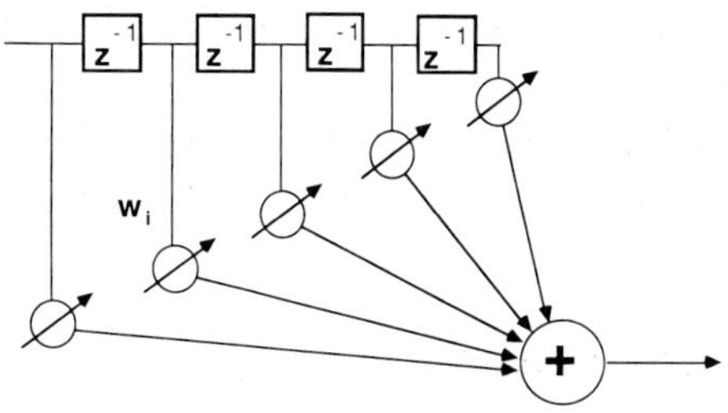

Fig. 13. Linear adaptive predictor computing predictions using a sum of weighted prior values. Unit delays are represented by z^{-1} and the variable weights by w_i.

Let's assume that the goal is to compute the best prediction of a target position $\hat{x}(t+\tau)$ using a linear combination of prior positions that minimizes the expected squared error,

$$E\{[(\hat{x}(t+\tau)-x(t+\tau)]^2\} \tag{16}$$

The form of the predictor is given by:

$$\hat{x}(t+\tau) = \sum_{k=0}^{n} w_k x(t-k) \tag{17}$$

where w_k are real numbers called weights. The predictor forms a moving average of prior samples of the target trajectory. If the random process describing the target trajectory is Gaussian then the linear predictor is, in fact, the optimal predictor. The relatively simple structure of the predictor, shown in Fig. 13, can be easily implemented and simulated on conventional computers. Similar structures have often been used as models of neurons in attempts to explain the computational ability of biological systems (McCulloch and Pitts, 1943; Rosenblatt 1961; Rumelhart and McClelland, 1986).

The problem is to compute the values of the weights. An exact computation of these weights solving the Wiener-Hopf equation is difficult, as I noted in section 2.2.3. (Stochastic systems), and not very useful if the statistical properties of system and signals vary in time. Fortunately, a number of algorithms have been proposed and used to predict signals whose statistical properties vary in time. The best-known application is the linear predictive coding (LPC) of speech signals (for a review see Makhoul, 1975). In a typical application for speech analysis (and synthesis) a new set of weights is computed for each frame (e.g., 20 ms of signal). The computation methods are based on algebraic operations on matrices which are sensitive to noise and require perfect memory and computational capabilities. Therefore, these methods are not attractive candidates for modeling prediction and anticipation in eye movements.

A method which is less sensitive to noise, errors and variations in time is the LMS algorithm originally proposed by Widrow and Hoff (1960). In their algorithm, which has been successfully applied to many adaptive-filtering and prediction problems, the weights are modified using a simple procedure. At each instant of time a prediction is generated which is then compared to the actual observed value. The error, defined as the difference between the predicted and observed values, is then used to modify the weights. In particular, the new weight at time t is computed by the following recursive relation:

$$w_k(t) = w_k(t-1) + \eta[x(t-\tau) - \hat{x}(t-\tau)]x(t-\tau) \quad (18)$$

The parameter η is a positive constant which governs the rate of convergence, and the difference $x(t-\tau)-\hat{x}(t-\tau)$ is the error in prediction during the previous instant in time. The multiplication by $x(t-\tau)$ has the effect of making the change in weight depend on the correlation of the error with the target trajectory. This algorithm can be shown to converge to the optimal linear moving average representation (Widrow and Stearns, 1985).

This type of model has been applied to the oculomotor system in the adaptation of the vestibulo-ocular reflex (VOR). For example, the original models of the cerebral function of Marr (1969) and Albus (1971) have been recently modified by Fujita (1982) to explain the VOR adaptation data of Gonshor and Melvill Jones (1976). Although there is a question about whether the VOR actually adapts in the way claimed by the authors (e.g., see Berthoz, 1985; Collewijn, 1989; Melvill Jones et al., 1988), the models can accommodate gradual adaptation. The applications of the adaptive models have been limited to account for changes in gain and phase lag observable over long periods (e.g., 30 days). Although the predictions of the models have not been explicitly tested, it is possible to find a set of parameter values so that the model of the adaptation process has a similar time course to that reported by Gonshor and Melvill Jones (1976). It should be noted that the particular realizations of these models were motivated by the assumptions about the likely physiological and anatomical constraints.

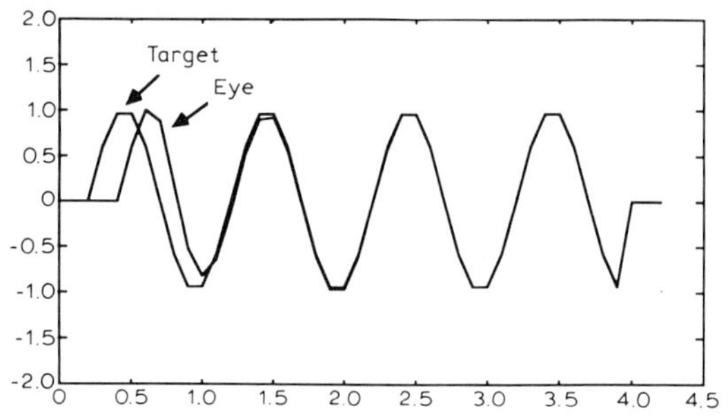

Fig. 14. The result of an LMS algorithm learning to predict and track a sinusoidally moving target. The linear adaptive filter consists of 10 delays and 10 variable weights. The trajectories are sampled every 200 ms. The learning is almost complete within one period of target motion.

The advantage of the LMS algorithm is its simplicity and robustness. The behavior of this model depends on the two aspects: (1) the parameter values (in particular the learning rate η in Equation 18 and the number of weights) and (2) the properties of the trajectory to be predicted. An example of the behavior of the LMS algorithm is illustrated in Fig. 14. In this example, the model is attempting to predict the movement of a target which is moving sinusoidally in one dimension. The graph in Fig. 14

demonstrates that a model of this type can learn to predict sinusoidal motion after being exposed to a few cycles of the target motion, and is consistent with the data in Fig. 7.

The second aspect that determines the behavior of the LMS algorithm is the type of the target motion. In particular, the model as presented here generates desirable prediction situations in which the target trajectory can be predicted by a linear combination of the previous samples (positions) of the trajectory. I will return to this approach based on linear adaptive filters in the last section of this chapter and consider extensions of this method to nonlinear systems. But for now I will close the basic description of the optimal control theory by discussing the predictability of trajectories. In particular, I am concerned with the question of how predictable are various so-called 'unpredictable' trajectories used in eye movement experiments.

2.2.7. Randomness of pseudo-random signals

Most of the 'predictable' target trajectories used in eye movement experiments are simple, periodic waveforms such as sine or square waveforms. Thus predictability is, for simplicity, associated with periodicity. A typical misconception resulting from this oversimplification is that aperiodic stimuli are not predictable. This is generally incorrect because (1) many pseudo-random trajectories are completely predictable, and (2) all physically realizable trajectories are predictable to some degree. I will discuss these two points in turn.

Experimenters frequently use pseudo-random target trajectories composed of a relatively small number of sinusoidal components. Such a pseudo-random trajectory is given by the sum

$$x(t) = \sum_{i=1}^{m} a_i \sin(\omega_i t + \Theta_i) \tag{19}$$

where the phase Θ_i, and sometimes the amplitude a_i, are random variables sampled for each trial from some distributions. The important question is, just how predictable or unpredictable are such trajectories? Unfortunately, predictability generally depends on the mechanism that represents the trajectory and computes the prediction. In the case of linear systems, signals are conveniently represented by a sum of sinusoidal components. The parameter of each component is determined by the Fourier transform. The Fourier analysis of a small portion of the trajectory, described by Equation 19, may provide good estimates of the parameters a_i and Θ_i. Therefore, after a short time, this type of signal is completely predictable. Similar analysis can be carried out assuming other forms of the predictor.

The intuition that trajectories with more sinusoidal components are less predictable is better interpreted in terms of complexity (cf. St.-Cyr and Fender, 1969b). That is, while additional components do not necessarily reduce predictability they increase the *complexity* of the trajectory. In some sense, one requires a more complex algorithm or larger number of samples to characterize the multicomponent waveforms. In accordance with the theoretical notions of complexity, in the sense of Kolmogorov-Chaitin (e.g., Chaitin, 1974), it is possible to define the complexity of a trajectory in a class of band-limited functions by the number of samples required to completely specify the signal. In this respect, the experiments purporting to study predictive capabilities are, in fact, discovering the ability of the oculomotor system to process signals differing in complexity.

The second point concerns the fact that even if the random component of the trajectory is derived from truly random white noise, so that any two distinct values are uncorrelated, a physically realizable target trajectory must usually obey a variety of physical laws. The effect of these physical laws can be represented by a band-pass filter. The result of the band-pass operation introduces correlation and consequently some predictability. In fact, the predictability of band-passed white noise is directly related to the impulse response of the filter.

In summary, this discussion shows that the predictability of the 'unpredictable' target trajectories is not an all-or-none phenomenon. Any empirical study of anticipatory behaviors must consider the potential predictability of all trajectories.

With this brief introduction to the theory of opti-

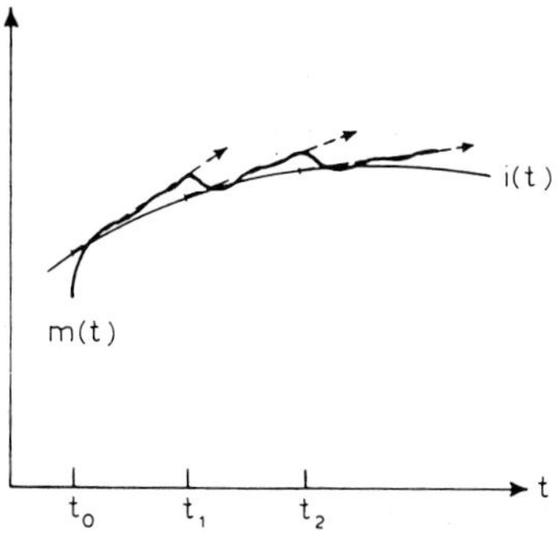

Fig. 15. Sequential tracking process using linear extrapolation. The controller follows a sequence of tangents to the system input $i(t)$, producing the system output $m(t)$. From Greene and Ward (1979).

mal control and signal prediction, I will now describe several applications of these approaches to behavioral data.

2.3. *Application of the optimal control theory to eye movements*

An adequate model of the predictive oculomotor behavior should take into account both the stochastic nature of the tracking task and the probabilistic knowledge that the organism has about its environment. In the previous section I have discussed several engineering approaches to building such models. These approaches consist of control systems which generate good control signals based on the extraction of statistical information from the inputs. The recursive methods which were discussed, the Kalman filter and the LMS algorithm, were accumulating information continuously about the correlations and crosscorrelations in the inputs and outputs. The information was used to adaptively generate better predictions and to improve tracking performance. It would appear possible to use these approaches to develop models of the oculomotor system, and in particular to describe its predictive behavior. Attempts to do this will be described below. Unfortunately, most of the attempts to use the optimal control theory to model the oculomotor behavior sidestepped the issue of information extraction and build models in which most of the

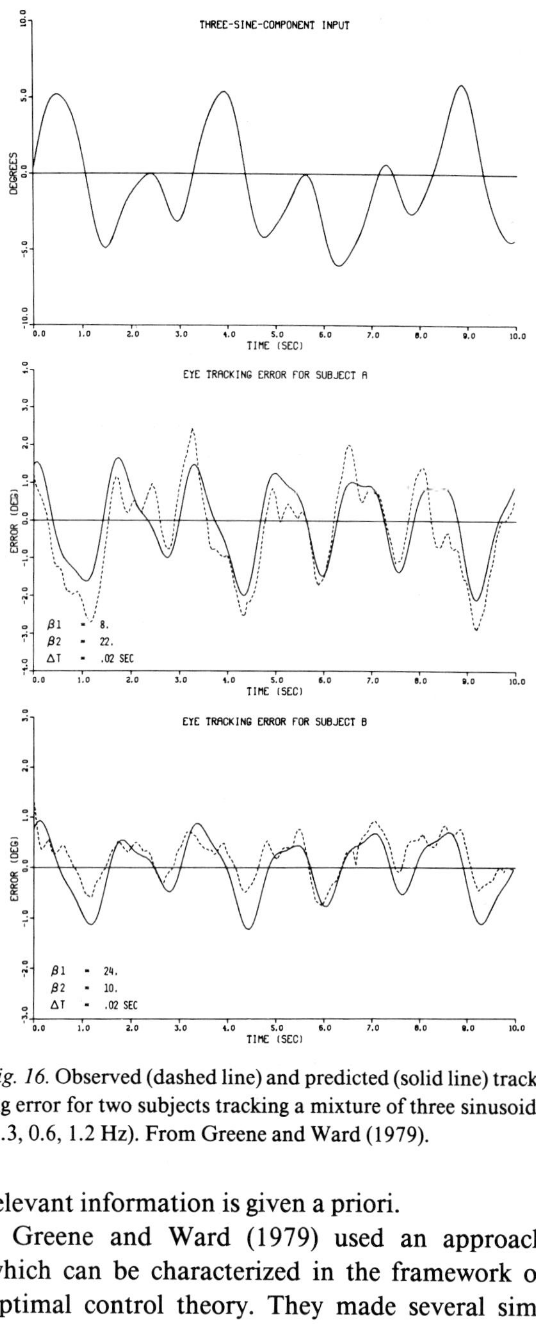

Fig. 16. Observed (dashed line) and predicted (solid line) tracking error for two subjects tracking a mixture of three sinusoids (0.3, 0.6, 1.2 Hz). From Greene and Ward (1979).

relevant information is given a priori.

Greene and Ward (1979) used an approach which can be characterized in the framework of optimal control theory. They made several simplifying assumptions. First, they assumed that the position error of the combined saccadic and smooth pursuit oculomotor system can be characterized by a second-order differential equation, similar to the model in Fig. 2 used in the previous examples. The input driving the second-order dif-

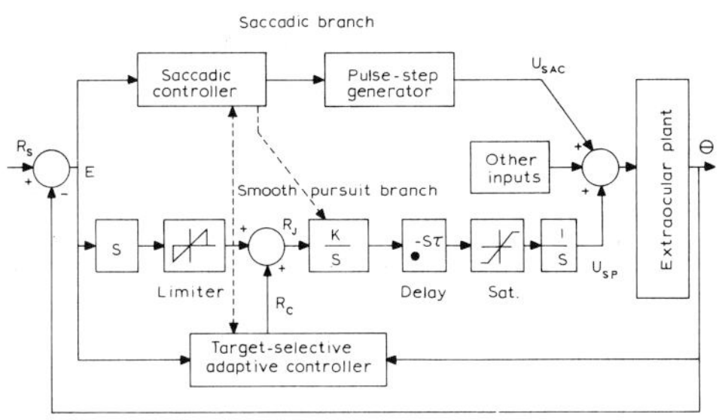

Fig. 17. Target Selective Adaptive Control Model. From Bahill and McDonald (1983).

ferential equation was the predicted target trajectory. Their second assumption, illustrated in Fig. 15, was to base the computation of predicted positions on a polynomial extrapolation of the target trajectory. In particular, the output of the predictor at time *t* was assumed to be a linear extrapolation of the target movement observed up to $t-\tau$:

$$v(t) = x(t-\tau) + \tau \frac{dx}{dt}(t-\tau) \tag{20}$$

Their third assumption was that the objective function consists of a linear combination of the sum of squared error, the squared first derivative and the squared second derivative. As a result of this objective function, their model, in addition to minimizing tracking error, also minimized the speed and maximized the smoothness of the resulting tracking trajectories. The minimization of functions such as speed and acceleration are typical constraints used by control engineers to represent constraints on available energy and torques. Greene and Ward (1979) then computed the parameters of their second-order predictor to minimize the objective function for particular target trajectories.

They compared their model to the eye movements of two observers tracking three single sinusoids and the combination of the three sinusoids. The fit was marginal in that the observers performed better than predicted by the model (See Fig. 16). While the applicability of this work is difficult to assess because of the limited types of stimulus that were tested, the model represented an interesting attempt to develop an adaptive approach modeling predictive oculomotor behavior. One particular contribution of interest is the inclusion of smoothness and acceleration components to the objective function.

In another attempt to characterize predictive eye movements, Bahill and McDonald (1983) compared the performance of observers to that of an adaptive control model. Their optimal control-theoretic model is based on a deterministic approach with complete knowledge of the fixed plant dynamics. The model consists of a plant (Westheimer, 1954), a typical smooth-pursuit branch (Young and Stark, 1963) and a simple saccadic branch that generated an accurate corrective saccade whenever the position error exceeded a fixed threshold (see Fig. 17). The predictive component was represented by a target-selective adaptive controller which could consist of either one of two different predictors. The first, and more successful, predictor was based on an idea, proposed previously by other investigators (e.g., Dodge et al., 1930), that various trajectories are stored in memory. When a target begins to move, the trajectory is recognized and the predictive signal is generated by recalling the exact trajectory from memory and modifying it to compensate for the system dynamics. While Bahill and McDonald did not adequately explain how the waveform is selected from three possibilities (sinusoids, parabolas or cubic), this model does track these specific target motions with minimal delays, as shown in Fig. 18. The second type of predictor they tested was a linear filter with three fixed weights. This predictor was less successful and appeared to generate more corrective saccades (see Fig. 18).

There are several problems with the model proposed by Bahill and McDonald. First, most of the predictive behavior was due to the memory subsystem, which was not described in much detail. A better description of the storage and retrieval would be necessary, because a critical issue in modeling predictive behavior with memory for trajectories is the process of retrieval of a specific memory of a target trajectory from a large number of possible trajectories. In some models of the memory sub-

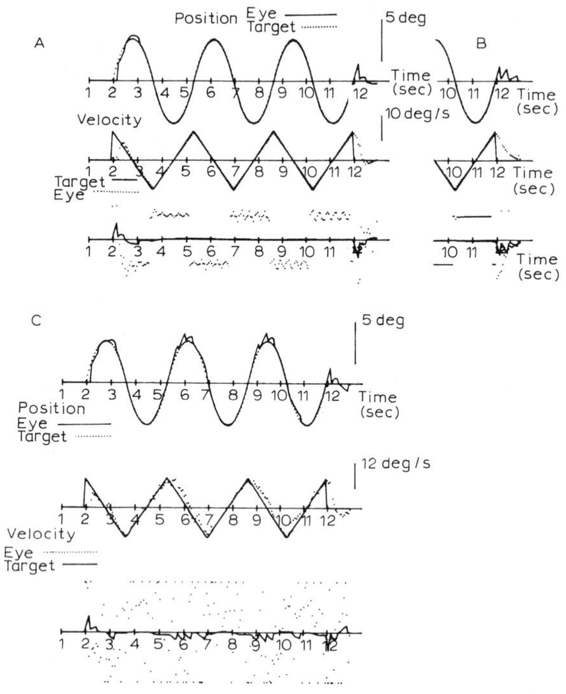

Fig. 18. (A) Target Selective Adaptive Control Model tracking parabolic motion. Gain (K, see Fig. 17) was 4. The top axis shows target (dotted line) and model (solid line) positions. The middle shows target (solid) and eye (dotted) velocities. The bottom shows position error (solid) and the signal R_j in Fig. 17. Time axis is labeled in seconds. (B) Termination of tracking after the gain had been reduced from 4 to 2. (C) The performance of the model with the difference equation predictor tracking parabolic target motion. From Bahill and McDonald (1983).

system the retrieval process might generate many false trajectories and therefore fail to account for human performance.

Another difficulty in assessing the model stems from the fact that the model generated a corrective saccade whenever the position error exceeded 0.5° or 0.3°. This is an arbitrary choice, given that human observers do not have to make saccades when they track (Puckett and Steinman, 1969). Moreover, saccades need not be systematically related to position error (Heywood and Churcher, 1981). To demonstrate the validity of the model would require a separate treatment of the saccadic and smooth pursuit components.

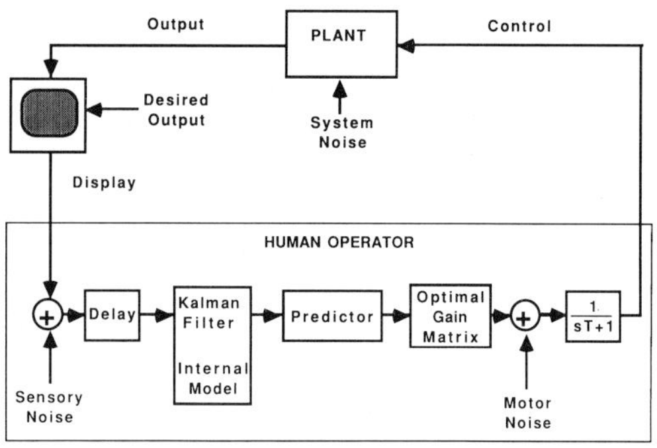

Fig. 19. An optimal control model of an operator. After Levison (1982).

2.4. Applications of the optimal control theory in other areas

The two models of the oculomotor system, described in the previous section, are based on deterministic control theoretic principles. There appears to have been little attempt to develop stochastic models of predictive eye movements. This is in contrast with theoretical and empirical research on manual tracking (McRuer, 1980; Kleinman et al., 1980). There have been several examples of stochastic prediction using a model based on the Kalman filter developed originally by Gai and Curry (1976a), which will be described in detail below.

Kalman filtering, described in section 2.2.5, is a linear prediction method which is used when the target trajectory is produced by a known linear system, but both the system behavior and the observations are contaminated by errors. This model has been successfully used to model the performance of human operators in a variety of monitoring tasks. Gai and Curry (1976a) used this model to describe human performance in detecting changes in the mean value of stimuli which are generated by a simple linear system. Curry and Govindaraj (1977) used the same model to characterize the performance of human pilots monitoring the behavior of automatic pilots during landing. This model was also used in describing how human operators detect changes in the characteristics of the linear system

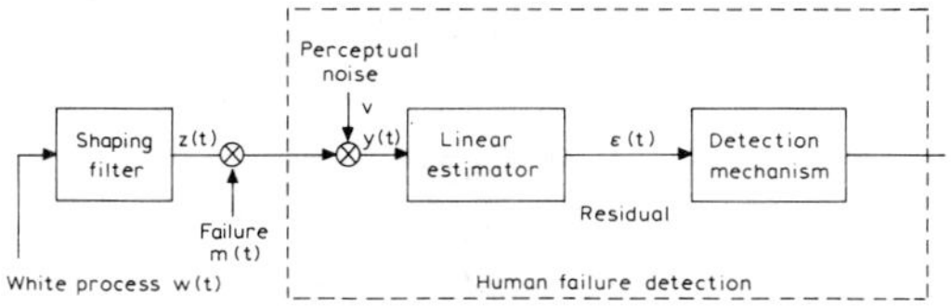

Fig. 20. Gai and Curry's (1976a) functional model of detection of 'failures'. The linear estimator is the Kalman filter. From Gai and Curry (1976a).

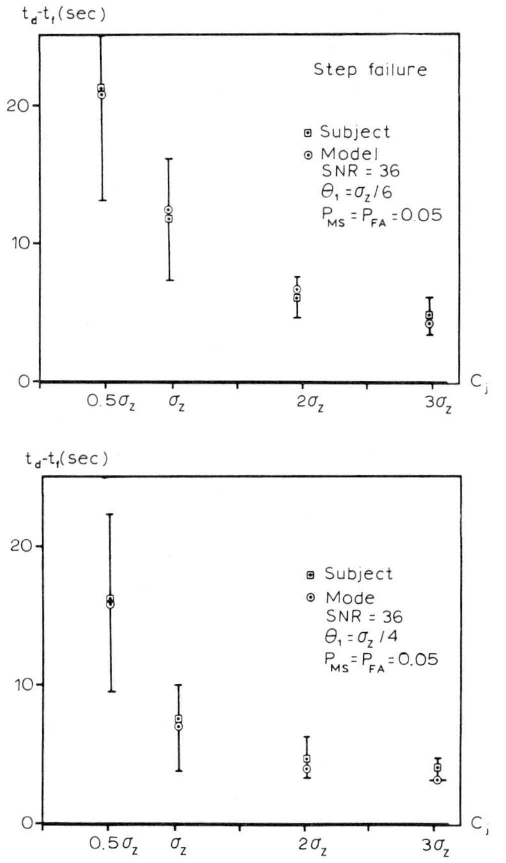

Fig. 21. A comparison between Gai and Curry's (1976a) model and the performance of two subjects, whose performance is shown in the top and bottom graphs, respectively. Detection time is a function of the standard deviation of the noise. After Gai and Curry (1976a).

that generated the stimuli (Curry and Govindaraj, 1977). A Kalman filter was also incorporated in a model of manual tracking by Kleinman et al. (1971). More recently, the Kalman filter was used as an essential component of a similar optimal control model studied by Levison (1982). In this model, shown in Fig. 19, the Kalman filter is used to model human operators' ability to estimate the state of the controlled system and use the resulting estimates to generate predictions.

Consider Gai and Curry's (1976a) approach in more detail. In their application of the Kalman filter, the subjects were asked to monitor the position of a randomly moving bar and to detect changes in its average position. These changes were described to the observers as 'failures'. The random motion was generated by a second-order, linear time-invariant system. Gai and Curry (1976a) examined the hypothesis that the observers were predicting the state of the observed process by a Kalman filter and using the difference between the predicted and the observed positions to decide whether a change had occurred (see Fig. 20). The average time required to detect the change in the average target position was taken as the measure of performance. The results from two subjects, as a function of the variance of the target motion, compared favorably with those of the model (see Fig. 21).

Although the success of Gai and Curry's (1976a) model indicated a potential for using the Kalman filter as a component of a model of human predictive behavior, there are at least three issues of concern in applying the model to eye movements. First, the mathematical complexity and the accuracy required for the proper operation of the model may be difficult to implement in some biological systems. Second, the oculomotor system would have to be able to acquire and maintain an accurate representation of the characteristics of the mechanism which generates the target trajectory, e.g., the physical laws governing the motion of the object to be tracked. So, there is a need for a description of a mechanism which would be able to identify, measure and store accurate information about the world. Finally, the Kalman filter technique is based on the assumption that the mechanism generating the trajectory is a linear system. This implies that the performance of the oculomotor system would deteriorate if the trajectory-generating system were nonlinear.

2.5. Limitations of the control theoretic approach

The control-theoretic approaches described so far appeared promising in a few restricted contexts. The classical control-theoretic models could account for some steady-state tracking phenomena, in particular, the improved tracking accuracy for continuous, periodic target trajectories. The modern control-theoretic approaches had the additional virtue of being able to learn to extrapolate target trajectories. However, there are at least three aspects of the predictive oculomotor system behavior which were not incorporated into these models:

(1) Learning. The models described so far did not explain how the oculomotor system learns to extrapolate trajectories. Instead, the models included assumptions about the appropriate system configuration and the values of the parameters for a given trajectory and task of the observer. These assumptions worked well in the examples I have described because each model was developed for a particular context and a specific experimental situation. The effect of context, e.g., the experimental task, was presupposed by the model builder, who fixed the structure of the model, decided which parameters could vary, and determined the values of these parameters. The underlying (and untested) assumption, needed to make the models more general, is that the observer would somehow have direct access to the contextual information and then correctly determine which aspects of the system to keep fixed and which to allow to change over time.

(2) Contextual information. Oculomotor prediction is not limited to trajectory extrapolation. For example, eye movements can be generated prior to the stimulus event (Dodge et al., 1930; Westheimer, 1954). The information used by the subjects to prepare such anticipatory responses is derived from the context of the experimental situation. A complete model of the predictive oculomotor behavior must include a way to make this type of knowledge available to the control model.

(3) High-level control. The oculomotor system is, to a large extent, under voluntary control. For example, a tennis player may choose to look quickly at his opponent rather than to continue to track the ball, or he may pursue the ball but introduce a deliberate lag in the anticipation of a change in direction. Thus, eye movements are, in part, determined by decisions to look at different points in visual space or decisions about how to pursue a moving target. In this respect eye movements resemble other voluntary movements, such as hand and finger movements. The control-theoretic approaches did not fully consider the contribution of the high-level decisions and control.

The role of learning, contextual information and high-level control give rise to important theoretical issues not considered by the mechanistic control-theoretic models. The question then is how to incorporate the three factors into the models of the oculomotor system. All three factors must be considered, because they all contribute to the subjects' performance. For ways to address this issue it is helpful to look at the results of research in visual, cognitive and motor processes, where similar questions about the role of prediction have been considered. In the next section I will describe some empirical and theoretical tools developed both to characterize anticipatory behaviors and to minimize their contribution to the measurement of visual and cognitive functions.

3. Models of decision-making and response generation

The goal of this section is to describe information-processing and decision-making models which might be able to characterize the effects of learning, contextual information and high-level control on eye movements. To the extent that such models can be borrowed from the study of visual and cognitive processes, they could then be integrated with control-theoretic models of the oculomotor system for a complete model of performance.

One reason that it is useful to turn to the study of visual and cognitive processes is that the role of learning, context and other high-level factors may be very similar in perceptual, cognitive and oculomotor research. In many cases, the only difference between the cognitive paradigms and those used in oculomotor research is the particular motor response mechanisms, i.e., a finger movement versus an eye movement. One might, therefore, expect that eye movements could be affected by anticipation in the same way as other motor responses. And, indeed, there is ample evidence that human responses in a variety of visual and cognitive tasks are affected by the tendency to anticipate future stimulus events. In the next section I will discuss how the expectation of a stimulus affects its detectability, and how manual response times are affected by a subject's preparedness. I will also discuss the customary approaches to modeling these anticipatory behaviors. A comprehensive model of the anticipatory behavior of the oculomotor system will have to include a consideration of decision-making mechanisms in the same way that other motor responses, such as reaching or pointing, need to include high-level decisions. The first step in modeling cognitive processes consists of task analysis, which tells a modeler what information is relevant to the task, and when this information is useful.

Task analysis Recall that to specify a problem in the control-theoretic framework one must carefully describe the inputs, the outputs, and the objective function. Similar information is required in order to characterize information-processing and decision-making models. This information can be obtained by performing a task analysis. In task analysis a complex behavior is broken into a set of small steps, or elementary operations, in the same way that a computer algorithm is divided into individual statements. By specifying the sequence of operations it is then possible to determine: (1) the information required to perform each operation, (2) the result of each operation, and (3) objective function, or the goal. This type of analysis then enables both the model builder and the experimentalist to characterize the availability and the quality of information as well as the capabilities of various components. This type of analysis can prevent omission of relevant contributing factors, facilitate the choice of appropriate theoretical assumptions, and help in the design of well-controlled experiments.

Example: Anticipation and the latency of saccades In the following example, unlike those considered in the previous section on control theory, the anticipatory effects are not derived by a simple extrapolation of a trajectory. Suppose that one would like to characterize the visual and motor processes required to generate the appropriate commands to execute a saccade. One possible observable measure is saccadic latency, i.e., the interval between the onset of a visual target and the onset of a saccade. The particular issue to be considered in this example is how saccadic latency varies depending on whether the fixation point is extinguished before or after the appearance of the saccadic target (Ross and Ross, 1980; Saslow, 1967). One could expect that the removal of the fixation point before presentation of the saccadic target would shorten the response latencies because it would cue the subject to expect the target to appear. Ross and Ross (1980) found that the average saccadic latency decreased with increasing warning interval, and that the offset of the fixation stimulus was a more effective warning than other sorts of signal, such as onset of a target, or the change in the shape of a warning stimulus. Their results show that the expectation about when a target is likely to appear affects the latency with which saccades are prepared and executed.

A straightforward interpretation of these results is difficult for two reasons that are apparent from an analysis of the task. The first concerns the possibility of anticipatory responses. To prevent anticipatory responses, Ross and Ross (1980) randomly varied the warning interval over trials. It is not obvious, however, that the observers were not able to make better predictions for longer warning intervals. The second difficulty arises from the possibility that an observer may be able to select a strategy to make shorter latency but less accurate saccades, in some conditions. To evaluate the impact of these concerns requires a model of the processes for generating responses which would incorporate the observers' experience, the effect of contexts, and the observers' objectives.

In the following sections I will briefly illustrate the theoretical and empirical approaches in three different areas of perceptual and cognitive processes directly relevant to oculomotor research: signal detectability, response times and probability learning. Each of these areas is related to a component of programming and execution of eye movements. The discussion of each of these areas will consist of three parts: (1) the empirical evidence for anticipation, (2) a theoretical approach to model anticipatory behaviors, and (3) the development of paradigms which may be less sensitive to the effects of expectation.

3.1. Signal detectability

Before the programming of an accurate saccadic eye movement, it is necessary to detect and localize the visual target. It is, therefore, likely that any anticipatory effects observed in target detection and localization will also affect the eye movements. This may be the case despite the fact that targets in eye movement research are usually well above their intensity detection thresholds.

I will illustrate the effect on the following example shown in Fig. 22. Suppose that the observer is asked to fixate, as quickly as possible, a peripheral target which can appear in one of two possible eccentric locations. The observer's task can be viewed as monitoring both locations and initiating his eye movement as soon as he detects a signal at one of the two locations. Although the target intensity is above detection threshold, the strength of the percept may increase over time, as shown in Fig. 22. In order to respond as quickly as possible, the observer must attempt to detect the target and its location when the percept is still relatively weak. In this manner, the process of detecting targets very quickly is similar to that of detecting signals near threshold. The question is how does prior knowledge or expectation affect such detection processes? To answer this question I will first consider empirical evidence from psychophysical research and then I will describe a theoretical framework called signal detection theory. The signal detection framework provides a way of distinguishing the effects of sensory processes from those which could be described as decision-making. In this respect, signal detection theory could serve as an example of how to integrate a mechanistic perceptual system with contextual information processing and high-level control.

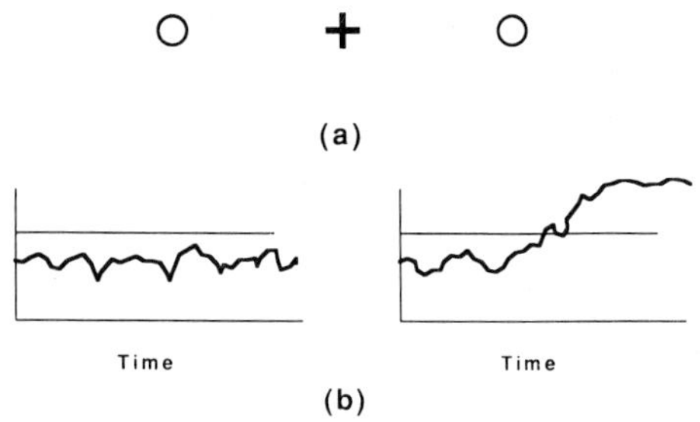

Fig. 22. Role of signal detectability in eye movements. The observer is to make an eye movement to one of two possible locations shown in (a), upon the appearance of a target in one of the locations. The cross represents the starting fixation position. The strength of the percept over time after the target onset is limited by the perceptual variability and the time constants (b). The decision regarding the onset and the presence of a target can be modeled by a threshold for detectability.

3.1.1. Empirical evidence: anticipation in signal detection

Anticipatory behavior in visual detection is apparent in experiments in which subjects are asked to report on each trial (by saying YES or NO) whether they saw a dim flash of light. In these YES/NO experiments, the experimenters presented a light stimulus of different intensity on each trial. The measure of performance is the probability of saying YES as a function of stimulus intensity. The threshold of visibility can be defined as the light intensity at which the probability of a YES response equals a fixed number, e.g. 50%.

The important empirical fact is that the measured thresholds depend on the prior probability of visible stimulus (e.g. Swets, 1961). Observers in such experiments appear to use the prior probability of stimulus to predict that a visible target may be present. For a given light intensity, the probability of a YES response is higher if the prior probability of a visible light was higher. The measured thresholds of even very careful observers are affected by anticipation. The presence of anticipatory effects can be readily demonstrated by completely omitting the stimulus on some trials and counting '*False Alarms*': YES responses given by subjects when no stimulus was present. As the probability of the stimulus presentation increases, so does the proportion of false alarms.

The probability of stimulus presentation is not likely to have a large effect on low-level sensory processes. Rather, the observed anticipatory effects are due to higher-level, albeit subconscious, decisions. If the goal is to determine the sensitivity of the perceptual system it is necessary to separate the effects of cognitive decision-making from those of sensory processes. The two effects can be separated using signal detection theory.

3.1.2. Signal detection theory

Signal detection theory, originally developed by engineers to characterize the performance of communication receivers, describes how the optimal decisions of a receiver should depend on the expectations specified by the prior probabilities of various signals. The theory was developed when radar engineers recognized that a given receiver can arbitrarily increase the proportion of a positive response by lowering its criterion for detection, but that this increase is accompanied by a commensurate increase in the number of false alarms. The important feature of the signal detection approach is the realization that even the responses of an optimal receiver, in the presence of noise, should depend on the prior probabilities in order to minimize the proportion of errors.

To formalize the signal detection theory, consider a detector that is designed to discriminate between two targets A and B whose prior probabilities are $Pr\{A\}$ and $Pr\{B\}$. In the signal detection theory the targets are represented by random variables X_A and X_B whose distributions $Pr\{X_A\}$ and $Pr\{X_B\}$, respectively, differ in their means, e.g. $E\{X_A\} > E\{X_B\}$. On each trial, the receiver must decide whether the signal $X=x$ came from the distribution of X_A or X_B. An optimal receiver minimizing the number of errors should respond A if

$$\frac{Pr\{X_A=x\}}{Pr\{X_B=x\}} > \frac{Pr\{B\}}{Pr\{A\}} \tag{21}$$

and B otherwise. The left-hand ratio of probabilities, or the *likelihood ratio*, is a function of the observed value x. The decision to respond A or B is made by comparing this likelihood ratio to the criterion specified by the right-hand ratio of the prior probabilities. Thus, the prior probabilities determine the decision criterion.The proportion of A responses is determined by proportion of trials in which X exceeds the criterion. The capability of discriminating A from B depends on the the separation of the distributions of X_A and X_B relative to the amount of variability. In particular, when the distributions of X_A or X_B are Gaussian, and equal in variance σ^2, then the measure of sensitivity d' is the distance between the means of the distributions normalized by the standard deviation:

$$d' = \frac{E\{X_A\} - E\{X_B\}}{\sigma} \tag{22}$$

This measure of sensitivity is independent of the criterion used by the observer.

To determine the sensitivity of a receiver, without making any assumptions about the distributions, requires the measurement of performance for many different criteria corresponding to different prior probabilities. The resulting plot of the probability of being correct as a function of false alarms, called receiver operating characteristic (ROC), represents the performance that is independent of prior probabilities. The area under this ROC curve can be used to represent the sensitivity of a receiver.

At this point we can make predictions about the behavior of the observer whose task was to look at a target which could appear in one of two possible locations (Fig. 22). His criterion at each potential location could be set in accordance with his subjective prior probability of a target at that location. If the experimenter emphasizes speed, the observer is going to make more mistakes, and generate faster but less accurate eye movements. The effects of the criterion can be assessed by manipulating the prior probability of each of the target locations.

3.1.3. Bias-free paradigms in signal detection

Signal detection theory facilitated the design of new paradigms which are potentially less sensitive to anticipatory effects. In one such paradigm, called two-alternative forced choice (2AFC), observers are presented with two stimulus alternatives and asked to choose one of them. The important aspect is that the two alternatives are statistically independent. For example, the observer may have to indicate which of two temporal intervals contained a dim light. If the target light is equally likely to be in either of the intervals, then the bias of an observer to choose one of the intervals has only a small effect on the estimate of the detection threshold. Note that the probability of selecting one or the other interval should not depend on the prior probability of stimulus presentation. Any bias with respect to the alternatives can be easily assessed by comparing the proportion of responses to each alternative. Another advantage of the 2AFC paradigm is that the observer is given a chance to view, on each trial, a stimulus without the target (one of the intervals on each trial). This paradigm, therefore, does not completely eliminate the biases due to prediction but has the potential of reducing its effects. Because of the continuous nature of the oculomotor response, using such paradigms may not always be possible in oculomotor experiments.

3.2. Response times

Response time, or the latency of a response, is commonly used to characterize various oculomotor processes. This is because it is assumed that the duration of response preparation is a good measure of the amount of processing necessary to make the response. That is, the latency of response is assumed to indicate the complexity of planning of responses such as finger movement or a saccade.

Response times always require theoretical assumptions in order to interpret experimental results. This is because the connection between the complexity of a process, or the difficulty of a task, and the duration of response preparation depends on the theoretical description of the process (e.g., serial stages, etc.). Thus, a theory of response times, whether explicit or implicit, always underlies the interpretation of response time data. In cognitive psychology there are many such theories, a well-developed methodology, and a large body of data (e.g., Sternberg, 1969; See Luce, 1986, for an extensive treatment of response times). These theories are directly applicable to anticipatory behavior, because some notion of prediction is usually an integral part of most of these theories. In the following three subsections I will describe the empirical evidence for the effects of prediction on response times, and provide a brief account of some models and experimental approaches to control the anticipatory effects.

Although the results of response-time measurements are more difficult to interpret than those of detection experiments, they are particularly relevant to eye movements because they involve the detection and recognition of signals, and the planning and execution of motor responses.

3.2.1. Anticipation in response times: empirical evidence

In a typical cognitive response-time experiment, subjects are asked to perform a task such as stimulus identification and to respond as quickly as possible and as accurately as possible. Using such paradigms, psychologists have studied human pattern-recognition processes, search and retrieval from memory, motor planning and attentional processes. Similar paradigms in oculomotor research might provide information regarding visual target acquisition, computation of target location and the planning of saccades.

Even the earliest researchers (e.g., Donders,

1868) noted that when subjects are instructed to be as fast as possible, they may generate anticipatory responses. They would respond either before the onset of the stimulus, or with very short latencies. These anticipatory responses are similar to the *False Alarms* observed in the detection paradigm. In fact, the faster responses are usually less likely to be correct. This phenomenon is called a speed–accuracy tradeoff. The speed–accuracy tradeoff is similar to the tradeoff between the proportion of hits and false alarms in the signal detection paradigm. Response latencies can also be affected by prior probabilities, instructions and feedback. The response latencies are also subject to sequential effects, that is, the response time on a given trial may depend on the immediately preceding trial or trials.

To the extent that subjects use predictive strategies, the distribution of the response times will be a combination of the anticipatory processes on one hand and the sensory, perceptual and motor processes on the other. Clearly, the anticipatory responses pose a problem to a researcher interested in sensory, perceptual and motor systems, who will therefore have to rely on theoretical models in order to distinguish these effects.

3.2.2. Models of response times

To distinguish the effects of anticipation from the underlying sensory, perceptual and motor processes requires a theoretical description for the anticipatory processes. A theory must account for both the response identity and its latency. One of the simplest methods to account for observers' behavior is based on finite-state models. I will illustrate the approach using one of the simplest examples of such models, called the fast-guess model (Ollman, 1966; Yellott, 1971).

Simple example: Fast-guess model In the fast-guess model the subjects' strategy is represented by two discrete states, A and G, shown in Fig. 23. In state A, the 'analytical' state, a subject is assumed to process and analyse the information presented in the stimulus. In state G, the 'guessing' state, the subject is assumed to respond randomly, without processing the stimulus. According to the model, both the response times and the response identities are random variables whose distributions depend on the state. Short, but inaccurate, responses are more likely in the state G, where the probability of a correct guess is given by p_G. In the analytical state A the probability of a correct response, p_A, is higher, but so are the latencies. Let the distribution of latencies conditional on the state S be given by $P\{T<t|S=G\}$ and the probability that the subject is in the guessing state be g. Then the proportion of correct responses is given by:

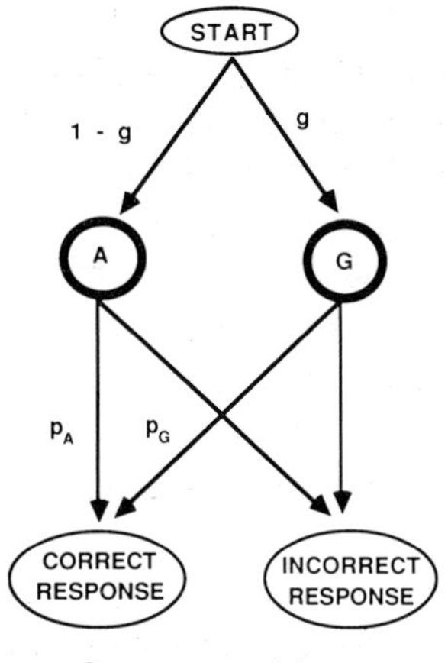

Fig. 23. A two-state fast-guess model.

$$P\{C\} = g\, p_G + (1 - g)p_A \tag{23}$$

and the distribution of latencies T is

$$P\{T<t\}=gP\{T<t \mid S=G\}+(1-g)P\{t<T \mid S=A\} \tag{24}$$

Experimental data are then used to estimate the parameters of the model. The parameter g is a measure of the proportion of anticipatory responses that may be initiated before the perception of the stimulus.

While this simple fast-guess model can account for some observed speed-accuracy data, it has some serious shortcomings. In particular, the model cannot represent responses based on partial (rather than all-or-none) information about the stimulus. This model can, however, be extended to include partially analysed stimuli by adding intermediate states. Another limitation of the fast-guess model described above is that it represents subjects only in their steady-state situation when the parameters do not vary over trials. It does not describe how predictive strategies are learned. (Ways to extend this model to deal with the issue of learning will be discussed in subsequent sections, beginning with 3.3.).

Other models There are many other models of response times based on different assumptions. A comprehensive review of the models and detailed analyses of their properties can be found in the book by Luce (1986). Many of these models are based on specific assumptions about the underlying processes. For example, one class of response-time models that relates the speed and accuracy of detection response is motivated by assumptions about the neurophysiological representation of information (Luce and Green, 1972). They assumed that the presence of a target is represented by an increasing firing rate and that an underlying process counts the number of neural spikes. A response is generated when this count exceeds a fixed criterion. This formulation is, therefore, a form of signal detection theory in that the observed anticipatory effects due to prediction can be treated by adjusting the criterion level.

A similar idea, in which the observer gradually accumulates information until he reaches a criterion, was described by Link and Heath (1975). They modeled the response-generation process as a random walk with two barriers. A point representing the instantaneous state of the observer is placed at a given position between two barriers. As the observer accumulates evidence this point moves towards the corresponding barrier. A response is triggered when the process reaches one of the barriers. Anticipatory behaviors are incorporated into the model by adjusting the starting position in accordance with the observer's expectations.

3.2.3. Response times: experimental control of anticipation

One way in which experimenters try to control anticipatory responses is to occasionally omit an expected stimulus or present an unexpected one. The trials on which an expected stimulus is omitted are called *catch* trials. Thus, in an experiment consisting of a series of trials with predictable stimuli and responses, the catch trials are those trials where the expectation is violated, for example, a stimulus is not presented at the expected time. If an observer responds on a catch trial, his response is interpreted as anticipatory, i.e. purely a result of prediction. The catch trials can be used to identify and, perhaps, discourage anticipatory behaviors. The proportion of anticipatory responses on the catch trials is often used to estimate the overall proportion of such responses. In the framework of the fast-guess model described above, catch trials can be used to estimate the probability g of being in the guessing state, and the response latency distribution associated with the guessing state.

3.2.4. Randomization of foreperiods

Another common attempt to control anticipatory responses is by randomizing the stimulus foreperiod. Recall that on each trial in a reaction-time experiment subjects receive a warning signal followed by the stimulus after a short delay (the foreperiod). The purpose of the foreperiod is to ensure a certain state of preparedness on the part of the subject. The problem with a foreperiod of constant duration is that the subject may learn to anticipate the stimulus. Therefore, experimenters randomize the durations of the foreperiods. But the fact that the foreperiod is a random variable does not mean that the target event cannot be predicted. In order to understand the effects of this randomization it is necessary to express the predictability of stimulus occurrence as a function of time. One way to do that is by using the hazard function to be defined below.

Consider a subject during the foreperiod awaiting the stimulus presentation, e.g., a step change in the target location. The predictability of this stimulus occurring can be expressed as the probability that the stimulus will be presented in the next instant of time, given that it has not yet occurred. The expression of the conditional probability as a function of the time is defined as the hazard function.

More formally, let $F(t) = Pr\{T<t\}$ be the probability distribution function of the time of occurrence of event A, e.g., a step change in target position and $f(t)$ its probability density function. The probability of the event occurring at time t, given that it did not occur prior to t, is given by the hazard function

$$H(t) = \lim_{\Delta t \to 0} \frac{Pr\{t<T\leq t+\Delta t \mid T\geq t\}}{\Delta t} = \frac{f(t)}{1-F(t)} \quad (25)$$

A uniform distribution is the one most commonly used in experiments to randomize the foreperiod. Unfortunately, the hazard function for the uniform distribution

$$H(t) = \frac{1}{1-t} \quad (26)$$

indicates that the predictability of stimulus occurrence is not at all uniform. This can be seen intuitively because if a stimulus has not occurred near the higher end of the interval of a uniform distribution it will almost surely occur in the next instant, as shown in Fig. 24.The results of an experiment with a uniformly distributed foreperiod will, therefore, result in a mixture of strategies. Trials with shorter foreperiods will include a smaller proportion of anticipatory responses than those with long foreperiods. The relevance of the hazard function to saccadic latency has been pointed out by Findlay (1981).

A more appropriate probability distribution function to use in order to render the hazard function constant is an exponential distribution. Thus if

$$F(t) = 1 - e^{-\alpha t} \quad (27)$$

then the hazard function is equal to $H(t) = \alpha$. As a result, the predictability of the stimuli will be uniform. The problem with the true exponential function is that it requires a small number of very long foreperiods. A truncated exponential distribution

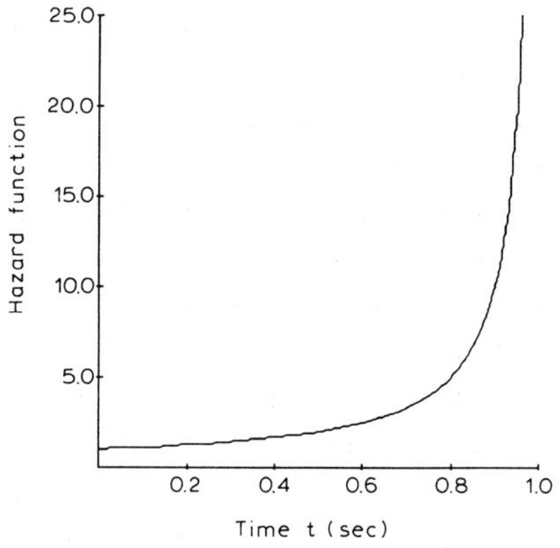

Fig. 24. The hazard function for uniformly distributed foreperiods over the interval 0–1 second.

with a small number of catch trials is sufficient for practical purposes.

3.3. Probability learning

As implied in the previous discussion of signal detection and response times, the prior probability of a stimulus event (e.g., a target presentation) can affect both the accuracy and the latency of eye movements. In the discussion of both of these topics I assumed that subjects somehow know the objective prior probability of stimulus. The theories associated with each paradigm then explained how subjects combine the prior probabilities with their percepts to generate responses. In this section I discuss how people make decisions that depend only on the prior probability and how to characterize subjective probability, which may change over trials, depending on a variety of contextual variables including the sequence of stimuli on prior trials. One important result of probability learning is that randomization of stimuli does not necessarily preclude anticipatory effects in human decision-making.

3.3.1. Probability learning: empirical evidence for anticipation

A great deal of evidence on predictive behavior has been gathered in experiments in which subjects were asked to predict a random event. In a typical probability learning experiment one of two stimuli are presented on each trial, for example, lights (e.g. LEFT or RIGHT). The sequence of stimuli was typically independent Bernoulli trials with fixed probabilities, $Pr\{RIGHT\} = p$. The subjects were asked to predict the identity of the next stimulus so as to maximize the number of correct predictions. Following each guess, they were shown the actual stimulus. The normative optimal strategy for maximizing the number of correct predictions is, of course, to select the stimulus with the highest probability every time. It was surprising to find that human subjects did not use the optimal strategy. Rather, the probability of their prediction matched that of the stimuli; i.e., the subjects were *probability matching*. For example, if the probability of the RIGHT light was $p = 0.75$, subjects predicted RIGHT light 75% of the time (Humphreys, 1939; Grant et al., 1951).

The discovery that subjects predicted the less probable stimulus on some trials poses a problem for the theories which are based on the assumption that people always behave as optimal decision-makers. One possible way to interpret this 'suboptimal' behavior within the framework of these theories is by assuming that, on some trials, subjects had higher subjective expectations for the less likely stimulus. The higher expectation can arise naturally owing to the well documented gambler's fallacy. According to the gambler's fallacy, the subjective probability of an event increases if that type of event has not occurred for some time. For example, consider a completely randomized sequence of two equally likely stimuli (e.g. LEFT, RIGHT). If, during the course of an experiment, the observer has seen four RIGHTs in a row he begins to expect and predict a LEFT stimulus on the following trial. Such behaviors may introduce complex sequential dependencies in responses that depend on subjects' expectations.

The degree of probability matching, as opposed to the optimal choice, was found to depend on a variety of experimental variables, including the instructions, the number of trials, the task and the payoff for correct predictions. Even when the sequences are completely unpredictable, subjects are likely to show sequential effects and probability matching. The data suggested that the subjects constructed complex hypotheses about sequential dependencies, and frequently had high expectations for specific stimuli on particular trials (Yellott, 1969). Similar results were obtained in various studies of the effects of expectations on smooth anticipatory eye movements (e.g. Kowler and Steinman, 1981). Therefore, completely randomized stimuli do not guarantee that the subjects will not make confident predictions on individual trials.

In the situations in which probability learning has been studied, subjects' decisions were based only on the prior probabilities, because the response on a given trial was required prior to stimulus presentation. But probability learning can also underlie prediction in situations requiring responses after the stimulus presentation, including those measuring the accuracy or the speed of detecting signals, because subjective probabilities affect the subjects' preparedness for one or another stimulus. The next section describes a theory which characterizes probability learning.

3.3.2. Models of probability learning

Efforts to model probability learning have a long history. Much of the work was based on stochastic learning theories developed in the 1950s and 1960s. The goal of the theorists was to develop models of the learning processes which would explain the fundamental principles of learning, and fit the data, including observed sequential dependencies, in the subjects' responses.

Most of the theories were based on variants of Markov processes. One such model, developed by Bush and Mosteller (1955), is called the *linear operator model* and describes the probability p_{n+1} of response RIGHT on trial n+1 by

$$p_{n+1} = \alpha p_n + (1 - \alpha)\lambda(s_n) \tag{28}$$

where α is a constant controlling the rate of learning, s_n is the actual stimulus on trial n, and λ represents *reinforcement* such that $\lambda = 1$ if $s_n = RIGHT$ and zero otherwise. If the stimulus *RIGHT* is presented on each trial with a constant probability π then, in the limit as $n \to \infty$, this model predicts probability matching in that $\lim_{n\to\infty} p_n = \pi$. A linear model that depends on only the preceding trial can be easily generalized to models in which p_n may depend on less recent trials. While models of the linear operator type are adequate in characterizing the average behavior, they are less effective in predicting the trial-to-trial sequential effects for individual subjects and the inter-subject variability (e.g. Yellott, 1969). Many other models were developed in order to characterize the various details and the reader can refer to many extensive reviews, e.g. Myers (1970).

A class of models with somewhat different sequential characteristics consists of finite state Markov models with a small number of discrete states. I will illustrate this approach using a simple two-state Markov model, proposed by Bower (1961) to characterize learning experiments. The 'hidden Markov process' model I will describe was proposed by Falmagne et al. (1975) to characterize sequential dependencies in manual reaction-time experiments. This model, which is very similar to the fast-guess model described above, is illustrated in Fig. 25. In their experiment subjects were asked to push one of two buttons to indicate the orientation (LEFT or RIGHT) of a visual stimulus. Before each trial a subject is assumed to be in one of these two states, *LEFT* or *RIGHT*. The probability of the subject remaining in a given state, or switching to the other state, depends on the stimulus actually presented on the trial. If, after a trial, the subject switches his state to that corresponding to the stimulus just seen, then this model will predict probability matching. Negative recency (the gambler's fallacy) obtains if the subject switches to the opposite state from the current stimulus.

The two-state Markov model for manual reaction time (Falmagne et al., 1975) described above was applied to anticipatory smooth eye movements (drifts in the direction of expected target displacement) by Kowler et al. (1984). In their experiment,

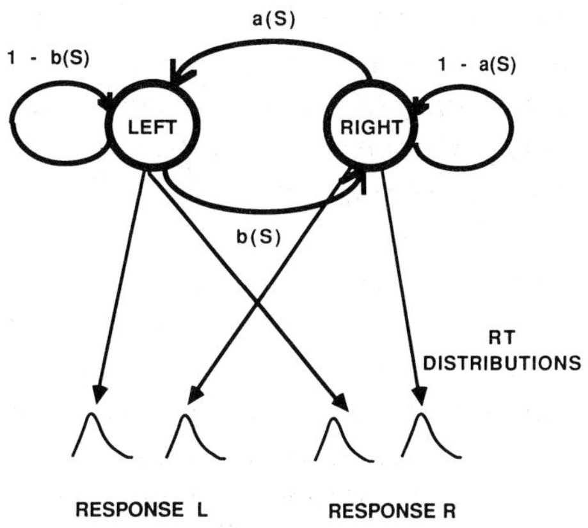

Fig. 25. The two-state Markov model of Falmagne et al. (1975) for manual reaction time. The state transition probabilities, *a* and *b*, depend on the stimulus *S*. The distribution of reaction times depends on the stimulus and the state.

observers viewed a target which would step from a central location either to the left or to the right. The probability of a rightward step was set to 0.65 or 0.35, and was constant over experimental sessions. They found sequential effects analogous to those found in the reaction-time experiments (Falmagne et al., 1975). Specifically, the velocity of the smooth anticipatory eye movement was higher to the right when the previous trials were rightward steps. The latency of rightward saccades was also shorter when the previous target steps were in the same direction as the step on the current trial. More recently, sequential effects were found for anticipatory smooth eye movements before expected ramp motions (Kowler, 1989).

The model of Falmagne et al. (1975) was used to account for the velocity of smooth eye movements prior to each expected step. According to this model, observers were assumed to be in one of two possible states before the presentation of the stimulus. The state (Right or Left) determined the observer's expected direction. Each state was associated with a different eye velocity distribution. The eye velocity distributions for the Right and Left states were biased towards the rightward or leftward motions, respectively. The transition between states was governed by a Markov process illustrated in Fig. 26. The Markov process was used to capture

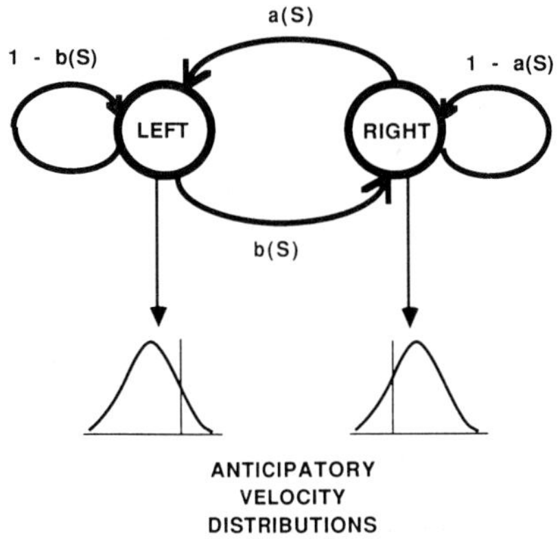

Fig. 26. A two-state Markov model of the effects of stimulus probability and prior stimulus sequences on anticipatory smooth eye movements. After Kowler et al. (1984).

the effects of the stimulus probability and the observed sequential effects. The model accounted well for the first-order sequential effects, although the authors noted that there were secondary sequential effects in those data which would require a more complex representation (e.g., more than two states).

To the extent that this model is successful, subjects' behavior can be characterized in terms of transitions between two states. Each transition, to switch or to remain in the same state, can be thought of as a 'decision', even if it is not made on a conscious cognitive level. The probability of switching states or remaining in the same state can be viewed as a result of a comparison of an internal random variable to a criterion. For example, if this internal variable exceeds a criterion, on a given trial, then the next state will be the *LEFT* state. The results of such decision processes are implicitly summarized by the state-transition probabilities. The model then provides an explicit probabilistic mechanism to represent the 'decision', or state transition, and its dependency on the previous state and stimulus. More recently, this type of hidden Markov model has been used to characterize more complex sequences, such as speech.

I included this model to illustrate how a finite-state model of human 'decisions' may be used to characterize eye movements. The model, however, does not specify how the state of preparedness is converted into the smooth eye movements. Consider, for example, the eye movements of an observer tracking an object whose velocity changes at predictable intervals. How would the anticipatory smooth eye movements made just before an expected change in target velocity combine with the smooth eye responses to the current ongoing target motion? Would the smooth eye movements resulting from anticipation be simply added to the smooth pursuit or would they modify the parameters governing the smooth pursuit? (See Kowler et al., 1984, for additional discussion of this problem.)

To combine two influences on smooth pursuit – anticipatory influences and sensory-motor influences – requires a combination of two large, apparently separate, classes of models. The first class of models, perhaps based on the control-theoretic concepts, may be able to characterize the ability to carry out continuous, low-level processes, such as the coding of velocity or the local extrapolation of trajectories. The second class of models, perhaps based on decision-theoretic concepts, characterizes discrete, inherently nonlinear aspects of prediction and anticipation. In order to describe eye movements in a variety of different contexts, including many simple laboratory experiments, the two classes of models should be combined. In the final part of this chapter I outline a framework which might be able to incorporate and integrate the low-level (control-theoretic) and higher-level (decision-making) approaches. This proposed framework is based on recent advances in adaptive pattern-recognition research.

4. Pattern-recognition approach

Both the control-theoretic and decision-theoretic models of prediction presented so far can be viewed as pattern recognizers. While there are many ways and frameworks for implementing various pattern-recognition schemes, I will describe an approach based on the language of adaptive networks. The motivation for this choice is that the language involving adaptive networks appears to be sufficiently powerful to implement both control-theoretic and decision-making models.

4.1. Prediction as pattern recognition

The generation of predictive eye movements has been, at least implicitly, viewed as requiring recognition of contexts, trajectories and mechanisms that generate target motion. For example, a reduction in the lag between the eye and the target during the pursuit of a sinusoidal target movement might be described as recognizing the frequency, phase and amplitude of the sine wave and then generating the appropriate tracking response. Similarly, predicting a future change in position might consist of recognizing a previous subsequence of movements and computing the subjective probability of the change in position. Thus, predictive mechanisms can be described as using the recognition of familiar aspects of a situation to generate an appropriate response. There are many situations in which the virtues of this description are quite obvious. Prediction of the motion of a small object seen in the sky will be different if the moving image is recognized as a fly rather than a Boeing 747. A small nearby fly would be expected to change its speed and direction much more rapidly than a large distant airplane.

Incorporating different types of predictive behavior into an oculomotor model requires the predictor to perform a general form of pattern recognition. In the following section I describe a specific class of adaptive pattern-recognition methods that appear particularly suitable for eye movements. If prediction is interpreted as a form of pattern recognition, one can expect to benefit from the vast amount of research in the field of pattern recognition. A detailed discussion of pattern-recognition concepts is beyond the scope of this chapter. See Duda and Hart (1973) for general background. In this section I will focus on an approach to pattern recognition that is related to the models of prediction discussed in the previous sections. In particular, a class of pattern recognizers implemented as adaptive networks can be seen as generalizing the linear prediction methods discussed in section 2.2.6.

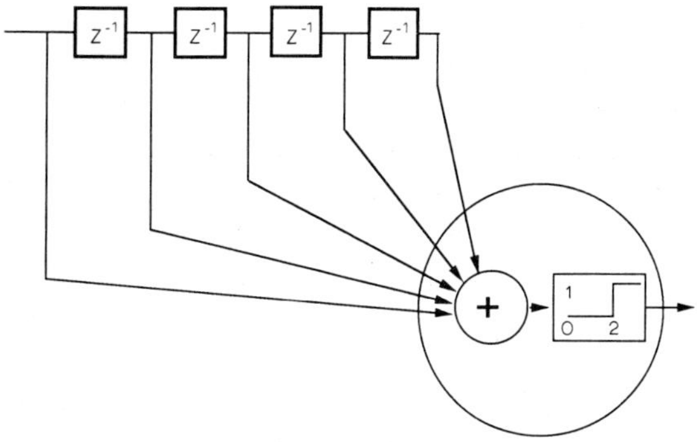

Fig. 27. A graphical representation of a linear threshold unit with 5 delayed inputs and a threshold equal to 2.0.

4.2. Adaptive networks for prediction

Consider the linear predictor shown in Fig. 13, where the prediction was computed by a linear combination of the previous points on the trajectory. Such a predictor is completely specified by the weights $\{w_i\}$, whose computation I discussed in section 2.2.6. In fact, the weights of this linear predictor can be computed recursively, and therefore the filter can be used as an adaptive system. This predictor has been extensively investigated by Widrow and his colleagues (Widrow and Stearns, 1985) and successively used in many signal-processing applications and models (Marr, 1969; Albus, 1971; Ito, 1985). An important feature of this structure for modeling the oculomotor system is that it can be used to perform categorization, and thereby to model decision-making processes. For example, if the output of the linear filter is transformed by a threshold function, as shown in Fig. 27, then the resulting mechanism can be used to assign target trajectories into one of two categories. In this example, the output of the thresholding device is '1' if the output of the linear predictor is greater than the threshold 2.0 and zero otherwise.

This mechanism, called a linear threshold unit (LTU), capable of classifying trajectories into two categories ('0' and '1'), is the basic building block of many pattern-recognition schemes and has been extensively studied (e.g., Nilsson, 1965; Rosenblatt, 1961; Minsky and Papert, 1969). Because of its popularity in different fields, this mechanism has many labels associated with it, including linear discriminator, perceptron, adaline (for adaptive linear element), threshold logic unit, and others. Many contemporary researchers consider the apparent similarity of the LTU to biological neurons as critical in modeling biological systems (e.g., Cooper, 1984; Rumelhart and McClelland, 1986) and refer to these models as artificial neuron and neural networks.

Since its introduction much research has been devoted to studying the capabilities and limitations of the linear threshold unit (e.g., Cover, 1965; Minsky and Papert, 1969). One particularly useful result for modeling eye movements is the availability of several algorithms, for example the LMS algorithm described earlier, for the adaptive adjustment of the parameters (weights) to perform the desired decisions (see section 2.2.6).

One limitation of the LTU is that it can discriminate only between those trajectories that can be recognized by a linear combination of variables such as the prior values (i.e. points, on a trajectory). These kinds of patterns are called linearly separable. This distinction between classes of patterns which can be discriminated by a single linear function and those which cannot is an important distinction made in the field of pattern recognition (Duda and Hart, 1973; Minsky and Papert, 1969). This is because constructing pattern recognizers for linearly separable problems is, as I noted above, a relatively simple computational problem. While some trajectories are predictable using linear predictors, there are those whose extrapolation cannot be accomplished by a linear threshold unit. Consider, for example the four trajectories in Fig. 28. The two trajectories with a horizontal initial portion at the bottom of the figure require a different prediction from the two oblique ones at the top. To generate predictions for each of these trajectories may require a nonlinear pattern-recognition mechanism.

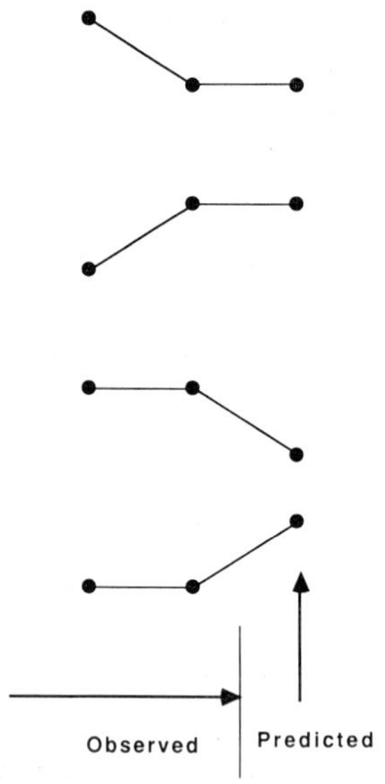

Fig. 28. A set of four target trajectories whose continuation is not predictable by a linear threshold unit. A multilayer network is needed to generate accurate predictions.

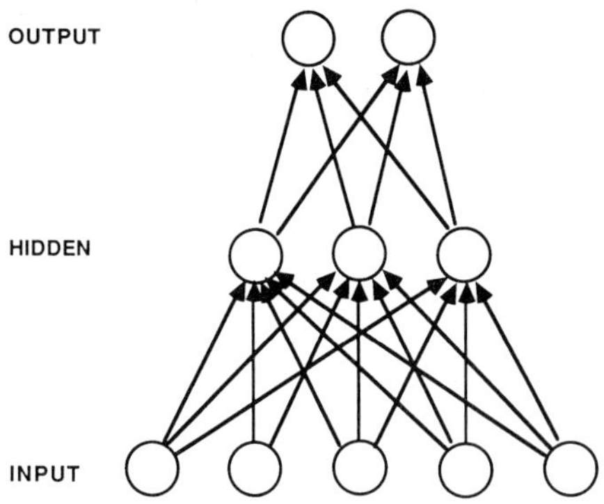

Fig. 29. An example of a two-layer network with 5 input units, 3 hidden units and 2 output units. Each unit is a memory-less nonlinear transformation of the sum of its inputs. Each connection is associated with a real-valued weight.

A useful generalization of the linear filters and the linear threshold units approach to problems that are not linearly separable is based on the notion of multilayer adaptive networks. The basic idea is to interconnect the linear threshold units into a network where the output of one LTU may be an input to another. An example of such a network is shown in Fig. 29.

A feed-forward adaptive network is an acyclic, directed graph with defined starting (input) and terminating (output) nodes (units). Hidden units are those which are labeled neither input nor output. Each directed arc is labeled by a real valued weight. A unit may, in general, be a dynamical system but in the simplest adaptive network a unit is defined by a memory-less, nonlinear function of the sum of incoming arcs. The value contributed by each arc is equal to the value of the originating unit multiplied by the weight of the arc. The activation of each unit is then the value of the nonlinear response function, as shown in Fig. 29.

This network structure is a generalization of the linear prediction considered in section 2.2.6. It differs from the linear prediction model in two respects. First, the activation of the units is a nonlinear function of their inputs. The second difference concerns the number of parameters. The number of parameters in a linear predictor (i.e., the number of weights), with a given number of inputs and outputs, is a product of the number of inputs (i.e., input dimension) and outputs (output dimension). In contrast, for given input and output dimensions, in a multilayer network there may be many more parameters, because there is no theoretical limit to the number of hidden units and therefore the number of connections. Each connection may represent a free parameter because each connection is associated with a weight.

The advantage of such networks is that they can perform more complex computations than the linear threshold units. For example, a two-layer adaptive network consisting of an input, hidden and output layers with an unlimited number of hidden units can represent any computable boolean function (Nilsson, 1965; Minsky and Papert, 1969). Moreover, a network consisting of three layers of interconnected LTUs can perform practically any computation (Kolmogorov, 1957).

As in the case of the linear prediction, a network requires finding an appropriate set of weights to perform a particular prediction task. In the case of a single LTU, the weights can be computed recursively using the Widrow-Hoff LMS rule, which minimizes the average squared error (see section 2.2.6). In contrast with the single LTU, or a linear predictor, the process of determining the value of all the weights (adaptation) in a multilayer network is more difficult. This is because the dependency of the output error on the weights connected to the hidden units is more difficult to estimate.

The recent revival of interest in the adaptive network technology is, in part, due to the development of a simple adaptation technique for computing the weights for the hidden units. The technique is based on the ability to compute the partial derivative of the output error with respect to any weight in the network. These derivatives can be computed if the response function of each unit is differentiable. Then, the weights of a multilayer network can be determined recursively by a generalization of the Widrow-Hoff rule used in the linear case. This class of methods, called *backpropagation*, approximates minimization of expected square errors by gradient descent (LeCun, 1985; Werbos, 1974; Parker, 1985; Rumelhart et al., 1986).

The main attraction of the adaptive networks is that a single structure can be used to model both linear and highly nonlinear systems. Unfortunately, a modeling approach based on adaptive networks has several shortcomings. The biggest current disadvantage of the adaptive networks is a lack of theoretical understanding. Consequently, the implications of various modeling decisions can be evaluated only by computer simulations. Another closely related difficulty is that the current adaptive procedures, such as backpropagation, may find solutions (weight values) that are local rather than global minima. The implications of the possibility of many locally optimal solutions must be carefully evaluated for each specific case. These shortcomings can sometimes be avoided by introducing additional constraints to the adaptive networks.

In the following two sections I will demonstrate that an adaptive network can incorporate both the mechanistic trajectory extrapolation and the decision-theoretic type of model. Although many aspects of the behavior of the networks are not well understood, I will illustrate the potential of the feed-forward adaptive networks to model some predictive phenomena by circumscribing the difficulties discussed above.

4.2.1. Continuous nonlinear control

The application of network-type architectures to the nonlinear estimation problem is not new. For example, Gabor et al. (1960) used an electro-mechanical analog of a two-layer network with nonlinear units for nonlinear estimation. Since the layered network model is frequently a generalization of the linear predictor it is not surprising that it can perform at least as well. It should also be able to make predictions for sequences that are not predictable by linear systems. To demonstrate this ability Lapedes and Farber (1987) used a layered network pattern-recognition model to successfully predict the trajectories of highly nonlinear chaotic systems. Lapedes and Farber compared different predictive methods on sequences generated by various nonlinear difference equations. An example of such a sequence is the classic logistic difference equation to compute the evolution of x in time, $x(t+1) = 4bx(t)[1 - x(t)]$, where b is a constant. Lapedes and Farber used multilayer networks with units whose nonlinear function had the form of a logistic function. They found that the predictive performance of a multilayer network exceeded several popular conventional techniques. It appears, therefore, that multilayer networks are potentially good candidates for nonlinear prediction and control.

Since in many predictive applications the predictor must be able to generate signals (e.g., recall a remembered trajectory), I will describe an approach to generating sequences using feed-forward networks. To produce sequences, the adaptive network must have a memory of its previous states and/or outputs. The idea of using the prior output as a part of the current input has been proposed by Jordan (1986) and is shown in Fig. 30. The structure of this network is similar to the structures of conventional digital sequential machines. The current state of the network is stored (delayed) and used as the input to compute the next state. The properties of the sequences are controlled by additional, external inputs to the 'plan' units. Jordan's network was designed to generate sequences to model and implement speech production. Since then, many other investigators have used this type of recurrent network to recognize and produce many different sequences (e.g., music). This type of network can be used to model anticipation in eye movement behavior.

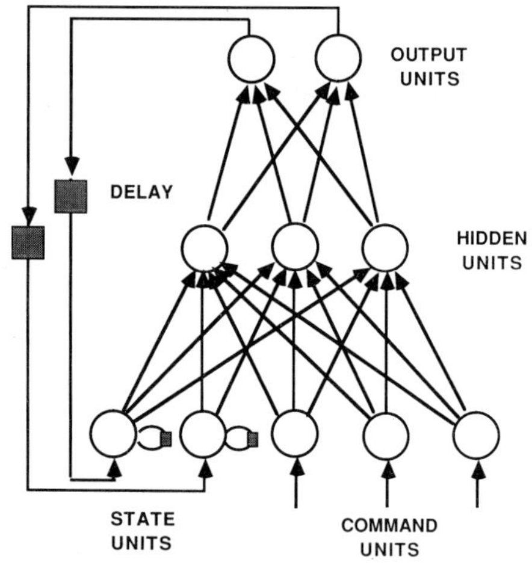

Fig. 30. A network capable of generating sequences. After Jordan (1986).

4.2.2. Application: anticipatory smooth eye movements

I will illustrate, using an example of anticipatory smooth eye movements, how a very simple, nonlinear, network can model behavior that has previously been modeled by a discrete Markov process (Falmagne, 1975; Kowler et al., 1984). This model, described in section 3.3.2, was used to represent anticipatory smooth movements generated by the subjects' expectation of target motion to the right or left. As I noted earlier, although the data were well characterized by the a two-state Markov process, there were no provisions for learning of the parameters (transition probabilities) from prior experience and the model was not explicitly integrated with the low-level aspects of the oculomotor system. In this section I illustrate how one might try to address both of these problems by using adaptive networks.

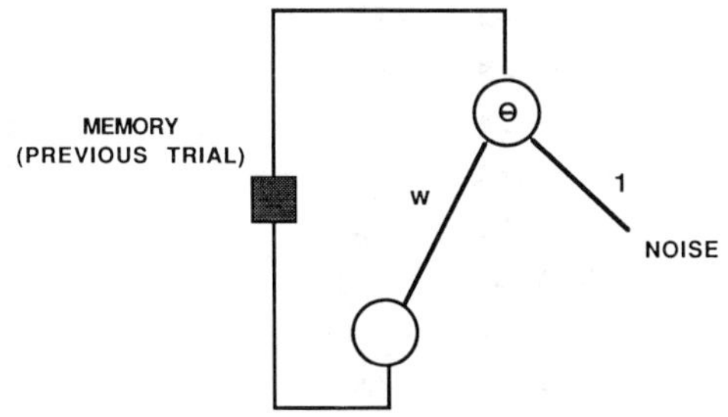

Fig. 31. A network implementation of a two-state Markov model with state-transition probabilities independent of stimulus presentation.

I will first discuss a simplified version of the model in which the state-transition probabilities are independent of the stimulus on current trial. In that case, the model can be implemented using a single-unit network model, shown in Fig. 31. The output of the unit represents the result of the subject's prediction of the direction of the stimulus motion for the next trial (*RIGHT* = +1 and *LEFT* = −1) and could provide an input for oculomotor control. The architecture of this model is similar to that proposed by Jordan (1986) (Fig. 30) for sequential problems. There are two inputs to the unit. The first input is the memory of the previous state ±1 multiplied by a weight w. The second input is a random variable ζ (noise, in Fig. 31) which represents the stochastic nature of this model necessary to model the stochastic behavior of humans.

The output of the unit $X(t)$ is computed, in this case by a threshold response function of the sum of the inputs. If the sum of the inputs is greater than a fixed threshold θ, the output is positive (+1), corresponding to a subject's expectation of a target motion to the right. Otherwise the output is negative (−1), corresponding to the leftward expectation. In this manner the network represents a model of a simple decision process to remain in the current state or to switch to the other state. The threshold θ and the weight w, together with the distribution of ζ, determine the transition probabilities. In the following analysis I demonstrate that this single-unit network can implement the simplified model. That is, there exists a set of parameter values, w and θ, such that the transition probabilities will be equivalent to the corresponding Markov process. I will then extend this simple model to the Markov model (Falmagne et al., 1975) used by Kowler et al. (1984).

If θ and w are selected so that

$$Pr\{\zeta - w < \theta\} = p_{LL} \tag{29}$$

and

$$Pr\{\zeta + w < \theta\} = p_{LR} \tag{30}$$

then this model is equivalent to a Markov process with transition probabilities specified by $p_{RL} = 1 - p_{LL}$ and $p_{LR} = 1 - p_{RR}$ where p_{ij} is the probability of a transition from state j to state i,

$$p_{ij} = Pr\{X(t+1) = i \mid X(t) = j\}$$

In this case, there is a unique solution because there are two variables and two linearly independent equations. The values of the parameters can be determined uniquely by specifying the distribution of the random variable ζ. For example, if ζ is normally distributed, with zero mean and unit standard deviation σ, then the values of the parameters are given by $\theta = (z_{LL} + z_{LR})/2$ and $w = (z_{LL} - z_{LR})/2$, where the variables z_{ij} represent the inverse of the normal probability distribution function $z_{ij} = \Phi^{-1}[p_{ij}]$, or so-called "$z$-scores".

For steady-state behavior this model is equivalent to that of a two-state Markov process. The critical advantage of this formulation is that the values of the parameters can be computed by learning from experience. Starting with some arbitrary initial values, and using a rule such as the Widrow-Hoff LMS rule, the network can update the parameter values and converge on those consistent with the experimental results. The advantage of this approach is that the network can be used to model the initial trials in the experiments when the learning of subjective probabilities and determination of the decision criteria are taking place.

This single-unit network is an implementation of a two-state Markov process in which the state-tran-

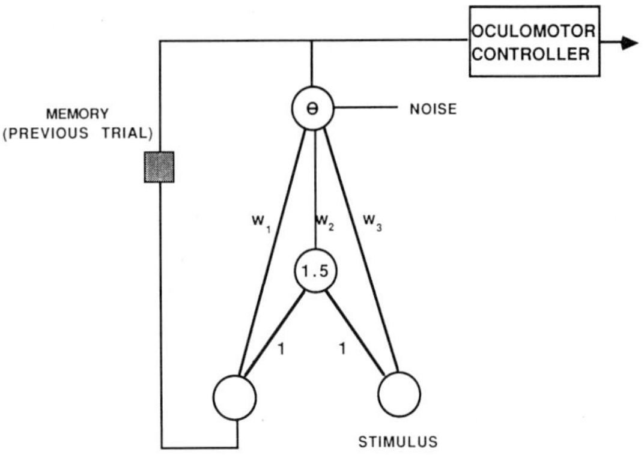

Fig. 32. A simple network that models the Markov process proposed by Falmagne et al. (1975) and used to model anticipatory smooth eye movements by Kowler et al. (1984). The hidden unit is assigned a threshold of 1.5.

sition probabilities do not depend on the stimulus. The decision to remain in one state or to switch to the other state is, in this case, a linearly separable problem, and can be performed by a single linear threshold unit. This is not true of the two-state Markov model (Falmagne et al., 1975; Kowler et al., 1984). A single unit cannot, in general, make decisions in such a way that all the appropriate state-transition probabilities are achieved. One way to see the difficulty is to compare the number of linearly independent equations (i.e., four) to the number of parameters (i.e., three). A complete model requires, therefore, at least two layers of linear threshold units.

One of the simplest minimal networks that can model the two-state Markov process (Falmagne et al., 1975; Kowler et al., 1984) is shown in Fig. 32. By the addition of a hidden unit, the network that was previously overdetermined became underdetermined. There are still four equations, one for each transition probability, but now there are seven independent variables. That means, in this case, that there are many different solutions which are equivalent with respect to the input-output behavior. To illustrate how this network makes decisions to predict leftward or rightward motions I selected a particular solution by fixing the weights associated with the hidden unit, and, thereby, the behavior of the hidden unit. In this network, shown in Fig. 32, the hidden unit H 'recognizes' the case when both the expected and the actual stimulus were rightwards motions. With this constraint, the system of equations has a single solution.

In this type of model, the values of the parameters are determined by updating the values of the parameters until the system reaches a steady state. When the parameters associated with the hidden unit are fixed (not allowed to update) the learning behavior of this network is the same as for a simple linear threshold unit. The parameters are learned in such a way that the steady-state values are approached exponentially. An exponential learning curve is quite reasonable for many types of human learning. When the parameters of the hidden unit are not fixed, then it is necessary to use methods such as backpropagation to perform the adaptation. Using the backpropagation adaptation method would require changing the response functions of each unit from a discontinuous threshold function to a monotonic function, such as the logistic function. Continuous outputs are desirable not only for the adaptation process, but also because the outputs in eye movement experiments (the velocity of anticipatory smooth eye movement or the latency of saccades) are continuous stochastic variables. However, to determine the appropriateness of this network for modeling anticipatory behavior would require experimental data on how people perform at the beginning of an experiment and how they change with additional trials.

In general, there are two advantages of the network-based implementation. First, the model has specific input and output signals and could, therefore, be interpreted as a signal processor. The inputs can be signals representing sensory events as well as results of higher-level cognitive operations. The activity of the output unit can be interpreted as a desirable control signal which can be used as an input to the smooth-pursuit oculomotor sybsystem. For the example above, the output of the unit can be used to determine the desired direction and magnitude of the smooth eye movement velocity. This then becomes the input to the optimal controller part of the oculomotor system. Such a network model can, therefore, be integrated with control-theoretic models describing lower-level processes in place of the predictive mechanisms of the sort postulated by Dallos and Jones (1963) and others. This approach opens the possibility of addressing specific questions about the nature of predictive abilities. For example, one could ask whether anticipatory behavior is better modeled by signals which are summed with the retinal error signal or, rather, as modifications to the system parameters, e.g. 'gain'. In the framework of adaptive networks it is possible to devise experiments to test such hypotheses directly.

The second advantage of the the network implementation is that the parameters of the model need not be known in advance. The values of the parameters can be determined by learning. For example, the transition probabilities mediated by the network weights can be learned from previous trials. That is, starting with some arbitrary values for the weights and thresholds, and using a simple learning algorithm (such as the generalization of the LMS rule), the network might converge to the desired values. Thus, unlike the model of Falmagne et al., which is limited to steady-state performance with the experimenter determining the parameter values, network models learn their parameter values to perform the prediction. The capability for learning and rapid adaptation is an essential component of prediction.

One disadvantage of using feed-forward networks is that our current theoretical knowledge about their behavior is limited. Among the issues which need to be further investigated are the representation of information (e.g., binary) and the effect of various network architectures. Another difficulty is related to the methods used to adapt a network and to find the values of the parameters that solve a specific problem. The commonly used back-propagation method is known to be susceptible to local minima and must be used with caution. Nevertheless, it is already possible to build network models which minimize these disadvantages. This can be achieved, as I have demonstrated above, by adding constraints to the architecture and by limiting the number of free parameters.

5. Conclusions

In this chapter I have reviewed some empirical and theoretical treatments of prediction and generation of anticipatory oculomotor behavior. The following summarizes several of the key points.

1. Many experimental results indicate that expectation and prediction can have considerable effect on both the saccadic and smooth-pursuit eye movements. Because of this, it is not wise to interpret most eye movement data without some consideration of prediction.
2. Randomization of experimental variables, such as the intervals between stimulus presentations, does not eliminate anticipatory behavior. Observers tend to make predictions even in completely unpredictable situations. Using pseudo-random signals composed of sinusoidal components in an attempt to eliminate anticipatory eye movements does not produce unpredictable target trajectories. Such trajectories may not be periodic and may appear to be quite complex, but may be, in fact, completely predictable.
3. Classical approaches to modeling anticipatory behavior using linear time-invariant systems were shown to be limited to characterizing the tracking of periodic signals, where anticipation reduces the phase lag. Adaptive approaches of modern control theory are capable of providing a better approximation to eye movement behavior, but they too are limited to the extrapolation of trajectories. It is difficult to generalize these models to incorporate prediction based on contextual information.
4. Decision-theoretic models, developed to explain performance in various perceptual and cognitive tasks, permit the use of contextual information in making decisions and generating responses. These models are useful for characterizing high-level processes but are not easily integrated with the low-level, sensory-mo-

tor mechanisms.

5. Models based on methods of pattern recognition might be able to integrate the high- and low-level processes. In this framework, the contextual information and prior target trajectories correspond to patterns to be recognized, and the prediction corresponds to a response. A particularly useful way to implement the pattern-recognition schemes is based on a language involving adaptive networks. Adaptive networks can implement a continuum of models, ranging from signal-processing mechanisms to categorization and decision-making. In addition, network-based models can incorporate learning and adaptation to changing environments and tasks. Using the language of adaptive networks, it might be possible to incorporate anticipatory behavior with models of the low-level oculomotor mechanisms.

Acknowledgement

This work was supported by a grant from the Air Force Office for Scientific Research, AFOSR-84-03-08, NASA NCC 2-269, and NASA NCC 2-307 to Stanford University. I thank Thomas V. Papathomas and Zygmunt Pizlo for making useful comments on the manuscript.

References

Albus, J.S. (1971) A theory of cerebellar function. Mathemat. Biosci. 10, 25–61.

Allum, J.H.J., Tole, J.R. and Weiss, A.D. (1975) MITNYS-II. A digital program for on-line analysis of nystagmus. IEEE Trans. Biomed Eng. 22, 196–202.

Bahill, A.T. and McDonald, J.C. (1983) Model emulates human smooth pursuit system producing zero-latency target pursuit. Biol. Cybern. 48, 213–222.

Berthoz, A. (1985) Adaptive mechanisms in eye-head coordination. In: A. Berthoz and G. Melvill Jones (Eds.), Adaptive Mechanisms in Gaze Control, Elsevier, Amsterdam, pp. 177–201.

Bower, G.H. (1961) Application of a model to paired-associate learning. Psychometrika 26, 255–280.

Bryson, A.E. and Ho, Y.C. (1968) Applied Optimal Control, Halsted Press, New York.

Bush, R.R. and Mosteller, F. (1955) Stochastic Models for Learning, Wiley, New York.

Chaitin, G. (1974) Information-theoretic computational complexity. IEEE Trans. Inform. Theory IT-20, 10–15.

Collewijn, H. (1989) The vestibulo-ocular reflex: is it an independent subsystem? Rev. Neurol. 145, 502–512.

Collewijn, H. and Tamminga, H.P. (1984) Human smooth and saccadic eye movements during voluntary pursuit of different target motions on different backgrounds. J. Physiol. 217–250.

Cooper, L.N. (1984) Neuron learning to network organization. In: M.S. Berger (Ed.), J.C. Maxwell, The Sesquincentennial Symposium, Elsevier, Amsterdam.

Cover, T. (1965) Geometrical and statistical properties of systems of linear inequalities with applications in pattern recognition. IEEE Trans. Electron. Comput. EC-14, 3, 326–334.

Curry, R.E. and Govindaraj, T. (1977) Human as a detector of changes in variance and bandwidth. Proc. 13th Annu. Conf. Man. Control 217–221.

Dallos, P.J. and Jones, R.W. (1963) Learning behavior of the eye fixation control system. IRE Trans. Autom. Control AC8, 218–227.

Dodge, R., Travis, R.C. and Fox, J.C., Jr. (1930) Optic nystagmus. Arch. Neurol. Psychiatr. 24, 21–34.

Donders, F.C. (1969) On the speed of mental processes. Acta Psycholog. 30, 412–431.

Duda, R.O. and Hart, P.E. (1973) Pattern Classification and Scene Analysis. Wiley, New York.

Falmagne, J.C., Cohen, S.P. and Dwivedi, A. (1975) Two-choice reactions as an ordered memory scanning process. In: P.M.A. Rabbitt and S. Dornic (Eds.), Attention and Performance, Vol. V, Academic Press, New York, pp. 296–334.

Fender, D.H. and Nye, P.W. (1961) An investigation of the mechanism of eye movement control. Kybernetik 1, 81–88.

Findlay, J.M. (1981) Spatial and temporal factors in the predictive generation of saccadic eye movements. Vision Res. 21, 347–354.

Fujita, M. (1982) Adaptive filter model of the cerebellum. Biol. Cybern. 45, 195–206.

Gabor, D., Wilby, W.P.L. and Woodstock, R. (1960) A universal non-linear filter, predictor, and simulator which optimizes itself by a learning process. Proc. Inst. Electr. Eng. July, 1960. Paper no. 3270M.

Gai, E.G. and Curry, R.E. (1976a) A model of the human observer in failure detection task. IEEE Trans. Syst. Man Cybern. SMC6, 85–94.

Gai, E.G. and Curry, R.E. (1976b) Failure detection by pilots during automatic landings: model and an experiment. J. Aircr. 14, 135–141.

Gonshor, A. and Melvill Jones, G. (1976) Extreme vestibulo-ocular adaptation induced by prolonged optical reversal of vision. J. Physiol. 256, 381–414.

Grant, D.A., Hake, H.W. and Hornseth, J.P. (1951) Acquisition and extinction of a verbal conditioned response with differing percentages of reinforcement. J. Exp. Psychol. 42, 1–5.

Greene, D.F. and Ward, F.E. (1979) Human eye tracking as a sequential input adaptive process. Biol. Cybern. 33, 1–7.

Heywood, S. and Churcher, J. (1981) Saccades to step-ramp stimuli. Vision Res. 21, 479–490.

Humphreys, L.G. (1939) Acquisition and extinction of verbal expectations in a situation analogous to conditioning. J. Exp. Psychol. 25, 294–301.

Ito, M. (1985) Synaptic plasticity in the cerebellar cortex that may underlie the vestibulo-ocular reflex. In: A. Berthoz and G. Melvill Jones (Eds.), Adaptive Mechanisms in Gaze Control. Facts and Theories, Elsevier, Amsterdam.

Jordan, M.I. (1986). Attractor dynamics and parallelism in a connectionist sequential machine. Proc. 8th Annu. Conf. Cognitive Sci. Soc. Erlbaum, Hillsdale, NJ.

Kalman, R.E. and Bucy, R.S. (1961) New results in linear filtering and prediction theory. J. Basic Eng. 83D, 95–108.

Keller, E.L. (1973) Accommodative vergence in the alert monkey. Vision Res. 13, 1565–1575.

Kleinman, D.L., Baron, S. and Levison, W.H. (1971) A control-theoretic approach to manned-vehicle system analysis. IEEE Trans. Autom. Control AC-16, 824–832.

Kleinman, D.L., Pattipati, K.R. and Ephrath, A.R. (1980) Quantifying an internal model of target motion in a manual tracking task. IEEE Syst. Man Cybern. SMC-10, 624–636.

Kolmogorov, A.N. (1941) Interpolation and extrapolation of stationary random sequences. Bull. Acad. Sci USSR Ser. Math. 5 (Transl: Rand Corp., Santa Monica, CA, RM-3090 PR, W. Doyle and J. Selin, 1962).

Kolmogorov, A.N. (1957) On the representation of continuous functions of many variables by superposition of continuous functions of one variable and addition. Dokl. Nauk. USSR 114, 953–956.

Kowler, E. (1989) Cognitive expectations, not habits, control anticipatory smooth oculomotor pursuit. Vision Res. 29, 1049–1057.

Kowler, E. and Steinman, R.M. (1981) The effect of expectations on slow oculomotor control. III. Guessing unpredictable target displacements. Vision Res. 21, 2, 191–203.

Kowler, E., Martins, A.J. and Pavel, M. (1984) The effect of expectations on slow oculomotor control. IV. Anticipatory smooth eye movements depend on prior target motions. Vision Res. 24, 3, 197–210.

Kuo, B.C. (1982) Automatic Control Systems, Prentice-Hall, Englewood Clifs, NJ.

Lapedes, A. and Farber, R. (1987) Nonlinear processing using neural networks: Prediction and system modeling. Technical Report, Los Alamos National Laboratory, Los Alamos, NM.

LeCun, Y. (1985) Une procedure d'apprentissage pour reseau a seuil assymetrique (A learning scheme for asymmetric threshold network). Proc. Cognitiva 85, Paris, 599–604.

Levison, W.H. (1982) The optimal control model for the human operator. Theory, validation, and applications (AF-FTCOTR-82-5). Proceedings, workshop on Flight Testing to Identify Pilot Workload. Edwards AFB, AF Flight Test Center.

Link, S.W. and Heath, R.A. (1975) A sequential theory of psychological discrimination. Psychometrika 40, 77–105.

Luce, R.D. (1986) Response Times, Oxford University Press, New York.

Luce, R.D. and Green, D.M. (1972) A neural timing theory for response times and the psychophysics of intensity. Psychol. Rev. 79, 14–57.

Makhoul, J. (1975) Linear prediction: a tutorial review. Proc. IEEE 63, 561–580.

Marr, D. (1969) A theory of cerebellar cortex. J. Physiol. 202, 437–470.

McCulloch, W.S. and Pitts, W.H. (1943) A logical calculus of the ideas imminent in nervous activity. Bull. Math. Biophys., 5, 115–133

McRuer, D. (1980) Human dynamics in man-machine systems. Automatica 46, 237–253.

Melvill Jones, G., Guitton, D. and Berthoz, A. (1988) Changing patterns of eye-head coordination during 6h of optically reversed vision. Exp. Brain Res., 69, 531–544.

Michael, J.A. and Melvill Jones, G. (1966) Dependence of visual tracking capacity upon stimulus predictability. Vision Res. 6, 707–716.

Minsky, M. and Papert, S. (1969) Perceptrons: An Introduction to Computational Geometry. MIT Press, Cambridge, MA.

Myers, J.L. (1970) Sequential choice behavior. In: G.H. Bower (Ed.), The Psychology of Learning and Motivation: Advances in Research and Theory, Academic Press, New York.

Nilsson, N.J. (1965) Learning machines. McGraw-Hill, New York.

Ollman, R.T. (1966) Fast guesses in choice reaction time. Psychonomic Sci. 6, 155–156.

Parker, D.B. (1985) Learning Logic. TR-47, Center for Computational Research in Economics and Management Science, MIT.

Puckett, J. de W. and Steinman, R.M. (1969) Tracking eye movements with and without saccadic correction. Vision Res. 9, 695–703.

Robinson, D.A., Gordon, J.L. and Gordon, S.E. (1986) A model of the smooth pursuit eye movement system. Biol. Cybern. 55, 43–57.

Rosenblatt, F. (1961) Principles of neurodynamics: Perceptrons and the theory of the brain mechanisms. Spartan, Washington, DC.

Ross, L.E. and Ross, S.M. (1980) Saccade latency and warning signals: stimulus onset, offset, and changes as warning events. Percept. Psychophys. 27, 251–257.

Rumelhart, D.E. and McClelland, J.L. (Eds.) (1986) Parallel Distributed Processing: Explorations in the Microstructure of Cognition, Vol. 1: Foundations Bradford Books/MIT Press, Cambridge, MA.

Rumelhart, D.E., Hinton, G.E. and Williams, R.J. (1986) Learning internal representations by error propogation. In: D. Rumelhart and J. McClelland (Eds.), Parallel Distributed Processing: Explorations in the Microstructure of Cognition, Bradford Books/MIT Press, Cambridge, M.A.

Saslow, M.G. (1967) Latency for saccadic eye movement. J. Opt. Soc. Am. 57, 1030–1033.

Shaw, M. (1983) Division of attention among spatial locations: a fundamental difference between detection of letters and detection of luminance increments. In: H. Bouma and D.G. Bouwhuis (Eds.), Attention and Performance X, Lawrence Erlbaum, Hillsdale, NJ.

Stark, L., Vossius, G. and Young, L.R. (1962) Predictive control of eye tracking movements. IRE Trans. Hum. Factors Electron. 3, 52–57.

St.-Cyr, G.J. and Fender, D.H. (1969a) Nonlinearities of the human oculomotor system: Gain. Vision Res. 9, 1235–1246.

St.-Cyr, G.J. and Fender, D.H. (1969b) Nonlinearities of the human oculomotor system: time delays. Vision Res. 9, 1491–1503.

Steinman, R.M., Haddad, G.M., Skavenski, A.A. and Wyman, D. (1973) Miniature eye movement. Science 181, 810–819.

Sternberg, S. (1969) The discovery of Processing Stages Extensions of Donder's Method. Acta Psychol. 30, 276–315.

Swets, J.A. (1961) Is there a sensory threshold? Science 134, 168–177.

Van den Berg, A.V. (1988) Human smooth pursuit during transient perturbations of predictable and unpredictable target movement. Exp. Brain Res. 72, 95–108.

Werbos, P. (1974) Beyond regression: new tools for prediction and analysis in the behavioral sciences. Doctoral dissertation (Economics), Harvard University, Cambridge, MA.

Westheimer, G. (1954a) Mechanisms of saccadic eye movement. Arch. Ophthalmol. 52, 710–724.

Westheimer, G. (1954b) Eye movement responses to a horizontally moving visual stimulus. Arch. Ophthalmol. 52, 932–941.

Widrow, B. and Hoff, M.E. (1960) Adaptive switching circuits. Inst. Radio Eng. West. Electron. Show Conv. Conv. Rec. 4, 96–194.

Widrow, B. and Stearns, S.D. (1985) Adaptive Signal Processing, Prentice-Hall, Englewood Cliffs, NJ.

Wiener, N. (1949) The Extrapolation, Interpolation and Smoothing of Stationary Time Series. Wiley, New York. Originally issued as a classified MIT Rad. Lab. report Feb. 1942.

Wilson G.T. (1972) Factorization of matrical spectral densities. SIAM J. Appl. Math. 23, 420–426.

Yasui, S. and Young, L.R. (1984) On the predictive control of foveal eye tracking and slow phases of optokinetic nystagmus. J. Physiol. 347, 17–33.

Yellott, J.I. (1969) Probability learning with noncontingent success. J. Math. Psychol. 6, 541–575.

Yellott, J.I., Jr. (1971) Correction for guessing and the speed-accuracy tradeoff in choice reaction time. J. Math. Psychol. 8, 159–199.

Young, L.R. and Stark, L. (1963) Variable feedback experiments testing a sampled data model for eye tracking movement. IEEE Trans. Hum. Factors Electron. 4, 38–51.

Eye movements and their role in visual and cognitive processes
E. Kowler, Editor

CHAPTER 3

The role of eye movement in the detection of contrast and spatial detail

Robert M. Steinman and John Z. Levinson

Department of Psychology, University of Maryland, College Park, MD 20742, U.S.A.

1. Introduction

1.1. Scope, goal and plan of this chapter

The role of eye movement in a variety of basic visual information processes, such as the detection of contrast, the detection of fine details and the discrimination of the positions of such details relative to each other, has a long history in visual science. Eye movements have been treated as beneficial, as detrimental, and as both beneficial and detrimental, depending on the nature of the visual stimulus. Eye movements have also been treated as irrelevant for understanding basic visual processing, on and off, during the last 125 years. This chapter traces out the reasons for such varying interest in the relationship between eye movement and basic visual information processing throughout this entire period. We adopted a long-term historical perspective because we feel that both, now highly specialized subjects, oculomotor control and visual information processing, as well as current understanding of the relationship between these specialized subjects, would benefit from a relatively detailed examination of prior attempts to work out the relationship between what the eyes do and what the human being can see. Reasons for ignoring the potential significance of eye movements in the past are as worthy of review as reasons for emphasizing their role. We base this claim on our belief that now that we have just entered a period in which eye movements are coming into prominence again, we are inclined to believe, based on the history of this area, that interest will last a decade or two to be followed by a period of neglect, once again, for seemingly plausible reasons. We hope that the reader will not interpret this last remark as simply the cynicism of older investigators. He will, we believe, come, as we have, to view the work in this area as exceptionally cyclical with peaks for and against an important role for eye movement, reflecting technical or theoretical developments in one or the other specialty. Other problem areas in visual science show analogous perturbations but we feel that they are more prominent here perhaps because those of us who specialize in vision or in oculomotor control tend to return to safer, more familiar ground once difficulties are encountered at the interface of these two relatively technical specialties. Those few who have tried to work on problems at this interface, bringing only expertise in one but not the other specialty area, have not, in our opinion, advanced far beyond their largely uninformed, initial assumptions about how eye movements interact with visual processing. It is for this reason that we undertook this chapter together: one of us (JZL) is a veteran visionary, the other (RMS) a veteran oculomotorist. We have tried, by working together on research at the interface of vision and oculomotor control, as well as by collaborating in writing this chapter, to provide some new information and also to provide the reader with a view of prior and present work that does not do violence to either of our specialties. If we have succeeded, we will have provided the reader with some insight into where this problem area has been, where it is, where it might profitably go and the problems likely to be encountered along the way.

Tracing out in some detail the history of what has become an interdisciplinary problem area over a period of more than a century required considerable selectivity in our choice of examples. We have neglected scores of interesting papers and failed to cite directly many very worthy investigations, investigators and their ideas. Our selection was dictated by knowing the end of the story we wanted to tell before we began and we chose our examples accordingly. The chapter reads as though it was historical, but it is history seen from a parochial point of view. Specifically, our 'history' sets the stage for our current work, in which it is proposed that eye movements play a very prominent role in basic visual information processing. This treatment is self-serving, but we tried to write the chapter in such a way as to encourage the reader to believe that we have treated antecedent developments fairly, albeit idiosyncratically. We tried to accomplish this in two ways: By referring the interested (or suspicious) reader to major contemporaneous reviews of the material under discussion and by adopting the practice of using quotations rather more extensively than is current practice. We adopted this practice not only because it allows the reader to judge for himself whether we are being fair but also because it avoids our being credited with the ideas of others – an outcome almost unavoidable in the currently popular writing style in which paraphrase is preferred to quotation.

We begin the chapter with a brief section describing so-called 'types' of eye movement and a brief treatment of the role each type might serve in visual information processing. Prevailing ideas about different types of eye movement and their implications for defining specific oculomotor 'subsystems' are derived from observations and classifications originally made by Raymond Dodge, a psychologist who began the objective, systematic study of human eye movement early in the present century (Dodge, 1901, 1903). Currently, it is popular to describe the oculomotor system as if it is composed of a number (at least 5) of independent 'subsystems', each of which has different velocity-amplitude characteristics, is controlled by different stimulus characteristics and serves a somewhat different function. This approach has influenced a great deal of oculomotor research since its introduction by Dodge. Currently, the value of this approach has begun to be questioned (Collewijn, 1989; Erkelens et al., 1989b) and it is likely to be replaced in future years by a simplification into only two subsystems, that is, a fast, jump-like saccadic subsystem and a smooth eye movement subsystem, whose action includes what is now described as the output of the smooth pursuit, slow control, optokinetic nystagmus, vestibulo-ocular response and vergence 'subsystems'. We have adopted current usage in our introductory sections and throughout the chapter because it makes it easier for the reader to evaluate the classical literature on our topic and also allows us to use quotations which would not be possible if the oculomotor material were treated in less conventional language. We expect that a good deal of the oculomotor terminology we have used will seem quaint in a few years. The ideas should, however, remain clear despite the fact that such distinctions as vergence, smooth pursuit, OKN, VOR and slow control may fall into disuse. The introductory sections, just below, also serve to define a number of terms and important concepts used throughout the chapter.

1.2. Eye movement characteristics and putative functions

The human eye rotates for a number of quite different reasons. Specifically, it may rotate in a rapid jump-like manner ('saccade') so as: (1) to bring the retinal image of an attended, but eccentric, stationary object to fall at the foveal center. Once the attended object is at the foveal center, the object is said to be 'fixated' or, less commonly, 'foveated'. Attention and fixation may remain coincident once fixation is established, or they may, once again, go their separate ways, establishing a complex set of asynchronous cognitive processes and visuomotor acts (see Kowler, Ch. 1 of this volume, and Viviani, Ch. 8 of this volume, for discussion of this complex interaction). The eye may also rotate smoothly so as: (2) to reduce the retinal image velocity ('slip') of an attended object which is moving in the visual field. When this occurs, the eye is said to be 'smoothly pursuing (tracking)' the attended object. Both saccades and smooth pursuits are usually observed in the oculomotor pattern when moving objects are tracked. This mixed style of tracking reflects a subject's desire to follow or to lead a moving object by combining 'catch up' or 'get ahead' saccades with smooth, retinal image slip-reducing, eye rotations – a strategy that can minimize tracking error if it is used cleverly. This mixed tracking strategy seems to be used by most, if not all, subjects, but it is not a hard-wired oculomotor characteristic. Simple instruction is sufficient to modify the manner in which saccades and smooth pursuits are mixed when a moving object is tracked (Puckett and Steinman, 1969).

The eye may also rotate so as: (3) to compensate for movements of the head and body, allowing the line of sight to remain near a fixated stationary object as the orientation of the fixator changes in space. These eye rotations are called 'compensatory' eye movements. They include (a) saccades which re-establish fixation of an attended stationary object displaced from the foveal center by head or body movement, (b) smooth pursuit of an attended stationary object when its image slips on the retina because of deficiencies inherent in the operation of (c) the vestibulo-ocular subsystem, which uses signals from the semicircular canals to produce smooth rotations of the eye opposite in direction to rotations of the head. These vestibularly activated smooth compensatory eye rotations serve to help maintain objectively stationary visual details relatively stationary on the retina as the head or body rotates. Such compensatory eye movements are frequently referred to as the 'VOR', an acronym derived from vestibulo-ocular reflex (or response).

Finally, (4) the eye rotates because it is not fused to the skull. This arrangement guarantees that the eye will rotate with respect to the skull despite the operation of the position- and velocity-sensitive biological 'control systems' that have evolved to compensate for movement of the head and body or for movement of objects in the visual field (Walls, 1962). Real biological control systems are certain to fall somewhat shy of perfection when they operate. These imperfections always produce some irreducible variability of eye position and velocity (oculomotor 'noise'). There is also, what we now consider to be a noisy, high-frequency small-amplitude eye movement that can be seen while a subject attempts to maintain fixation with his head immobilized on a biting-board. These tiny eye movements are called 'physiological nystagmus' or 'high-frequency tremor'. These tremors, which can only be observed with the most sensitive recording instruments, have been ascribed to incomplete tetany of the extrinsic oculomotor muscles during maintained fixation (e.g., Cornsweet, 1956). Discussion of attempts to establish the functional significance of the various kinds of eye movement, described above, constitutes a large part of the content of this chapter.

1.3. Eye movements and the fovea

Eye rotations, regardless of their origin and purpose, have considerable significance for basic visual processing. A good deal of this significance arises from the fact that the human retina is exceedingly heterogeneous in its functional properties. A foveate animal, such as ourselves, must be able to orient its eye with respect to the direction of objects in space and to maintain the eye's orientation exceedingly well because our best detail vision depends on specialized tissues (very densely packed cone receptors) found only at the center of the floor of the fovea – a region occupying less than 0.02% of the retinal surface area (Polyak, 1941). The presence of such a tiny highly specialized fovea guarantees that a very high degree of oculomotor skill will evolve so that a foveate animal, for example, such disparate creatures as a chameleon or a human being, is able to make use of its specialized foveal cells to discriminate fine details in the visual environment (see Walls, 1962, and Steinman, 1975, for elaboration of this point).

1.4. Eye movements as sources of neural transients

There are additional reasons for taking eye rotations seriously when considering basic visual processing. Eye rotations might be beneficial for the detection of contrast or spatial detail by producing changing or transient retinal stimulation. Changing or transient stimulation might help, or might even be required, to prevent photochemical depletion, neural fatigue or adaptation. Transient stimulation might actually be required to generate such basic physiological events as afferent bioelectrical potentials or lateral inhibitory processes in the retina or higher visual centers. Alternatively, eye rotations might be detrimental to basic visual processing because they could create, or allow, excessive retinal image motion. Such retinal image motion could smear the 'proximal stimulus' (the distribution of light on the retina where the transduction of physical to biophysical messages takes place). However, commands to generate eye rotations might initiate efferent or associative neural processes which serve to elevate detection thresholds, and thereby reduce the visual significance of the smear or retinal blur caused by high-velocity eye movements (see Matin, 1974; Volkmann, 1986; or Sperling, Ch. 7 in this volume, for reviews of research on 'saccadic suppression' – the name given to threshold elevations observed before, during and following a saccade).

All of these potentially beneficial and detrimental effects have been described in the visual psychophysical literature. All call attention to the potential importance of eye movement for visual processing. All have been studied and discussed, with varying enthusiasm, for more than a century. Important trends in the development of ideas about the relationship between eye movement and basic visual processing will be traced out next. Current thinking about this relationship, as in other areas of visual science, sometimes fails to take antecedent mistakes and progress into account. Our review includes this old material, partially for completeness but also because it will be shown later that many very old ideas bear directly on recent and current work.

Ideas about the relationship of eye movement to basic visual processing had well-established roots by the time visual science entered the final quarter of the 19th century. Like most areas in visual science in this period, very clear alternative positions were available. Alternatives, proposed clearly and authoritatively by H. von Helmholtz (1866), were traditionally contested and/or elaborated by E. Hering (1899, 1920). Their antagonistic relationship can be found in the subject matter of this chapter as well as in many other problem areas. Consider first Helmholtz's treatment of 'visual acuity'.

2. Helmholtz's treatment of visual acuity

2.1. The retinal mosaic and intensity discrimination

As early as 1866 Helmholtz pointed out that the finite size of the light-absorbing retinal elements, which were already believed to be the rods and the cones on the basis of psychophysical experiments (Brindley, 1960, p. 151), could place a theoretical limitation on the ability to discriminate details in an extremely fine pattern. Imagine the fovea to be stimulated by two mathematical point-images. In this *hypothetical* case it is apparent that the ability to discriminate two discrete points requires their separation to be at least as large as the diameter of one of the visually sensitive retinal elements. If the separation were smaller, only a single element would be stimulated and discrimination would be impossible. There would be no physiological basis for the perception of the gap between two mathematical point-images if the gap were smaller than a retinal element. In Helmholtz's words: "The light which falls upon a single sensitive element can produce only a single light sensation, within which it is impossible to distinguish whether individual parts of the element are strongly illluminated, others weakly illuminated" (p. 215). In other words if we could test with infinitely small points or their extension as infinitely thin lines, retinal element size would place a limit on acuity. This limit, as Helmholtz knew well, applied only to hypothetically thin stimuli and that once acuity is measured with real points or real lines, the ability to discriminate detail could be appreciably better than this 'theoretical' limit imposed by the retinal mosaic. Real stimuli always have appreciable extent in the proximal stimulus, guaranteeing a gradient of light stimulation which will fall on a number of elements, particularly near the central fovea where these elements are densely packed. According to Helmholtz, when real stimuli are used to measure visual acuity, acuity is limited by the capacity to discriminate intensity, not by the size of the retinal elements.

2.2. Elaboration of Helmholtz's ideas

Helmholtz's emphasis on intensity discrimination in limiting visual acuity was picked up and elaborated by Hartridge (1922) and Hecht (1927) more than 60 years later. Intensity discrimination theories of visual acuity subsequently came to be known as 'static' theories (Falk, 1956). They were called static because they ignored the potential importance of eye movements. The proximal stimulus was treated as though it were stationary. This treatment implies one or more of the following assumptions: (1) visual information is sampled only within relatively brief intervals during which the test stimulus cannot move far or fast, (2) oculomotor compensation for movement of the stimulus or the body of the observer is virtually perfect, producing effectively stationary test stimuli in the presence of motion, or (3) oculomotor noise is too small to have visual consequences. Much more will be said about each of these possibilities later. Static theories can be contrasted with 'dynamic' theories of visual acuity which are based on Hering's ideas (1899). Dynamic theories emphasize the role of eye movement. Ultimately, they develop to the point where eye movement is treated as a *necessary* condition for visual acuity. Hering's ideas and their development will be described later after elaborations of Helmholtz's approach have been presented.

Many authors since 1866, during the early years of the current century as well as more recently, have been under the mistaken impression that Helmholtz proposed an anatomical limit for real, as well as for hypothetical, acuity targets. For example, Hartridge (1922) implied that he may have made this mistake by saying that "One assumption has been made in the past, namely that the finite diameter of the foveal cones sets a maximal limit to the resolving power of the eye, and various calculations of the performance of the eye under different circumstances have been made on this basis" (p. 52). Hartridge does not attribute this idea specifically to Helmholtz, nor to anyone else for that matter, but it seems likely that its basis is Helmholtz's treatment of hypothetical test stimuli. Le Grand (1967, p. 106) made a clear attribution of this idea to Helmholtz more recently. Hartridge went on to elaborate Helmholtz's treatment of real acuity stimuli by calculating the illumination differences on adjacent foveal cones produced by particular test stimuli and relating the calculated intensity differences to the likelihood that such differences would be sufficient to be perceptually discriminable. His calculations of retinal light distributions include aberrations and other errors expected in a biological optical system such as the living human eye. In short, Hartridge's often-cited paper is an elaboration of Helmholtz's intensity discrimination approach to the limit of visual acuity. Byram (1944) subsequently pointed out that Hartridge's calculations could be in error by as much as a factor of two because Hartridge used Rayleigh's equations intended for a square aperture on image formation in the human eye, whose aperture is round. Hecht (1928) will make the same mistake with more modest consequences (15%) a few years later. A clear understanding of Helmholtz's (1866) priority for his treatment of the acuity limit-intensity discrimination question has not, however, been completely lost from the secondary vision literature. It reappears from time to time where the persistent misinterpretation of Helmholtz is duly noted and criticized (e.g. Wilcox and Purdy, 1933, or Walls, 1943). The retinal mosaic-acuity limit idea is often, but not always, falsely attributed to Helmholtz. It kept reappearing periodically for more than a century probably because it could be made to serve a useful didactic purpose (e.g. Senders, 1948; Riggs, 1965; or Le Grand, 1967). More recently, textbook treatments of spatial vision tend to ignore the retinal mosaic-acuity limit idea when they discuss the problem in terms of contrast sensitivity and the 'spatial modulation transfer function' – an approach brought from optical engineering by Schade (1956). The retinal mosaic and the functional significance of the fineness and symmetry of its cytoarchitecture have been the subject of renewed interest very recently (see Yellott, 1983; Hirsch and Hylton, 1984; Williams, 1985; for representative research).

3. Hering's approach to spatial vision

3.1. The direction, as well as the number, of perceived details

Consider next Hering's approach to the problem of visual acuity. His approach came to lean heavily on the role of eye movement in the hands of subsequent theorists. Consider first the traditional definition of visual acuity commonly found in the literature of Hering's day. This definition, 'visual acuity is the capacity to perceive fine details' (e.g. Hofmann, 1920), was usually 'operationalized' (studied empirically) by measuring the smallest separation, in visual angle, at which two neighboring objects could be resolved in the sense that two objects, rather than one object, were perceived. Secondary source treatments of visual acuity, starting with Helmholtz's first edition (1866) of his *Treatise on Physiological Optics*, traditionally include accepted values of visual acuity which had been measured up until that time with a variety of different test stimuli. Fixed stars, parallel lines of the same width, parallel lines with wider and narrower intervals, white squares separated by a black grating, spider webs and rod gratings were some of those mentioned in Helmholtz's original compilation. Tables of acuity values with such different test stimuli permeate the vision literature on acuity. Hartridge (1922), for example, continued this tradition and added new test results for such stimuli as absorption bands, and black and bright brass wires to the list of tasks. By the time Senders (1948) published her review article on visual acuity, stereoscopic acuity and vernier acuity had become traditional members of the list.

These were important additions. They highlight a distinction made by Hering almost 50 years earlier. Hering (1899) distinguished two kinds of detail vision. In this he was influenced by a report of Wülfing (1892), who measured what we now call the vernier displacement threshold of the offset contained within a dark bar ('vernier acuity') and found it to be only a few seconds of arc – very much better than anyone's ability to perceive two objects when they are separated by a gap of only a few seconds of arc. Hering was already familiar with Volkmann's (1863) demonstration that differences in the width of bars as small as 7 seconds of visual angle could be discriminated when the two bars were seen at the same time. Such delicacy of detail vision, about an order of magnitude better than the ability to discriminate gaps, led Hering to propose distinguishing resolving power (*Auflosungsvermogen*), the capacity measured in the traditional visual acuity task, from the space sense (*Raumsinn*), the capacity to distinguish differences in spatial position as measured in vernier, stereo and size estimation tasks. Interest in Hering's *Raumsinn* was rekindled recently by Westheimer (1981), who has been studying what he calls 'hyperacuity', i.e., the capacity to perceive position differences much smaller than the smallest retinal element. Hering's *Raumsinn* is a quite remarkable capacity, not only because of its delicacy, but also because it has been known since the turn of the century to be insensitive to blurring, intensity and appreciable motion. Hering (1920) also anticipated another currently important characteristic of visual acuity when he emphasized the importance of contrast in the perception of detail. Hering, as well as Helmholtz, was well aware that imperfections in the dioptrics of the normal human eye degraded the quality of the proximal stimulus and proposed that such degradations could be overcome by contrast effects produced by antagonistic neural processes – a quite modern view. He said: "The retinal image of every contour line, even when seen with perfect accommodation, is blurred. But our 'inner eye' has the power to create in the psychological visual field (providing that the intensity of the imperfect line-image is sufficient) a sharp boundary between two contiguous colors – thereby producing sharply-contoured elements in the retinal image. Our visual system owes this power to interaction of visual areas. The retinal image is always blurred; but, like the photographer who retouches a defective print, this interaction corrects the picture of external objects" (p. 154).

3.2. Weymouth's development of Hering's ideas

Hering's influence on dynamic theories of visual acuity can be seen first, and most explicitly, in the work of Averill and Weymouth (1925). These authors began by pointing out that thresholds [vernier and stereo] "far below the known size of the retinal elements" have been measured but "no satisfactory explanation has been offered of the way in which the delicacy of a perception might exceed the retinal grain" (p. 147).* They go on to propose that the idea of the position of a straight line is a complex percept based on at least three factors; namely, mutual effects of adjacent retinal elements, the averaging of successive stimulus patterns on the retinal mosaic caused by the continual occurrence of small eye movements, and the combining of similar stimulus patterns from each of the eyes. They propose that the visual system employs a statistical method, which uses signals from a large number of retinal elements, to calculate a percept based on what they call the 'retinal mean local sign'.

3.3. An experimental test of Hering's ideas

Averill and Weymouth (1925) acknowledged that their proposals were anticipated by Hering (1899) – a fact that Weymouth, Andersen and Averill (1923) had overlooked in an earlier brief report. They go on to point out that Hering, despite his clear, but neglected priority, gave no empirical support for his ideas – a situation they set out to remedy. Averill and Weymouth (1925) describe an ingenious simulation experiment in which they attempted to reproduce the stimulating conditions they believed would occur during a vernier task in a living eye. First, they made a replica of a portion of the fovea centralis (magnified 350x) by drilling many fine holes in a thin sheet of aluminum. The placement and density of these holes were carefully contrived to imitate the receptor surface as it was believed to be at the time. Light from an optically distant source passed through this perforated diaphragm and fell on a frosted glass screen which was viewed by a 'reagent' (observer). The projected spots of light represent the visually sensitive elements of the fovea. Objects placed between the perforated diaphragm and the screen will cast a shadow on the screen, cutting off some of the 'retinal elements' from the light. This situation is intended to simulate a proximal stimulus, where some retinal elements are stimulated while others are not. Opaque, inverted V-shaped objects were used to cast the object-shadows. These objects were attached to a motor-driven eccentric cam which was used to simulate the effect of eye movements by oscillating the shadow used to simulate the proximal stimulus. The inverted V-shaped objects were of two types. One could have an offset on one of its edges at a variable position along a contour. The other type had a uniform contour. The reagent's task was to report the presence and position of the offset, if any, and to give a confidence rating about his report. He

* In this, Averill and Weymouth, like many others, seem to be unaware of Helmholtz's original treatment of the relationship of visual acuity to the capacity to discriminate intensity differences rather than to the size of retinal elements, see section 2.1.

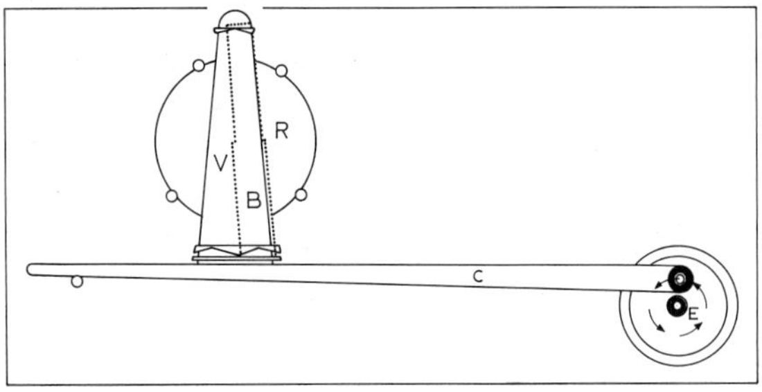

Fig. 1. Diagram of apparatus. R, replica of fovea (Fritsch) on an aluminum disc, cones being represented by minute perforations (see Fig. 2 for details). V, inverted V-shaped shield used to produce the image-shadow. B, brass rod with offset (dotted) held in such a position that its broken edge projects just beyond the margin of the shield. C, wooden cross-bar to which the shield is attached. The cross-bar and shield move in an elliptical path whose horizontal diameter is 8 mm (5 cone diameters) and vertical diameter about one-third as great. E, motor-driven eccentric which produces oscillation of the cross-bar and shield in an elliptical path. (From Averill and Weymouth, 1925)

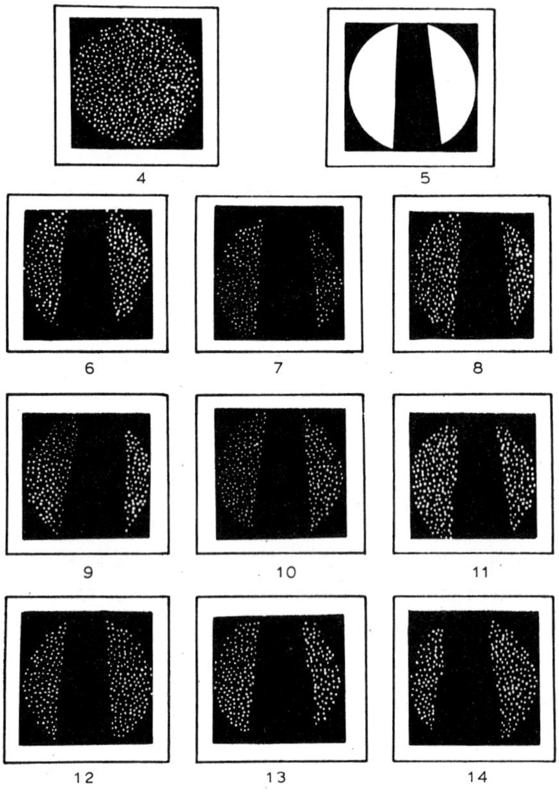

Fig. 2. (4) Diagram of retinal mosaic after Fritsch. Note the irregular arrangement of the cones and the great variation in inter-conal distances. This diagram is a replica of the perforated aluminum disc. (5) Appearance of the image shadow with displacement along the left margin and with the wider portion above the offset. (6–14) Representations of the retinal field as observed by the subject (reagent), who was required to judge the presence of an offset and its location when an offset was present. For example, in (14) there was a relatively large offset on the left which was wider in the lower part of the retinal field. (From Averill and Weymouth, 1925)

did this when the shadow of the V-shaped object was seen while it was stationary and also while it was moving so as to simulate fixational eye movements as they understood them to be at the time (see Figs. 1 and 2 for illustration of their technique).

They found: displacement thresholds far smaller than the 'retinal elements' (the projected spots of light); thresholds were lower when 'eye movements' (oscillations of the V-shaped object) were present than when the V-shaped object was stationary; thresholds were lower when longer objects were viewed (this allowed more retinal elements to contribute to the average); and short exposures with both eyes were better than short exposures with a single eye, demonstrating the role of binocular summation in 'the delicacy of perception of offsets'. Averill and Weymouth (1925) concluded by claiming to have shown that relative motion between the retina and an image greatly increases the delicacy of visual perception.

The 'dynamic' theory of visual acuity was launched empirically by this experiment, which made the approach seem plausible despite somewhat indirect tests. Further progress with the dynamic approach had to wait more than 20 years to gain prominence after Selig Hecht's static theory had fallen out of favor and a physiological variant of dynamic theory was proposed by Talbot and Marshall (1941) and Marshall and Talbot (1942). Hecht's commanding position in the development of visual science and his static theory of visual acuity will be presented next.

4. Hecht's static photochemical theory

4.1. The man

Selig Hecht (1892–1947) was "one of the most vivid scientific figures of his time; a pioneer in the development of general physiology in this country [USA]; and for more than two decades leader in his chosen field, the physiology of vision" (Wald, 1948). Hecht's approach to visual problems was physicochemical. The origin of this approach is traced by Wald (1948) in his obituary of Hecht, where Hecht is described as having been profoundly influenced by three factors, namely, the birth of the science of photochemistry, which occurred near the turn of the century, Jacques Loeb's treatment of animal phototropism, with its source in ordinary physicochemical processes, and the publication of Arrhenius's book, 'Quantitative Laws in Biological Chemistry', in1915 while Hecht was a graduate student at Harvard. Hecht favored biochemical, over neurophysiological, explanations of visual processes whenever possible, applying peripheral, biochemical explanations to potentially complex central visual processes (e.g. color), as well as to potentially simple, retinal visual processes (e.g., dark adaptation). Present-day visual biophysicists, undoubtedly wiser for having had such an influential, but only fleetingly successful, intellectual antecedent, tend to be less ambitious. Hecht's theory of visual processing was very broad in scope as well as parsimonious with respect to the number of required explanatory principles. For example, Hecht explained absolute sensitivity to light, the discrimination of brightnesses and the detection and discrimination of spatial details by reference to the concentration of photopigments in the rod and cone receptors and to the distribution of the thresholds of these receptors. Only the first of these problems – the absolute threshold for light (Hecht et al., 1942) – is still held to be amenable to photochemical explanations, but, even here, at the very beginning of visual processing, neural reorganization associated with dark adaptation has added a significant neurophysiological embellishment (Barlow et al., 1957). Hecht's approach was taken very seriously in his day – the simplicity and wide-reaching scope of the approach undoubtedly adding to its influence. Hecht employed classical Fechnerian psychophysical techniques with experienced human observers (his collaborators and himself) in most of his work. Ascidians, clams, bees and flies also served as his subjects.

4.2. Hecht's theory

Hecht's (1927, 1928) theory of visual acuity is an elaboration of Hartridge's (1922) approach, which, in turn, is derived, without attribution, from Helmholtz's idea that visual acuity is limited by the ability to discriminate differences in light intensity. Hartridge advanced this idea by calculating the light distribution in the retinal image of an optical device, such as the human eye, when it is presented with a variety of conventional acuity targets and comparing such light distributions to acuity thresholds measured with these targets. Hartridge concluded that the limit of acuity was determined by the ability to discriminate intensity. His calculated limit was about 5–10%. Hecht, adopting a similar approach, concluded that the limit of intensity discrimination and, therefore, the limit of visual acuity was about an order of magnitude better.*

Hecht's elaboration of the Helmholtz-Hartridge idea went far beyond demonstrating that the exquisite delicacy of spatial vision could be limited by a similar sensitivity to intensity differences. He developed a general theory, encompassing the full range of variation of acuity with a variety of differences in stimulating conditions, related these variations to the functional density of the retina complete with its two kinds of receptors, and explained all of these phenomena at the level of the

* See Hecht and Mintz (1939) for the 'minimum visible' acuity limit, that is, the ability to make out the presence of a dark bar against a moderately intense background, where the threshold was found to be about one half second of arc – a value that was calculated to correspond to an intensity difference across adjacent receptors of about one half of one percent with this type of display.

chemistry of the photopigments. Hecht's grand scheme could only seem to succeed by being selective with respect to the data it was willing to consider and by being indifferent to or, perhaps, naive about the desirability of statistically testing the goodness of fit of data to theory. A discussion of Hecht's theory of acuity and traditional criticism of the theory will be presented next (see Senders, 1948, for a more complete and particularly fine review of Hecht's theory published near the end of its useful scientific life).

Hecht's theory begins by recognizing that the human eye is not a perfect optical device and the presence of chromatic aberration, spherical aberration and diffraction guarantee that the distribution of a point of light will be spread when it is imaged on the retinal surface. The retinal image of an acuity target is considerably more diffuse than the calculated geometrical image of the same acuity target. He goes on to assert that the ability to discriminate details reduces to the ability to discriminate differences in intensity in this diffuse retinal image. Next, Hecht calls attention to the established fact that intensity discrimination improves with the intensity of the stimulating light and proposes that if acuity is actually an intensity discrimination, acuity should improve in the same manner. In other words, the functions for the intensity difference threshold ($\Delta\ I/I$)/intensity function and the visual acuity (1/minimum angle resolved)/intensity functions should be similar in form. Hecht supported this point in his 1928 and later papers by showing that the log of visual acuity plotted against the log of stimulating intensity is similar in form, that is, sigmoidal, to plots of $\Delta I/I$ against the log of the stimulating intensity. Hecht pointed out that Helmholtz had previously suggested that the poor visual acuity measured at low intensities of background stimulation (the shallow lower limb of this sigmoidal function) might be related to the coarseness of intensity discrimination under these conditions. Hecht goes on to consider why this might occur. He credits König with realizing that this lower limb might reflect the operation of rods in the periphery at low levels of illumination, but not before pointing out that Broca supposed that the connection between retinal elements and nerve fibers might not be fixed and that the number of retinal elements which communicate with each nerve fiber might vary with the intensity of illumination – an idea rather ahead of its time. Hecht claims credit in his 1928 paper for realizing that the lower limb in the acuity-intensity function is the rod limb while the rest of the function describes activity of the cones. He encourages the reader to confirm this simply by looking at an acuity target in low illumination, where the reader will note that fixation is eccentric, causing the target to fall on the peripheral retina where the highly light-sensitive rod receptors are located. Fig. 3 (top) reproduces the acuity-intensity functions Hecht used to develop his theory.

Hecht develops his ideas by pointing out that: "the fineness of detail which a surface can register depends on the number of receiving elements present in a unit area of the surface. In other words, its resolving power varies in inverse proportion to the average distance between the centers of the sensitive elements. This is very evident in such a case as the photographic plate. The retina is a surface of this kind since it is composed of discrete rods and cones which function as individual units or groups of units. The way in which visual acuity varies with illumination indicates the way in which the resolving power of the retina varies. A low visual acuity means that the average distance between the retinal elements is large; whereas a high visual acuity means that the distance is relatively small. To account for the large variation of visual acuity with illumination, one must suppose that the number of sensitive units per unit area of retina can and does vary nearly a hundred-fold. But the number of rods and cones in the retina is fixed anatomically. Therefore it is necessary to assume that the number of these elements is variable functionally" (pp. 259–260). Hecht next assumes that the thresholds of these sensitive retinal elements are not the same; rather, they vary in the "manner of populations" (p. 260).

Hecht's last assumption, that is, that receptor thresholds are normally distributed is illustrated in

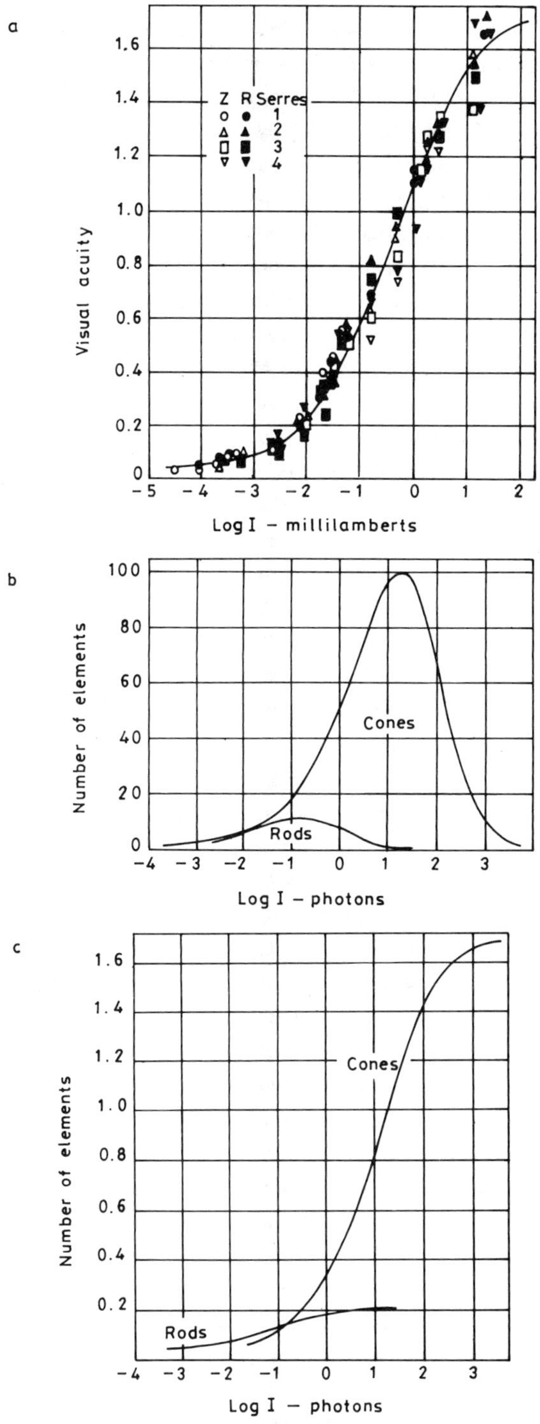

Fig. 3. (a) Relationship between visual acuity and illumination. Data of Roelefs and Zeeman re-plotted by Hecht. (b) Distribution of thresholds of rods and cones. (c) Statistical distribution of the sensitivity of rods and cones. (From Hecht, 1928)

Fig. 3 (middle), which reproduces his assumed threshold distributions. The 'functional density' of the retina can be estimated by summing the rod and cone threshold distributions for each potential illuminating intensity plotted in Fig. 3. Functional density (the integrated curve) is illustrated in Fig. 3 (bottom). **N.B.** Hecht emphasized that he is assuming that a level of stimulating intensity will be reached where the functional density asymptotes (saturates), that is, the number of cones stimulated to threshold no longer increases as intensity increases. This assumption clearly implies that visual acuity will cease to improve at these high levels of stimulation. This counter-factual prediction will, along with other problems, eventually make trouble for Hecht's approach. Hecht next goes on to test his theory quantitatively by using Reeve's data on the effect of stimulating intensity on pupillary diameter to correct König's acuity-intensity data. This correction is necessary once one wishes to estimate the actual retinal intensity associated with the König's measurements of visual acuity because König did not control for pupillary diameter. Hecht makes similar corrections for Roelofs and Zeeman's data and also examines the acuity data of two completely color-blind subjects (described by König and Uhthoff) whose eyes should only show the rod limb of the acuity function. In all cases there is excellent agreement between the calculated and observed relationships between illumination and visual acuity (see Hecht's, 1928, Tables I and II).

4.2.1. The unit retinal area

An appreciation of this relationship and Hecht's treatment of it requires brief discussion of his treatment of what he calls the 'unit retinal area'. His unit retinal area is "a minimal retinal area which contains the equipment for recording the various properties such as intensity perception, color vision, visual acuity, and the like, usually ascribed to the retina as a whole" (p. 275). Hecht bases his estimate of the unit retinal area on König's brightness discrimination data, in which König found 572 discriminable steps over the complete range of intensities to which the eye can respond: in other words,

572 just noticeable differences (JNDs), assuming, of course, that one JND (a mental unit) is equal to the difference threshold (DL), measured in physical units, at each level of stimulating intensity.* Hecht, on the basis of his work on intensity discrimination, asserted that 30 of these 572 steps are based on rod function and the remaining 542 are based on cone function. This number, 542, then, represents the number of cones that must be contained in the unit area of the rod-free part of the fovea, that is, the minimal foveal unit area is at least this large. According to the acuity-intensity discrimination theory, this minimal unit retinal area, which is based on intensity discrimination data, should be able to mediate all visual acuities as well because intensity discrimination provides the basis of visual acuity. Hecht supports this analysis by pointing out that the unit retinal area, based on König's acuity data, would be 0.04 mm^2, which, according to Helmholtz, would contain 540 cones (cone density in the fovea was believed to be 13500 per mm^2 at that time) 'the same number as that derived from intensity discrimination' (Hecht, 1928, p. 276).

The next step was to show that intensity discrimination, which could explain visual acuity, was "a necessary consequence of the photochemical system" action (p. 269) that Hecht had developed to explain dark adaptation. The general form of this photochemical system can be summarized as follows:

$$S \underset{\text{dark}}{\overset{\text{light}}{\rightleftarrows}} P + A$$

where S is a sensitive substance, P and A are decomposition products and also precursors of S.

The sensitivity of each retinal receptor depends on the concentration of decomposition products necessary to generate an action potential in the nervous element monitoring the state of the receptor.

* This equality of JND and DL is a common assumption, going back to Fechner (1860), but it is worth noting that it is only an assumption – the JND and the DL are quite different entities – the former is mental; the latter, physical.

The total number of active elements is a linear function of the concentration of decomposition products. It follows that the number of active elements can be described by the following equation:

$KI = x^2/(a—x)$, where a is the initial concentration of photosensitive substance S, x is the concentration of the decomposition products (A and P), I is intensity and K is a constant.

The final form of Hecht's quantitative treatment of visual acuity in his photochemical system was presented by Hecht and Mintz in 1939. The following treatment of the acuity-intensity relationship is based on the equations presented in that paper.

$\Delta I/I = c[1+1/(KI)^{1/2}]^2$, where c is the minimal value of $\Delta I/I$ at the highest value of I, and K is the reciprocal of the intensity at which $\Delta I/I$ is 4 times the minimal value. This represents the photochemical equation as applied to intensity discrimination data, but the minimum angle resolved (the acuity threshold) can be viewed as a function of $\Delta I/I$ and therefore: $a = b' \Delta I/I$, where a is the visual angle and b' is a constant.

Then: $a = b[1+1/(KI)^{1/2}]^2$ where $b=b'c$. The b fixes the curve on the ordinate and K fixes it on the abscissa.

4.2.2. Summary of Hecht's theory

Briefly, Hecht's theory of visual acuity can be summarized as follows: the density of active receptor elements in the retinal mosaic sets the limit on visual acuity; the larger the number of active elements per unit retinal area, the better the acuity. The number of receptor elements is, obviously, fixed by the anatomy of the retina, so the variation in acuity observed, when acuity is tested on different background illluminations, must be produced by variations in the number of anatomical elements that are functionally rather than anatomically present, under a given set of illuminating conditions. Individual retinal elements respond differentially to the same amount of photochemical decomposition compounds. A few have very low thresholds, a few very high thresholds, while most thresholds cluster near the middle. In other words, thresholds are normally distributed. The intensity of the stimulating light determines the amount of photochemical decomposition. This relationship between stimulating intensity and the concentration of decomposition products predicts both intensity discrimination and the discrimination of visual angles in the acuity task. In other words, visual acuity is based on intensity discrimination.

4.3. Criticism of Hecht's theory

Hecht's theory was criticized on three grounds, namely, some of the facts used as basis of the theory were not correct, the theory was insufficient to account for some well-established facts and, finally, the theory was not the only or the best interpretation of the facts. In short, when all was said and done, there really was not a great deal of lasting merit in the acuity theory other than its simplicity and breadth. We will next give examples of some of the problems which brought it down.

First, there were problems arising from facts known in Hecht's day. Hecht makes much of the 'excellent' quantitative agreement between the number of cones in the 'minimal unit foveal area' and the number of discrete steps (JNDs) of intensity discrimination across the range of lights to which human vision responds. This quantitative agreement is the heart of his intensity discrimination theory of visual acuity. It rests on Helmholtz's (1896) estimate of 13500 cones per square millimeter in the fovea. In 1941 Polyak provided a better, more modern estimate of 55000 cones per square millimeter. This density is for the foveal floor. The cone density in the central bouquet of the foveal floor, whose diameter is about 20 minutes of arc, is still greater. The foveal bouquet would be the likely preferred fixation position when the absolutely best acuity is desired, providing, of course, that the intensity of the target background is sufficient to stimulate the densely packed cones found in this retinal region. So, within 2 years of Hecht and Mintz's (1939) definitive quantitative confirmation of the intensity discrimination–acuity theory, the minimal retinal unit area in the central fovea (the 0.04 mm^2) claimed by Hecht (1928), on the authority of Helmholtz, to contain 540 cones was actually shown to have more than 2000 cones. Recall that 540 cones was within 2 cones of the number needed to account for König's number of JNDs of intensity discrimination (namely, 542) so as to bring intensity discrimination into agreement with the fineness of grain of the retinal receptor mosaic required to resolve details of acuity targets. This, of course, is only a quantitative disagreement, but a factor of more than four was considered by some sufficient to raise serious doubts about the soundness of the underlying idea that visual acuity is based exclusively on intensity discrimination.

There were additional problems. The number of JNDs of intensity depend on the conditions under which the difference thresholds (DLs) are measured and also on the statistical convention used to calculate the DLs used to estimate the JNDs. The particular conditions König used, the size of his test field and/or his exposure duration, for example, affected the size of his DLs. DLs measured with fields of different sizes or durations would give different values. These facts imply that the splendid quantitative agreement emphasized by Hecht is actually a coincidence based on König's particular choice of conditions rather than on a general relationship between visual acuity and intensity discrimination. Other problems were clearly evident before the sudden untimely death of Hecht in 1947. Byram's (1944) criticism of Hartridge's (1922) use of Rayleigh's equations for a square aperture on the round pupil of the eye applies to Hecht's calculations of retinal light distributions of acuity targets as well as to Hartridge's. Byram calculates Hecht's error with the minimum visible dark bar used by Hecht and Mintz (1939) to be smaller, however, only about 15% – a modest difficulty when compared to the factor of four error in estimating the number of cones in the minimal foveal unit area. The similarity of the form of the $\Delta I/I$ vs. I and VA vs. I functions, so important to Hecht's formulation, as well as the exact retinal light distribution of his acuity targets, can also be questioned. The acuity function seems to be stable or to continue to improve even at the highest intensities measured, whereas intensity discrimination does deteriorate at high levels of intensity as Hecht believed (see Walls, 1943, p. 493, for a review of these facts in the context of Hecht's theory).

There is also reason to wonder about the adequacy of Hecht's photochemical theory to explain facts well-established when the theory was first proposed. The decline of interest in Hecht's theory in the 1940s derives, in part, from his making a poor guess about what he could choose to ignore in the interests of developing his theory of acuity within the limitations of the simple biochemical model he preferred. Hecht chose to ignore the role of eye movements in visual acuity – a problem that had already received serious attention when he began working on his general biochemical theory of visual processing. It continued to interest other investigators during the period from 1921 to 1942 while Hecht was extending his ideas to encompass visual acuity as well as adaptation, intensity discrimination, color and the absolute threshold. Weymouth and his co-workers had published their dynamic theory of visual acuity, based on Hering's idea of the mean local retinal sign, at about the same time that Hartridge was publishing his acuity–intensity discrimination paper that Hecht would build upon within a few years. Hering had emphasized the importance of eye movements and the mean local sign to explain how a straight line can appear straight despite the fact that it is imaged on a receptor mosaic believed at the time to contain cones arranged in a rather haphazard spatial configuration. Fig. 4, taken from Walls (1943), ilustrates Averill and Weymouth's development of Hering's idea as applied to the perceived straightness of edges.

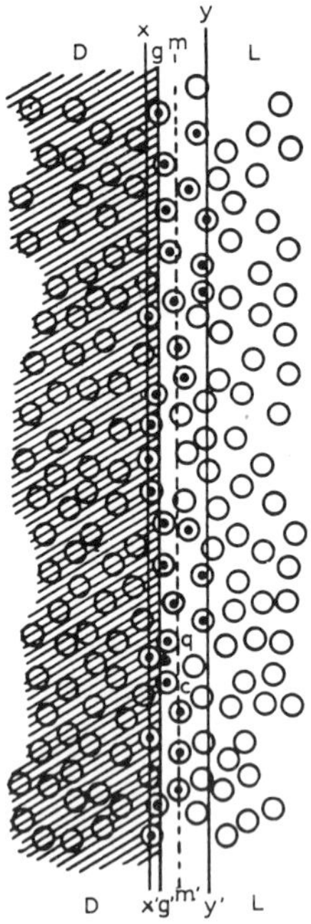

Fig. 4. Illustrates Weymouth's theory of vernier and stereoacuity. The diagram shows retinal conditions at the margin of a stimulated area. D–D is in darkness, L–L is illuminated. The geometrical margin of the image is g–g′. The cones are shown as circles. Cones a, b and c (near the bottom of region g–g′) have local signs whose 'center of gravity' is amidst them, tending to pull b to the right. This action among all of the cones cut by g–g′ smooths the percept of the contour despite the raggedness of the line of cones concerned. Furthermore, normal nystagmus shifts g–g′ back and forth between the extreme positions x–x′ and y–y′, so that m–m′ represents the center of gravity of all the points stimulated, and is the 'local sign' of the percept. The localization of this percept is independent of such factors as the size of one cone. (From Walls, 1943)

Hecht ignored this problem of how the sharpness and straightness of a straight line can be perceived when its proximal stimulus would be expected to contain offsets and jagged edges. This was a good thing to ignore. This 'problem', taken seriously by visual scientists in the first half of the present century, is analogous to the problem of how the proximal stimulus, known to be an inverted image of the distal world on the retina by the beginning of the 17th century, is perceived as upright. It is hard at this point in time to understand why perceived straightness continued to worry people long after the phenomenology of the upright ceased to be troublesome. It is not obvious why anyone would expect the physiological correlate of a perceived straight edge to be a straight edge in the receptor mosaic any more than that the physiological correlate of an upright world need be an upright image on the retina. Hecht's failure to worry about this problem does not seem to discredit his work despite Walls's (1943) contrary claim. There were, however, other, more serious questions about the sufficiency of

Hecht's approach that were worth considering. For example, Averill and Weymouth (1925) had shown that visual acuity depends on the length of the test stimulus up to some critical value of about 30 minutes of arc. It is difficult to imagine how a photochemical theory such as Hecht's can deal with such a fact. Hecht used long stimuli in his acuity experiments (e.g., wires subtending about 9–14 degrees of arc in Hecht and Mintz, 1939), but avoiding the effects of target length in this way does not solve the problem for a photochemical theory introduced by the fact discovered by Averill and Weymouth and used to support their dynamic theory.

Even more important to Hecht's theory was its inability to handle the effects of adaptation on visual acuity. Retinal adaptation has a clear photochemical basis and the failure of Hecht's theory to deal with the influence of this variable did a great deal to undermine the theory. The critical experiments on adaptation were done by Craik (1938, 1939). According to Hecht's theory, visual acuity depends on the intensity of the stimulating light and intensity differences in the retinal light distribution produced by the acuity target. Acuity will be best when the intensity of the stimulating light is sufficient to exceed the threshold of even the least sensitive receptors, providing the receptors are ready to catch quanta because their bleached photopigments have been allowed sufficient time to regenerate completely. So, the best acuity will be obtained when an intense stimulus is delivered to a dark-adapted eye. This is not the case. Craik found that acuity is best for a given level of test intensity when the eye is adapted to the test intensity before acuity is measured. Acuity suffers markedly when it is tested in a dark-adapted eye with even moderately intense backgrounds.

Hecht's receptor 'recruitment' proposal, the term he used to describe the increases in functional density attributed to the normal distribution of receptor thresholds, was also criticized on physiological grounds as soon as modern single unit recordings from visual neurons became available. There were also experiments by Senders (1949) and Nachmias (1958) showing that acuity depends on the subjective brightness, rather than the intensity, of the background field – another result not amenable to a simple photochemical explanation.

There is another class of criticism that is particularly germane to our treatment of Hecht's theory. Remember, we undertook a rather detailed examination of Hecht's photochemical theory for two rather different reasons. The first was because his theory was the most developed of the static theories of acuity, that is, theories that ignore eye movements. An appreciation of the most complete static theory sets the stage for an appreciation of theories that make eye movement a necessary requirement for acuity. The second reason we chose to go into such depth was because Hecht's quantitative theory was very influential in its day and criticism of this theory contributed to the development of an awareness of modeling issues in the contemporary visual science community that is often lacking in the much younger contemporary oculomotor community. An appreciation of such issues needs to be developed in the oculomotor community if we are to approach the level of theoretical sophistication that was apparent in our parent discipline 40 years ago. Specifically, how should one go about testing a model? Consider Senders treatment of this question in 1948.

"Hecht says that the distribution of sensibilities in the manner of populations is fundamental to his theory of visual acuity. The basis of this distribution is the photostationary state equation. Hecht feels justified in arriving at this conclusion because the photostationary state equation curves 'fit' the obtained data. This question of curve-fitting deserves extensive consideration, but only a few words will be devoted to it here. What is the most acceptable criterion of goodness of fit? In general, there are three main classes of criteria: (a) inspection, (b) statistical (e.g. least squares) and (c) parametric analysis. Each type of criterion is suitable to some types of data, and in a practical sense may be inapplicable to others.

"Essentially the same curve may be obtained from totally different equations. Crozier, for example, has pointed out (1937) the complete formal identity of the log logistic and the photostationary state equation as used by Hecht. In many cases, the curves predicted by the photostationary state equation and those predicted by the normal probability integral are so similar as to be indistinguishable by any visual criterion, and a statistical criterion is sometimes also inadequate. In such a case, the most suitable way to distinguish between the curves is by an analysis of the parameters of the function... When Hecht says that his curves fit his data, he means that a good visual inspection fit is obtained. In the absence of further analysis, this cannot be taken to mean that the photostationary state equation describes the data better than any other." (pp. 491–492)

Senders goes on to show that Crozier, her main doctoral advisor at Harvard and an undergraduate and graduate school classmate of Hecht's at CCNY and Harvard, had shown (1937) that Hecht's treatment of visual acuity as a special case of intensity discrimination was often arbitrary and not the best interpretation of the functional relationships observed.

5. Marshall and Talbot's new dynamic theory

5.1. Hartline's influence

Soon after Hecht's static theory of visual acuity had been confirmed in its final quantitative form by Hecht and Mintz (1939), Talbot and Marshall (1941) and Marshall and Talbot (1942) introduced a new dynamic theory that would dominate research on visual acuity for more than 20 years before it was replaced by the application of Fourier optics to the problem of spatial vision. The Marshall-Talbot dynamic theory placed emphasis on three things, namely, the cortical magnification factor, averaging in the visual cortex of signal transients generated in the fovea, and generation of these transients by tremor of the fixating eyeball. The appearance of this theory in the early 1940s was timely in large part because Hartline (1938, 1940) had just demonstrated phasic, as well as tonic, discharges from the ganglion cells of the frog retina – discharges to changes in stimulation, as well as discharges that began when a light came on and continued as long as the light was present, albeit at a diminished frequency. The latter kind of response, which was the only kind of response that had been observed in the compound eye of the horseshoe crab, was not tuned specifically to transients and would not, therefore, have led theories in the direction of a new, physiologically grounded, dynamic theory of visual acuity. Alternatively, the new transient neurons discovered by Hartline in the frog, which has a simple eye with a retina somewhat like the human being's, could and did provide the impetus for the development of such a theory. Neurons that signalled when a light came on and/or when the light went off were clearly capable of being driven by lights and shadows that were moved in and out of their receptive fields by eye movements. Hartline (1938) introduced the term 'receptive field' of a neuron in the same paper in which he reported the discharges in response to changing stimulation – terminology and observations at the core of modern visual neurophysiology.

The Marshall-Talbot theory was reviewed rather sceptically by Walls (1943) soon after its appearance. It was reviewed somewhat more sympathetically by Senders (1948), whose main criticisms were directed largely to Hecht's theory (see above), and subsequently by Falk (1956), whose review of visual acuity is largely devoted to criticisms of the Marshall-Talbot theory near the end of its useful life. These reviews, as well as the source papers, provided the material used in the following discussion and the reader is directed to them for additional details.

5.2. Walls's scepticism about the Marshall-Talbot theory

Walls (1943) introduced his criticism of the Marshall-Talbot dynamic theory by way of his discussion of the earlier publications of Weymouth and his associates (see sections 3.2 and 3.3), who had based their dynamic theory on Hering's idea of averaging 'retinal local signs'. (Walls's approach to this material was very clear and we will base our treatment of the Marshall-Talbot theory on his paper.) Hering introduced the idea of retinal local signs as processes which could compensate perceptually for irregularities assumed to be present in the spatial distribution of the receptor elements making up the retinal mosaic. The average of such retinal local signs can provide the physiological correlate of a straight-looking edge from the jagged edge of stimulation assumed to be present in the proximal stimulus. The concept of average local retinal signs can also provide a mechanism for abstracting the very tiny offsets in a proximal stimulus that are produced by a vernier acuity target (see Walls's illustration of Weymouth's theory reproduced in Fig. 4).

Weymouth used the assumed irregularities in the retinal mosaic coupled with the involuntary, continuous oscillations of the eyeball (physiological nystagmus) to facilitate the resolution of such details as straight edges and vernier offsets. This was accomplished by assuming, as Hering did, that each retinal receptor element had a unique directional local sign, whose activity would produce the percept of a point of light in a unique direction in visual space. When two such adjacent elements were stimulated, the perceived direction would be the spatial directional average of the local signs of each of the elements. Jagged edges in a proximal stimulus caused by irregularities of the retinal mosaic would be averaged out in this way. Differences in such averages could also provide reliable indications of offsets in vernier acuity targets. In short, characteristics of the receptor grain do not, in themselves, limit the perception of spatial details once average directional local signs, rather than discrete unrelated activity of individual receptor elements, provides the physiological correlate of the perception of the sharpness or position of spatial details. The longer the contours over which the local signs could be averaged, the larger is the number of elements contributing local signs to the average; the larger the number of elements contributing to the average, the sharper the edge. A larger number of elements allows greater reliability of the averages, increasing the likelihood of detecting any offset that might be present in the edge. These benefits derive from ordinary statistical considerations – averages are more likely to be accurate and differences in these averages can be estimated more reliably when sample size is increased. Confirmation of this theory can be had by showing that acuity improves as length of contour increases and also that acuity improves as exposure duration increases because increasing exposure duration allows more time for the tremor of the eyeball to contribute samples to the calculation of the average local signs. The former prediction was confirmed by Weymouth and his coworkers (see section 3.3), but their confirmation of the effects of exposure duration on acuity were more ambiguous theoretically as well as less clear-cut experimentally. The theoretical significance of exposure duration for dynamic theories of visual acuity would remain uncertain for many years until exposure duration could be varied with acuity targets stabilized on the retinal surface. This procedure permits unconfounding the contribution of the number of independent elements contributing to a particular sample with the contribution of the effects of the same sampling elements acting for longer periods of time (see Riggs et al., 1953, discussed in section 6.2.1, for the answer to this question).

The dynamic theory of Marshall and Talbot was much more elaborate than the dynamic theory of Weymouth and his coworkers. Part of the interest it engendered probably came from its complexity. If the visual system and the brain are complex, theories of their function should also be complex. Not everyone was prepared to adopt this view. Consider their theory as described by Walls (1943).

Marshall and Talbot came to the problem of visual acuity from their work on the physiology of the visual system and "erected a ponderous machinery with which they can explain almost everything that happens in vision. It is based upon supposed anatomical relationships and to an even greater extent upon such neurophysiological phenomena as recovery cycles, multiplication of paths, reciprocal synaptic overlap, facilitation, channeling, funneling, and peaking. These matters are most difficult for all but a chosen few – not including the writer – to comprehend fully. One tangible experimental fact is that two minutes of arc of the Rhesus monkey fovea (= ca. 9 μ) project to one linear millimeter of the visual cortex. Talbot and Marshall believe that the effective ratio of cortical ganglion cells to foveal cones is at least 600:1, which could account for vernier and stereo-thresholds very much smaller than those actually observed – whose smallness is already so frightening" (Walls, 1943, p. 502).

Walls often showed himself to be a man of considerable prescience and good taste in his numerous publications (e.g., he was not terribly keen about Hecht's theory either). The best Walls could manage to say about the Marshall-Talbot theory is that it is essentially the Weymouth version of "Hering's local signs pulled up to the *cortical* visual cells (where it probably always belonged) in order to account for the precision of spatial localization" (Walls, 1943, p. 502).

5.3. Assumptions of the Marshall-Talbot theory

If Hecht's theory of acuity could be criticized because it seems to be overly simplified, the Marshall-Talbot theory cannot be criticized for the same reason. To illustrate, seven mechanisms are assumed to be necessary to explain performance in the various kinds of acuity task, ranging from the minimum visible dark bar, through gaps and gratings and back to the stereo and vernier task. These 'mechanisms' include (1) diffraction by the pupil, which produces a statistical spatial distribution of light from every point in an acuity target; (2) physiological nystagmus, which applies the graded light distribution produced by diffraction at the edges of the pupil to the receptors; physiological nystagmus, itself, follows a statistical distribution; (3) reciprocal overlap between neural pathways, which provides a mechanism for increasing a gradient of excitation and producing peaks in the gradient of excitation because of temporal summation; (4) the neural recovery cycle, which can amplify or depress the level of excitation, depending on when in the recovery cycle the stimulus is presented; (5) multiplication of cells in the visual pathway in the sense that each retinal receptor projects to a distribution of cortical cells rather than to a single cell (it does not always do this by means of the same pathways; in other words, the specific population of cortical cells is a random variable); (6) threshold mechanisms in all of the cells in the pathway which can pass more or less of the information received; and, finally (7) an operating range of neural activity that covers about two log units of intensity, depending on the level of adaptation. The level of adaptation may be determined by photochemical processes. The total number of impulses arriving at the cortex is a function of the number of receptors active at that level and the number of impulses delivered by each receptor to the next level. The number of these impulses is determined both by the intensity of the stimulus and by the way these impulses are modified by other events in the visual pathway. These impulses may be facilitated, inhibited, peaked, etc. This menu was proposed as sufficient to develop a complete theory of visual acuity. Fortunately, this theory was built on estimates of the fineness of the receptor grain and the size and frequency of physiological nystagmus, which provided the transient stimulation-generating samples for the cortical averaging process. We say 'fortunately' because it will prove possible to remove the underpinnings of the scheme without getting into the nitty gritty of its other assumed mechanisms.

5.4. An example of how the theory worked

We next describe how this theory worked before getting into the experimental difficulties it encountered once visual scientists were able to give up their war-related research and return to basic science. Some essential features of the theory are illustrated diagrammatically in Fig. 5, which reproduces a figure from Falk (1956).

Fig. 5 shows the proximal stimulus of a bipartite field made up of a light and a dark half. The curve is the intensity distribution of the border between the light and dark halves. The slope of the distribution

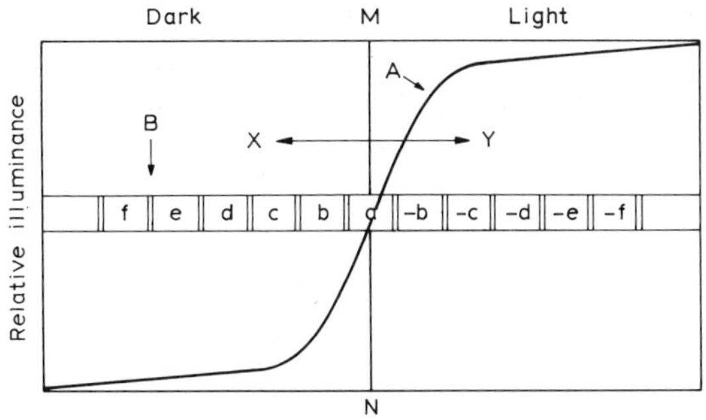

Fig. 5. The distribution of illuminance on the retina across the geometrical boundary (MN) separating Light and Dark halves of a field. See the text for details. (From Falk, 1956)

is caused by diffraction and aberrations of the edge in this proximal stimulus. The distal stimulus would be an intensity step, containing an abrupt transition from the light to the dark side of the stimulus (the MN border in Falk's figure). B is the foveal cone distribution in which cones have a center-to-center distance of 1.5 μm (a retinal distance corresponding to about 19 seconds of visual angle). The distance XY represents the average amplitude of physiological nystagmus as it was believed to be by Marshall and Talbot, that is, about 2 minutes of arc, which would contain about 6 cones. XY marks the limits of tremor for cone *a* whose stimulation by the blurred border of MN is represented by the light distribution curve A. As physiological nystagmus vibrates the retinal light distribution back and forth across cone *a*, cone *a* will receive the greatest rate of change in illumination because it lies on the steepest part of curve A. Cone *b* receives a lower rate of change and would, therefore, generate a lower rate of neural firing. The relationship between firing rate and rate of change of illumination proposed by Marshall and Talbot had been observed in the eccentric cell of the lateral eye of the horseshoe crab by Hartline and Graham (1932). These authors had also demonstrated that firing rate depended on the amount of illumination. It was these two factors, the combination of differential rate of change of illumination and the amount of illumination across the cones, that create a gradient of firing rates, which is peaked in the center of the row in the example illustrated in Fig. 5. Cone size is important in this theory, unlike the Hering-Weymouth theory, which averages local signs in order to produce the physiological correlate of an edge. Marshall and Talbot were quite specific about the importance of the relationship of cone size to the retinal light distribution, going so far as to point out that: "Smaller receptors would be useless, because though traversing the optical gradient oftener, they would gather proportionally less brightness differential. The limiting retinal factor in acuity seems to be the relation of receptor width to the highest optical *gradient* in a moving pattern, rather than the average static differential illumination on one cone, compared with its neighbors." Multiplication of pathways and reciprocal overlap on the way to the primary visual area in the cortex produce additional sharpening of the peak produced in this way in the retina, as does the 'neural recovery cycle', which favors the successful centripetal travel of the signal peaks as compared with signals arising from other receptors.

5.5. Criticism of the Marshall-Talbot theory

5.5.1. Byram's criticism

Criticisms of the dynamic theory of Marshall and Talbot were as diverse as the backgrounds of the critics. Consider for example, Byram (1944), who approached the problem of acuity from the viewpoint of a physical scientist, and developed a Hartridge-Hecht variety of static theory in which 'energy rate discrimination', rather than 'illumination discrimination', which he correctly attributed to Helmholtz, provided the basis for the discrimination of details in the retinal light distribution produced by an acuity target. In Byram's words, Marshall and Talbot "use a neuro-physiological approach in which most of the emphasis is on the post-retinal system. According to this point of view, neural mechanisms play an important role and visual acuity and contour recognition are achieved to a large extent in the visual cortex and associated systems. They point out that the grain of the cortex is in effect much finer than the grain of the retina and attribute certain accomplishments of the visual system, such as the perception of vernier offset, to both the fineness of the cortical grain and the operation of certain neural mechanisms. This would mean that the cortical image and the test object would have in common certain energy differentials which would be lacking in the retinal and photochemical images. In view of the physical concept of entropy, it is hard to see how the energy in the cortical image could be in a more highly organized state, with respect to the test object, than the energy in the retinal image. This would be equivalent to obtaining a sharp enlargement from a blurred photographic negative by manipulating the focusing mechanism of the enlarger so as to obtain an 'equal and opposite blur" (pp. 736–737).

5.5.2. Empirical tests of the theory

Entropy can proceed slowly in science, as well as in the Cosmos, and the Marshall-Talbot theory was still under serious consideration, albeit with continuing scepticism, 12 years later, shortly after one of its most basic assumptions, namely, an explicit quantitative functional relationship between cone density at the foveal center and spatial and temporal characteristics of physiological nystagmus, had been discredited in a number of difficult, carefully executed, experiments (Ratliff and Riggs, 1950; Riggs and Ratliff, 1951; Ratliff, 1952; Barlow, 1952; Ditchburn and Ginsborg, 1953). Marshall and Talbot had used the measurements of physiological nystagmus provided by Adler and Fliegelman (1934) to construct their theory. Adler and Fliegelman had used an optical lever with a plane mirror mounted at its fulcrum on the eye to measure fixational eye movements, apparently without appreciating the angular amplification factor of two inherent in this kind of optical arrangement. They reported that the average amplitude of physiological nystagmus was more than 2 minutes of arc – a value that would permit the proximal stimulus produced by an acuity target to flutter over more than 6 foveal cones once cone-to-cone separation in the foveal bouquet was known to be less than 1/4 minute of arc. Polyak (1941) had published such values for the primate retina precisely when such measures of cone density were needed by Marshall and Talbot to support their dynamic theory. Polyak's views of the potential for reciprocal overlap in the afferent pathways arising in the central fovea, however, did not offer direct support of this aspect of their theory (Polyak, p. 431). Adler and Fliegelman had also reported that the frequency of physiological nystagmus was high, ranging from 50 to 100 Hz. This range of frequencies seemed capable of synchronizing with the neural recovery cycle.

Ratliff and Riggs (1950) corrected Adler and Fliegelman's data for their neglect of the optical lever's amplification factor. This reduced the amplitude of physiological nystagmus, actually observed by Adler and Fliegelman, to about one minute of arc. Physiological nystagmus with an amplitude of only one minute of arc would sweep an acuity target image over about 3 foveal cones on average – a rather small sample of receptor elements from which to calculate reliable transient peaks signalling illumination differences – the essential requirement for all later processing proposed in the Marshall-Talbot theory. Fixational eye movement characteristics present additional difficulties for the theory once allowance is made for drifts of the eye and fixational microsaccades, both of which would move critical features of the proximal stimulus onto new receptors – shifts that would broaden the peak of the average transient generated by the moving stimulation. In electrical jargon, DC shifts in average fixation position, produced slowly by drifts or abruptly by microsaccades, would blur the peaks generated by physiological nystagmus, the relatively fast AC component in the fixational eye movement pattern.

Even more troublesome, however, were Ratliff and Riggs's (1950) measurements of physiological nystagmus, which they reported to have a median amplitude of only 17.5 seconds of arc and a frequency ranging from 30 to 70 Hz. The distribution of amplitudes was such that nystagmic movements as large as one minute of arc were rare. The somewhat lower frequency observed by Ratliff and Riggs was not an insurmountable problem because Marshall and Talbot had not worked out the quantitative details required to synchronize physiological nystagmus and the neural recovery cycle. The difference of almost a factor of 7, however, in the average amplitude of physiological nystagmus was critical. Seventeen and a half seconds is about the diameter of a foveal cone in the central bouquet where acuity is best. Physiological nystagmus, the high-frequency fixational eye movement so essential to the dynamic theory of acuity, was actually found to be so small that it seemed unlikely to have any functional significance whatsoever. It would allow the intensity distribution of an acuity target to sweep back and forth over only a single cone – precisely the situation described by Helmholtz almost a century earlier to be incapable of providing the nervous system with a signal indicating a difference in the stimulation in one or another part of the proximal stimulus. Barlow (1952) and Ditchburn and Ginsborg (1953) confirmed Ratliff and Rigg's values, Barlow agreeing with these authors that such results cast doubt on the Marshall-Talbot theory. Ditchburn and Ginsborg, however, thought that although such values did not support the theory, they were, nevertheless, compatible with the theory. This seemingly odd interpretation probably stems from Ditchburn's early committment to an important role for fixational eye movements in visual processing – a preference that would persist and become increasingly difficult to maintain in later years (see Ditchburn, 1980; and Kowler and Steinman, 1980; for an exchange of letters on this point couched in terms of the functional significance of fixational microsaccades – the miniature fixational eye movements that Ditchburn chose to emphasize when he abandoned the functional significance of physiological nystagmus).

5.6. Motor theories of perception after Marshall-Talbot

By the middle of the 1950s, the Marshall-Talbot dynamic theory, which made small high-frequency tremor a necessary condition for visual acuity, was fatally compromised by new measurements of fixational eye movements. These measurements required the development of very sensitive, accurate eye movement measuring instrumentation. This instrumentation was soon elaborated so as to stabilize the retinal image of visual targets – a development that ushered in an era in which a lot of effort was expended in the study of the role of transient stimulation in initiating and maintaining the visibility of simple and complex visual displays. Most of this work was done within a relatively loose theoretical framework. Lessons learned from the fate of the Hecht static and Marshall-Talbot dynamic theories of visual acuity and their derivatives, for example, Jones and Higgins (1948), had apparently tempered enthusiasm for attempting elaborate general theories of basic visual processes as well as compromising physiological nystagmus as an important contributor to basic visual processing. The treatments of more complex visual processes were also influenced by these new measurements of fixational eye movements. For example, Osgood's (1952, 1953) use of what he called the 'statistical theory' to explain 'figural aftereffects' (Köhler and Wallach, 1944) died along with its explanatory base. Osgood's 'statistical theory' was based on the Marshall-Talbot treatment of physiological nystagmus. By the mid 1950s, researchers interested in the role of eye movement in basic visual and more complex perceptual processes, such as the perception of form or size, began to confine interest to the functional significance of saccades and drifts. Only work on basic visual processes will be reviewed in this chapter. Hebb's motor theory of form perception (1949) and Festinger's (1971) 'efferent readiness' theory of visual extent will not be covered (see Steinman, 1976, or Murphy et al., 1974, for a review of this work, and Steinman, 1986b, for comments on more recent efforts; Skavenski (Ch. 5 of this volume) reviews the role of eye movement in the perception of direction and Wallach (Ch. 6 of this volume) reviews the role of eye movement in the perception of motion and shape).

6. Stabilized image research

Experiments with stabilized images were very prominent in the study of spatial vision from their introduction by Ratliff and Riggs in 1950 until the mid-1960s when the new direction of visual science became the application of Fourier analysis to optical problems ('Fourier Optics'). Schade (1956) was the harbinger of this approach for spatial vision, but earlier instances of its use have been cited (cf. Le Grand, 1967). The application of Fourier Optics to temporal factors in vision was pioneered by de Lange (1952, 1954, 1958), followed shortly by Levinson (1960). The application of Fourier Optics to spatial vision – the topic of this chapter – began with studies of image formation by the human eye (Westheimer, 1960), moved inwards to consider the relative importance of neural, as well as optical, factors in limiting spatial resolution (Campbell et al., 1966), and then extended the approach by making psychophysical measurements of the 'spatial modulation transfer function' (the Spatial MTF; currently called the Contrast Sensitivity Function (CSF)) of the human visual system by Campbell and Robson (1964). Thinking of the visual system as a spatial frequency analyser gave rise to the 'channel hypothesis' introduced by Blakemore and Campbell (1969). This hypothesis treats the visual system as though it contained a limited number of band-pass filters tuned to different portions of the spatial frequency distribution. This hypothesis seemed far-fetched to many, perhaps most, visual scientists active at the time. In retrospect such wide-spread scepticism seems unwarranted. The channel hypothesis, despite its novelty, only assumed that the physiological processes underlying spatial vision in the visual system are analogous to the kinds of processes long believed to serve color vision and qualitative dimensions in other sensory systems. To illustrate, a limited number of independent channels, assumed to be only three in both the Young-Helmholtz and Hering theories, had accumulated a good deal of empirical support in the century since the introduction of a 'channel hypothesis' in color vision by Helmholtz, who extended J. Müller's (1826) Doctrine of Specific Nerve Energies to 'hue' – the qualitative dimension in the visual modality. The channel hypothesis also brought theories of spatial vision into line with theories of auditory pitch discrimination. Helmholtz's (1863) auditory 'place' theory assumed a large number of independent neural channels, each tuned to a different temporal frequency of air pressure change, to explain the human being's capacity to discriminate several thousand pitches.

Once viewed in this broad historical perspective, the channel hypothesis, which flowed quite naturally from the attempt to use Fourier Optics in the study of spatial vision, fits in with a long tradition of 'labelled line' sensory theories going back at least to J. Müller. The channel hypothesis will be described in greater detail later after research from the initial period of image stabilization has been reviewed. At this point it is sufficient to note that the shift to Fourier Optics from traditional ways of studying visual acuity forced a change in thinking about spatial vision. In traditional approaches it had been appropriate to pit static theory against dynamic theory – static theories emphasized spatial factors and largely ignored temporal factors; dynamic theories included both but placed greatest emphasis upon the temporal changes caused by physiological nystagmus. This dichotomy ceased to be aesthetically pleasing by the late 1960s because both spatial and temporal properties of visual stimulation were intimately bound together when the new theoretical paradigm was adopted. The relative importance and interactions of these factors, however, in the search for the physiological underpinnings of spatial vision constitute an important area of current concern.

6.1. Early stabilized image research

Most of the specific interests and techniques of the scientists working with stabilized images during the almost 20 years that intervened between the first accurate measurements of the fixational eye movement pattern, which did the Marshall-Talbot theory in, and the beginning of interest in the channel hypothesis can be traced to three sources; Riggs in the USA, Ditchburn in England and Yarbus in the Soviet Union. Developments during the first 10 years were summarized in an unusually perceptive review by Fiorentini (1961) and reviewed again by Heckenmueller (1965) towards the end of this period of greatest initial interest. The material which follows is based, in part, on these reviews. Both reviews provide descriptions of the stabilizing techniques as well as summaries of the visual effects produced by stabilization.

6.1.1. Dependent variables in early research

The two main dependent variables in stabilization research were: (1) the 'disappearance time fraction', i.e. the proportion of time a stabilized image was visible during an experimental run, usually 30 or more seconds in length; and (2) unrestricted phenomenological reports of the appearance of critical features during stabilization. Both have serious methodological limitations. The first cannot be used conveniently to test quantitative models of visual function for reasons described below. The second can be even more troublesome. Phenomenological reports are readily influenced by expectations of the subjects. Such reports can produce reliable scientific information only when done by unusually discerning observers, otherwise providing masses of what, in the long run, amounts to useless speculation. Examples of the latter can be found in the stabilized image literature, where phenomenological reports, widely cited as supporting Hebb's and Gestalt theories of perceptual grouping, were subsequently shown to be more parsimoniously interpreted as response biases inherent in the linguistic constraints on open-ended verbal reports about ambiguous visual stimuli (see Steinman, 1976, for references and comments on this topic, which is beyond the scope of this chapter).

These dependent variables were used frequently in early stabilization research because of severe limitations on the length of experimental sessions. This restriction made it awkward to use traditional psychophysical methodology (see, for example, Woodworth, 1938, Ch. 17). Fechner's Method of Constant Stimuli was, and remains, the generally preferred traditional psychophysical method. This method bases its threshold estimate on hundreds of *independent* observations made in experimental sessions, typically lasting 2 or 3 hours. Such lengthy sessions are usually repeated a number of times to verify the reliability of the estimated threshold. Thresholds estimated in this way have calculable probable errors based on normal curve statistics. A large number of studies have demonstrated the appropriateness of normal curve statistics for the treatment of such independent psychophysical observations. More efficient 'interactive' procedures with known probability interpretations of their threshold estimates have come into use during the last 20 years, e.g. double random staircases, but neither the techniques nor appropriate statistical treatment had been worked out when stabilization research started (see Penner, 1978, for an introduction to the newer methods). The psychophysical procedures with unambiguous statistical treatment, available during the 1950s and early '60s, required a number of long experimental sessions. Contact lenses, fitted so as to be suitable for stabilization, could not be worn for more than 40–60 minutes and normally are not inserted more than once in 24 hours. Yarbus-type suckers placed even greater restrictions on wearing time. Such methodology does not readily lend itself to 'proper' psychophysical threshold measurement. It was these restrictions, rather than indifference to methodology, that encouraged the use of the disappearance time fraction and unrestricted phenomenological reports in most of the early stabilization research. 'Thresholds' are often reported in the old stabilization literature but they are usually based on the length of time a critical feature was visible, for example, the threshold was "the contrast at which the targets would be seen during 50% of the [30 second] viewing period" (Krauskopf, 1957*). The relationship of this kind of threshold measure to thresholds derived from large sets of independent tests with calculable probable errors has not, to our knowledge, been worked out. Ignorance of this relationship makes it risky to use the 'threshold' data from early stabilization experiments to test quantitative visual theories that were based on thresholds measured in traditional ways.

6.2. *Important early results with stabilized images*

The old stabilization literature contains some important generalizable facts about the relationship between eye movement and the perception of contrast and spatial detail. We will describe a few papers from this period in some detail. These papers were chosen because they introduce important ideas and have clear implications for the relationship of eye movements to spatial vision. The reader is directed to the reviews, cited above, for discussion of additional papers in what became a relatively voluminous literature in the period between 1950 and 1965 despite the difficult research methodology.

6.2.1. *Effect of exposure duration on stabilized vision*

Riggs et al. (1953) reported results of a short flash threshold experiment, as well as results from a 50% disappearance time experiment, in which the width of a dark line against a lighted background was varied under normal, stabilized and exaggerated movement conditions. The main results of this seminal experiment have stood the test of time. They also contain an observation, which will be replicated by other investigators, whose significance will not be appreciated for 27 years.

Two 'minimum visible' dark bar visual acuity experiments were reported. The dark bars were images, projected on a magnesium-oxide-coated screen, of wires, oriented vertically, whose visual angles ranged from about 6 to 93 seconds. In the first experiment the disappearance time fraction was measured during one-minute viewing periods. Fractions were measured under three conditions,

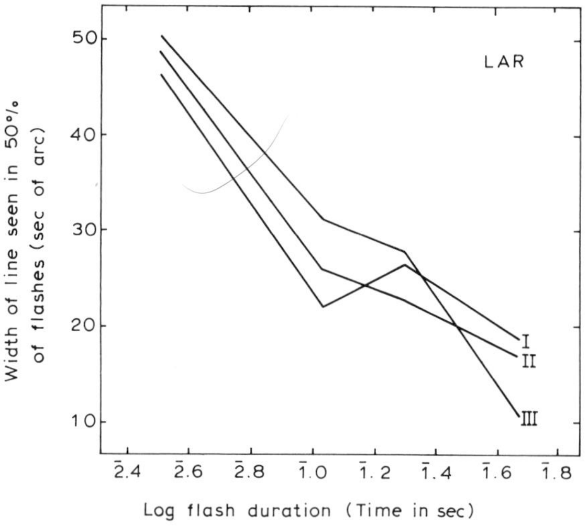

Fig. 6. Width of a line seen during 50% of flashes as a function of flash duration under viewing conditions I (stabilized), II (normal) and III (exaggerated motion, i.e., twice normal). The subject was L. Riggs. (From Riggs et al., 1953)

namely, (I) a horizontally stabilized (compensated) wire seen against a homogeneous, moderately intense (5 ft-L) background, (II) normal, that is, unstabilized viewing of the same stimuli, and (III) twice-normal image motion while viewing the same targets. The results, in the words of the authors, were as follows:

"In Condition I, the 'compensated' condition, the black line target was clearly seen when it first appeared. The subject was surprised by the fact that the line was always at the center of the field regardless of eye movements. Soon, however, the line began to fade out. Finally, it disappeared altogether, so that the projected image seemed to consist only of a bright circular field. Occasionally, the bright field also disappeared; in these intervals the subject saw only the stationary annulus [an unstabilized surround used to keep the stabilized central test area from drifting beyond the operating range of the contact lens optical lever stabilizing apparatus]. A fine black line usually disappeared during the first few seconds of viewing, and failed to reappear later. Heavier lines took longer to disappear and often reappeared from time to time during one minute of

---

* Krauskopf was aware of the fact that thresholds inferred from disappearance-time fractions were not necessarily the same as thresholds measured in traditional psychophysical experiments and provided the rationale he used for drawing this inference. The reader should consult his paper for a description of the assumptions underlying his inferred relationship.

steady fixation.

"In Condition II, the 'normal' condition, the fading of the image did occur for the fine lines, but the lines reappeared sporadically. Heavier lines seldom disappeared.

"In the 'exaggerated' condition, Condition III, there was scarcely any disappearance of even the finest lines. The impression was that the target was 'locked in place' so that steady fixation was effortless, automatic" (p. 498).

In their second experiment flashed targets were used to measure 50% frequency of seeing thresholds. This was a genuine threshold experiment, rarely attempted in this early period. It suffered from limitations imposed by wearing tight-fitting contact lenses. Only 432 judgments for one of the subjects (the senior author) were obtained in two experimental sessions in which there were 18 experimental conditions (6 line widths and 3 viewing conditions) each of which was replicated 24 times – a modest number for estimating a threshold from a psychometric function based on Fechner's Method of Constant Stimuli (100 or more replications for each of the 18 conditions would probably have been obtained if the contact lens had not restricted the length and number of experimental sessions). Four flash durations were used, namely 34, 110, 213 and 472 ms (5 to 7 durations would probably have been used if a contact lens had not been worn).

The results of this flash experiment, summarized in Fig. 6, were described as showing "no striking differences for short flashes among the three experimental conditions. Consistently, however, the 'compensated' image of condition I yielded the best seeing for the shortest flashes. The 'exaggerated' condition, III, begins to excel at exposure durations beyond 0.2 sec. It is of interest to note that in all cases the intermediate Condition II [normal viewing] yields results which lie between those of Conditions I and III" (p. 500).

The conclusions drawn from these experiments are as follows:

"1. Vision is impaired under conditions such that the retinal image of an object remains essentially motionless with respect to the retina. During prolonged viewing under these conditions single-line test objects gradually disappear from view. The rate of disappearance is related [inversely] to the angular width of the line.

"2. Normal involuntary eye movements prevent the disappearance of test objects during long periods of observation. Exaggerated movements of the retinal image [twice as fast as normal movements] are even more effective in preventing the disappearance of images.

"3. In the case of short exposures (less than 0.10 sec) of test objects, the above relations appear to be reversed. Vision is poorer under conditions of normal or exaggerated motion than under conditions of reduced motion of the retinal image" (p. 501).

These conclusions were based on the following considerations. The disappearance of the stabilized target after prolonged viewing is "consistent with the theory that under uniform stimulation conditions each photoreceptor may attain a stationary state in which a minimum number of impulses are initiated in the retina". With shorter exposure durations the situation becomes more complex. When exposure durations are set at or below 10 ms, drifts are too slow to be significant and physiological nystagmus allows the eye to move through only about 5 seconds of visual angle. This discussion rested on a prior fixational eye movement experiment in which Riggs and Armington (1952) had shown that the eye was virtually stationary during 10-ms intervals and only moved about 25 seconds of visual angle during 100-ms intervals (these values would soon be confirmed by Riggs et al., 1954, as is shown in Fig. 7).

With flashes shorter than the exposure interval known as the 'critical duration' (an interval of about 100 ms in which the intensity of the stimulating light and its exposure duration are reciprocally related) the light–time product was held to be the primary determinant of the ability to see a detail. Acuity improved as the light–time product increased with durations shorter than the critical duration because 'the differential responses of stimulated and unstimulated retinal elements [in the proximal stimulus of an acuity target] might be

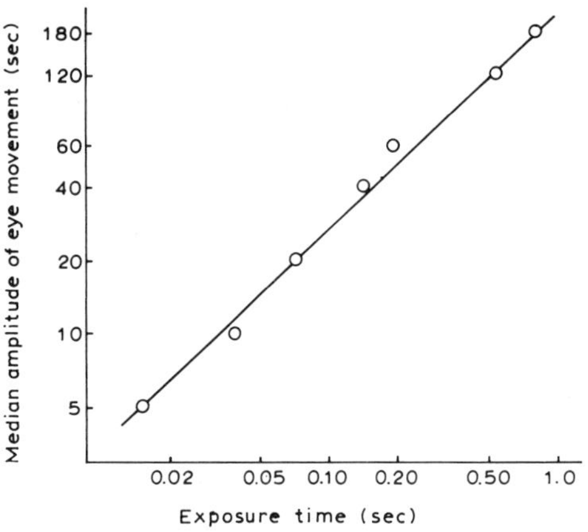

Fig. 7. The median extent of motion of the retinal image as a function of exposure time. (From Riggs et al., 1954)

expected to increase with exposure duration'. This explanation can be sufficient, providing the stimulus remains on the same retinal elements. Cone diameter in the central fovea is only about 18 seconds of visual angle, which means that target details would remain on the same receptors during about two-thirds of the critical duration. Stabilization would be expected to be beneficial for acuity once the exposure duration is sufficient to allow the unstabilized image to begin to move onto new receptors – a result consistent with Ratliff (1952), who reported that eye movements could be detrimental (stabilization helped) when a grating target was exposed for 75 ms. With exposures longer than the critical duration (100–500 ms), there is no longer reciprocity of intensity and time, and the eye can move through a couple of minutes of arc. Here, stabilization is only beneficial up to about 200 ms. Beyond 200 ms *exaggerated* motion of the retinal image leads to the best acuity. When exposure duration is longer than a half second, "eye movements, and even more those of double the amount in Condition III, clearly serve to maintain prolonged seeing. Hartline's experiment on the frog retina lends support to the idea that motion of the retinal image may serve to trigger 'on' and 'off' responses of individual retinal units. . . A brief, but inadequate summary of these points might be to the effect that eye movements are bad for acuity but good for overcoming the loss of vision due to uniform stimulation of the retinal receptors" (p. 501).

Riggs et al.'s (1953) interpretation of their results was described in some detail because it calls attention to two questions that continue to be of interest. First, why does the visual system perform better with exaggerated retinal image motion than with normal retinal image motion? Most, if not all, visual scientists like to believe that evolutionary pressures have tuned physicochemical and physiological processes rather exactly to psychophysical function. Why are normal fixational drift eye movements too slow by a factor of two to be consistent with this popular teleological belief?

Second, Hartline (1938, 1940) reported that only 50% of his frog units were phasic 'on-off'; the units Riggs et al. (1953) credited with maintaining vision with normal, unstabilized input. Prolonged failure to stimulate these units was held to cause the target to disappear. Note, however, that 20% of Hartline's remaining units were tonic 'on' units, similar to the units invariably observed in the horseshoe crab. They burst shortly after stimulus onset, pause and then continue to fire at a reduced rate as long as the stimulating light is present (the other 30% were called 'off' units, bursting when the light went off). Why were Riggs and his coworkers not puzzled by the failure of these tonic units to sustain vision when the image was stabilized? A possibility, not discussed by Riggs and his coworkers, that will come to be of interest subsequently is that the complete disappearance of a stabilized image depends critically on having low-contrast and/or low-intensity test stimuli. Both were modest in their experiment. Such conditions might have rendered the sustained 'on' unit responses subliminal, permitting complete disappearance of the stabilized portion of their display. The question of whether high-luminance, high contrast, foveally centered stabilized targets ever disappear completely will be encountered periodically in subsequent research. This question is still unsettled. We will discuss it further after we have considered the first publication in which the effect of motion, controlled by the experimenter, was imposed on a stabilized acuity target image – currently, a much-touted technique for studying spatial vision.

6.2.2. Motion imposed on stabilized images

Krauskopf (1957) was the first to publish detailed results of this kind of research (he credits Cornsweet and Riggs with a prior report at an Eastern Psychological Association Meeting in 1954). The logic behind this and subsequent work is the desire to control, and thereby simplify, the waveform, frequency and amplitude of retinal image motion while concurrent psychophysical measurements of spatial vision are made. If this can be done, the effect of retinal image motion on spatial vision can be understood. Once such knowledge is at hand, it may then become possible to understand the functional significance of the various motions observed in the natural fixational eye movement pattern.

Krauskopf used the Riggs et al. (1953) contact lens optical lever technique to stabilize his targets. The stabilized targets could be oscillated in a controlled manner by mounting a mirror in the stabilizing optical path on a galvanometer which could be driven by a signal generator. Targets consisted of a bright bar of variable width (10 sec arc, 1, 4 or 8 min arc of visual angle) presented at the center of a 1 degree diameter circular background field of 20 ft-L. This background field was enclosed in a 10 ft-L unstabilized annulus, which prevented the line of sight from drifting outside the range of the optical stabilizing system and also served as the fixation stimulus – the subject being required to maintain his line of sight at its center during tests. The 'contrast' of the test bar (the ratio of its brightness [photometric intensity] to the brightness [photometric intensity] of the background field) was the dependent variable used to estimate 'the 50% contrast threshold'. This 'threshold' was based on the percentage of time a particular target was reported as visible during a 30-s test interval (such threshold estimates require assumptions about the relationship of 'disappearance-time fractions' to 'frequency of seeing' measures; see above). The frequency of the imposed sinusoidal oscillations was varied (1, 2, 5, 10, 20 or 50 Hz) as was the peak-to-peak amplitude of these oscillations, which were 30 sec arc, 1, 2 or 4 min arc of visual angle.

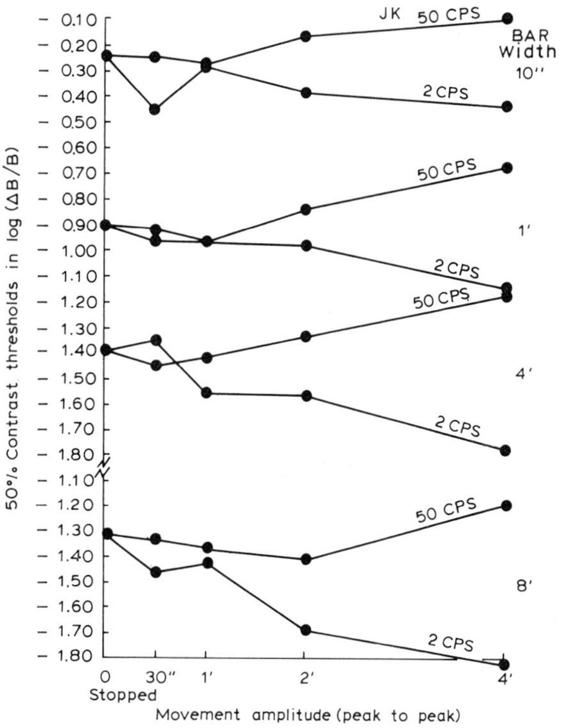

Fig. 8. Fifty percent contrast thresholds as a function of amplitude of vibration of 2 and 50 Hz for four bar widths, ranging between 10″ and 8′ of arc. There were four determinations for each datum point. (From Krauskopf, 1957)

Krauskopf found that "the effect of low-frequency motion [1 and 2 Hz and, to a lesser extent 5 Hz] was to improve seeing while higher frequency [10 Hz and above] had a generally detrimental effect. The curves suggest quite strongly, however, that motions at amplitudes below 1 minute of arc had little effect" (p. 743). He goes on to conclude that "The results of the present experiments as well as those of Cornsweet and Riggs (1954) suggest that the disappearance of stopped [stabilized] images during prolonged viewing is the result of the removal of the low-frequency components of normal retinal image motion. The present results suggest that oscillations at frequencies below 10 cps [Hz] may be constructive if they are of sufficient amplitude. The critical amplitude appears to be in the neighborhood of 1 min of arc (peak-to-peak). High frequency motion on the other hand appears to have detrimental effects. Again it seemed in the present experiments that the amplitude of these motions had to exceed 1 min of arc to have a demonstrable effect on the contrast thresholds" (p. 744). He goes on to point out that "it is dangerous to generalize from experiments with externally controlled sinusoidal motion to the normal fixation case" but ventures, nevertheless, to suggest that physiological nystagmus, whose amplitude is mainly below 1 min of arc, is not likely to be visually effective – a conclusion he treats as consistent with the earlier brief E.P.A. report of Cornsweet and Riggs, who imposed variable-amplitude 30, 50 and 70 Hz sinusoidal oscillations on a stabilized target. Krauskopf did not attempt to extend his results showing that low-frequency imposed motions were visually beneficial to the role of low-frequency fixational eye movements because he adopted the then-current view that "the low-frequency components are much more irregular [than physiological nystagmus]", and ended his elegant paper by leaving open the possibility that these low-frequency movements, along with fixational microsaccades, "may well be beneficial to maintenance of vision": both assumptions will continue to be the subject of some controversy many years later (see Ditchburn, 1980; Kowler and Steinman, 1980).

6.2.3. Exposure duration revisited with a variety of target types

Keesey (1960) examined the effect of stabilization and exposure duration (7 durations, ranging from 20 to 1280 ms) with three types of dark target presented on a lighted background (a single dark bar, two dark bars, one above the other in a vernier arrangement or multiple equally-spaced dark bars, in effect, a square-wave grating). The single dark bar was produced by a thin wire stretched across an aperture filled with collimated light. The grating and vernier targets were photographic negatives which could be mounted in the same aperture. The single bar would have very high contrast; the other targets somewhat less, depending on the photographic film and processing technique used to reproduce the 'opaque' portions of the test stimuli. The intensity of the 58 min arc diameter circular test field and its matched unstabilized annulus was not specified, but it was likely to be at least as high (20 ft-L) as in the Krauskopf (1957) report, described above, which used rather similar optical arrangements, that is, the test field was presented in Maxwellian view (a lens formed an image of the test field at the entrance pupil of the eye).

There were important methodological advances in this doctoral thesis (L. Riggs was chief advisor) in addition to the use of different kinds of acuity target presented with relatively high contrast on backgrounds of relatively high light intensity. Namely, traditional acuity thresholds were estimated by determining the threshold size of the critical spatial detail (the angular subtense of the single dark bar, of the vernier offset or of the bars making up the grating) by means of a 'forced-choice' Constant Stimulus Method. This means that the subject was forced to report a particular property of the test target on each trial. For the single line, its presence at any time during a test exposure was required to be reported, in other words, a single forced 'yes' or 'no'. For the vernier stimulus, the direction, right or left, of the lower segment was required; for the grating its orientation, horizontal or vertical. This kind of psychophysical methodology is still considered to be the optimal way of measuring thresholds, with the exception of the single line target, where its orientation would probably be varied in the same manner as the grating. These were, and remain, very ambitious experiments because a tightly fitting scleral contact lens had to be worn in sessions long enough to make measurements with normal, as well as with stabilized, targets – the design optimal for making valid inferences about effects of stabilization. The difficulties were not simply confined to running many long sessions under uncomfortable conditions. Using target orientation in the forced-choice procedure with the grating required that stabilization had to be achieved on the vertical, as well as on the horizontal, meridian – most previous and subsequent work with stabilized grating targets is less ambitious, confining itself to gratings with vertical bars and stabilization exclusively on the horizontal meridian.

It is not entirely clear from the publication that these stringent demands were completely met. The number of tests of each type of target were not described nor were the total number of replications so it is not possible to determine the number of tests contributing to each of the thresholds reported. There were probably only a modest number because the author found it desirable to report an 'additional' experiment to verify the main result. In this experiment only "two stimuli around threshold size were presented 60 times [in itself a modest number for this kind of measurement] for each of the exposure durations of 0.20, 0.75 and 1.00 sec" [7 durations were used in the basic experiment]. An additional complication can be seen in the fact that only tests with the vertical grating were used for estimating thresholds because there "was often a difference in thresholds between vertical and horizontal orientations of the grating lines." It is possible that these differences arose from the fact that stabilization was less complete on the vertical meridian (the meridian critical for a grating with horizontal lines) than on the horizontal meridian, where vertical lines are the critical detail. We suspect this because one of us knows from personal experience (Steinman, 1965) that it is difficult to orient a contact lens mirror to be exactly orthogonal to a line parallel to the line of sight even when it is 5 or more mm in diameter and mounted on a ball and socket joint at the end of a stalk cemented to the contact lens. It is difficult to imagine how this adjustment would be made and maintained from session to session with the 1.5-mm-diameter mirror embedded in the surface of the contact lens – the arrangement used in Keesey's experiments.

Quibbling aside, the results reported were very orderly, particularly for the single dark bar target. Keesey's graphs for this condition for both of her subjects are reproduced in Fig. 9, where it can be seen that stabilized and normal viewing were affected similarly by exposure duration across the entire range studied. It is also clear that acuity

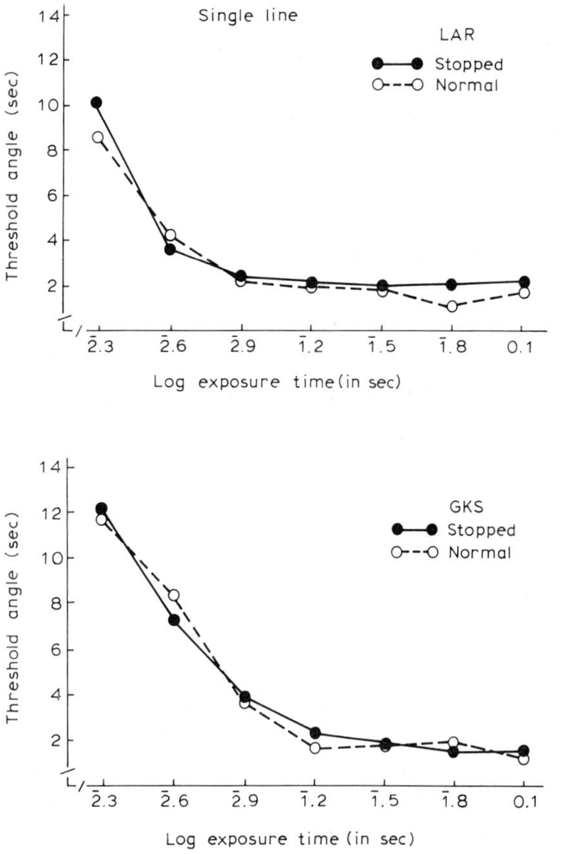

Fig. 9. Threshold curves for detection of single black lines as a function of log exposure time under stabilized (stopped) and normal viewing conditions. (From Keesey, 1960)

asymptotes to its best value at about 200 ms. Keesey "noted that for the relatively short stimulus durations used in this study no disappearance of targets was reported. A few isolated exceptions were the disappearance of very fine lines during the 1.280 sec exposure time with the stabilized image condition" (p. 772). Her results with the vernier and grating targets led to the same conclusion although the performance of her second subject, GKS, was less orderly than LAR with these test stimuli. At this point once it had been shown that acuity was the same with stabilized targets as it was when normal eye movement was permitted, it was possible to conclude that "acuity is mainly based on the discrimination of the spatial pattern of retinal illumination, regardless of any temporal changes of intensity pattern on the receptor cells" – clearly, a complete refutation of dynamic theory, Weymouth as well as Marshall-Talbot.

6.2.4. But were retinal images really stabilized?
Barlow (1963) was not convinced that they were and published a paper which stirred up appreciable controversy, both about the appearance of stabilized images and about the merits of alternative methods of stabilizing images. Prior to his report, both facts and methods had seemed to be relatively well-established. Barlow undertook his research because he felt that the results obtained by the main groups investigating stabilized images (the groups led by Ditchburn, Riggs and Yarbus) "are not in good agreement" with each other or with "information available as to what happens when a pattern of light is held unchanged on the retina". He pointed out that a variety of entoptic images (percepts arising from features located within the eyeball), such as the shadows of small retinal blood vessels made visible by moving a small point source of light or by light shining through the sclera, only remain visible for very short periods when the conditions required to render them visible in the first instance are maintained. Other entoptic phenomena such as Maxwell's spot and Haidinger's brushes show similar characteristics. The disappearance of such intrinsically stabilized images is rapid, complete and persistent. Observations such as these suggest that steady, unchanging stimulation produces only a short-lived percept which can only be reinstated by changing the stimulation once the initial percept has faded. Barlow also pointed out that the situation with visual afterimages is similar. They lose their fine details and then fade out completely. Periodic blinks or flashes of light are required to bring them back into view once they have disappeared. These well-known properties of entoptic images led Barlow "to the clear expectation that any arbitrary pattern of light held stationary on the retina will fade and cease to be visible within a few seconds of first presentation, but only Yarbus's results fit in with this." Both Ditchburn's and Riggs's group had reported that stabilized images disappear relatively slowly and reappear periodically, results at variance with the expectation from both entoptic phenomena and Yarbus's reports (1957a,b).

Very different stabilizing techniques were being used. Both Ditchburn and Riggs used a tight-fitting scleral contact lens to place a mirror at the fulcrum of an optical lever designed to stabilize targets located in the optical path. Their optical instruments usually incorporated provisions for convenient control of critical properties of test stimuli, such as their contrast, size or motion. These instruments were also typically laid out so as to make it convenient to alternate normal with stabilized viewing of the same target. Their research scleral contact lenses were fitted so as to rest on the limbus (the margin of the cornea and sclera). Pressing such lenses into place establishes suction between the lens and the eye, sometimes making the lens hard to remove after it has been worn for a half hour or so.

Yarbus's method was completely different. He used a rubber 'sucker' to establish negative pressure in a lightweight aluminum cone ('cap') whose base had serrated edges that rested on the margins of the cornea near the limbus. A high-power ('short focus') positive lens, mounted at the apex of the cap, allowed the subject to see a focused stimulus object located very near the eye. These stimulus objects were stabilized by attaching them to the aluminum cap by means of a girder. When the eye moved, the object moved with it, providing, of course, that the girder was rigid and the aluminum cap stayed in place on the eye (see Barlow, 1963, for additional details, or Yarbus, 1967, for a complete treatment of his method and findings). Yarbus's method, unlike the contact lens optical lever, does not allow convenient control of properties of test stimuli, but it may have at least one distinct advantage, namely, it stabilizes the stimulus far better, at least according to Barlow. Unfortunately, Barlow's conclusion rests on experiments in which he confounded characteristics of these quite different methods – a problem (explained below) that Riggs and Schick (1968) would subsequently suggest contributed importantly to Barlow's conclusion. Barlow's paper, however, includes a number of important observations about the appearance and possible physiological underpinnings of stabilized images as well as a number of criticisms of Yarbus's method. For these reasons Barlow's paper will be described in some detail despite the fact that his rejection of the scleral contact lens does not apply to its use in an optical lever.

Barlow prepared scleral contact lenses of "the type ordinarily used for stabilized image work, with a close fit at the limbus." He then painted an artificial pupil on the perspex (acrylic) contact lens, and molded the corneal portion so as to form a 40 D supplementary lens. A short aluminum tube, which was cemented around the pupil, was extended on one side to form a girder used to hold a target in focus 25 mm in front of the eye. These additions to the scleral lens, particularly the aluminum tube and girder with a target at its end, seem certain to apply much larger, potentially dislodging, forces on the contact lens than a beam of light falling on a small mirror at the fulcrum of an optical lever – the method introduced by Riggs and Ditchburn. Barlow's modifications of the Yarbus sucker cap were more modest, but important nevertheless. The basic cap was similar to Yarbus's. It was made of aluminum and had a rubber sucker glued over a hole pierced near its narrow anterior end. The cap carried a girder which was used to mount targets 15 – 25 mm in front of the eye. The main differences were the kind of short-focus lens (Barlow's were planoconvex with the flat side towards the target) and the fact that the cap was filled with a 1.5% solution of $NaHCO_3$ rather than with air, the filler used by Yarbus. The fluid filling made Barlow's caps heavier than Yarbus's (350 rather than 100 mg) but their optical quality was reported to be much better than could be achieved by following Yarbus's method.

An afterimage technique was used to examine the effectiveness of the two types of stabilizing method, first qualitatively, then quantitatively. The quality of stabilization was examined by making a persistent afterimage in the shape of an arrowhead by presenting a brief intense light in Maxwellian view through an aperture mounted on the contact lens or sucker cap. An occluder which had covered a portion of the visual field when the afterimage was made was then removed, exposing a transilluminated aperture in the shape of an arrowhead with its point facing and lined up with the point of the afterimage. If the contact lens or sucker cap did not move relative to the eye, the two points of the arrowheads should stay in alignment despite movements of the eye. Barlow found that relative movements were "unmistakenly detected" during attempts at maintained fixation, as well as when the subject looked around, when the contact lens was used to stabilize the transilluminated arrowhead. Relative movements were much less with the sucker cap and when they occurred "they are most often caused by the rim. . . touching the eye-lid." During large eye movements with the sucker cap, relative motion was observed, but at the end of each large eye movement the original relationship was restored.

Quantitative estimates of the effectiveness of stabilization were obtained by making two afterimages of a target, separated by several seconds, under conditions in which a failure of stabilization would produce a displacement of a feature in the composite afterimage whose extent could be measured psychophysically. Barlow accomplished this by mounting a target with a long straight edge on one or the other stabilizing device and first produced an afterimage of one half of the edge, waited 4 or 5 seconds, and then produced an afterimage of the other half of the edge. If the stabilizing device did not change position on the eye during the interval, an afterimage with a single continuous straight edge would be seen. If, however, the device changed position on the eye in the interval, the second afterimage would be offset from the first and a single long straight edge would not be seen. The size of the offset of the edge in the composite afterimage would indicate the extent to which the stabilizing device had slipped during the 4- or 5-s interval. A rotatable polaroid was used to deliver light to each half of the straight edge independently without disturbing the location of either the target or its stabilizing device.

When both afterimages had been made, the subject removed the stabilizing device from his eye and adjusted the projected image of a step of variable size to be the same size as the offset seen in his composite afterimage. The subject viewed the projected variable-step display and his composite afterimage simultaneously on a screen located at about arm's length. Using this technique, the estimated r.m.s. deviation of the contact lens relative to the eye was more than 3 minutes of arc. The sucker cap was much better. Its r.m.s. deviation was well under 1 minute of arc. Barlow concluded that "the full-fitting type of contact lens does not stabilize the image adequately" and proceeded to use his version of the Yarbus sucker cap to study the appearance of stabilized images. He also discussed a number of potentially important artifacts associated with this device. This discussion of artifacts will be summarized next because they bear on Yarbus's prior work and also because they provided a useful guide for subsequent investigators who used a Yarbus-type sucker cap (most notably Gerrits and his collaborators).

6.2.5. Artifacts in Yarbus's method

Before considering Barlow's concerns with potential artifacts in Yarbus's method, it is worth noting that Barlow reported that his version of the Yarbus sucker cap was not perfectly fixed upon the eye. Its variability (r.m.s. deviation) during 4- or 5-s intervals was somewhat more than a half minute of arc. Barlow's sucker cap performed much better than his scleral contact lens carrying the same loads, but the sucker cap only reduced retinal image motion. It did not eliminate retinal image motion entirely. How good does stabilization have to be before it is good enough to guarantee that functionally effective transient stimulation, sufficient to drive visual neurons, has been eliminated? Barlow did not deal with this question explicitly. His discussion, however, assumes that his version of Yarbus's method, unlike the method of Riggs and Ditchburn, would be good enough. Later, we will describe Arend and Timberlake's (1986) recent theoretical calculations, which show that Barlow's assumption, made by other contemporary and subsequent investigators as well, was unwarranted.

Barlow's other concerns, concerns which encouraged him to modify Yarbus's method, stem primarily from optical considerations. The inner surface of the supplementary lens mounted at the end of a sucker cap "steams up very rapidly unless the lens is first warmed, and this only delays it for about ½ minute." Also, the suction used to hold the cap to the eye changes the shape of the cornea. Changes in the shape of the cornea change the focus of the eye. If the target is in focus when the sucker is first attached, it will be out of focus somewhat later. Barlow eliminated both problems by filling his sucker cap with a solution of bicarbonate. Chromatic aberration can also be a problem with a sucker cap. It is is not significantly greater with a Riggs- or Ditchburn-type of scleral lens optical lever than with the unencumbered eye because this method does not require a short-focus supplementary lens. Chromatic aberration becomes a problem, however, when a short-focus lens is added to the optics of the eye, an eye which already has some chromatic aberration, because "its own aberration will be added to that of the eye, and is liable to become the limiting factor [in resolving details]. The additional error is greater the shorter the focal length, which is why lenses at ca. 20 mm have been used rather than 5–10 mm as favoured by Yarbus" (p. 42). Barlow used a zinc-crown glass planoconvex supplementary lens with its curved surface immersed in $NaHCO_3$ to reduce the chromatic aberration introduced by the positive surfaces of the glass. Yarbus sometimes used pinhole apertures to reduce aberrations, but Barlow points out that this technique severely compromises image quality because of diffraction effects.

There are other potential artifacts which cannot be easily circumvented with the Yarbus sucker cap. Barlow mentions trans-scleral light, which could reduce the contrast in the stabilized image. Trans-scleral light can be reduced with a scleral contact lens simply by painting the scleral portion with an opaque substance such as several coats of black acrylic paint. With a sucker cap the sclera is completely exposed and trans-scleral light could reduce contrast in the retinal image, depending on its intensity and the optical arrangements used to illuminate the target. Reducing contrast could have important consequences for the time-course and ultimate appearance of a stabilized image. It is probably worth noting, before going on to report Barlow's description of the appearance of stabilized images free from misting and serious optical aberrations, that he procured these improvements by adding appreciably to the forces applied to the sucker cap. His fluid-filled cap was 3 times heavier and the lever used to support the target was 2–4 times longer than Yarbus's.

6.2.6. The subjective appearance of stabilized images

Barlow, having convinced himself that previous reports were suspect because of either poor stabilization or poor optical quality and that he had reduced or eliminated both problems, undertook to provide a description of the appearance of stabilized images. His description is somewhat at variance with previous reports. In his words: "When one inspects an image of good contrast and optical quality, moderate retinal illumination (say 1 to 100 Trolands) and as well stabilized as we are able to achieve, it is seen with full clarity only for the first few seconds, at the end of which time it lacks some of the fine detail and contrast of the original. There is then a period of a minute or so during which its appearance fluctuates, disappearing and regenerating in a way that will be described later. Finally these fluctuations die out, leaving a stable appearance or a fog or grey sky with ill-defined dark and light clouds in it corresponding to the white and black parts of the original image. This final state, a very blurred, very low contrast version of the original image, seems to persist without fluctuation for as long as conditions are held unchanged. On the occasions when it has disappeared, the cornea has been found to be misted, or the lens smeared, on removing the contact lens [sucker cap]" (p. 43).

"In summary then, stabilized images both fade and regenerate, but they do not fade completely, for after several minutes a cloudy, low contrast form of the original persists, and they do not regenerate completely, for there is an initial 'blurring' or loss of detail and contrast that is never regained" (p. 45).

The main differences with previous reports were his failure to observe complete disappearance of all features of the stimulus, the persistent blurring of sharp details, which did not sharpen when the stimulus regenerated, and regeneration itself. His observations were most at variance with those of Yarbus, who had described complete disappearance without reappearance. The main differences with Riggs's and Ditchburn's groups was their observation of the reappearance of fine details and high contrast following regeneration. Barlow felt that these differences called attention to shortcomings in their scleral contact lens method. Barlow was able to repeat his observations after homatropinizing the eye, which showed that his observation of blurring and regeneration was not caused by fluctuations in accommodation of the crystalline lens. The differences with Yarbus are ascribed to the poor optical quality of Yarbus's stimulus, with some emphasis on trans-scleral light, both of which could reduce the contrast of Yarbus's displays. Barlow believed that Yarbus's failure to observe regeneration and to achieve complete disappearance resulted from the poor quality of Yarbus's stabilized retinal images. Barlow next has to explain his failure to satisfy his own criterion for achieving adequate stabilization, namely, the failure to observe complete disappearance, which he initially described as a characteristic of all entoptic phenomena. These intrinsically stabilized images disappear rapidly and completely (see section 6.2.4). He ascribes the failure to meet his initial criterion to the fact that the details in the entoptic percepts are very small, of low contrast and in some instances arise outside the central fovea – in many ways the same kind of reasons he uses to explain Yarbus's result which is congruent with the expectation from observations of entoptic phenomena.

Barlow next offers neurophysiological speculations for a number of his observations. He suggests a 'diffusion process' in the retina of the kind proposed by Brindley (1962) to account for the blurring and loss of detail observed in the stabilized image. A 'two-channel hypothesis', that is, 'a dual system of fibres connecting eye and brain' is proposed to explain other observations. The first is a rapidly adapting [transient] channel which signals changes in illumination in small retinal regions relative to the average signal arising from larger regions. "These units would signal an approximation to the spatio-temporal derivative of the light, $-\delta(\delta^2 i/\delta x^2+\delta^2 i/\delta y^2)/\delta t$, and would have properties similar to the on-centre and off-centre units of the cat's retina . . . The second channel is a slow- or non-adapting channel [sustained] which would serve as the mechanism subserving the 'dim clouds' which appear after prolonged stimulation, and are correctly related to real luminance of parts of the visual field" (p. 49).

6.2.7. Krauskopf's ring-disk experiment

In the same year that Barlow published his paper comparing the Yarbus and Riggs-Ditchburn stabilization methods, Krauskopf (1963) reported an experiment in which he showed that stimulation by a moving edge was critical for maintaining perception of the color within the region circumscribed by the edge. Krauskopf traced his interest in this problem to observations by Liebmann (1927), who had reported that equally bright patches of different color were unstable when viewed for prolonged periods, and to Ditchburn and his coworkers (Ditchburn, 1957; McCree, 1960; Clowes, 1962), who had reported that stabilization had different effects on lights taken from various parts of the visible spectrum. Krauskopf did his experiment by using a Lummer-Brodhun cube from a *Macbeth Illuminometer* to produce a ring of one color surrounding a disk of another color. Four relatively narrow-band chromatic stimuli, selected from the long, middle and short wavelength portions of the visible spectrum, were employed. A Riggs-type optical lever stabilized the light passing through the Lummer-Brodhun cube. A field stop (aperture), which was placed near the outer edge of the approximately 2 degree stabilized test field, destabilized the outer edge of the ring surrounding the disk. Neutral density wedges were used to match the luminance of the chromatic stimuli under normal fixation conditions, that is, conditions in which the ring and disk were not stabilized. All possible combinations of the four wavelengths as rings and disks were used. Each ring-disk combination was presented for 30 seconds, the subject pressing a key whenever he saw the disk and releasing the key whenever the disk disappeared. A disappearance-time fraction, based on these key-presses, provided the dependent variable Krauskopf used to evaluate reports that effects of stabilization varied with spectral locus.

Krauskopf "found that when the image is stabilized, the inner boundary which is stabilized disappears, the central disk taking on the color of the annulus. Thus in a case in which the observer saw initially a red disk on a green annulus he reported that after disappearance he saw a large green disk. . . Another mode of appearance was reported when the disk luminance was greater than that of the annulus. Under this condition the observer reported that the border between the disk and the annulus became uncertain and irregular in shape. The simplest description of the result is that the central color seemed to spill out through the border and invade the annulus" (p. 742). His analyses of the disappearance-time fraction data did not permit any simple generalizations about effects of stabilization on combinations of colored lights selected from different parts of the visible spectrum.

6.2.8. Gerrits's elaboration of Yarbus's method

Gerrits, De Haan and Vendrik (1966) introduced important refinements of the stabilization technique developed by Yarbus. They eliminated two of Barlow's criticisms of Yarbus's method, namely, fluctuations of accommodation and the accumulation of water on the inner surface of the air-spaced compensatory lens which Yarbus mounted on his sucker cap. Fluctuating accommodation would allow the target to come in and out of focus, making it less and then more likely to disappear when stabilized. Reports of fluctuating target appearances could be caused by fluctuations in accommodation rather than from more central visual processes associated with stabilization. Similarly, water condensed on the inner surface of the high-power compensatory lens would reduce the contrast of the test stimulus, making it more likely to disappear rapidly when stabilized and to remain invisible throughout a subsequent long period of stabilization. In short, condensed water could lead to reports of complete and persistent disappearance, which would not be observed if water had not accumulated during the experimental run. The first problem was eliminated, as Barlow had suggested, by instilling a mydriatic drug into the eye. This has the effect of dilating the pupil as well as almost eliminating changes in accommodation of the crystalline lens. The second problem was eliminated by flowing warm water, which kept the compensatory lens near body temperature, through a tube wrapped around the cone of the sucker cap.

Gerrits et al. (1966) also made a number of other elaborations of the Yarbus-Barlow technique. For example, they used a threaded tube, rather than an aluminum lever, to mount their target objects on the sucker cap. The threaded tube allowed the observer to make fine adjustments in the focus of the test object so as to render its image subjectively sharp. They also used ingenious hydraulic drivers to impose linear unidirectional and random motions on a test object mounted on the sucker cap. In subsequent research Gerrits and Vendrik (1970) developed a miniature synchronous electric motor, which was mounted on the sucker cap and used to impose rotational and 'jumping' motions. They also began to take care to eliminate trans-scleral light, which reduces target contrast, in line with another of Barlow's (1963) suggestions (see Fig. 10 for diagrams of this remarkable instrumentation).

As the reader might suspect, the instrumentation illustrated in Fig. 10 was heavy (almost 10 g by 1970) and Gerrits and his coworkers found it necessary to make observations only while in a supine position; these devices would move around and even fall off if the observer sat up. Inconvenience and unsuitability for a wider variety of visual stimuli eventually led to the retirement of the elaborate instruments diagrammed in Fig. 10. Gerrits and Vendrik (1972, 1974) devised a replacement by mounting the end of a fiber optic bundle on their version of the Yarbus-type sucker cap. The bundle, which provided a visual field subtending about 13 degrees of visual angle, contained 160000 fibers, each fiber subtending about 1.8 minutes of arc (about 5 times the diameter of a cone at the foveal center). Individual fibers had been dissected free of the relatively stiff protective outer plastic sheath for a distance of several centimeters so as to permit a reasonable range of eye movements when the dissected end of the fiber optic bundle, which was cemented into a metal band, was inserted into a tube mounted at the end of the sucker cap. The other end of the fiber optic bundle 'looked at' the face of a TV display upon which a variety of stationary or moving test stimuli could be presented. The weight and stiffness of the dissected end of the fiber optic bundle was such as to require the observer to maintain a supine position. It is important to note that in all the research with the fiber optic bundle the diameter of the individual fibers "is larger than the visual resolution of the cone system (fovea). Therefore the moving contours of the stimuli used had to be located out of the fovea, where individual fibers were no longer observable" (Gerrits and Vendrik, 1974, p. 176). Stabilization of targets confined to the foveal floor, or even more importantly to the 20 min arc foveal bouquet where the retinal mosaic is at its finest, has never to our knowledge been accomplished with the Yarbus-type methodology, the methodology believed by some to be capable of the best possible stabilization, at least since Barlow's report. More will be said about this later in section 6.2.10.

6.2.9. Main observations of Gerrits and his coworkers

They reported that "once the perception of a stabilized image has disappeared it does not come back as long as the subject is capable of preventing large rapid eye movements. Trained subjects can achieve an uninterrupted absence of perception for at least ten minutes" (Gerrits et al., 1966, p. 434). In

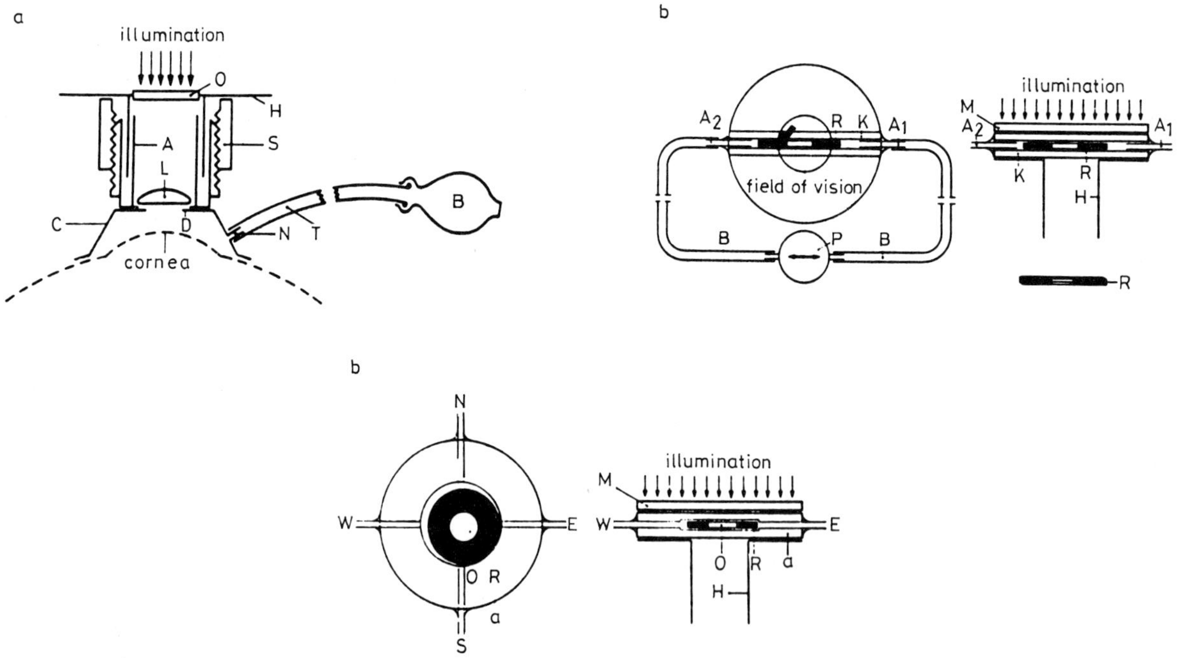

Fig. 10. (a) A standard cap sucked onto the eye (not drawn to scale). The object holder, H, with the object, O, can be changed during the experiment. The weight of the cap is 2.2 g and the object in its holder adds another 0.5 g. A is a non-reflecting black tube, B is a bulb, C is a dural cone, D is a diaphragm, L is a 50 diopter lens, N is a connector, S is a screw and T is a flexible tube. (b) System used to obtain movement in one direction of a stabilized object. The weight of the object in its holder is 2.1 g. A_1, A_2 are tubing connectors, B are flexible tubes, K is an acrylic (perspex) channel, M is an opaline plate, P is a volume pump and R is an acrylic (perspex) rod. (c) System used to obtain random movements in all directions of an otherwise stabilized object. The weight of the object in its holder was 2.7 g. N, E, W and S are four inlets. R is a black annulus, O is a hole, M is an opaline plate and G is an acrylic (perspex) leader. (From Gerrits et al., 1966)

their next experiment with the synchronous electric motor mounted on the sucker cap (Gerrits and Vendrik, 1970), they studied the effect of motion imposed on a stabilized target. They operated the motor in ways that they believed imitated "the drift, the saccadic and the tremor movements of the eye, and studied their influence on perception. It was found that drift-imitating movements regenerate (fill in) a disappeared object. The movements imitating saccades and tremor were never effective in restoring vision" (p. 1455). These conclusions seem reasonable for drifts and tremor, but are less clear with respect to a role for saccades. Gerrits and Vendrik (1974) made quantitative estimates of the drift motions optimal for preserving perception in a subsequent experiment in which they used their fiber optic stimulating bundle. They found that mean drift-like image speeds of about 22 minutes of arc per second were optimal for preserving the perception of a stabilized object. They duly noted that this speed, "which is very effective in preserving perception, is higher than the mean speed of [natural] eye drifts (1–6′/sec)" (p. 178). Remember that Riggs et al. (1953) also found that doubling (in their case) 'natural' retinal image motion was more effective than natural image motion in preserving perception (see section 6.2.1). We will encounter this mysterious fact again before its significance is appreciated.

By 1978 Gerrits found himself at variance with other investigators with respect to the effect of such stimulus properties as the order of fading in the peripheral and foveal retina, the importance of boundaries in the stabilizing field, the number of cycles and duration of tests when the target was a spatial frequency grating. His discussion of this problem is useful because it calls attention to persistent problems in stabilized image research – problems that are still unresolved. He pointed out that discrepancies between stabilized image researchers with respect to details of stimulus properties are often found in experiments in which the investigators also fail to obtain fading for long periods of time. He fears that such "discrepancies can be understood by an incomplete, insufficient stabilization (Barlow, 1963). One should be very careful before attributing effects to [targets stabilized on] foveal cells: an extremely high degree of stabilization is demanded to prevent conclusions to be drawn from small artefacts some of which prove to be very effective in the foveal area but remain invisible in the periphery. The difference in movement sensitivity [between the fovea and the periphery] is even a common observation in non-stabilized conditions. It is very easy to limit voluntarily one's eye movements, the larger amplitudes can be suppressed. As a result the image fades in the periphery, in the areas containing the largest elements [receptive fields] (Troxler's effect). After a short training smaller and smaller amplitudes of eye movements can be suppressed too, also by naive subjects (Winterson and Collewijn, 1976), even down to the microsaccades (Steinman et al., 1967, 1973). This results in further shrinkage in the visual field, down to the fovea. An image with contours in the foveal area never fades by voluntary effort because it is impossible to suppress the remaining miniature eye movements, e.g., the drifts. The influence of these, particularly effective in the foveal area, can only be fully cancelled by excellent stabilization. However, when no stimulus contours are present in the foveal area, e.g., in the case of a large stimulus covering the fovea, even the foveal (filled-in) brightness percept can be made to fade by voluntary effort. The percept is restored by a saccade of large amplitude" (pp. 239–240).

Gerrits, Stassen and van Erning's (1984) recent extension and summary of almost 20 years of research on stabilized images in Nijmegen concluded that "drifts are capable of preserving the perception of stimuli in and around the fovea but not stimuli with contours far outside the fovea". It is important to realize, however, that their conclusion of the necessity for saccades with large stimulus patterns, whose edges fall far away from the fovea, is based on observations made while the observer was lying as still as possible with his head supported artificially. We shall see later that this methodologically imposed constraint, immobility of everything except the eyeball, in stabilized image research obscured important properties of normal visual processing until very recently.

Before we close this section on the Nijmegen School of Stabilization, we feel that it is important for the reader to realize that no instrumentation so far devised has freed the stabilized image investigator from making a great many subjective decisions about the merit and purity of particular observations. Much of the stabilized image research literature rests on the finesse and skill of the observer, almost always one of the investigators. In many instances the observation of stabilized images developed into a highly stylized performing art. This was particularly true when subjective reports, rather than thresholds, provided the primary or only basis for discussion and theory (our nervousness about the role of artistry in visual science was discussed in section 6.1.1). Gerrits and his coworkers were aware of the highly subjective nature of many of their reports and went out of their way to give the reader indications of the kind of observational skills and judgement upon which their reports were based. Consider, for example, the following quotation from the method section of Gerrits (1978) in which he describes the use of the fiber optic stimulator:

"Most of the results to be described have been obtained from two highly trained subjects; one investigated these effects for 2 years, the other for 4 years. A number of other subjects participated occasionally in the experiments. When the cap is sucked on the eye of the subject, the image of the object does not, in most cases, fade within a few seconds after the light is switched on. The subject starts to bring the image in focus and thereafter looks for the most comfortable yet satisfactory position of his head as well as his eyes in his head. He changes his line of sight until no on- and off-borders (caused by small shifts of the cap over the eye) are generated any more and the image fades easily. Small shifts causing destabilization will occur if the object holder touches the subject's nose or eyebrow, if the small rubber tubes supplying warm water and the underpressure [suction] exert a pulling force on the cap and, particularly, when an unquiet subject moves his eyes too much. Just by looking to the relative position of the on- and off-borders a trained observer is able to correct a wrong direction within a few minutes and to keep this most comfortable" (Gerrits, 1978, p. 227).

The instrumentation in Nijmegen never progressed to the point where less skill and training was required. To illustrate, Gerrits et al. (1984) report that "The stiff protecting mantle of the fiber bundle was removed over a length of 30 cm in order to allow the bundle to follow the subject's eye movements. These eye movements did not affect the position of the image on the subject's retina as long as the suction cap adhered well to his eye. The optic fiber bundle had, however, a small braking effect and therefore could cause slippage.

"To enable the subject to distinguish between a percept generated by a genuine stimulus movement or by an unwanted slippage of the suction cap, a small black disc at the end of a non-moving stalk was placed in front of the color TV display. This disc functioned as a control spot relative to the moving square [the stabilized test target upon which movement would be imposed] and enabled the center of the square to be projected onto the fovea before the onset of the movement of the square" (pp. 447–448).

6.2.10. In defense of the contact lens

Barlow's (1963) paper on stabilization methodology did not force the contact lens into retirement despite the impetus it provided for Gerrits and his coworkers to undertake a long line of research based on the sucker cap method introduced by Yarbus. Barlow's comparison of the stability of the contact lens and the sucker cap was fair only when both of these devices were used to hang a relatively heavy optical stimulator at the end of a lever which extended a centimeter or two in front of the eye. Contact lenses were first used in this way by Ditchburn and Pritchard (1956). Their method had begun to gain popularity because of its relative simplicity when Barlow undertook his study. Barlow did not test Riggs's optical lever stabilization technique, in which only a lightweight mirror is mounted on or within the surface of the scleral contact lens. Free-standing optical elements provide the compensating path required for image stabilization in the Riggs-type apparatus. These arrangements meant that the forces applied to the contact lenses were very small as compared to the forces applied to the contact lens in the Ditchburn-Pritchard-type apparatus tested by Barlow. Riggs and Schick (1968) pointed out this limitation in Barlow's experiment when they borrowed his afterimage method to measure the stability of a scleral contact lens when it is used at the fulcrum of an optical, rather than mechanical, lever (see section 6.2.5).

They modified Keesey's (1960) visual acuity apparatus (see section 6.2.3) to allow vernier-offset measurements between an afterimage and a stabilized image. The configuration of these two images was arranged so as to provide a vernier acuity test target in which vernier acuity could be used to estimate changes in the position of the contact lens. The vernier acuity test target consisted of a dark rectangular afterimage, whose long side was vertical, and a stabilized dark bar of the same size and shape. The afterimage was made by viewing a strobe-flash through a bar-shaped aperture while the aperture was in vernier alignment with the stabilized dark bar. The horizontal alignment of the stabilized dark bar with respect to the afterimage could be adjusted by the subject so as to eliminate any observed offset in their vertical alignment. Data were considered to have merit during trials in which the dark negative afterimage was sharp and the vernier alignment was good at the beginning of the experimental run (the aperture and dark bar were aligned by the subject just before he fired the strobe). Experimental runs lasted as long as the afterimage remained clear (20 to 80 s after the strobe-flash). The afterimage was kept visible by flickering the background field illumination about once each second. If the contact lens moved with respect to the eye during the experimental run, the adjustable dark bar, which was stabilized by reflection from the contact lens mirror, would change its vernier-offset relative to the afterimage. The subject's task was to adjust the offset, whenever necessary, so as to bring the configuration back into vernier alignment.

Control measurements, made with a real unstabilized bar substituted for the afterimage, showed that the vernier tracking error (standard deviations of offset corrections for offsets introduced by the experimenter rather than by contact lens slippage) was less than 11 seconds of visual angle for each of the three subjects. This level of precision was clearly adequate for the proposed measurements of contact lens stability, which, based on Barlow's report (1963), should be 5 to 16 times larger (see section 6.2.4). Riggs and Schick's (1968) main measurements consisted of offset-error position corrections of the stabilized bar relative to the afterimage. These measurements were made while the subject attempted to minimize large eye movements – the mode of viewing subjects would employ during a typical experiment on stabilized images (see section 6.2.8). Data were also collected when the two more experienced subjects made saccades of known magnitudes (up to 6 degrees), the subject making alignment adjustments before and after each saccade. In this experiment the stability of the contact lens was inferred by calculating the differences between measurements made before and after saccades. Measurements were also made over extended periods of time by substituting an unstabilized bar for the afterimage and tracking the vernier relationship between the stabilized and unstabilized dark bars for a half hour with offset corrections made every 3 minutes.

Each subject made about 50 tracking records and the median standard deviations of image displacements were about 23 and 25 seconds of arc for the two more experienced subjects and about 35 seconds of arc for the less experienced subject. The average shifts in image displacement were slightly smaller. The shifts in image displacement associated with voluntary saccades were also less than a minute of arc. The long-term drift of the position of the contact lens was slow. Its speed ranged from about 6 to 15 seconds of visual angle/minute. Riggs and Schick (1968) suggested that the continuance of slow drift of the contact lens over long periods of time can be "explained in part by the fact that the eyeball changes shape over extended periods of wearing a tightly fitting lens". The authors go on to discuss the "extent to which numerous earlier studies of eye movements and stabilization may have been affected by errors of the magnitude reported" when they, conservatively, take the magnitude of contact lens slippage to be about half a minute of arc for relatively short-term stabilization. They conclude that error of this magnitude "is not sufficiently large to be of much significance in work with stabilized images" (p. 165). Their conclusion rests primarily on the report of Krauskopf (1957; see section 6.2.2) and Riggs et al. (1961), who reported that motions of the retinal image smaller than 1 minute of arc are not sufficient either to prevent disappearance of a stabilized target or to cause regeneration of a stabilized target which has disappeared. They also cite work by Ditchburn and his coworkers in support of the conclusion that retinal image motions smaller than one minute of visual angle have no consequences for vision.

Riggs and Schick include important comments on the expected appearance of entoptic phenomena in their paper. They note that complete disappearance of entoptic images, whose images are intrinsically stabilized, does not provide convincing evidence that failure of complete disappearance and periodic re-appearances of mechanically (extrinsically) stabilized stimuli does not necessarily result from imperfect stabilization. The differences associated with the fate of images stabilized with intrinsic and extrinsic techniques can be explained by other facts, most notably the poor focus, low contrast and extrafoveal location of most entoptic images. All of these factors would facilitate rapid and persistent disappearance of entoptic images. Such effects would not be expected when well-focussed, high-contrast targets are presented at the center of the fovea with an extrinsic stabilization technique (Barlow, 1963, had already called attention to such considerations).

So, having first shown that Barlow's (1963) rejection of the contact lens for stabilization was restricted to a special case in which large inertial forces were applied to the contact lens, Riggs and Schick (1968) went on to conclude, on the basis of prior contact lens optical lever research, that stabilization good to only one minute of arc is sufficient to study the effect of target motion on visual processing. This conclusion left open the possibility that complete, persistent disappearance of an intense, stabilized foveal target with good optical properties may not be characteristic of visual system performance (Barlow's, 1963, conclusion). Riggs and Schick (1968) did not comment either on Barlow's reported failure to achieve complete disappearance of a stabilized image which met these criteria, or on the contradictory report of Gerrits et al. (1966) in which complete, persistent disappearance was, once again, suggested to be the sine qua non of effective stabilization – a claim that Gerrits and his coworkers would continue to make in subsequent experiments published during the next two decades. The final fate of an adequately stabilized, intense, well-focussed, high-contrast display presented to the central fovea remained uncertain as the stabilization technique entered the 1970s – the third decade of research with stabilized images. At this time emphasis shifted away from tests of stabilization techniques towards the development of rather elaborate quantitative theory, which attempted to relate eye movements to basic visual processing. A step in this direction had been made ten years earlier by Bryngdahl in 1961.

7. Fourier Optics and the role of eye movements in spatial vision

We have already referred to the introduction of what we called 'Fourier Optics' into the analysis of visual system function shortly after techniques were developed to do research with stabilized images (see section 6). By way of reminder, Schade (1956) and de Lange (1957, 1958) were responsible for initiating this initial interest; the former providing an example of how linear systems analysis might be used to describe spatial factors in vision, the latter providing experimental evidence of the power of these techniques, as well as an example of how they might be used to study the operation of temporal factors in the human visual system. Their approach was immediately taken up by others and by 1959 Levinson had used Fourier Optics to show that in a "flicker-fusion experiment there is more to flicker than meets the eye" (p. 919). Levinson supported his timely dictum by Fourier-analysing the harmonic content of a complex pulse-sequence of flashes and thereby explaining puzzling aspects of Brown and Forsyth's (1959) experiment with flickering lights. Levinson's analysis of the Brown and Forsyth data led him to suggest that at fusion threshold all but one of the Fourier components of the flickering stimulus (the fundamental) were below threshold – a conclusion consistent with the treatment of flicker introduced by de Lange in his doctoral dissertation. Within a year, however, Levinson (1960) had found a flicker waveform (the addition of a near-threshold second harmonic of suitable phase) which showed that flicker threshold did not always depend exclusively upon a single fundamental Fourier component. Fourier Optics was proving to be a powerful tool for the study of temporal factors in vision, so much so that, within the decade, Levinson (1968) had developed and tested a multistage linear low-pass filter model of the response of the visual system to flickering lights. The application of Fourier Optics to temporal factors in vision had considerable merit. Could it also be used to analyse and model the spatio-temporal variations inherent in visual stimulation now that we knew that the eye was in continual motion despite all efforts to maintain fixation?

7.1. Bryngdahl's linear filter model of eye movement and visual acuity

Bryngdahl's (1961) paper was entirely theoretical. He described the impetus for his work as "recent developments of eye-movement recording techniques [provide] a way for an examination of the information channel between the eye and brain. Questions in this field can be treated by either information theory or linear filter theory" (p. 1). Bryngdahl chose the latter.* He built his theoretical treatment on the then-new understanding of the fine-grain characteristics of the fixational eye movement pattern and on recent demonstrations of the effect of artificial motion imposed on stabilized images. Both had been worked out by Riggs and Ditchburn and their coworkers during the preceding decade (see sections 6.2.1 to 6.2.3). Bryngdahl also leaned heavily on de Lange's (1957, 1958) treatment of the perception of flickering lights. Bryngdahl approached eye movements at the level of single cones as events designed to cause variations in the intensity of the stimulating light – variations essential to maintain the visibility of acuity test targets and to enhance the contrast of differences in the light distributions of acuity targets. He began by pointing out that "the visual system works logarithmically for large variations at low frequencies [of sinusoidally time-modulated illumination]. . . [but] for limited variations *the system appears to work linearly* [his italics]. The frequency characteristic for cone seeing (attenuation characteristic) shows a filter action for intermittent light [after de Lange]. The response function has a maximum at about 10 c.p.s. [Hz]. This opens a way to determine the constants of the visual transfer [function] and to explain a correlation between eye movements and CT-curves" [contrast sensitivity functions] (pp. 3–4).

A detailed treatment of Bryngdahl's model would occupy much more space than the subsequent success of the model would justify. The model is highly speculative, resting in large measure on details of the transduction process about which Bryngdahl freely admits "almost nothing is known" (p. 9). Nevertheless, the model does propose an eye movement-based contrast enhancement mechanism. In subsequent work Gilbert and Fender (1969) claimed that Bryngdahl's (1961) paper "has shown that the prediction [of such a contrast enhancement mechanism] was quantitatively plausible" (p. 192). We are not convinced that Bryngdahl actually succeeded in doing this and suggest that the interested reader should study Bryngdahl's model himself. It is sufficient, here, to appreciate that his treatment was consistent with a number of features that had already been observed in the eye movement and stabilized image research. In this he sets the stage for numerous subsequent efforts to correlate eye movement features with contrast detection and visual acuity.

The main relationships that he inferred from his calculations, which were consistent with the empirical work of others, were as follows: (1) "flicks [saccades] are capable of supporting normal vision", (2) "the amplitude of high frequency motion had to exceed 1 min arc in order to have a demonstrable effect on the contrast threshold" [i.e., only very rare large-amplitude components of physiological nystagmus would have visual consequences], and (3) because "the critical resonance frequency is

---

* Information theory (Shannon, 1948) has not figured prominently in the development of modern visual science, particularly when compared with the enthusiastic adoption of Fourier Optics by the visual science community. Information theory had a brief period of influence in higher-order processes such as form perception (e.g., Attneave, 1957), but very little influence on theories of more basic visual processing. Ditchburn and Drysdale (1973a,b) provide an exception in that they used information theory in their analysis of visual information obtained from flashes and from afterimages. St.-Cyr and Fender (1969) provide an exception in the eye movement literature. These authors attempted to explain very short phase-lags observed during smooth pursuit of predictable, relative to pseudorandom, target motions from an information theoretical approach. Kowler and Steinman (1979) and Kowler et al. (1984a) showed that there were historical as well as empirical problems with St.-Cyr and Fender's ill-conceived attempt.

known to be about 10 c.p.s. [Hz] (the eye movements try to make this signal as large as possible)... this frequency is transduced by the *drift* [his italics] for 1 sec arc targets" [i.e., acuity for a minimum visible dark bar depends on slow drifts] (p. 13). Another way to think about this third point is to realize that with high spatial frequencies slow drift eye movements could provide flicker in the critical resonance range of about 10 Hz. Bryngdahl's treatment of the correlation between eye movement and contrast sensitivity explicitly reduces the motion of inhomogeneities in the retinal light distribution to a problem of resolving temporal variations produced by motions of this light distribution. This approach simplifies the problem because it eliminates the need to consider target velocity qua velocity – a spatio-temporal interaction. Only temporal factors need be understood. Unfortunately, this simplification would be tested and rejected by subsequent researchers (see section 7.2.4).

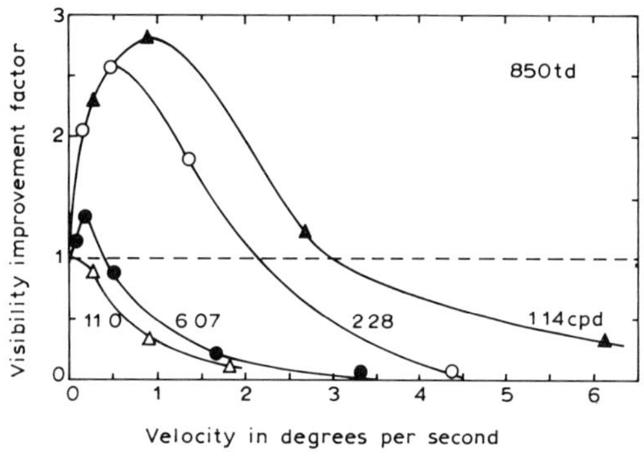

Fig. 11. Visibility improvement factors for four spatial frequencies as a function of the velocity of the grating. The average retinal illuminance was 850 trolands. (From Van Nes, 1968)

7.2. Enhancement of visibility by motion

7.2.1. Van Nes's observations at low spatial frequencies

Van Nes (1968) reported "evidence for enhancement of visibility by regular motion of retinal images" just as Fourier Optics began to dominate the research activities of the visual science community. His evidence was obtained by comparing the contrast sensitivity of a human observer to stationary and to moving sinusoidal spatial frequency gratings. The observer's task was to maintain fixation at the center of a 2.4° × 1.2° television monitor which displayed a sinusoidal grating of a particular spatial frequency and average luminance. The psychophysical contrast threshold for the grating was measured by varying the modulation of the grating from trial to trial. The grating either remained stationary or moved at a constant velocity on a given trial. Trial duration was left to the discretion of the subject, most judgements being made in less than 15 s. The retinal illuminance of the display was varied over a ten-fold range from 8.5 to 850 photopic Trolands. The average light level of the display proved to be an important variable in Van Nes's experiments; the most important results were observed most clearly only at the highest light level. Van Nes's 850 td retinal illuminance was equivalent to about 130 mL at the entrance pupil of the eye – a value more than 3 times higher than the light levels likely to have been used in the experiments in which motion was imposed on stabilized images described in section 6.2. His highest light level was also almost 3 times higher than the light level used in more recent studies of retinal image motion imposed on a stabilized spatial frequency display (Kelly, 1979a,b).

Van Nes used the Method of Limits, which he had found to be much more precise than the Method of Adjustment when used to measure psychophysical contrast sensitivity thresholds (Van Nes and Bouman, 1967). Spatial frequencies were varied from 0.64 to 11 cycles/° and constant velocity motions were varied up to a maximum of 13°/s. The main measurements were made with horizontal gratings moving vertically, but similar results were obtained in a smaller set of observations when the gratings were vertical and the motions were in the horizontal direction.

Van Nes found that "for low spatial frequencies and low velocities but rather high retinal illuminances, the grating thresholds for moving patterns were lower than for stationary patterns". He reported this "enhanced visibility as a 'visibility-improvement factor': the ratio of grating-threshold modulation at zero-velocity to grating-threshold modulation at velocity, *v*, for a given spatial frequency" (p. 369). Fig. 11 reproduces Van Nes's graph of the visibility-improvement factor at 850 td as a function of spatial frequency with grating velocity as parameter. In this figure, factors smaller than 1 mean that motion was detrimental and factors greater than 1 mean that retinal image motion was beneficial. Spatial frequencies of about 1 and 2 cycles/° benefited from retinal image motion when velocities were as high as 3°/s. Higher spatial frequencies, about 6 cycles/°, which were just beyond the peak of the human contrast sensitivity function, only benefited very slightly from motion and only when velocity was very low, below 0.5°/s. Visibility-improvement factors could be quite large for the lower spatial frequencies. For example, a 1 cycle/° grating required only a third of the modulation to be visible when it moved at 1°/s compared to when it was stationary, the condition in which retinal image motion was provided exclusively by normal fixational eye movements.

7.2.2. Assumptions about fixational eye movements

There is an important assumption underlying all research of this kind. Namely, it is assumed that the eye does not smoothly pursue when a subject is asked to maintain fixation of some stationary visual reference in the presence of a moving, structured visual background. Reflexive smooth pursuit eye movements, should they occur in this kind of experiment, would *reduce* the velocity of the grating's motion on the retina. If such reflexive smooth pursuit eye movements had been made in the Van Nes experiments, the visibility-improvement factor reported for low spatial frequencies during grating motion would actually have been obtained with lower retinal image velocities than he assumed, as were the visibility decrements caused by the retinal image motion of higher spatial frequency gratings. Without knowing what the eye is actually doing during experiments of this kind, it is difficult to draw firm conclusions about the effects of retinal image motion on contrast sensitivity. Conclusions rest entirely on the observer's subjective impression of the stability of his fixation, that is, he experiences the grating as moving while he experiences his line of sight as fixed with respect to the edges of the rectangular TV display, which in Van Nes's experiments were small enough to be almost entirely confined to his fovea. Such impressions, compelling as they are, could be misleading because the perception of motion of a particular visual stimulus need not be associated with displacements of its retinal image and retinal image motions arc not necessarily correlated with perceived motion. For example, the perception of the 'induced motion' of an objectively stationary object is caused by the motion of visual frameworks around the object, and objects show 'position constancy' with respect to the environment when the retinal position of the image of the object is changed when the eyes move (see Wallach, Ch. 6 of this volume, for a discussion of the relationship of eye movement to the perception of motion).

This problem, the unknown contribution of eye movements to the retinal image velocity of a grating target, encouraged the development of instrumentation that would permit experiments of the kind reported by Van Nes, but avoid assumptions about the stability of fixation in the presence of moving grating targets (see sections 9 and 10 and Kelly, 1979a,b, for the direction these developments took.) The development of such instrumentation was not really necessary because moving gratings, particularly moving gratings whose contrast is near threshold, do not stimulate a smooth pursuit reflex, which captures the line of sight, when stationary objects are present in the field of view (Murphy et al., 1975; Kowler et al., 1984; Kowler, Ch. 1 of this volume), but it was not at all obvious, when Van Nes first reported his contrast threshold measurements, that eye movements had not contributed to his results.

To summarize, the Van Nes experiment was important in two ways for the development of our contemporary understanding of the role of eye movement in the detection of contrast. First, it showed that retinal image motion aids the visibility of low spatial frequencies while it hinders the visibility of high spatial frequencies. The former was news. The latter had been appreciated for a long time (see Crook, 1937; Ludvigh, 1948; for influential antecedent experiments). It also called attention to the potential importance of controlling eye movements during experimental procedures of this kind just as Fourier Optics began to be used widely to study spatio-temporal factors in human vision.

7.2.3. The role of eye movement in the 1970s – a necessary nuisance

At this point in time, eye movements were viewed primarily as an obstacle to be overcome rather than as a potential mechanism for enhancing visual acuity – the way eye movements had been viewed during the Marshall-Talbot decade. Most visual scientists no longer viewed eye movements as providing a mechanism for enhancing acuity by 'dithering' the target, but the status of eye movements had improved over what it had been in the pre-dynamic, static period of Selig Hecht. The eye movement recording and image-stabilizing experiments, which had removed the behavioral underpinnings of the Marshall-Talbot theory, had contributed new importance to the functional significance of eye movements for visual processing. It was now widely accepted that normal fixational eye movements (drifts and/or microsaccades) provided the retinal image motion required to preserve normal vision, complete with fine details, by producing transient stimulation – the kind of stimulation that had figured prominently in theories of visual processing ever since 1938 when Hartline reported a preponderance of 'on-off' phasic responses in frog retinal ganglion cells (see section 5.1). Physiological nystagmus was out but larger, lower-frequency eye movements were in.

Despite the generally accepted view that eye movements were necessary for the maintenance of normal vision, it was clear that eye movements could be an obstacle to research on spatio-temporal factors because eye movements could interfere with, or be confounded with, the control of stimulation to the retina. This became increasingly important when the traditional way of minimizing the effects of eye movement in psychophysical experiments by keeping test exposures very short, below 150 ms, were shown to produce undesirable transients, in themselves capable of clouding results as profoundly as uncontrolled eye movements (see, for example, Estevez and Cavonius, 1976).

For reasons such as these, it seemed clear, at least to some investigators, that it might be safest to do Van Nes's kind of experiment without making assumptions about the quality of the observer's fixation while he observed moving gratings. This could be done by imposing motion on a grating stabilized on the observer's retina. Once the display was stabilized, the observer could view it for as long as he wished while he adjusted its contrast to threshold or made judgements about the visibility of the grating as its contrast was varied by the experimenter. Renewed interest in this possibility represented a return to the kind of experiments that Krauskopf had initiated in 1957 and extended to contrast sensitivity in 1962, in which he imposed motion on a stabilized acuity target. In all his work, Krauskopf had stabilized the targets on his retina by means of a contact lens optical lever. This means of stabilization placed constraints on his experimental procedures (see section 6.2.2). Renewed interest in this kind of research took the form of trying to develop techniques to stabilize test targets with respect to the retina without using any attachments to the eye. Stabilization without attachments to the eye would have the obvious advantage of permitting long experimental sessions during which traditional psychophysical techniques could be used to provide very reliable estimates of threshold values. Attachment-free stabilizing instrumentation would also allow the participation of relatively large numbers of subjects because they would not have to wear tightly fitted, impermeable, research contact lenses. Such lenses can be uncomfortable, and can degrade visual acuity when they are worn for more than a half hour because they deprive the cornea of the oxygen it requires and normally obtains from its contact with air (Murphy, 1978, found that before oxygen depletion causes corneal clouding, research contact lenses can have minor beneficial effects on contrast sensitivity in emmetropic, as well as in myopic, observers. See section 6 for a description of early stabilization research, including problems arising from time-limitations inherent in this technique which make it hard to use during threshold experiments).

Attachment-free stabilizing instrumentation eventually achieved a degree of useful refinement. Data on the effect of retinal image motion on contrast sensitivity obtained with such new instrumentation will be described in section 9.3 after a new role for eye movement in theories of visual processing and new knowledge about the 'natural fixation pattern' have been described (here, 'natural' means the fixational eye movement pattern observed when the subject's head is not stabilized artificially). Before moving on, however, it is worth mentioning that Van Nes appreciated the fact that his observations 'were comparable' to Krauskopf's (1957) in that they both showed a beneficial effect of image motion on visibility. Krauskopf had oscillated a bright vertical bar sinusoidally and found a visibility improvement factor of 1.4 when its frequency was 4 Hz and its peak-to-peak amplitude was 12 minutes of arc. This beneficial, sinusoidal image motion would have a peak speed of about 5°/s and an average speed of about 3°/s. Krauskopf reported beneficial effects with oscillations as high as 5 Hz where peak and average speeds would be even higher, about 6 and 4°/s. Oscillation frequency had to exceed 8 Hz before motion became detrimental. Beneficial retinal image speeds such as these will interest us later when we consider 'natural retinal image motion' caused by imperfections inherent in oculomotor compensation for motion of the unrestrained head. Remember, however, that there were important differences between the Van Nes and Krauskopf experiments. Krauskopf's stimulus, a bright bar contained all spatial frequencies and its average light level was probably much lower, less than a third of the average light level of Van Nes's sinusoidal spatial frequency display. Recall that Van Nes found the greatest visibility improvements only with low spatial frequencies and high light levels – with spatial frequencies below 6 cycles/° and 850 td illuminating the retina. Higher spatial frequencies were adversely affected by motion. A truly 'comparable' finding, therefore, would require Krauskopf's bar to be seen without its sharp edges when its visibility was improved by target oscillation, that is, its high spatial frequencies would be missing from the percept. There is no mention of this in the published report and we have no way of knowing whether it underwent such appropriate changes in appearance. Recall also that Van Nes's grating moved at constant velocity; it always moved in the same direction. Krauskopf's targets oscillated sinusoidally. The difference in these patterns of motion may have important consequences for the effect of retinal image motion on visibility, as will be pointed out in section 8.2 when Kelly's measurements are compared with ours.

Research on the relationship of retinal image motion to contrast sensitivity was a timely undertaking in 1968, with Ercoles and Zoli reporting that constant-velocity motion of a bright Landolt ring, seen as a luminance increment on a bright background, enhanced the visibility of gaps in the ring of various sizes when target speed was about 2–3°/s. This visibility improvement, to use Van Nes's term, was observed both when the ring was presented at the fixation point and also when it was displaced 1–2° vertically from the fixation point. A decade earlier, Fiorentini and Ercoles (1957) had shown that sinusoidal oscillation of a test field at 1–3 Hz enhanced the visibility of Mach Bands – results similar to Krauskopf's in the same period.

Westheimer (1965) and Lit (1968) published representative reviews of the status of research and theories of 'visual acuity' during the early years of Fourier Optics. Both made reference to Fourier Optics but both still dealt mainly with the traditional problems of visual acuity present in Helmholtz's influential treatment of the subject a century earlier. To illustrate, slightly over 1 of the 13 pages of Westheimer's text is devoted to 'Fourier Theory and Resolution' – most of it sceptical about its application in visual science, while Lit devoted about the same space in his 23 pages of text.

7.2.4. Eye movements in Arend's model of spatio-temporal processing

In 1973 Arend published a theoretical paper on differential and integral operations in the human visual system in which eye movement was afforded a major role. Arend's treatment of spatio-temporal processing represents the most recent attempt, to our knowledge, to use eye movements in a general theory that includes the perception of brightness, color and contour in a single model. Arend's model will be described in some detail, more because of its novelty and scope than because of its influence on the visual science community in the decade and a half since it was published. Our discussion will emphasize his treatment of the role of eye movements only with respect to the detection of contrast and contour. His treatment of their role in the discrimination of hues and in the perception of absolute levels of hue and brightness is beyond the scope of this chapter.

Arend ascribes the source of his interest in this problem to the preceding two decades of research on stabilized images in which "experiments have consistently shown that the retinal stimulus must continually change over time if color perception is to continue ['color', as used here, includes the hue, brightness and saturation of a light]. In normal viewing, if the stimulus light itself is not temporally modulated, the principal source of temporal changes on the retina is excursions of contours on the retinal surface as the eye moves. Under these extremely common stimulus conditions, image-movement-generated responses carry essential information to the central visual system about the light falling on the retina... The pattern of temporal changes on the retina is a function not only of image characteristics, that is, the spatial rate of change of the stimulus illuminance and chromaticity but also of the pattern of motion of the image relative to the retina, a pattern dependent upon both eye movements and movements of objects within the external object distribution itself" (p. 374). This idea is shown schematically in Figs. 12 and 13.

The stages in the model up to the box labeled

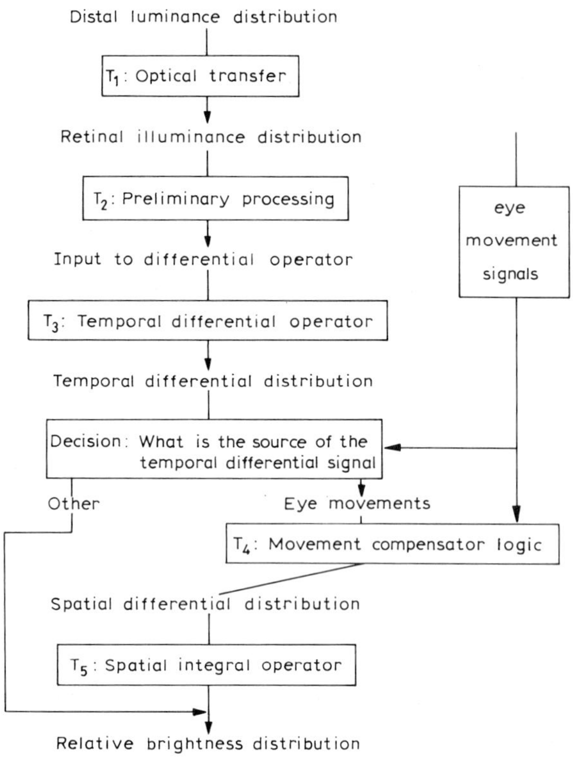

Fig. 12. Arend's (1973) block diagram of the stages of processing and intermediate spatial distributions of responses for responses generated by movement of a retinal image. See the text for an explanation.

DECISION in Fig. 12 are described as "not radically different from previous models" (p. 378). We concur and will only summarize them very briefly here. Arend's treatment of the early stages of visual processing would currently be called a retinal 'center-surround organization, opponent process' model. Models of early retinal processing of this kind are derived from ideas developed by Ernst Mach towards the end of the 19th century. Ratliff (1965) brought Mach's ideas back to prominence as he developed models of lateral inhibition in the compound eye of the horseshoe crab. Arend was well aware of Ratliff's influences and cites them accordingly. Such models are also derived from Kuffler's (1953) observations of the functional properties of the retinal ganglion cells of the cat. This influence can be seen in the theoretical weight-

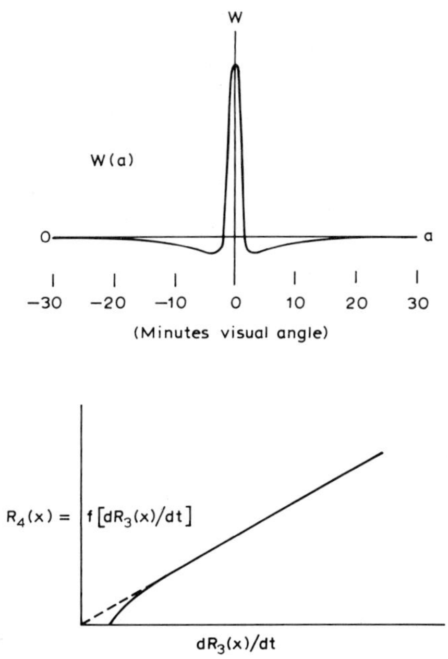

Fig. 13. (Top) Weighting function for a transfer from the luminance distribution to $R_3(x)$. The abscissa represents distance on the retinal surface in units of visual angle, *a*; the ordinate is *W*(*a*). (Bottom) The function relating $R_4(x)$ to $dR_3(x)/dt$. The solid line is this function. The dotted line is the extrapolation of the line, $R_4(x) = kdR_3(x)/dt$. See text for an explanation. (From Arend, 1973)

ing function plotted at the top of Arend's model shown in Fig. 13 where inhibitory flanks are shown adjacent to an excitatory central region. For Mach (and Arend), what mattered for seeing was not only retinal illumination, an obvious retinal requirement, but it was also necessary to have the second derivatives in *both space and time* of the retinal illumination.

In Fig. 12 the OPTICAL TRANSFER and PRELIMINARY PROCESSING boxes refer to optical, photochemical and neural processing. These processes are assumed to be modeled by an approximately logarithmic transformation followed by lateral inhibition of the kind proposed by Ratliff (1965, pp. 77–142) to account for Mach bands and related phenomena. The equation for these processes on a single dimension along the retinal surface is:

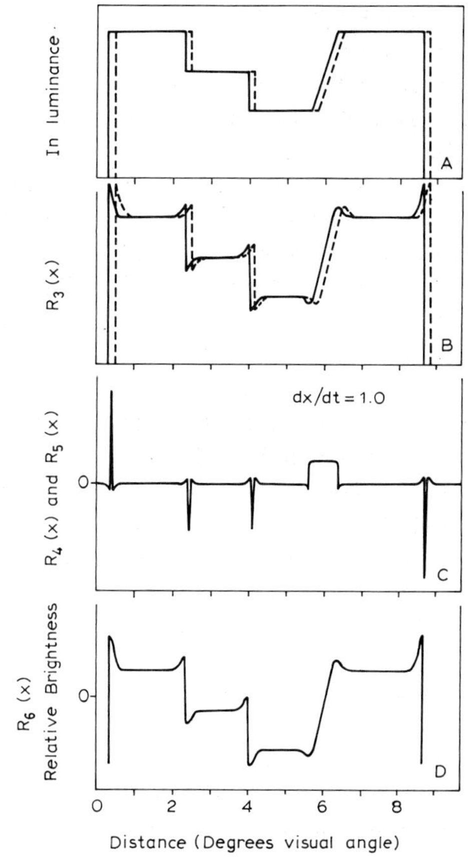

Fig. 14. Stages of processing of the spatial distribution of ln*L* is shown in part A of the figure. The solid line in part B shows the $R_3(x)$ for values of *x* along the abscissa at an instant when the eye is moving so as to displace the R_3 distribution towards lower values of *x*. The dotted line shows $R_3(x)$ a moment later after a displacement. Part C shows $R_4(x)$, and assuming that $dx/dt = 1$, $R_5(x)$, Part D shows the relative brightness distribution, $R_6(x)$, obtained by integrative processing of $R_5(x)$. (From Arend, 1973)

$$R_3(x) = \int_{-\infty}^{+\infty} W(a)\ \ln L(x-a)da$$

where $R_3(x)$ is the value of response distribution at Location *x*, *W*(*a*) is the value of the line response function shown at the top of Fig. 13, at point *a*, and *L*(*x–a*) is the luminance at location *x–a*. It is assumed that the temporal properties of box, T_2: PRELIMINARY PROCESSING, are complicated and, for simplicity, it is proposed that the luminance term in the equation above is a running average of the luminance taken over 10–20-ms intervals. In other words, it is assumed that there "is temporal as well as spatial blur". T_3 is the TEMPORAL DIFFERENTIAL OPERATOR. It represents the phasic response properties of the visual pathways which may be due to either a "passive adaptive process" or to "some active, opponent process". T_3 is described by the function:

$$R_4(x) = f[dR_3(x)/dt]$$

where $R_4(x)$ is defined in the same way as $R_3(x)$, $dR_3(x)$ is the momentary temporal rate of change of $R_3(x)$, and f is the function shown at the bottom of Fig. 13. Arend includes an important feature of his model in Fig. 13, which is not singled out for emphasis in his text. Namely, he shows the rate of change of the luminance distribution on the retina dropping to zero, close to but not at the origin of the abscissae. This means that he is assuming that there is a threshold velocity below which things will not be seen; some motion of the luminance distribution on the retina is assumed to be essential for vision. We will consider his justification of this assumption later when we evaluate the model, and it is sufficient here for the reader to notice that it is explicit and important to the success of his model. This velocity threshold provides the basis for cxplaining perceptual 'filling in', one of the main predictions of the model proposed in this paper. The same assumption will be made in all of Arend's subsequent work, which continues to emphasize the assumption of a velocity threshold and, thereby, Arend's persistent insistence on transient stimulation as the progenitor of all visual processing, an insistence likely to favor an important role for eye movement in visual processing (see section 9.5 for Arend and Timberlake's recent computation of the probable upper limit of this velocity threshold and Krauskopf's stabilization experiment described in section 6.2.7 for an example of 'filling in').

The later stages of the model, starting with the box labeled DECISION, are more novel and also of greater specific relevance to the topic of this chapter. The DECISION box is "required to separate eye-movement-related R_4s from R_4s produced either by object motion or by temporal modulation of the external stimulus". The proposed basis for the separation is "the temporal correlation between eye-movement-generated R_4s and responses specifying the pattern of movement of the eye" (p. 378). Arend does not describe the basis upon which retinal and extraretinal sources of position information ("inflow and/or outflow" signals) actually allow us to discriminate the motion of our eyes, head and body from motions of objects contained within the visual scene (see Wallach, Ch. 6 of this volume, and Skavenski, Ch. 5 of this volume, for a treatment of this and related problems). Instead, Arend simply makes reference to the fact that we can discriminate self-motion from object-motion reliably and, therefore, assumes that the information required for such discrimination "is available within the visual system". Having made this assumption, it becomes possible to go on to assume that "those R_4s not temporally correlated with eye movement signals undergo transformations different from T_4 and T_5, [transformations] which distort their information" (p. 378). Arend considers "temporal changes of the retinal stimulus not produced by eye movements beyond the immediate scope of this paper" (p. 392) and provides only a relatively terse treatment of how they might be included in a subsequent more elaborate model that includes such stimulation. In essence, he proposes that the rate of motion of objects relative to their backgrounds could provide the same kind of information about temporal changes as is provided by the generation of eye movements (the interested reader should consult pp. 392–393 of Arend's paper for details of his treatment of this problem. We will not go into it in any detail here because it is germane to the perception of motion and position constancy rather than to our topic, the perception of contrast and detail).

Next, we return to details of Arend's model, considering only eye-movement-generated responses.

T_4: MOVEMENT COMPARATOR LOGIC in Fig. 12 is a process in which eye-movement signals are used to evaluate the spatial differential responses (R_4) with which they are correlated temporally. Every R_4 that is above threshold is associated with a unique $dR_3(x)/dt$. Because the rate of eye movement which produces $R_4(x)$ is known, $dR_3(x)/dx$ may be determined by:

$$R_5(x) = R_4(x)/(dx/dt) \approx kdR_3(x)/dx$$

where dx/dt is the momentary rate of movement of the image relative to the retina, and k is the slope-constant of the linear portion of the function, f. An approximation symbol is used because of the threshold in this function.

T_5 is a discrete analogue of indefinite integration. Its output can be computed by arbitrarily assigning a value of zero to the output of the integration, $R_6(x)$, at any specific x. Then:

$$R_6(x+d) = R_6(x) + R_5(x+d)$$

where d is a very small unit increment of x. $R_6(x)$ is a relative brightness distribution with interval scale properties. The computation does not necessarily involve a 'scanning' mechanism that sweeps the distribution of R_5 over time. The brightness scale could be constructed by means of simultaneous operations. The initial arbitrary assignment of zero to the integration output, which was made for the purpose of computation, can be reassigned to an identifiable locus in the visual field, specifically, the locus whose R_6 value is the midpoint of the range of the R_6 distribution.

7.2.5. Predictions of Arend's model

The performance of Arend's model, when presented with step-changes of luminance across the retinal surface, is illustrated in Fig. 14. The spatial luminance distribution is stationary with respect to the physical world but its position changes on the retinal surface as it is "viewed with careful voluntary fixation" (p. 379). Such a displacement of the light distribution is represented by the differences between the solid and dashed lines shown in Fig. 14A. Fig. 14B–D shows the successive responses of the successive processing stages of the model which are produced by this kind of displacement of the stimulus. Fig. 14D represents the predicted relative brightness distribution resulting from the processing schematized in Fig. 12. This predicted brightness distribution resembles the actual appearance of a light distribution with such spatio-temporal properties inasmuch as it shows characteristic border-enhancement effects, that is, peaks and troughs, which correspond to the bright and dark bars perceived near regions of abrupt changes in luminance distributions. These peaks and troughs had, until recently (Ratliff, 1984), been widely believed to be caused by the operation of lateral inhibitory sensory processes at *abrupt* luminance borders, the same kind of inhibitory sensory mechanisms believed to be responsible for the perception of bright and dark Mach bands in retinal regions where there is a change in the rate of luminance change (that is, they were an example of the visual system responding to the second derivative of the retinal light distribution, Mach's original explanation of his bands). This property in a retinal light distribution is represented in Fig. 14A, which includes one typical Mach band stimulus (the relatively gradual slope drawn, one step-change in, on the right side of the abscissae).

Arend goes on to support his model mainly with reference to results from stabilized image experiments, primarily results of Yarbus and Gerrits and his co-workers, who reported that complete disappearance of stabilized targets will occur once stabilization is complete and that nothing will be seen as long as the stabilized image is not disturbed. He also demonstrates that his model predicts the appearance of the Craik-O'Brien-Cornsweet illusion. This illusion consists of creating the perception of an 'artificial contour' between areas of equal luminance. The artificial contour consists of an abrupt edge of luminance flanked by luminance gradients, which are below threshold, and return the luminance to the same level on each side of the abrupt edge. The percept is of an ordinary edge, that is, a contour separating two areas of uniform, but different, brightness. It is an illusion because these areas actually have equal luminance. Arend's model predicts this illusion and similar perceptual effects rather well, at least with respect to their qualitative properties. Effects such as these all require that "for a carefully fixating subject... there is a threshold spatial rate of change which must be present for any spatial brightness change to be perceived at that location" (p. 381). For Arend, image motions which exceed this threshold rate of change are provided by motions inherent in the eye movement pattern of the subject when he fixates carefully.

7.2.6. Evaluation of Arend's model

Arend's model, as might be expected, was particularly successful in explaining phenomena acknowledged to inspire its development, namely, 'artificial contours' in the Craik-O'Brien-Cornsweet illusion, and, more generally, 'filling-in' phenomena of the kind described by Krauskopf (see section 6.2.7). His explanation of these phenomena is derived largely from the assumption of a retinal image velocity threshold below which visual neurons are deprived of the stimulation they require to transmit information. Here it is assumed that *all* visual neurons signal transients, all are incapable of signalling the presence of a *stationary* discontinuity in the retinal light intensity distribution. This assumption can be viewed as controversial – it was not compelled by all data available when the model was proposed (see below).

Arend's model not only rested on a potentially controversial assumption, its support was entirely qualitative; for example, a demonstration that the perception of an 'artificial contour' can be predicted for an extension of the Craik-O'Brien-Cornsweet illusion. Quantitative estimates of the assumed retinal image threshold velocity were not provided, nor were specific eye movement characteristics associated with 'careful voluntary fixation' related to an estimate of this velocity threshold. There are hints, implicit in Arend's selection of results from the stabilized image research literature, which suggest that the threshold velocity might be rather low – probably in the range of retinal image velocities that would be generated by drifts, rather than by microsaccades, during 'careful voluntary fixation'. A selection of drift-like velocities for generating visual information in the model, a selection quite different from Ditchburn's (1973, 1980) life-long preference for the occasional, high-velocity transients produced by fixational microsaccades, would have been prescient because current thinking favors the continual, lower velocities associated with drifts (see section 6.2, or Ditchburn, 1980; Kowler and Steinman, 1980). But our inference that Arend actually preferred drifts over microsaccades as the functionally significant fixational eye movement is only a guess, because Arend avoided explicit treatment of fixational eye movement characteristics in his model. In this respect, Arend's model is very different from the Marshall-Talbot model, which proposed a specific fixational eye movement, physiological nystagmus, as the functionally significant behavior. Their proposal included specific assumptions about the dynamic properties of this high-frequency fixational tremor, as well as assumptions about its amplitude relative to the grain of the retinal mosaic. Unfortunately, the breathing-space Arend gained by being vague about the functional significance of particular fixational eye movement characteristics makes it difficult to evaluate how the model works during what Arend calls 'careful voluntary fixation'. Are the retinal image velocities typically produced by fixational drifts suprathreshold, or is effective stimulation confined to the very brief, infrequent transients produced by fixational microsaccades, or are all fixational eye movements equally effective once they exceed the velocity threshold? These, and other possibilities, are left entirely open.

Other features of Arend's model can be evaluated more directly. Arend's paper contains a footnote of considerable importance – a footnote in which Arend completely discounts Barlow's (1963) description of the appearance of the visual field after stabilization has been maintained for several minutes. Barlow observed what Arend (1973) describes as "residual hazy gradients of brightness in the field, roughly corresponding to the distribution of illuminance of the retina" (p. 375) (see section 6.2.6

for Barlow's description). Arend ascribes this observation to Barlow's failure to achieve adequate stabilization. Arend rests his interpretation of Barlow's result on "the weight of evidence against this view", specifically citing Yarbus's and Gerrits's reports of complete, persistent disappearance of their stabilized images. Here, of course, Arend is ignoring some important facts. Namely, Barlow had shown that Yarbus's technique (1) had very poor optical properties, producing a good deal of chromatic and other aberrations which precluded sharply focussed target images, and (2) allowed water, condensed from the air in contact with the cornea, to accumulate on the inner surface of the air-spaced compensating lens attached to the front of the sucker. Such fogging-up of the compensating lens greatly reduces the contrast in the retinal image of the target, as does the addition of trans-scleral light, which can find its way to the retina if the stimulating light is intense and the sclera is not screened. Yarbus did not screen the sclera. In short, Yarbus's technique was elegant in its simplicity but it was crude. It reduced the image quality and contrast of the stabilized retinal image to such an extent that, from Barlow's point of view, it produced conditions favorable for complete, persistent disappearance for much the same reasons that entoptic phenomena, such as retinal blood vessels, disappear and remain invisible. They are also of low contrast and fuzzy. They fade easily and remain invisible because of these properties. The trick in stabilization research is to find out what happens when a well-focussed, high-intensity, high-contrast target is stabilized and confined to the central fovea where cellular density is highest and receptive fields are very small.

Gerrits and his co-workers recognized the second flaw in Yarbus's technique and went to great lengths to eliminate condensed water in their elaboration of Yarbus's method, in the process loading down the sucker with tubing to circulate warm water around the air between the cornea and the compensating lens. They did not, however, satisfy all of Barlow's objections to the method. Gerrits and his co-workers also never succeeded in providing a retinal image with excellent optical quality (they always used simple, air-spaced compensating lenses and often permitted appreciable trans-scleral light as well) nor did they study targets stabilized on and confined to the central fovea. All of their stabilized targets had a relatively coarse grain and/or extended into perifoveal retinal areas where the complete disappearance of a somewhat degraded visual stimulus would be much more likely to occur than with a stimulus of better optical quality confined entirely to the central fovea. In short, Arend's complete rejection of Barlow's observation of a degraded but persistent visual stimulus after stabilization, in our view, rested rather clumsily on a controversial interpretation of the literature on vision during stabilized viewing. (See sections 6.2.4–6.2.9 for additional details of the Barlow-Yarbus-Gerrits research on the appearance of stabilized images. The situation has not changed since 1973 when Arend first published his model. We still do not know what would happen to the appearance of a high-contrast, high-luminance target, with 'normal' optical quality, which was stabilized, perfectly, and confined to the foveal center.)

It is hard to understand why Arend was, and has been throughout the ensuing years, so committed to discounting completely a role in visual perception for the 'sustained, non-adapting neural processes, carrying information about the retinal illuminance distribution' (Arend, 1973, p. 375), which were implied by Barlow's result and posited by him. This is particularly puzzling when it is remembered that the modern emphasis on phasic responses in the visual nervous system can be traced, from the Marshall-Talbot theory on down (see section 5), to Hartline's (1938, 1940) recordings from frog retinal ganglion cells which included a population of tonic units (20%), whose responses would provide precisely the kind of non-adapting sustained responses Barlow's observations would require (see section 5.1). It is true that Hartline reported more phasic units (50%) in these seminal papers, but it is unclear why the potential visual significance of these tonic units should be discounted *entirely*. Arend, in our view, seems to have sought simplicity in his model at the expense of plausibility. But, as we shall see, Arend went on to show recently that sustained units, should they have functional significance for visual processing, would only come to operate *alone* at retinal image velocities far below a value likely to obtain in any natural viewing condition or even under the best possible stabilizing conditions (see section 9.5).

To summarize, Arend afforded eye movements a critical role in the detection of spatial detail. Their importance stems from Arend's insistence on transient stimulation of phasic visual neurons as the exclusive source of significant visual input; such neurons are completely blind to stationary illumination gradients. This idea is incorporated in the model by the assumption of a retinal image velocity threshold. Also central to Arend's model is the idea that the visual brain must be able to distinguish between retinal image velocity signals associated with movements of the eye, head and body and retinal image velocity signals generated by motions of external objects. In other words, the visual brain must be able to distinguish between intrinsic and extrinsic sources of inescapable temporal and spatial blur. This is accomplished by feeding an eye movement signal into a 'comparator', which manages somehow to separate eye-movement-produced transients from other transients. The way the brain might accomplish this is not described. Arend's support for the idea rests entirely on perceptual accomplishments which are themselves still in need of additional psychophysical observations that suggest plausible neurophysiological explanations (see Skavenski and Wallach, this volume, for the current status of work on this problem.) The relationship of the proposed retinal image velocity threshold to characteristics of normal fixational eye movements was also left open.

These are large matters to leave unresolved. The model, notwithstanding these important omissions, has merit in our view, primarily because it is a 'dynamic' model, and as such encouraged consideration once again of the importance of eye movement to theories of spatial vision. As we shall see in later sections, the importance of incorporating some kind of dynamic processing of retinal image motion produced by eye movement continues to be an important problem – we will argue later, *the* most important current problem. In this, Arend, in our view, was clearly on the right track. Unfortunately, his model does not describe the functionally significant input to the comparator logic or how the comparator operates – both descriptions are required to allow us to move beyond an insistence on the need to consider eye movement, either to drive phasic units as Arend supposed or, more likely from our point of view, to keep wildly fluctuating binocular retinal images in some kind of functional registration so that details of edges can be extracted from these inputs, which are varying, very appreciably, in space and time.

7.2.7. Motion can enhance the visibility of low spatial frequencies

Shortly after publishing his model, Arend (1976) showed that retinal image motion can be beneficial for the detection of low spatial frequency sinusoidal gratings. His experiment was similar to Van Nes's (1968) earlier report, which had already shown that retinal image motion made it easier to see low spatial frequency gratings (see section 7.2.1). The main difference between the two experiments was the manner in which the grating was moved on the retina. Van Nes moved the grating, Arend moved the eye. A comparison of some of the details of the two experiments will be helpful before dealing with their significance for our topic. Namely:

Van Nes required the subject to maintain fixation at the center of the stationary 2.4° × 1.2° TV display while a sinusoidal spatial frequency grating remained stationary or drifted at a constant velocity, ranging from 0 up to 13°/s (effects of image velocities up to 39°/s were reported previously by Van Nes et al., 1967). The grating was drifted either up or down on a given trial while its contrast threshold was measured by the Method of Limits at 1 of 3 luminance levels, spanning a hundred-fold range. The Method of Limits, with contrast steps of 0.1 decade, was used because the Method of Adjustment had been found to be much less precise in a prior experiment with monochromatic sinusoidal gratings (Van Nes and Bouman, 1967). Van Nes et al. (1967) reported substantial detrimental effects of imposed, relatively low velocity drifts (>0.5°/s) on relatively high spatial frequency gratings (>6 cycles/°). None of Van Nes's reports was cited by Arend, who also failed to take note of Krauskopf's work on image motion (1957, 1962, or sections 6.2.2 and 7.2.3), work that Van Nes credited as the first demonstration of a beneficial effect of relatively low velocity retinal image motion on visibility as well as providing an early, accurate indication of the detrimental effects produced by faster image motions.

Arend's subjects fixated a luminous spot when it remained stationary at the center of a 3° × 4° display or smoothly pursued the spot when it moved back and forth, horizontally, at a constant speed; speed varied from trial to trial up to a maximum of 5°/s. The display contained a spatial frequency grating whose contrast was set to threshold by the Method of Adjustment. The subject made two kinds of threshold setting during smooth pursuit when spatial frequency was 5 cycles/° or higher. One setting was made at the middle of each track when eye speed would be expected to be fastest. A second setting was made near turnabouts when the eye would be expected to be pursuing more slowly, either slowing down or speeding up. All experiments were performed only with a single, relatively low, space-average luminance (about 7 mL). This light intensity was near the lowest level used by Van Nes, who, you will remember, had obtained his most striking results at his highest light level, about 130 mL.

Inferences about retinal image velocity in both the Arend and Van Nes experiments depended entirely on assumed characteristics of maintained fixation and smooth pursuit under conditions that had not been studied when their research was performed (see section 7.2.2 for a discussion of this point). Arend, for example, assumed that fixating a stationary spot at the center of more-or-less structured backgrounds (gratings with different numbers of 'bars') or smoothly pursuing the spot when it moved back and forth across one of these backgrounds would lead to essentially normal fixational or smooth pursuit eye movement patterns. Both assumptions did, in fact, prove to be reasonable when they were tested in eye movement experiments (Murphy et al., 1975), but they were by no means obvious before these experiments were performed. Even now, we know that these assumptions are not applicable to all subjects – an occasional subject with poor eye movement control slows down his smooth pursuit and increases his saccade rate when the pursuit target moves across a highly structured background (Collewijn and Tamminga, 1984). Van Nes had an analogous problem. He was forced to assume that a subject could fixate at the center of a relatively small, stationary frame and avoid pursuing a grating when it moved within the frame. Van Nes's assumption also proved to be reasonable when tested in eye movement experiments but, once again, this outcome was fortuitous, inspired entirely by subjective impressions about the fixational eye movement pattern under rather special experimental conditions (see Kowler et al., 1984; Kowler, this volume, for a discussion of maintained fixation and smooth pursuit in highly structured visual fields).

There is, however, an additional and even more fundamental assumption about the relationship of eye movements to visual processing that is raised by the Van Nes and Arend experiments. This assumption is not confined to their research; it permeates the visual science literature. Recent developments have brought it into question. Note that in both experiments it was assumed that paying attention to maintaining fixation at the center of a TV display, while *at the same time* paying attention to the visibility of striations within the grating (Van Nes's experiment), or paying attention to smoothly pursuing a spot moving back and forth across a grating, while *at the same time* paying attention to striations within the grating (Arend's experiment), does not influence the threshold measurements of contrast. It was also assumed that paying attention to the contrast of the displays did not influence the stability of fixation or the effectiveness of smooth pursuit. This assumption can be described in the terminology of cognitive psychology as follows: attentional resources can be allocated fully and independently to a visually guided oculomotor task and to a visual psychophysical discrimination task when they are performed simultaneously. Khurana and Kowler (1987) tested and rejected this assumption recently (see Kowler, this volume, for details). The conclusion of their research, once again, in the terminology of cognitive psychology can be described as follows: attending to visual stimuli for purposes of visual information processing and, *at the same time*, attending to another visual stimulus in order to exercise oculomotor control draws on the same reservoir of attentional resources. In other words, visual attention is unidimensional. 'Looking' in order to see and 'looking' in order to move the eye are not independent cognitive capacities. The significance of these experiments goes far beyond the scope of our chapter. Potentially, they have broad implications throughout visual psychophysics. Whenever an observer is asked to fixate or to pursue a visual feature extraneous to the subject matter of the particular psychophysical investigation, his performance on one task may affect his performance on the other. The magnitude and generality of such oculomotor and psychophysical interactions must still be determined (see Murphy, 1978, experiment 3, p. 527, for a fine example of this interaction reported 9 years before its significance was fully appreciated).

Despite these potential ambiguities in the interpretation of the role of retinal image motion in contrast sensitivity, the main results of the Van Nes and Arend experiments have proven to be relatively robust in the light of present knowledge – a fact that encouraged us to include them in this chapter. A somewhat detailed discussion of the goal and significance of Van Nes's experiment was presented in section 7.2.1. A similar treatment of Arend's (1976) experiment is presented next.

7.2.8. Image motion and the shape of the CSF

Arend undertook his experiments in order to clarify the mechanism responsible for the shape of the spatial MTF function in the light of "the discovery of psychophysical visual mechanisms responsive to narrow bands of spatial frequency (Blakemore and Campbell, 1969; Sachs et al., 1971), [which had become a problem when] Graham [1972] demonstrated with adaptation techniques that changes of MTF shape, resulting from temporal modulation, may not be attributed to drastic changes in the tuning of the narrow band channels... While some of the variation of thresholds for stimuli of different spatial frequencies may be attributable to differences in the structural properties of the underlying psychophysical channels, it is clear that factors which do not reflect differences among the channels may also affect the shape of the MTF (e.g. optical blur). It is essential, therefore, that other possible sources of variation be examined in detail; the only current means of obtaining psychophysical evidence concerning the relative sensitivities of channels tuned to different spatial frequencies is progressive correction of the spatial MTF for mechanisms common to all the channels" (Arend, 1976, p. 1035) (see sections 6 and 7 for the 'channel hypothesis' in Fourier Optics).

Arend (1973) had already pointed out in his model paper (described in section 7.2.4) that the temporal rate of change of retinal illuminance would be such a factor that should affect the shape of the spatial MTF. The shape of the spatial MTF is 'strongly influenced' by temporal variations, particularly for spatial frequencies below the region of maximal sensitivity to contrast, i.e., 3–6 cycles/°. Once allowance is made for differences in sensitivity to the temporal rate of change of the retinal illumination gradient, low spatial frequency 'channels' do not differ in peak sensitivity. Thus, the well-known, progressive loss of sensitivity to increasingly coarse gratings need not, in itself, be an indication of differences in contrast sensitivity. It could indicate just as well that all low-frequency 'channels' require the same *amount* of contrast to reach threshold, but this contrast threshold depends on temporal, as well as on spatial, variations of contrast, and that temporal variations must occur more rapidly when spatial frequency is lowered.

Arend (1976) made two assumptions about these temporal variations. First, temporal variations are assumed to be essential for vision. This assumption is based on the somewhat controversial fact (see section 7.2.6) that all visual images (including intense, high-contrast visual targets confined to the central fovea) will fade completely and remain invisible when all temporal variations are prevented by an effective image-stabilizing technique. It is also assumed that these temporal variations must exceed some *temporal* threshold value. In Arend's words, "the temporal change of retinal illuminance must exceed a criterion magnitude if the subject is to detect spatial nonuniformity or pattern of any spatial frequency" (p. 1035). Three additional assumptions are made in order to explain the "linear decline of contrast sensitivity commonly found at low spatial frequencies with steady stimulus presentation" (p. 1035). First, it is assumed that there is a monotonic relationship between the response of the visual system in a local retinal region to the rate of change of the illumination falling upon this local retinal region. Second, it is assumed that there is a *spatial pattern* threshold, that is, the detection of the spatial pattern occurs when the local response exceeds some criterion level. Finally, it is assumed that, in Arend's words, "the population of eye movements of a subject, viewing sinusoidal stimulus patterns near the contrast threshold, is approximately independent of the spatial frequencies of the patterns, at least when the subject is fixating a small spot" (p. 1035).

This last assumption is quite important for developing the role of eye movements in the detection of contrast because it leads to the conclusion that the decline in sensitivity for low spatial frequencies should be ascribed to characteristics of fixational eye movements. "If the population of eye movements is constant across spatial frequencies, the stimulus modulation amplitude must be increased in direct proportion to reductions of pattern spatial frequency if the same level of response is to occur. As a result there is a linear rise of threshold with decreasing spatial frequency, a prominent characteristic of the steady-state MTF. According to this model, then, the rise of threshold with decreasing spatial frequency merely reflects the steeper spatial slope of high frequency sinusoidal patterns relative to lower frequency patterns" (p. 1036). In short, once it is assumed that eye movement characteristics do not adjust themselves to the spatial frequency of the grating being viewed, low spatial frequencies may not produce the suprathreshold temporal and spatial variations required for detecting the striations in the coarse grating pattern.

Of course, the argument given above can only explain why very low spatial frequencies require more contrast than higher spatial frequencies. When spatial frequencies are relatively high (i.e., above the peak sensitivity region usually found to lie between 3 and 6 cycles/°), contrast must also be increased. When sinusoidal spatial frequency gratings as high as 50–60 cycles/° are viewed through the normal optics of the eye, striations cannot be seen at any contrast level. When this occurs, it is said that the 'high-frequency cutoff' of the spatial MTF has been reached. At relatively high spatial frequencies progressively more and more contrast is required. Arend ascribes part of this loss of sensitivity at high spatial frequencies to eye movements, explaining that "even the limited eye movements of fixation will produce rapid, multiple-cycle temporal changes at all points on the retina illuminated by the display" (p. 1036). Here, he is proposing that eye-movement-produced temporal blur adds to spatial blur caused by diffraction and other optical characteristics of the normal human eye (inherent dioptric errors). These aberrations become important when high spatial frequencies are viewed. Arend's main results are summarized in Fig. 15.

Visibility improvements were observed with spatial frequencies as high as 5 cycles/° when the stationary display was moved on the retina by smoothly pursuing a point that moved across the display at 0.5°/s. This improvement was relatively modest, about 0.05 log units, a bit more than 10%. 'Visibility improvement', here, as in Van Nes's experiments (see section 7.2.1), refers to increased contrast sensitivity produced by moving the grating of a

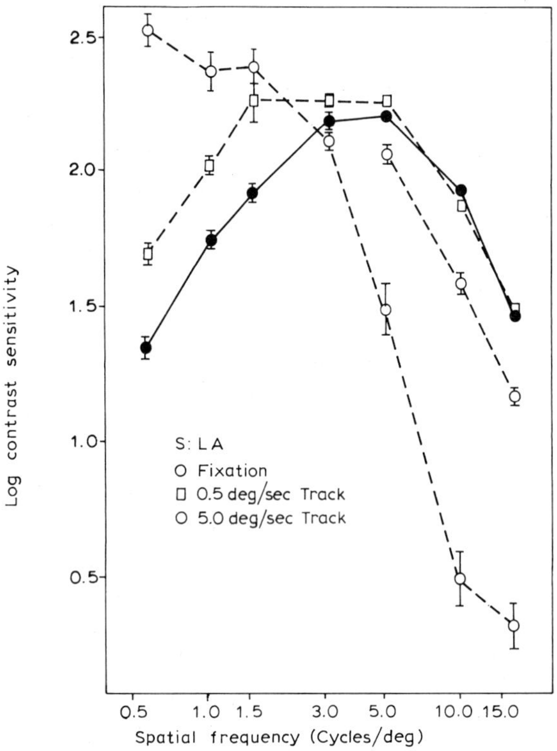

Fig. 15. Mean log sensitivities for seven spatial frequencies at three rates of target motion, namely, a stationary target (filled circles), 0.5°/s (open squares) and 5°/s (open circles). Contrast sensitivities are larger by 2 log units than those published in Arend (1976) due to a labeling error in his original figure. (From Arend, 1976)

particular spatial frequency on the retina relative to the contrast sensitivity observed with the same grating when its movements on the retina were produced exclusively by fixational eye movements. The improvement was about the same when thresholds were measured with the 3 cycle/° grating but increased to about 0.35 log units, a factor of 2.25, when spatial frequency was reduced to 1.5 cycles/°. At 1.5 cycles/° and below, the improvement in visibility reflects the progressively greater loss of sensitivity to fixated gratings relative to the sensitivity to gratings moved relatively slowly on the retina (0.5°/s). Still larger improvements in visibility, actual increases in sensitivity to low spatial frequency gratings rather than reduced decreases in sensitivity, were observed when the grating moved faster, that is, when nominal smooth pursuit velocity increased to 5°/s. At this velocity the improvement with 1.5 cycle/° grating was about 0.49 log units, a visibility improvement factor greater than 3. It increased further to about 0.65, a factor of 4.4, with 1 cycle/°, and further still to 1.2 log units, more than a factor of 10, with the 0.5 cycles/° grating. We are inclined to be somewhat sceptical of this last value because Arend's display only subtended 4° of visual angle, which means that Nyquist's criterion for estimating the frequency of a sinusoid was just met when the grating's spatial frequency was only 0.5 cycle/°.

The situation at 1 cycle/° is less ambiguous but here we note a somewhat troublesome difference in the results reported by Arend (1976) and Van Nes (1968). Namely, Van Nes's greatest visibility improvement was observed when a 1.14 cycle/° grating drifted at about 1°/s. This improvement was substantial (0.64 log units), essentially the same as Arend's greatest improvement once his lowest spatial frequency is ignored for reasons described just above. There were, however, very large differences in the conditions under which each author obtained his maximal improvement. Van Nes only got his large improvement when the space-average luminance of his display was at its highest level (about 130 mL). He obtained no measurable improvement when his display was set to be near the level Arend used (7 mL). Furthermore, Van Nes reported his maximum improvement when the 1.14 cycle/° grating drifted at 1°/s. This grating showed virtually no improvement when it drifted at 3°/s and suffered an appreciable adverse effect of motion when velocity was only 6°/s. Arend reported his maximum improvement with his 1 cycle/° grating when it moved at 5°/s. At 0.5°/s, the visibility improvement was less than half as great. There are, then, some clear differences in the outcomes of these experiments. Detailed speculation about possible reasons for these differences, such as differences in the way in which retinal image motion was produced or the effects of large differences in retinal illumination levels, will not be attempted here. Many variables could be responsible. Arend (1976, p. 1040) devotes considerable space to a discussion of the potential importance of the number of cycles in the grating displayed, and to the size of the display, including the diameter of its homogeneous surround, when he compares his results with other reports. Rather, we will call attention to other features of interest in Arend's summary graph. These features will be emphasized in subsequent sections when we reproduce contrast sensitivity functions measured in the presence of known 'natural' retinal image motion (see section 8.2). Note the large adverse effect of imposed image motion on contrast sensitivity when spatial frequency was at or above the 3–5 cycle/° peak of the spatial MTF. Five degree/second motions were very detrimental above 3 cycles/° with the high-frequency cutoff lying somewhere in the region of 10 to 15 cycles/°. Sensitivity falls by 1.6 log units, a factor > 40, as spatial frequency increases from 3 to 10 cycles/°. The crossover spatial frequency, that is, the spatial frequency where image motion helped below and hindered above, occurred at 3 cycles/°. This spatial frequency represented the lower end of the region of peak sensitivity observed during fixation or when the relatively slow 0.5°/s motion was pursued.

Arend provided a very nice demonstration figure which permits the reader to examine for himself the beneficial effects of image motion on low spatial frequency sinusoidal gratings and at the same time to examine the detrimental effect of the same motion on high spatial frequency gratings. His demonstration plate is reproduced in Fig. 16. It will be used to illustrate these phenomena now and will be used later to illustrate a number of related points. Place this figure, which contains the sum of a relatively low and a relatively high spatial frequency sinusoidal grating, at arm's length and fixate the small centered dark square (hold it in only one arm, leaving the other arm free to provide a moving stimulus). You should be able to see a relatively high spatial frequency sinusoidal grating clearly and a much lower spatial frequency grating, somewhat vaguely, at the same time. The figure contains about 10 cycles of the easily seen, high-frequency grating to a single cycle of the harder to see, coarse grating. At arm's length (about 75 cm) the entire display subtends about 11° horizontally and about 8° vertically. At this distance the low-frequency component of the display is about 0.4 cycles/° and the high-frequency component is about 4 cycles/°. The high frequency is near the peak sensitivity of the spatial MTF and the low frequency would fall just below the lowest spatial frequency Arend studied – the region receiving the greatest benefit from imposed motion (see Fig. 15).

Fixate the tip of your finger (or the end of an unsharpened pencil) and hold it at arm's length so that it rests just at the surface of Fig. 16. Now, move your finger tip back and forth from one side of the figure to the other at about 5°/s. It will take about 2 seconds to get across when you move your finger tip at the correct speed. Now, shift your attention to the appearance of the grating as you pursue your finger tip. Shift attention when your finger tip is near the center of the figure where your eye movements should be up to speed. Be sure, while you shift your attention to the appearance of the grating, that you are smoothly pursuing the tip of your finger and also be sure that your finger is moving back and forth, uniformly, at the correct speed. When you have this just right, the low spatial frequency component of the grating will stand out as broad dark bands. The high spatial frequency component, which stands out quite clearly when you fixate the small centered dark square, appears blurred while you smoothly pursue your finger tip and attend to the, now prominent, dark bands. These effects illustrate, quite compellingly, the visibility improvement retinal image motion can produce for low spatial frequencies while retinal image motion interferes with your ability to see relatively fine gratings – the findings first reported by Krauskopf (1957, 1962), and confirmed by Van Nes (1968) and then by Arend (1976).

Now that you have made these observations yourself, you will probably have been struck by how hard it was to know exactly what you were doing while you made them. Actually, you probably noticed that the broad dark bands popped out when you were not at all sure that you had the conditions exactly right. It is not easy to attend to how each of

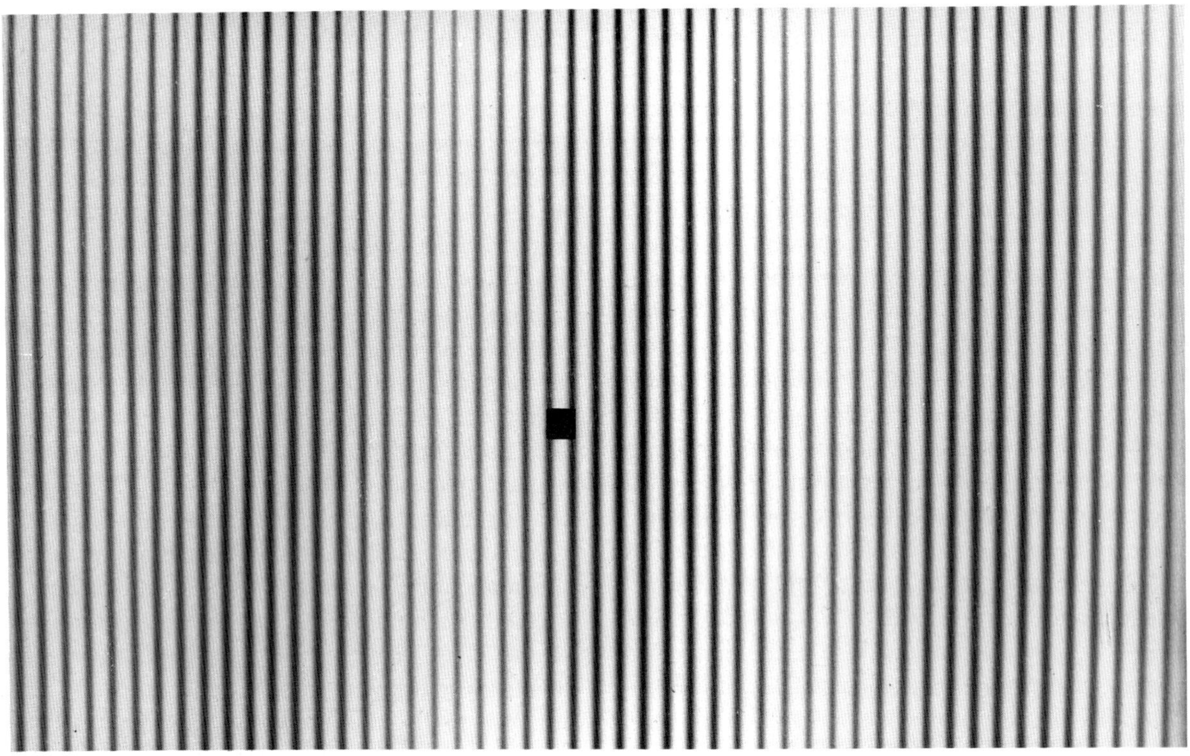

Fig. 16. Photograph of the sum of two sinusoidal spatial frequency gratings. See the text for the manner in which this figure should be viewed. (From Arend, 1976)

the two spatial-frequency components look while you attend to pursuing smoothly at the same time. Concerns such as these were raised, just above, when we alluded to recent experiments by Khurana and Kowler (1987) on the allocation of attentional resources between visual information processing and oculomotor control. Putting aside this still unanswered problem, it was well-established by 1968 (Van Nes) that retinal image motion can affect the detection of both low and high spatial frequencies, helping one and hurting the other.

How do these well-established experimental observations, which establish relationships between image-motion and the visibility of patterns of different spatial frequencies, relate to the visual processing of spatial patterns in everyday life? Specifically, is the effectiveness of oculomotor compensation for movements of the head sufficient to explain how we maintain pattern vision over the range of retinal image motions the human being typically encounters? We will consider this possibility first in the relatively simple case in which the observer's head is supported as he tries to make out details in a moving target by tracking the target with smooth-pursuit eye movements (one of the compensatory oculomotor behaviors). Here, we ask over what range of target velocities is the effectiveness of smooth pursuit sufficient to keep the residual retinal motion (retinal slip velocity) of the target image low enough for its details to be discerned? Once this question has been answered, we will then consider the more complex, but more natural situation, in which the observer is free to move about. In this situation, the observer can use both visual and vestibular signals to drive the full gamut of his oculomotor compensatory repertoire. Here, we would expect, on teleological grounds, that he would stabilize the retinal image of objects which catch his interest just enough to be optimal for vision, that is, to allow sufficient retinal slip to facilitate his detection of the low spatial frequency content, while at the same time keeping retinal slip low enough to preserve sufficient high spatial frequency content to allow the moving retinal images to provide good signals about the significance of the distal objects.

7.2.9. Slip limits contrast sensitivity during smooth pursuit

Murphy (1978) showed that retinal slip limits contrast sensitivity during smooth pursuit by making psychophysical contrast threshold measurements concurrent with accurate recordings of smooth-pursuit eye movements. In one condition, the subject tracked a constant-velocity motion of a 1.36° × 1.36° sinusoidal grating display which moved in synchrony with a 2-bright-point acuity test target located at its center. The acuity test target was adjusted to threshold (for both subjects, a 4′ separation between two bright points of light) just prior to the measurement of the threshold contrast of the grating. The composite test grating–fixation target display could be moved, horizontally, within a 5.38°-wide part of the CRT face where the raster was set to the same space-average luminance as the grating. An acuity target was used as a guide for fixation in order to establish and maintain the subject's crystalline lens focussed at the plane of the grating, which provided poor cues for accommodation when its contrast was near threshold. The moveable test portion of the display contained 7 cycles of a 5.14 cycle/° grating, whose contrast could be adjusted to threshold. A high criterion for 'threshold' was used, that is, the subject was required to set contrast so as to establish a "just visible pattern of bright and dark bars" rather than the lower criterion in which the subject sets threshold until he sees a "smudge (frequently described as an inhomogeneity in the display)" (p. 524). Murphy's high-criterion instruction was similar to the instruction given by Van Nes and Arend to their subjects, that is, they required the threshold to be set to 'stripes' or 'striations'.

A contact lens optical lever was used to record eye movements, a choice which allowed very accurate indications of smooth pursuit velocity but severely restricted the length of experimental sessions (see section 6.1.1). This restriction encouraged the use of the Method of Adjustment because of its relative speed, despite the fact that this psychophysical method was known to be influenced by starting-point biases and could be influenced readily by the subject's knowledge about the likely (or desired) outcome. Murphy went to some lengths to prevent such influences from contaminating his threshold measurements, e.g., the relationship between physical settings of the subject's potentiometer and the contrast it delivered was changed from trial to trial, and his subjects were not given any information about their performance ('receive feedback') while the experiments were under way.

Murphy included elements of both the Van Nes and the Arend experiments in his design (see section 7.2.7), that is, he produced retinal image motion by moving the grating and also by moving the eye. There were, however, three important differences between his and the previous experiments: namely, (1) Murphy used only a single spatial frequency, 5.14 cycles/°, a value near the high end of the region of peak sensitivity of the typical subject's spatial MTF, (2) he recorded his subjects's eye movements very accurately rather than making assumptions about the likely characteristics of their eye movements, and (3) his grating and fixation target moved together while the contrast of the grating was adjusted to threshold – this procedure might have simplified cognitive aspects of his subject's task, relative to the cognitive demands of Arend's task, because attention to smooth pursuit (a visuomotor task) was not divided between it and the concurrent visual psychophysical task (a visual pattern threshold judgement) as much as it was divided under the conditions employed by Arend. Arend left the grating stationary and the subject tracked the fixation target back and forth across the grating. The subject in Murphy's tracking condition (half of his trials) set the contrast of a moving grating while he pursued a special feature at its center which moved in precisely the same way as the grating.

The other half of Murphy's trials were similar to Van Nes's in that in both experiments the subject maintained fixation on a stationary target while he set the contrast of a moving grating to threshold. There were differences, however; namely, Murphy's subject maintained fixation on a centered 2-bright-point acuity target while Van Nes's subject maintained fixation at the estimated center of a 2.4° × 1.2° display with only the edges of the display, which fell on perifoveal retina, available to maintain fixation. Fixation was probably maintained better under Murphy's fixation conditions than under Van Nes's condition (see Steinman, 1965), particularly when grating contrast was relatively high (Murphy et al., 1975). The pattern of grating motion was also different in the two experiments. Van Nes drifted his grating at constant velocity in only one direction (mainly up) while Murphy's constant velocity oscillations went back and forth horizontally. This difference in the patterns of retinal image motion might be quite important – a possibility considered later when we discuss issues in current research.

When the subject fixated the stationary target and the grating oscillated in Murphy's experiment, the effect of retinal image motion on the contrast threshold could be related directly to the speed with which the grating moved. Murphy could do this because he found that "the moving grating did not interfere with the ability to maintain a steady line of sight" (p. 526). Specifically, when the grating was moved at speeds which ranged from about 0.5°/s up to about 2.4°/s drifts of the eye during maintained fixation ranged only between 0 and 0.07°/s. Moreover, no correlation between the direction of grating motion and the direction of drift was observed at any grating speed when the subject maintained fixation on a stationary target while the grating moved.

In Murphy's other condition in which the subject pursued the grating, which oscillated along with the fixation target at its center, retinal image motion was produced by the failure of the eye to exactly match the velocity of the moving composite display (the grating with the acuity target at its center). In other words, the retinal image of the composite display slipped during smooth pursuit because smooth pursuit did not stabilize the display on the retina perfectly, even when the display moved in a highly predictable pattern. When Murphy performed these experiments, the now well-established fact that there is usually appreciable retinal image slip during smooth pursuit was still somewhat controversial, a circumstance which contributed in part to Murphy's interest in this experimental condition (see Kowler, this volume, for current concerns about smooth pursuit, which have taken a very different turn during the past decade). Murphy was able to achieve useful values of retinal image slip by setting the peak-to-peak amplitude of the moving display to about 3.5° and its speed to values ranging from 0 up to about 7°/s. These smooth-pursuit conditions produced retinal image motions (slip speeds) ranging from 0 to over 1°/s. Murphy's graph showing retinal image speed as a function of target speed is reproduced in Fig. 17. The results he obtained when image motion was imposed on a grating, while fixation was maintained on a centered stationary fixation target, are also reproduced in Fig. 17.

Murphy found that retinal image motions which were produced by moving a grating while fixation was maintained on a stationary target or by slip of the display during smooth pursuit had the same effects on contrast thresholds. In both cases, retinal image motions up to almost 2°/s had only very modest adverse effects, allowing Murphy to conclude that "it is possible to see pattern despite appreciable retinal image motion" (p. 529). Westheimer and McKee (1975, 1978) published similar observations for Landolt C and hyperacuity targets (vernier acuity and stereoacuity) at about the same time.

8. Natural retinal image motion

8.1. Its origin and probable extent

Why do human beings have this capacity to tolerate appreciable retinal image motion? A decade ago, it was rather widely believed that compensatory eye movements usually made tolerance of retinal image motion unnecessary, providing only that the full repertoire of compensatory eye movements was available. Availability here implies not merely a normal oculomotor system, it also implies that this sytem is provided with the stimulation, necessary and sufficient, to allow the oculomotor system to operate in a natural way. The experiments described thus far did not meet this condition because they precluded natural oculomotor compensation by immobilizing the head on chin rests or biteboards. Under these conditions, only smooth pursuit could be used to reduce the retinal image motion of moving displays. Saccades could also be used to correct position errors, which accumulated as eye speed lagged behind target speed, but velocity errors (retinal image slip) would persist because smooth pursuit was only able to keep up with relatively slow motions of the target. Even when target motion was relatively slow, smooth pursuit could only provide partial compensation because it often 'overcompensated' by starting to move or by changing direction *before* the target started to move or to change direction. Both of these anticipatory actions produce or increase retinal image slip rather than reduce slip (see Chs. 1 and 2, this volume, for discussion of these 'predictive' properties of smooth pursuit).

Other sources of oculomotor compensation come into play once the head is free from artificial supports. Once the head is free, the effectiveness of natural oculomotor compensation can be observed because the VOR can come into play as accelerations of the head, acting on the fluid and hair cells in semicircular canals, generate neural signals proportional to the angular velocity of the head. These signals can drive the eye in the direction opposite to the direction of the head and thereby compensate for retinal image motions that would be produced when the head rotates. The VOR was assumed to operate synergistically with smooth pursuit. Smooth pursuit handled the relatively slow motions of images on the retina while the VOR took care of the faster, higher frequency, motions resulting from head movement. The scheme just described was entrenched in the neuromythology of previous decades because of the coherent, user-friendly, textbook-ready, message it contained. Like all mythology, however, the synergy of smooth pursuit and vestibulo-ocular response rested on common-sense beliefs rather than on verified observations. In this common-sense (ostensibly 'theoretical') oculomotor world, the oculomotor system, operating in its natural mode, could, by itself, eliminate the need for tolerance of retinal image motion except under relatively extreme conditions of natural bodily movement. In this period, it was customary to demonstrate the 'virtual perfection' of compensatory eye movements (Wilson and Melvill Jones, 1979, p. 287) by asking the reader to make the following kinds of observations.

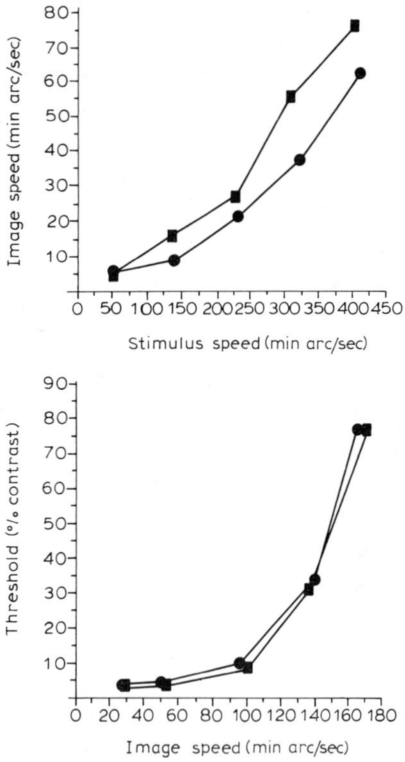

Fig. 17. (Top) Mean retinal image speed during smooth pursuit as a function of stimulus speed. The circles show subject RMS, the squares subject EK. (Bottom) Mean contrast threshold for a pattern when fixation was maintained on a stationary target and the grating moved. (From Murphy, 1978)

First, hold this book at arm's length with both hands and fixate a section of text at the center of the page. Now, move the book left and right at constant velocity through a comfortable angle (probably about 20 or 30°). First, try to keep your eyes centered in your head and your head as still as possible as you move the book. Note how quickly the text blurs, as retinal image motion smears the details in the proximal stimulus.

Having noted this effect, now allow your eyes to smoothly pursue the text as you continue to move it left and right. Note particularly the extent to which you can make out fine details near the center of your eye tracks when your smooth pursuit velocity would be at its highest and, consequently, the retinal image slip would be at its lowest value because your eye has reached its best possible speed and has not yet started to slow down in anticipation of your intention to reverse the direction of the moving book. Now, move the book left and right, faster and faster, reducing amplitude as you increase frequency, until the text blurs at the center of each track despite your best effort at smooth pursuit. You will find that you cannot move the book very fast and change direction very frequently before the text blurs despite your best efforts at smooth pursuit.

Now, having convinced yourself that you have a pretty good idea of the extent to which smooth pursuit can compensate for the motion of objects in the physical world, hold the book still at the center of your visual field and start oscillating your head about its vertical axis, all the while maintaining fixation of some portion of centered text. Move slowly at first and reduce the amplitude of your head oscillations as you increase their frequency. Keep speeding up, all the while trying to blur the text to the same extent it blurred when the text, rather than the head, was moving. Remember always to note what you see when your head is near the center of each oscillation.

You should now be convinced that oculomotor compensation can be virtually perfect until quite violent motions of the head are made. You will see motion, a jitter of the text when your head oscillates very rapidly. The best way to get very high frequency motions is to clench your teeth and strain the muscles of your jaws and anterior part of your neck and upper chest (tense your platysmas muscles). When you do this, you will notice that the finest details in the text will remain sharp until its jitter is near its maximum possible, naturally produced, value. The difference between moving the book with the head still and moving the head with the book still is the difference between compensation by smooth pursuit alone and compensation by the VOR supplemented by smooth pursuit. Observations such as these left oculomotor specialists (including one of us, RMS) feeling very smug. It was their system, the system they had chosen to study, which allowed human beings to see as they moved about in the real world. The belief that eye movements prevented unwanted retinal image slip made it plausible for the visual scientist to study vision conveniently after stabilizing his subject's head. In other words, observations and discoveries made with the head immobilized will generalize to the 'real world' precisely because of the effectiveness of oculomotor compensation. There was good reason for such oculomotor chauvinism 10 years ago; there is much less reason today now that the degree of oculomotor compensation has actually been measured rather than being inferred from informal perceptual observations of the kind just described.

8.1.1. Requirements for studying natural image motion

Some of the difficulties inherent in the development of techniques to make these kinds of measurements accurately and precisely in both space and time were not fully appreciated when this line of research began. Mistakes were made. The most embarrassing, in retrospect, was the failure to appreciate the extreme sensitivity of Robinson's (1963) magnetic field sensor coil technique to translations of the head within the small, usually about 0.6 meter, simple Helmholtz coils used by all in the 1960s and 70s (see Steinman, 1975, 1976; for measurements of head and eye movements with the sensor coil that confounded head translations with head and eye rotations).

The requirements for making accurate, translation-free measurements, while allowing head movement, were quite demanding. All prior work done with the head supported artificially had shown that the accuracy and precision of maintained fixation was of the order of 2–6 minutes of arc and that saccades, the fastest of the compensatory eye movements, had peak speeds ranging from about 5°/s to more than 500°/s when saccades shifted gaze from 6′ (the size of the average fixation microsaccade) to 75° (the size of the largest possible saccade that will bring the line of sight to fall directly on a small, very eccentric target). Performance such as this required an eye movement recording technique with accuracy and precision better than 1 minute of arc and bandwidth in the neighborhood of 200 Hz or better. It also required that rotations of the eye and head could be measured, unconfounded with spurious signals arising from translations of the head in space, at least when the targets were relatively far from the eye. When targets are far, translations of the head do not require the eye to rotate appreciably in order to maintain fixation (see Steinman et al., 1982, for details of this relationship).*

The difficulties inherent in making valid measurements of oculomotor compensation emerged quite quickly when the first measurements of fixation were made with the head free from artificial restraints (Skavenski et al., 1979). These authors found it necessary to build Helmholtz coils 2 meters on a side (3 times larger than customary), locate the 2 cm region of relatively homogeneous magnetic flux within these large coils, and provide a framework to confine the subject's free head within this small homogeneous region while recordings were made. After all these modifications of the Robinson magnetic field sensor coil technique, it was only possible to study oculomotor compensation while the subject maintained fixation on a target at optical infinity while he sat or stood *as still as possible.* Natural oculomotor compensation, even in this most limiting condition, was far from perfect, as is illustrated in Fig. 18. The recordings reproduced in Fig. 18 show eye and head position relative to an earth-fixed coordinate system. If the head or the eye did not change orientation with respect to this coordinate system, the position traces would not change position in these records. Note that the horizontal and vertical head traces did not change position; they produced horizontal straight lines when the head was supported by a biteboard. The horizontal and vertical eye traces were also relatively straight and only varied moderately in this condition. The variations which can be seen in the position of the eye traces are produced by the fixational eye movements described and discussed throughout the earlier parts of this chapter.

The story was quite different when the head was removed from the biteboard and the subject tried to sit or to stand as still as possible. The head moved a great deal on both meridians. The eye traces moved less than the head but they moved more than the head when it was supported by a biteboard. This shows that there is oculomotor compensation for small, irrepressible head movements. If there was no compensation whatsoever, the eye and head traces would move together, in the same direction and by the same amount. Compensation was not complete. The eye moved when the head was free. Complete oculomotor compensation would have produced eye traces that looked like traces of a head supported by a biteboard. The eye movement records reproduced in this figure may be interpreted so as to represent motions of the fixation target on the subject's retina as readily as they can be interpreted so as to represent movements of the eye with respect to earth-fixed coordinates. This important fact was established by Ferman et al. (1987), who discussed and examined empirically all known and

* We have just begun to study natural compensatory eye movements properly, i.e., so as to infer retinal image motion accurately from recordings of eye position when the head is free and the targets are nearby. Such inferences require techniques for measuring head translations to about 0.1 mm. It is not impossible to make these measurements but it is not a trivial undertaking and it must still be done. See Steinman (1986b) for a description of the development of the revolving magnetic field–silicone annulus sensor coil technique currently being used to measure eye and head orientation in free-headed human subjects, viewing distant targets, and Collewijn et al. (1990a) for the first accurate measurements with the head free and the target nearby.

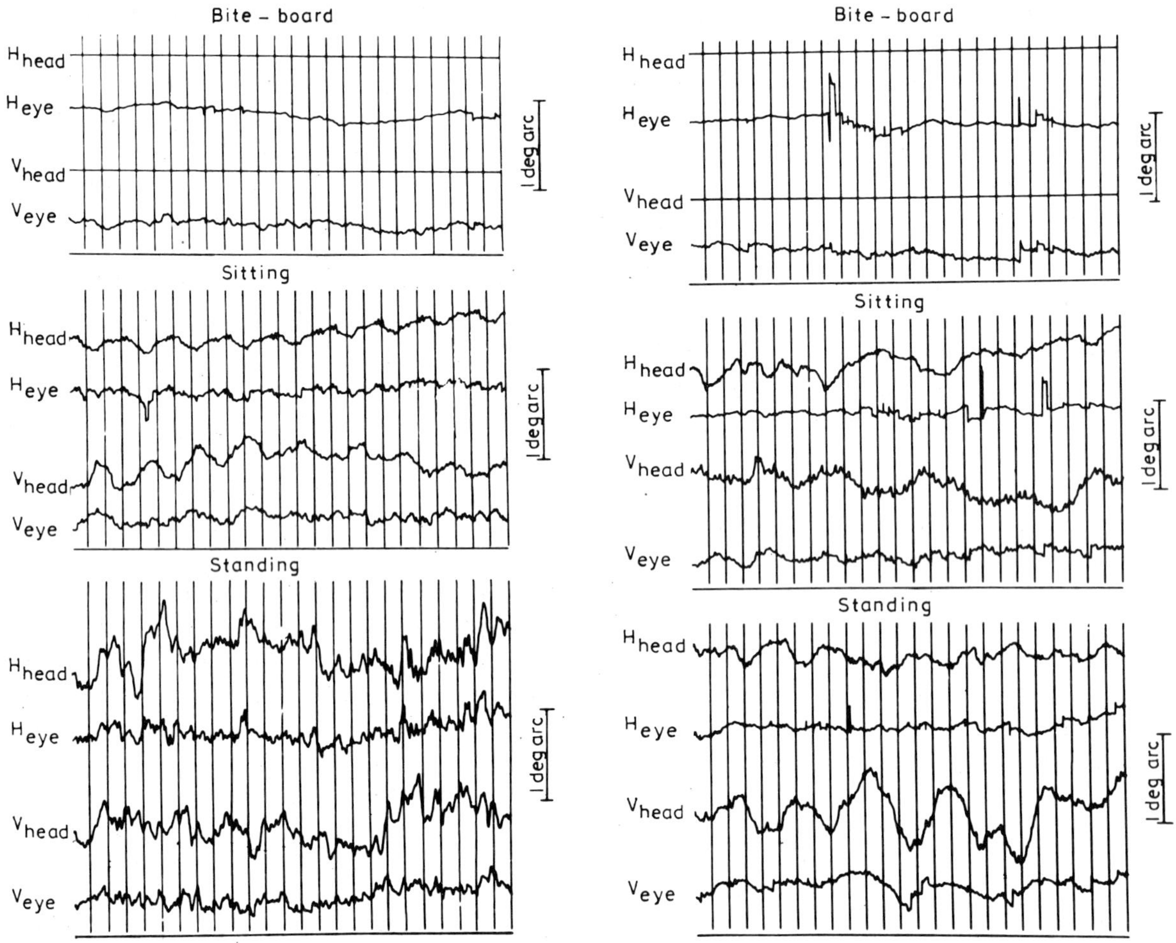

Fig. 18. Representative horizontal (H) and vertical (V) head position and gaze (retinal image position) of subject AAS (left) and subject RMS (right) while they fixated a target at optical infinity with their heads supported on a bite-board, or while they were sitting or standing as still as possible. Records begin on the left. The vertical time-lines show 1-s intervals and the vertical scales on the right side of each record show 1 degree of visual angle. Upward changes in these position traces signify rightward or upward rotations. (From Skavenski et al., 1979)

suggested potential artifacts in such recording methods. Before the Ferman et al. report, this claim was questioned by some (Duwaer, 1982; Stark, 1983).

Quantitative analyses of the retinal image motion observed in this experiment showed that motion increased, over measures obtained with the head supported on a biteboard, by factors of 2–4 when the head was free and retinal image stability depended entirely on compensatory eye movements. Compensatory eye movements corrected only a modest portion (on average, about half) of these irrepressible natural head movements. Skavenski et al. (1979) also measured the VOR to very small amplitude (0.5° and less) passive sinusoidal oscillations (0.1–15 Hz) and reported that compensation was better than when the subject remained as still as possible but still far from perfect (at best about 75%). Taken together, these results encouraged Skavenski et al. (1979) to conclude that "the degree of compensatory oculomotor response is actively adjusted downwards so as to guarantee sufficient retinal image motion to prevent perceptual fading when the body is relatively stationary and is actively adjusted upwards, so as to guarantee sufficient retinal stability to prevent blurring when the body moves actively. Seen this way, the goal of oculomotor compensation is not retinal image stabilization, but rather controlled retinal image motion adjusted so as to be optimal for visual processing over the full range of natural motions of the body" (p. 675). But what is optimal? This had actually been known, at least with respect to the optimal lower limit, since Riggs et al.'s (1953) influential early study of the effects of image stabilization on vision. In 1979, however, the fact that it was known had not yet been appreciated (see section 6.2.1).

Ten years ago, eye movement data obtained with the head stabilized on a biteboard were treated as if they represented an ecologically 'normal' oculomotor activity, that is, a behavior honed by evolutionary pressures to some value that would be optimal for vision. There was, however, long-standing, often replicated, evidence from stabilized image research that should have raised concern about this assumption. Before the Skavenski et al. (1979) report, the average 'normal' fixational drift speed on a single meridian was taken to be about 5′/s, the observed average value of intersaccadic drift (difference in eye position between the end of one saccade and its position at the beginning of the next saccade). Intra- and intersubject fixational saccade rates of the experimenters, who served as the main subjects in these contact lens optical lever experiments, ranged from 2/s to 0.5/s and lower, which means that that the estimate of 'normal' 5′/s drift speed was based on long sampling intervals, 500–2000 ms or more (5–20 times the length of the 'critical duration' for visual processing, i.e., the interval during which the intensity and duration of stimulation can substitute completely for one another). Estimates of fixational drift speeds based on somewhat more appropriate, shorter, sampling intervals (200 ms) gave slightly higher values (e.g., 6.5 to 9′/s in Nachmias, 1959, 1961; Steinman, 1965). Skavenski et al. (1979), with the still shorter sampling interval of 50 ms, obtained average drift speeds of about 14′/s with the head on a biteboard and 2–4 times that value when the head was free.

But which among these values was the 'normal' retinal image speed with respect to optimizing visual processing? Here, we can turn to results of stabilized image research. Recall the three conditions in the Riggs et al. (1953) experiment in which the effect of exposure duration on visual acuity was examined (section 6.2.1). Tests were made under normal, stabilized and 'exaggerated' image motion viewing conditions. They found that once exposures were longer than 200 ms, exaggerated image motion (twice 'normal' in their experiment) was clearly optimal for vision. 'Normal' fixational drift eye movements (i.e., drifts with the head on a biteboard) were *too slow*. Krauskopf (1957) made similar observations. He imposed oscillatory motion on a stabilized acuity target and also reported that higher than 'normal' retinal image motion was better than 'normal' motion, but, like Riggs and his co-workers, Krauskopf did not discuss the implications of this finding for natural visual processing (see section 6.2.2). The beneficial effect of higher than 'normal' fixational drift-like eye movements, imposed during stabilized viewing, permeates the stabilized image literature from 1953 until 1978, but it was only after Skavenski et al. (1979) had measured fixational eye movements under natural conditions that their significance became apparent. (See Kowler and Steinman, 1980, for a review of the history of this problem and a discussion of the visual significance of the new notion of 'normality'.) At present it seems most appropriate to infer 'normal' fixational eye speed for both the visual and oculomotor systems from the relatively high retinal image speed observed during natural oculomotor compensation, when the head is free, rather than to continue the older practice of inferring 'normality' from the relatively low speeds observed when the head is immobilized on a biteboard. This speed, observed with the head off the biteboard while a subject tries to sit as still as possible, is the *lowest* natural limit. It provides a reasonable estimate of the least amount of retinal image motion ordinarily available to provide transient stimulation to visual neurons. There is no deficiency of retinal image motion once the head is free despite intentions to remain as still as possible. But human beings rarely sit as still as possible. Most useful activity is accompanied by appreciable movement of the head and body. How effective is oculomotor compensation under these conditions?

8.2. Vision in the presence of natural retinal image motion

8.2.1. The extent of retinal image motion during active head movement

The first accurate measurements of this kind were made by Steinman and Collewijn (1978, 1980). They were made binocularly – a serendipitous undertaking which had unforeseen consequences for our understanding of binocular visual processing because each eye performed quite differently, an outcome that could not have been anticipated from the literature available a decade before. The significance of head movement for binocular oculomotor and visual performance is described by Collewijn and Erkelens (this volume) and will be mentioned from time to time only briefly in this chapter.* We will emphasize retinal image motion and its visual consequences only for a single viewing eye. Steinman and Collewijn (1980) asked the subjects (themselves and two co-workers in the Rotterdam laboratory) to maintain fixation on a distant object (5 or 35 kilometers away) while oscillating the head about its vertical axis at progressively increasing frequency; essentially the same thing the reader was asked to do as his last observation in section 8.1. There were only two differences. First, the reader maintained fixation on the nearby text while the subject in Rotterdam looked at a distant target. Second, both the reader and the subject in Rotterdam were asked to notice what he saw while the head oscillated, but the subject in Rotterdam wore binocular silicone annulus sensor coils (Collewijn et al., 1975) and his binocular, horizontal eye and head movements were recorded by means of a revolving magnetic field sensor coil monitor (Collewijn, 1977). The main results obtained in Rotterdam are illustrated in Fig. 19.

The four rows of position vs. time graphs show representative performance of each of the four subjects studied. The columns show head frequency, increasing from left to right. The data were actually collected during a continuous 30-s trial in which the subject started oscillating his head very slowly (leftmost graphs), continued to increase head frequency, reducing amplitude as he did so (the middle graphs), finally achieving his maximum head frequency with very much reduced amplitude, which is shown in the performance at the extreme right. These data were grouped into 3 separate graphs merely for convenience of plotting. These recordings show head and eye positions with respect to an earth-fixed coordinate system, which means that the significance of these records is the same as the significance of the records shown in Fig. 18 taken from Skavenski et al. (1979). There are only three differences: (1) the head movements in Fig. 19 are scaled down to 1/10th of their value because the subject moved his head through relatively large angles rather than kept it as still as possible, (2) recordings were only made of movements along the horizontal meridian and (3) binocular, rather than monocular, eye movements were recorded.

Virtually perfect compensation would cause the eye traces to approximate horizontal straight lines. Such lines were seen from time to time in *one* of the subjects's eyes. Note, for example, seconds 5 to 10 of subject RS's right eye in the record on the left and the first 4 seconds of subject LK's left eye, also on the left. In these instances, and in similar instances

---

* Discussions of binocular eye movements and their consequences for stereopsis, stereoacuity, fusion and 'hysteresis' can also be found in Collewijn et al., (1990b). A discussion of the precision of monocular and binocular gaze with a free head and its potential significance for vision can be found in Steinman et al. (1982). In this review, it was argued that natural failures of oculomotor compensation have more significance for binocular than for monocular vision, which had already been shown to tolerate retinal image motions up to about 2°/s (Westheimer and McKee, 1975; Murphy, 1978; see section 7.2.8).

in subjects studied subsequently, the compensation in the companion eye was always far short of perfection. This guaranteed considerable variation of the retinal position of the target image in at least one of the eyes and also guaranteed considerable variation of the absolute disparity between the retinal images present in each of the eyes. In other words, the oculomotor vergence response was not stable. The retinal image of the fixated distant target in one or the other or both eyes moved while the subject maintained fixation, binocularly, on an object whose distance and direction relative to the subject were not changing. Retinal image motion within each eye arose from both under- and overcompensation of head rotations. In these records (as in Fig. 18), undercompensation occurred when the eye trace moved in the same direction as the head trace and overcompensation occurred when the eye trace moved in the opposite direction. The reader should inspect the eye traces in Fig. 19 closely and note the degree of complexity and inconsistency over time of the binocular retinal image motion patterns that subjects tolerate, or perhaps even prefer, when they move their heads while using both eyes. The inter- and intrasubject variation of oculomotor compensatory activity, illustrated in Fig. 19, is characteristic of all subjects studied thus far. Subjects, despite all of these perturbations of the positions of their retinal images, reported 'normal vision', by which they meant that the perceived visual world was unitary and that fine details within it remained clear and stationary. It was only at the highest possible frequency of head movement that some jitter and slight degradation of fine detail was noticed. Try it yourself now that you know what is likely to be going on on your retinas. Use a distant target because it eliminates the need to consider translations of your head (see footnote on p. 177).

8.2.2. Residual image motion is the goal of oculomotor compensation

Collewijn et al. (1981, 1983) showed that the compensatory subsystems *prefer* appreciable retinal image slip by requiring the oculomotor system to adapt to novel optical arrangements (magnifying or minifying spectacles) that changed the amount of eye rotation required to compensate for a head rotation of a given size. "These adaptation experiments were undertaken to determine whether the observed departures from virtually perfect compensation arose from limitations inherent in the compensatory subsystems or from the desire of the compensatory subsystems to maintain retinal image motion at some nonzero value that might be optimal for vision" (Collewijn et al., 1981, p. 312). This second possibility had been raised as was noted above (section 8.1) by Skavenski et al. (1979) when they reported the first accurate measurements of natural retinal image motion, that is, image motion measured with the head free from artificial supports (see section 8.1). Collewijn et al. (1981) showed that the adapted compensatory response reestablished the deviation from perfect compensation that was characteristic of the individual subject when either no or normal minifying spectacles were worn in the case of myopic subjects. This occurred despite the fact that the optical arrangements required the compensatory eye movements to encounter a state in which the retinal image had zero slip during head oscillation. In the words of the authors, "it is important to realize that when we pushed the compensatory subsystems from their natural low gain to an unnatural high gain, gain moved through values that would have allowed virtually perfect stabilization of the retinal image. Had virtually perfect stability been the goal of the compensatory subsystems, they should have stopped adapting at this time. They did not. This result permits us to conclude that the compensatory subsystems seek some appreciable nonzero retinal image speed rather than virtually perfect image stability (p. 327)... We must now study individual visual capacities with known gaze velocities [retinal image slips] and show that the gaze velocities preferred by an individual are optimal for that individual's visual requirements" (pp. 328–329).

8.2.3. Visual psychophysics with known natural retinal image motion

The first actual psychophysical measurements,

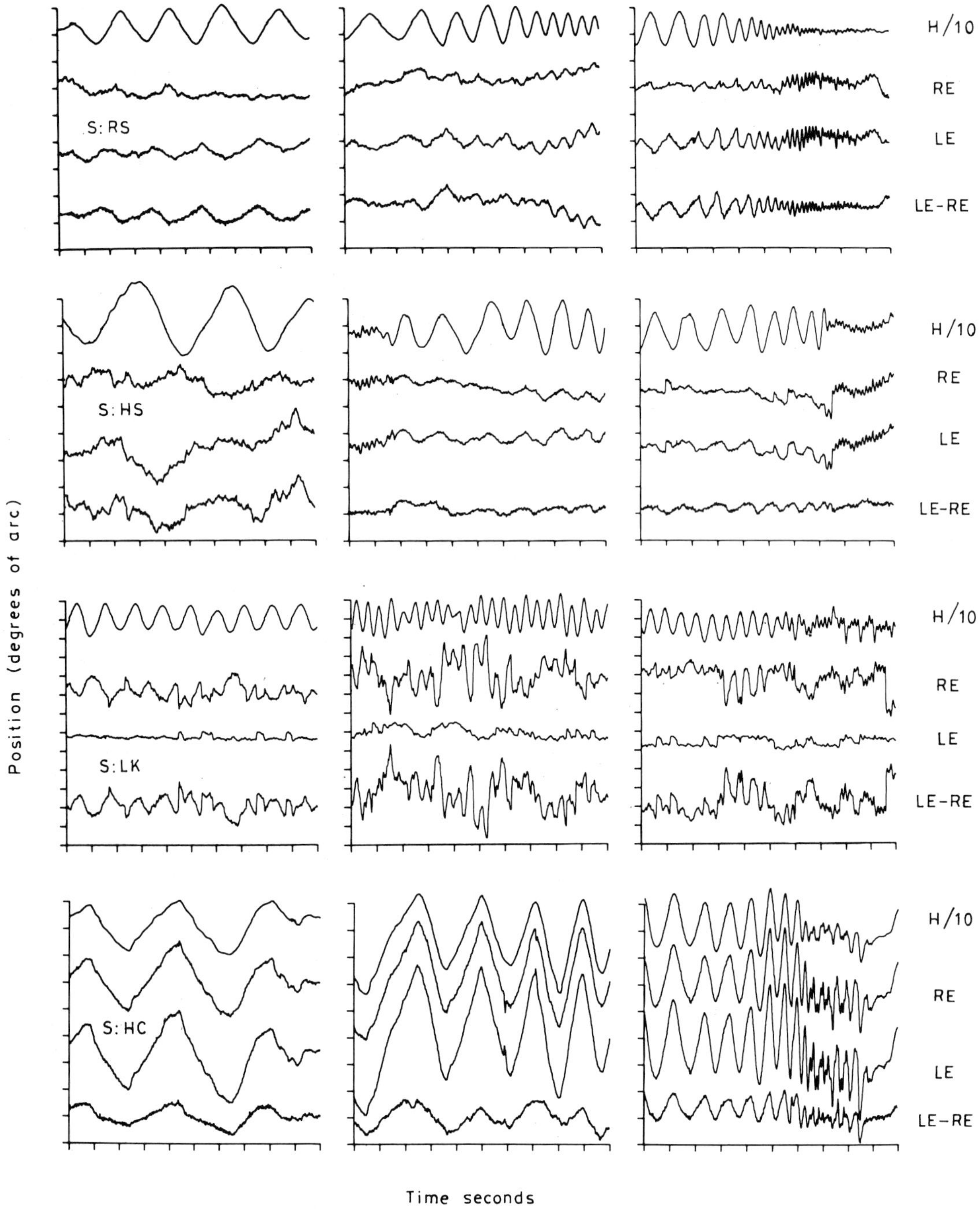

Fig. 19. Representative recordings of horizontal head (H) and binocular gaze (retinal image position) of four subjects while they fixated a distant target and oscillated their heads about the vertical axis. Each of the 12-s records begins on the left, and tick-marks on the abscissa indicate 1-s intervals. Tick-marks on the ordinate indicate 1 degree of visual angle. The movements of the head have been scaled to 1/10 of their actual value and the trace LE–RE signifies vergence eye movements, with convergence shown by upward changes in position. Upward changes of the right eye (RE), left eye (LE) and scaled head traces (H/10) signify movements to the right. (From Steinman and Collewijn, 1980)

rather than informal introspective descriptions, of stereoacuity and contrast thresholds in the presence of natural retinal image motion produced by head movements of the sort studied by Steinman and Collewijn (1980) (section 8.2.1) were reported by Steinman et al. (1983, 1985). These reports also included demonstrations which showed that random dot stereograms could be fused during violent head movement and also that fusion persisted despite heroic efforts to break fusion by shaking the head. Here, we will discuss only the work on contrast sensitivity, considered to be based primarily on monocular processes – binocular contributions to the detection of contrast are believed to arise exclusively through probability summation, essentially the parallel processing of two independent monocular processes. (The reader should consult Collewijn and Erkelens, this volume, for a discussion of the role of eye movement in unique phenomena such as fusion, stereopsis and stereoacuity, and Collewijn et al. 1990b, for a treatment of binocular processes when the head is free from artificial restraint.)

These experiments (Steinman et al., 1983, 1985) rested on previous information about the retinal image motion of three very experienced, eye movement subjects (namely, Collewijn, Kowler and Steinman), who had served in the adaptation experiments described just above. Their monocular contrast sensitivity was measured under three conditions: (1) with the head supported by a biteboard, (2) while they oscillated the head about its vertical axis through an angle of about 34° at 0.33 Hz, or (3) oscillated the head through the same angle at 1.33 Hz. Timing was paced by a metronome. Such oscillations were known to produce retinal image speeds that ranged from about ⅔ to 3°/s in these subjects under these conditions. Subjects were instructed to make their contrast judgements (determine whether they could they see the grating pattern) near the center of each swing of the head when retinal image speed would be at its highest value, essentially the same instruction Arend had used when he used smooth pursuit to move a grating across the retina (see section 7.2.8). A variant of the Method of Adjustment was used in which the subject indicated verbally whether contrast should be increased or reduced, continuing to indicate the change that should be made, until satisfied that contrast was set to its threshold value. This variant of the Method of Adjustment was used because the subject was too busy to twiddle a potentiometer knob and at the same time: (1) keep time with the metronome, (2) keep the size of head movements within the desired range and (3) make judgements about the appearance of the display near the center of each swing of the head.

Here, the reader surely realizes that the subject was required to do something akin to what the reader was asked to do in section 8.1, differing only in that: (1) the experimental display contained a sinusoidal spatial frequency grating which was far away (about 6 m), rather than the text in this book which was held at arm's length, and (2) the frequency of head movement was kept uniform in the experiment while contrast was varied until threshold was reached for the particular spatial frequency under test, rather than keeping contrast at the same, relatively high level (black letters on a white page) and varying the frequency of the head movement from very slow to as fast as possible while the reader judged the clarity of the text in a complex display, containing a wide range of spatial frequencies. The contrast sensitivity functions obtained for each of the subjects are reproduced in Fig. 20.

Steinman et al. (1985) reported that "the results for all three subjects were qualitatively similar. Head movement, with its concomitant retinal image motion, produced a need for more contrast at high spatial frequencies and reduced the need for contrast at low spatial frequencies. The crossover in the functions (where moving the head causes high-frequency attenuation and low-frequency enhancement of contrast sensitivity relative to the function obtained with the head on a chin rest) occurred at about 10 cycles/degree for subjects EK and RS and at about 6 cycles/degree for subject HC. Note, however, that the deleterious effects of image motion on high spatial frequencies were modest for all three subjects, the differences in all cases being less than a factor of 2 of contrast. Also note that the extrapolated high frequency cutoffs for each of the subjects would be well above 30 cycles/degree" (Steinman et al., 1985, pp. 227–228). These results are illustrated in Fig. 20, as is the average of these results (geometric means), which is also compared with the effects of retinal image motion on contrast sensitivity modeled by Kelly (1979b) for the same retinal image speeds. (Kelly's experiments will be described in detail in section 9.) Kelly's model was derived from threshold data, obtained with his eye, when constant-velocity unidirectional motion was imposed on a sinusoidal, relatively low spatial frequency display (<13 cycles/°), which had been stabilized on his retina by means of a *Double Purkinje Image Tracker, Stage III.* This, then-novel, non-invasive eye position monitor will be described and evaluated after the results of the naturally imposed and artificially imposed retinal image motion on contrast sensitivity have been compared. In other words, after effects of slip of the retinal image of the display during head movement have been compared with the effects of drifting a stabilized display.

There were several differences. Kelly's extrapolated high-frequency cutoffs would lie between about 9 and 18 cycles/°, whereas the Steinman and coworkers's extrapolated high-frequency cutoffs all fall above 40 cycles/°. Furthermore, Kelly's crossover points occur below 3 cycles/°. Steinman and coworkers's crossover points were above 6 cycles/°. Both of these results differ by at least a factor of 2, which led Steinman and his coworkers to conclude that the differences had potential theoretical implications.

In their words, "there are a number of important differences between our experiments that could contribute to the difference in results. Kelly imposed constant velocity displacements of the gratings – his stimulus moved continually in only one direction. Kelly's relatively low contrast sensitivity at high spatial frequencies and his relatively low crossover frequencies may reflect the effects of retinal velocity adaptation caused by continually moving the stimulus in the same direction. In other words, his constant-velocity technique could prevent normal processing by the visual system. Our free-head movements were periodic, resulting in retinal image motions of about the same frequency as the head. These periodic oscillations are the normal inputs to the visual system, which, even with the head restrained on a biteboard, occur, more or less sinusoidally, at frequencies predominantly in the range 2 to 5 Hz. Even such small-amplitude (<10′ peak-to-peak) oscillations are sufficient to prevent fading of targets located in the central fovea. Increasing the oscillation amplitudes by head movements improves contrast sensitivity at low spatial frequencies. But, of course, large-amplitude oscillations cannot but degrade the visibility of high spatial frequency gratings. The loss in acuity that we have found for image motion obtained with oscillatory head movements should be compared with the loss found with comparable oscillatory image motion imposed on a stabilized display" (p. 228).

Steinman et al. (1985), after discounting differences in the light levels and viewing conditions (binocular vs. monocular) in their and Kelly's experiments, suggested that image motion might be processed differently when it is associated with head movement than when motion is imposed while the head is immobilized. They speculated that the vestibular signal might provide the basis for a visual neural remapping that keeps track of changes of the position of details contained in the retinal image caused by the normal insufficiencies of the compensatory eye movements. The subject's visual system 'knows' about the motions of the head from the vestibular signal, already accepted as providing the oculomotor system with the information it requires to control compensatory eye movements. If the visual system also 'knew' the individual's preferred degree of retinal image slip (the 2–8% normal individuals allow reliably, albeit idiosyncratically), the visual system would be in a position to make allowance for the retinal slip expected to be associated with a head rotation of a given size. In effect, slip in the neural message would be less when the slip results from normal characteristics of com-

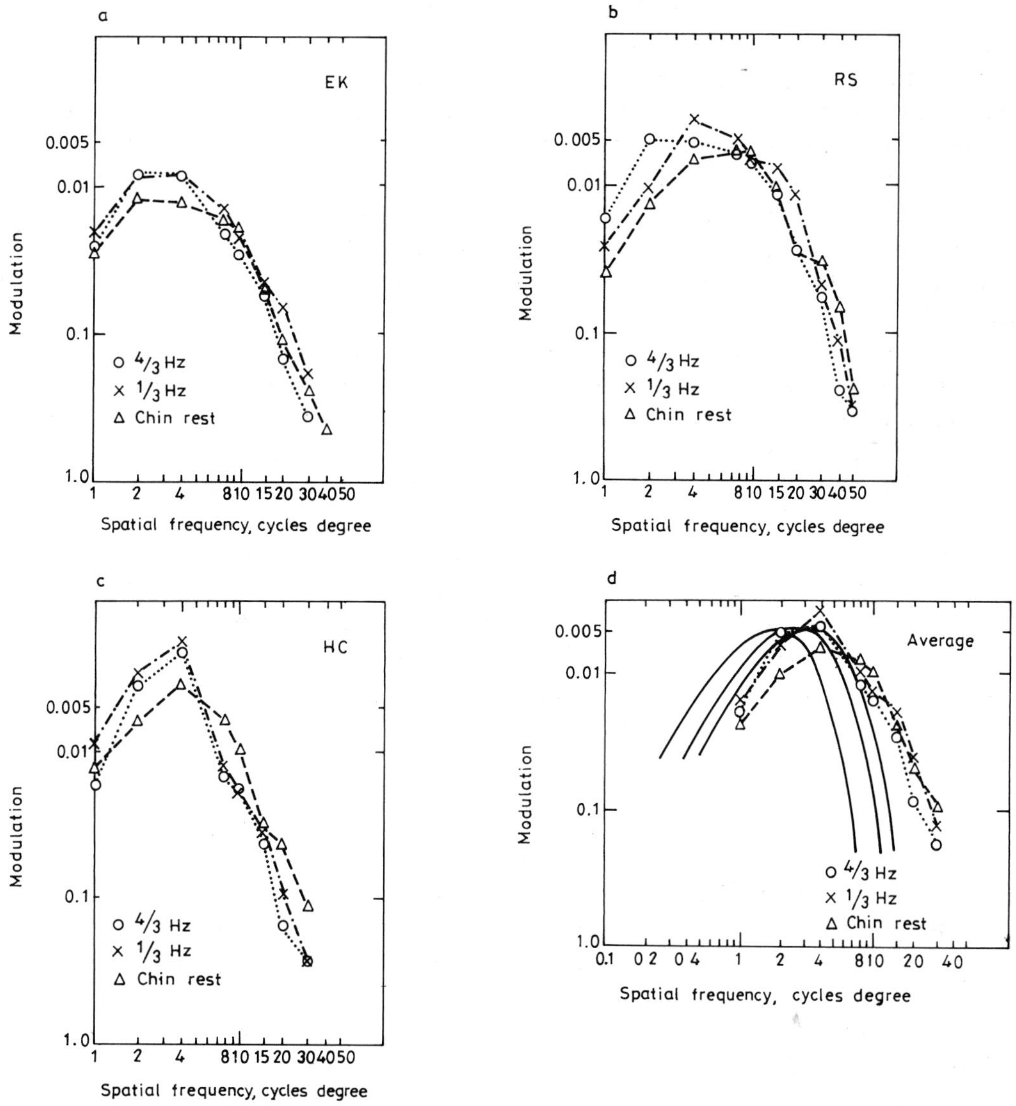

Fig. 20. Threshold grating contrast-modulation settings as fractions of 100% contrast at various spatial frequencies. Three frequencies of head oscillations about its vertical axis were used, namely, near 0 with the head supported by a chin-rest or oscillating at 1/3 and 4/3 Hz. (a) shows the CSFs obtained under these conditions for subject EK, (b) for subject HC and (c) for subject RS. (d) shows their average CSF (the geometric mean) as broken lines. Values and extrapolations from Kelly's model of the spatio-temporal transfer surface are shown as solid lines. These hypothetical functions are based on unidirectional motion of similar speed imposed on a grating 'stabilized' with a Stage III SRI eyetracker. See the text for a discussion of these functions. (From Steinman et al., 1985)

pensatory eye movements than when slip is generated by moving the visual stimulus while the head is immobilized. If this were to be the case, the well-known detrimental effects of image motion on high spatial frequency components of visual displays would be less when the slip is associated with concomitant head movements than when vestibular signals produced by head acceleration are not available. If additional principles do not come into play, the proposed mechanism for tolerating head-produced retinal image slip might, however, reduce the well-known visibility improvement for low spatial frequencies – an effect that was demonstrated originally when the head is stationary and the display is moved.

The reader should recognize that this is an elaboration of the 'comparator' function Arend (1973) included in his model described in section 7.2.4. Arend assumed there was such a comparator because the human being can distinguish between changes in retinal image position produced by rotations of his eye and changes in position produced by movements of external objects. Steinman et al. (1985) are proposing that vestibular information may have particular significance for the processing of retinal image motion under natural conditions. This change in emphasis is a natural outgrowth from the demonstration that virtual perfection of vision cannot be accounted for by the virtual perfection of oculomotor performance. There is, however, an interesting difference between the conclusions of Steinman et al. (1985) and the model of Arend (1973). Namely, Arend distinguished between the effects of image motion produced by moving the object and the effects of image motion produced by moving the eye. But Murphy (1978) had already shown that effects of image motion produced either by moving the object (stimulus) or by smooth pursuit were equivalent.

It was possible at this point in time to believe that the differences between the effects of retinal image motion reported by Kelly (1979b) and by Steinman et al. (1983, 1985) most probably arose from differences in their experimental procedures. Kelly (1979b) imposed an unnatural pattern of retinal image motion on his stabilized spatial frequency display, that is, a constant-velocity unidirectional drift, whereas Steinman et al. (1983, 1985) used the natural retinal image motion arising from imperfect oculomotor compensation associated with oscillations of the head. These natural, rather sinusoidal, retinal image motions consisted of relatively low frequency oscillations (most below 5 Hz). This experiment involved a potentially important artifact, notwithstanding the advantage it gained by using a natural pattern of retinal image motion: the subject might have ignored the instruction to make threshold judgements only near the middle of his head oscillation and actually made judgements when retinal image speed was low shortly before or shortly after the head changed direction at the end of each swing. Judgements made near turnabouts could produce very modest differences between thresholds obtained with an oscillating, as compared with a stationary, head at the high spatial frequency end of the CSF. An explanation along these lines would hardly be flattering to the dedication and competence of the three highly experienced subject-experimenters who served in the Steinman et al. experiment, to say nothing of its potential implications for their integrity. This possibility is being raised here not because we consider it to be a likely explanation of the failure to find large effects of natural retinal image motion on the contrast thresholds for high spatial frequencies but, rather, because such concerns had been expressed, and even supported experimentally, in the literature. Arend (1976) engaged this issue when he produced retinal image motion by smoothly pursuing a point that moved back and forth across a stationary spatial frequency display. He reported that he could measure reliable thresholds and that they were very much higher when he explicitly tried to make his judgements while the moving point was near the center of the display than when he tried to make his judgements near turnabouts, where his eye should have been moving more slowly (see Fig. 15 and section 7.2.7).

An artifact like this can explain how the bars in a relatively low contrast *high* spatial frequency display can be seen while the head moves but it muddies up simple interpretations of the observed beneficial effects of retinal image motion on thresholds for *low* spatial frequencies. Recall, Steinman et al. (1983, 1985) reported crossovers of the moving and stationary CSFs at 6–10 cycles/degree, while Kelly (1979b) reported crossovers at 2–3 cycles/degree. This means that the subject in the Steinman et al. experiment had to make threshold judgements, reliably, at two different parts of the head trajectory. He had to shift his threshold judgement interval from the ends to the middle of the head trajectory when the test grating was changed from a high to a low spatial frequency. Such a dual observational strategy would permit: (1) lower thresholds with low spatial frequency displays when the head moved than when the head was stationary and (2) similar thresholds with high spatial frequency displays when the head moved and when the head was stationary. The reader can get some feel for the ease with which this kind of dual observational strategy can be adopted and maintained by oscillating his head while fixating at the center of Fig. 16 (Arend's demonstration plate, which contains both a high and a low spatial frequency). Note the appearance of the low spatial frequency near the center of your head trajectory and also the appearance of the high spatial frequency when you change the direction of your head movement. The reader should also consider whether a subject using this dual observational strategy would be likely to be using these two different observational intervals, both reliably and inadvertently. In other words, try to form an opinion, based entirely on the subjective impression you form while engaged in this task, about the likelihood that a subject might consistently shift his observational interval without realizing that he was doing so. This may allow you to anticipate the outcome of an experiment (described in section 10) in which a subject making contrast threshold judgements while moving his head was prevented from using this kind of dual observational strategy.

In summary, Kelly's results are suspect because he used an unnatural pattern of retinal image motion, while Steinman and his colleagues's results are suspect because, despite the fact that they used a natural pattern of retinal image motion, they turned control of the experiment over to the subject, who might have been careless or cheated while making his observations. These issues are not completely resolved but some progress has been made. The final two sections of this chapter review this progress. The first will review both technical and theoretical developments underlying modern image-stabilization work.

9. Stabilized image research without attachments to the eye

9.1. A new technique for retinal image stabilization

In section 6, the development of techniques for stabilizing retinal images was described, from their introduction by Ditchburn, Riggs and their coworkers in the 1950s to their use in the hands of Gerrits and his coworkers, well into the late 1970s. All of these techniques were 'invasive', that is, they required attachments to the eye by means of either a tightly fitted scleral contact lens or a Yarbus-type sucker. It was pointed out in section 6.1.1 that all such techniques placed serious time-constraints on the investigators, constraints that precluded psychophysical methods for estimation of thresholds, or at least compromised the manner in which they could be used. An appreciation of the importance of this limitation encouraged Cornsweet and Crane to develop a stabilizing instrument which did not require attachments to the eye. This kind of instrument would make it possible to run long psychophysical sessions with the position (and therefore motion) of the retinal image of the test stimuli completely under the control of the experimenter. Their stabilization technique made use of what has come to be called the SRI Double Purkinje Image Tracker.

The Tracker has gone through five 'generations' or 'Stages' since its development began in 1967. It became a useful research instrument in its Stage III configuration after about 10 years of development. The subsequent two Stages concentrated on changes intended mainly to make it easier for inexperienced personnel to use the instrument. The development of the SRI tracker is described in two instrumentation publications (Cornsweet and Crane, 1973; Crane and Steele, 1978), neither of which provides detailed *quantitative* treatments of such important features as its frequency response, cross-talk between horizontal and vertical channels or the noise spectrum of its voltage output. Both of these publications do, however, describe quite clearly the problems to be overcome in the development of an instrument of this kind and the potentially effective solutions to these problems that have been incorporated into the instrument at its several stages of development. These publications, however, only provide selected eye movement records to illustrate the useful properties of the instrument. The reproducibility of these properties, within and between subjects, is not addressed quantitatively. The properties illustrated can be difficult to approximate in routine practice. The instrument can be used, but its performance and susceptibility to a variety of artifacts depend to no small degree on the characteristics of each subject's eye and the subject's ability to minimize head movement (even when the head is supported by a biteboard). Appreciation of these limitations, discussed in detail in the following sections, depends on the instrumentation skills and knowledge of the normal eye movement pattern that the experimenter brings to his evaluation of the SRI tracker from work with other 'state of the art' eye position monitors (viz., contact lens optical levers or the silicone sensor coil stationary or revolving magnetic field techniques).

9.2. Basis of our opinion of the SRI tracker

The sections which follow contain evaluative comments that call attention to technical limitations, which may be considered controversial by some Eyetracker users. Our comments are based on our personal experiences, and the personal experiences of our collaborators and acquaintances who have worked with Stage III or later instruments. In most cases, problems in using the instrument and its inherent limitations have not been emphasized in published papers. In our view, it is desirable to emphasize these problems here because inferences based on stabilization experiments done with the SRI tracker, as well as inferences based on all other available stabilization results, depend critically on the technical limitations of the device used to track movements of the eye. We believe that the problem of reliably stabilizing retinal images almost completely for periods of more than a very few seconds, without attachments to the eye and in the presence of natural behaviors (i.e., blinks, saccades and inescapable, albeit modest, changes of head position on a biteboard), has yet to be solved. **N.B.**, we are not proposing that the tracker cannot be useful in oculomotor or stabilized image research. Rather, we are calling attention to the inherent limitations in the use of the eyetracker as a stabilizing tool, and to the possibility that recent versions of the instrument, which have made it relatively simple to use, have risked increasing the likelihood of confusing artifacts with valid observations. We do not dispute that the SRI Double Purkinje Tracker, beginning with Stage III, has been used effectively in a number of publications, concerned both with eye movements and with stabilized retinal images. As noted earlier in section 6.2.10, the inability to obtain or to maintain perfect stabilization does not preclude drawing inferences about the effects of retinal image motion from observations made with a less than perfect instrument.

One central problem is that the validity of these observations rests primarily on the committed, highly experienced, subject's ability to separate observations that count from observations that must be discounted. This fact means that in SRI tracker stabilization research, just as in all previous stabilization research, experienced stabilized-image investigators must serve as subjects if relatively reliable results are to be obtained. In short, technology has not yet overtaken art in stabilized image research. We believe that the reader will find this view implicit in our quotations from the publications of Kelly – the SRI tracker's main champion and primary user for stabilized image research.

9.3. Retinal image stabilization with a Stage III SRI tracker

In this section, we will first describe the principle of operation of the SRI tracker and then describe an experiment (Kelly, 1979a) in which its relative effectiveness for image stabilization was reported. This section will show that inherent limitations make the Eyetracker useless for measuring sensitivity to high spatial frequency stabilized gratings even by highly sophisticated and committed subjects. This section will be followed by a discussion of recent theoretical and experimental work by Arend and Timberlake (1986), who claim that it may never be possible to stabilize images completely enough to drive 'on' ('sustained') neural units exclusively in a living eye (see sections 5.1, 6.2.4 and 7.2.6).

The SRI tracker measures changes in the distance between the first Purkinje image (the light reflected from the front surface of the cornea) and the fourth Purkinje image (the light reflected from the concave surface of the back of the crystalline lens). When a collimated beam of near infrared light is incident on the cornea, the convex surface of the cornea forms a virtual image (the first Purkinje) of its source within the eye. The location of this virtual image is nearly coincident with a real image (the fourth Purkinje) of this source formed by the concave posterior surface of the crystalline lens. Each of the reflecting surfaces forming the first and fourth Purkinje images is at a different distance from the center of rotation of the eye, which causes the distance between them to change as the eye rotates. "For small angles, this distance is a linear function of the rotation of the eye" (Kelly, 1979a, p. 1267). If the eye translates rather than rotates, the distance between the first and fourth images does not change. The degree, size and locations of the regions of approximate linearity of eye rotation indications depend on the anatomical structures of each subject's eye – these features vary within, as well as between, subjects. Calibration factors, within the same subject, can vary by about 10% between sessions. Some eyes are not suitable for use with this instrument – they cannot be brought into or maintained in a useful alignment for a variety of reasons, for example, very faint fourth images or subclinical cataracts.

The main virtue of the Eyetracker, and its great superiority over other non-invasive instruments, which use only the first Purkinje image or the amount of light diffusely reflected from the limbus, is its potential for separating signals arising from head translations from signals arising from eye rotations. As indicated above, in the SRI tracker, the distance between the first and fourth Purkinje images does not, in principle, change when the head or eye translates. It changes only when the eye rotates. In practice, the distance between the first and fourth images can change quite a bit whenever the tracker makes a focus adjustment, made necessary by a head movement (head rotations and translations cannot be completely eliminated by even the best combined biteboard and forehead supports).* The SRI Double Purkinje Tracker should make it possible to run large numbers of inexperienced subjects in lengthy psychophysical experiments with stabilized images because stabilization is accomplished without attachments to the eye. This eliminates the need for attaching tight-fitting, scleral contact lenses, suckers, or silicone annuli (described later) to the eye and for instilling topical anesthetics – procedures closely scrutinized by institutional committees for the protection of human subjects. In practice, however, considerable skill, cooperation and knowledge are required of the subject in stabilized image experiments and the investigators have continued to serve as the primary subjects for this kind of research. In the experiment to be described next (Kelly, 1979a), the subjects

* This is a significant problem in Stage IV and V instruments, which were designed to adjust focus of the first and fourth images as head position varied over a relatively large range – an 'improvement' in the direction of user-friendliness found to be less than completely successful by users who had made their own tests of tracker performance. Some such users have circumvented this problem by discounting data obtained during experimental intervals in which an appreciable change in focus was made by the tracker (e.g., 1 mm, personal communication A.A. Skavenski).

were L.A. Riggs, U. Tulunay-Keesey (see sections 6.1–6.2), and two SRI researchers, M. Clark and D. Kelly. All were highly experienced stabilized image researchers and would, therefore, be accustomed to selecting meaningful results, i.e., what they felt were steady-state thresholds in the presence of unavoidable artifacts, specifically, threshold changes produced by destabilization associated with blinks, saccades and head movements, and, as we shall see in the next section, even heartbeats.

Highlights in the SRI tracker stabilized-image literature will be illustrated by means of quotations from the publications of Kelly – its primary user. This is the same approach we took when the results of 'invasive' stabilization experiments were described in sections 6.2.4., 6.2.5 and 6.2.8–10. Quotations will also, as in previous sections, contain interleaved and footnoted evaluative comments. We begin with Kelly's description of how he used his SRI tracker to stabilize spatial frequency displays, and compared its performance to published data obtained with traditional invasive methods.

"We have found that the subject's task is easier (and his data are less noisy) if we stabilize only that aspect of the stimulus that is directly involved in his judgements. The eye tracker measures both horizontal and vertical eye movements, but we only use the horizontal signal to stabilize the image, since our targets contain only vertical lines. The same psychophysical method was used for moving or stationary gratings, stabilized or unstabilized. The subject found his steady-state threshold contrast by adjusting a multiturn potentiometer [Fechner's Method of Adjustment, see section 6.1.1]. He was instructed to choose whatever criterion he thought he could best remember and reproduce for all spatial frequencies and experimental conditions (rather than, e.g., adopting a 'high' or 'low' criterion level). Our unstabilized viewing technique was the same one used in previous studies... the subject... was permitted to move his eye 'normally', in any way that helped him see the target. He was instructed to judge his threshold in the *steady state* [Kelly's italics], i.e., to take enough time for each setting so that he felt the result would not change if he took longer. With this procedure, onset transients have no effect, and the contrast threshold is quite large at very low spatial thresholds... The same procedures were used in the stabilized condition, with one important exception. Since our purpose was to study the effects of normal eye movements by eliminating them as completely as possible, the subject was instructed to cooperate with the stabilizing equipment, rather than try to defeat it ... a blink or a large saccade can disrupt the stimulus with any type of stabilizer*. After a few practice trials, most subjects learned how to find a steady-state threshold in less than half a minute. Even with experienced subjects, however, it always took longer to reach steady state in the stabilized than in the unstabilized condition... In any stabilized-image technique, the movements of the retinal image produced by the apparatus should match the corresponding movements of the retina. In our experiments, this correspondence is very sensitive to small errors and must be adjusted as precisely as possible. The adjustment also varies between subjects... the optimum gain of our stabilizer varies from subject to subject, because it depends on the optical geometry of the subject's cornea and lens... Each subject must establish his own optimum setting, which he does in the following way:

"With the eye tracker controlling the position of a vertical line, the subject first adjusts the stabilizer as well as possible by voluntary fixation. Using two unstabilized fixation marks, he attempts to make

* This may no longer be true. A silicone annulus sensor coil, which can signal eye orientation when placed in a suitable magnetic field, will, unlike a research contact lens, a Yarbus-type sucker or the SRI tracker, follow the eye during saccades of all sizes (Steinman et al., 1982; Collewijn et al., 1983) and also during blinks made with the eye open or closed (Collewijn et al., 1985). In principle, this device could provide very effective long-term stabilization. So far, it has only been used for long-term stabilization of the vergence component of binocular eye movements (see Collewijn and Erkelens, this volume). The effectiveness of the stabilizing device used in conjunction with the annulus in these experiments has not yet been described sufficiently to allow comment on its potential for eliminating virtually all image motion during saccades and blinks.

the stabilized line move from one fixation mark to the other, as he looks from one to the other. To achieve this condition, he uses a knob that controls the gain and one that controls the bias of the eye-movement signal; i.e., one knob merely translates the stabilized line across his visual field to the desired position, while the other magnifies or minifies the effect of his eye movements on the position of the line. The task is not difficult but gain settings made in this way are seldom repeatable to better than about 10%. The reason for this lack of precision seems to be that the subject's line of sight is seldom where he thinks it is... once gain has been roughly set by the voluntary-fixation method, it can then be optimized much more precisely by means of an afterimage technique. Again the subject views a vertical line, which is considerably brighter than the rest of the CRT screen. Now if the line were turned off, he would see a prominent dark line at the same position (due to the fatiguing of that region of his retina). This negative afterimage provides a retinal landmark that can be used to adjust the gain, by comparing the positions of the bright and dark lines (i.e., the stimulus and the afterimage). While viewing the stabilized, bright line, the subject swings his eyes back and forth over a small, horizontal excursion of a few degrees... Now if the gain is perfect, the dark line [the afterimage] will not be visible... With this technique, or variations of it (e.g., using a step instead of a line), an experienced subject can repeat his optimum gain setting to better than 1%*... The factors that keep a stabilized image at or below threshold are in such delicate balance that almost any disturbance, a large saccade or even a loud noise, can disrupt our measurements. If the subject is aware of the source of destabilization, he can simply refrain from making a judgement until his steady-state returns" (Kelly, 1979a, pp. 1269–1271).

Kelly goes on to compare his stabilized and unstabilized CSFs with results obtained in three other experiments, two of which used contact lens optical levers and the third of which used a limbus monitor, hardly believed by anyone to be capable of beginning to stabilize a target. He reported that the best results of the contact lens optical lever stabilization experiments showed stabilization reducing contrast by factors of only 5 or 6 near the 2–4 cycles/° peak of the CSF, whereas his SRI tracker produced a reduction in contrast by a factor of 20 in both his and Riggs's eyes. The SRI tracker, in his hands, was capable of much better stabilization than had been reported in the experiments chosen for comparison with the contact lens optical lever, one of the two traditional invasive stabilization techniques. In Kelly's words "our threshold-elevation ratio is an order of magnitude greater than any of the others... moreover, we can mimic the results of others simply by decreasing the precision of our stabilizer... thus it would seem that we have achieved more precise stabilization than any of the other techniques" (p. 1272). Note, however, that, even with the SRI tracker, displays only lost contrast when stabilized. It seems here that Kelly has a confirmation of Barlow's (1963) main result, which is described in section 6.2.6, that well-stabilized displays with good optical properties and high contrast, lose contrast and high spatial frequency content, rather than disappear completely as Yarbus and Gerrits had claimed (see sections 6.2.4, 6.2.8 and 6.2.9).

Kelly next attempts to explain the reasons for the reduction of contrast after stabilization in terms of a 'sensitivity mask' – a kind of neural, rather than photochemical, afterimage which develops when patterned stimulation remains in the same place on the retina. "It takes about 10 s for the sensitivity mask to form or to dissipate – i.e., to reach steady state – with any stabilized, high-contrast stimulus... it is the sensitivity mask that makes sta-

* The reader should recognize that Kelly has adapted the afterimage technique, used by Barlow (1963) and then by Riggs and Schick (1968) to evaluate the effectiveness of various stabilizing methods, to help him optimize stabilization gain settings. It should be noted, however, that it has been shown recently that there are serious problems with using the perceived location of an afterimage to infer eye positions or retinal image motions, despite the superficially compelling logic of this procedure (see, for example, Ferman et al., 1987; or Collewijn et al., 1990b for similar failures of nonius line procedures).

bilized images disappear" (p. 1273). He then measures the CSF of this mask by creating afterimages of spatial frequency gratings and then varying the contrast of the display so as to bring the bars back to threshold after they have faded. Given the admitted difficulty of establishing and maintaining 'steady-state' thresholds (quoted above), it is clear that making these measurements was an arduous, as well as tricky, task. CSFs were obtained, however, allowing Kelly to point out that in this kind of measurement, in which a 'sensitivity mask' is overcome by a contrast increment, "the more steadily the stimulus is held in position during mask formation, the higher the resolution of the mask. We sometimes use this high [spatial frequency] cutoff as a final criterion for our stabilizer gain setting. The fact that some subjects can resolve a 12 cycle/° afterimage [of a grating] argues that the noise in the eyetracker must be less than the (2.5′) width of one bar in this grating" (p. 1273).

This last point is important for our present, and future, discussions, because it calls attention to the influence of tracker noise on the high-frequency cutoff of the CSF. 'Tracker noise' is actually determined both by characteristics of the instrument and by idiosyncratic characteristics of each subject's eye. The former can be estimated more or less accurately by recording reflections from an appropriately configured artificial eye. The latter cannot. It can only be estimated from behavioral measurements, at best capable of suggesting the lower limit for stabilization noise measurements. The significance of this limitation in inferring visual functions from 'stabilized' data can be illustrated by considering Kelly's sensitivity mask CSFs for himself and his colleague, M. Clark (see Fig. 10 in Kelly, 1979a). Kelly's high-frequency cutoff was about 12 cycles/°. Clark's high spatial frequency cutoff was about 7 cycles/°, almost a factor of two lower than Kelly's cutoff – in itself as high as any reported tracker-stabilized high-frequency cutoff. So, two subjects stabilized with the same instrument and participating under presumably identical experimental conditions showed very different high spatial frequency cutoffs, a fact which "argues that the noise in the tracker" can be very different in different subjects (see quote from p. 1273 just above). Now look at the high-frequency cutoffs of the CSFs reproduced in Fig. 20. All range from more than 30 cycles/° up to about 50 or 60 cycles/°. These are normal expected values for an unstabilized CSF, i.e., the high-frequency cutoffs measured in many subjects in many laboratories. This means that SRI tracker noise in the living eye, inferred from Kelly's measurement of the CSF of the sensitivity mask, attenuated the high spatial frequency response of his visual system by a factor of 3 and attenuated the high-frequency response of Clark's visual system by a factor of 8, assuming only that Clark's unstabilized high-frequency cutoff falls in the normal range as Kelly's cutoff does (see DK's unstabilized data plotted in Kelly, 1979a, Fig. 6).

The implications of tracker noise, as measured in the living eye, and its potential influence on the shape, as well as on the high-frequency cutoff, of the CSF, will be considered further after we have reviewed a recent paper by Arend and Timberlake (1986) in which the importance of SRI tracker noise figured prominently once again. Arend's interest in the significance of noise during retinal image stabilization was kindled, at least in part, by Kelly's (1979a) concluding remarks: "It is not certain that maximum threshold elevations much greater than our ratio of 20 could be obtained with still more precise stabilization. The only way to be sure of this would be to increase the precision and try the experiment, which was not possible at this writing. On the other hand, our stabilized thresholds seem to be tuned to the sustained receptive fields of the fovea. If these sustained responses cannot be silenced even by perfect stabilization, then we may already have reached the point of diminishing returns" (p. 1273). As early as 1973, Arend had proposed a model of contour perception which had depended on Yarbus's and Gerrits's results to discount the significance of 'sustained' retinal neural responses (see sections 7.2.4–7.2.6). Kelly's conclusion was contrary to this claim, which encouraged Arend and Timberlake to determine, on the basis of Kelly's (1979b) measurements of threshold motions imposed on a stabilized display, the minimum amount of retinal image slip that would be sufficient to drive 'transient' retinal neural units. Only displacements below this limit would properly fall in Kelly's region of 'diminishing returns' – the region within which better stabilization could not affect vision because 'sustained' retinal elements would take over visual processing.

9.4. What is psychophysically perfect image stabilization? Do perfectly stabilized images always disappear?

Arend and Timberlake (1986) raised these two questions in the title of their paper, which set out to evaluate and extend Kelly's (1979a,b) reports. Two things of particular relevance to this goal had happened in the intervening 7 years. First, the SRI tracker had advanced to Stage IV, claimed by its developers to have half the noise of the Stage III instrument used by Kelly. Second, Steinman et al. (1985) had reported effects of retinal image motion on contrast sensitivity to both high and low spatial frequencies quite different from those Kelly had observed and had suggested that these differences might have been caused by Kelly's use of unidirectional, constant-velocity retinal image motions, which do not resemble the natural oscillatory retinal image motions associated with fixation when a human being sits still or moves his head. Arend and Timberlake attempted to resolve this and related problems in a paper whose text, as well as title, began with a question. Namely,

"Does spatial pattern vision require temporal change of the retinal image? Definitive experiments on this question must involve temporally constant retinal stimuli, i.e., stabilized retinal images. Three decades of stabilized-image research have not provided a clear answer. Virtually all researchers have reported that stabilization raises luminance-grating contrast thresholds, but some report that residual detection of high contrast luminance gratings remains, in the form of either continuous visibility or fluctuating appearance and disappearance. On the other hand, several researchers using elaborate suction contact-lens stabilization report that even high-contrast, high luminance patterns disappear completely" (p. 235). Such introductory remarks should seem familiar to the reader, as should Arend and Timberlake's claim that "Kelly argued that all important retinal-image motion had been eliminated in his experiments. Accordingly, he attributed his residual contrast sensitivity to psychophysical mechanisms capable of detection of a stationary retinal image in the absence of temporal modulation from any source . . . It is difficult to assess adequacy of stabilization. If one's stabilized pattern disappears, one obviously has a strong argument that all temporal changes important for perception of the particular pattern under that particular prevailing experimental condition have been eliminated. If the pattern does not disappear, arguments for stabilization adequacy rest on descriptions of technique . . . In order to attribute residual pattern detection to static [sustained or tonic] psychophysical detectors, one must convincingly argue that all psychophysically significant motion of the retinal image has been eliminated. What is the smallest psychophysically meaningful retinal image motion? There has been no defensible criterion for judging the psychophysical importance of residual motion except image disappearance. Some of Kelly's observations indicate that the visual system is sensitive to extremely small local temporal-luminance changes . . . drifting an otherwise stabilized luminance grating at a constant velocity of 0.012°/s [43″/s] . . . raised contrast sensitivity by more than 0.5 log unit over a broad spatial-frequency range. Assuming a summation time for contrast thresholds of about 0.1 s, the patterns move only one fifth of the intercone distance [within the 20′ diameter foveal bouquet] in one critical duration. A 100% contrast grating need move even less than these threshold gratings to produce identical local temporal changes" (p. 235).

Arend and Timberlake go on to use a Stage IV, SRI tracker to replicate some of Kelly's (1979b) results for motion imposed on a drifting, stabilized spatial frequency grating and to develop "a method for calculating threshold *retinal-image motion* [their italics] as a function of grating contrast and spatial frequency from existing flicker data". They also try, less successfully as we shall see, to test this method empirically in new psychophysical experiments.

Arend and Timberlake's (1986) comparison of their contrast sensitivity results with Kelly's (1979b) is reproduced in Fig. 21. Both sets of results are for constant-velocity, unidirectional, drifting spatial frequency displays. The maximum reductions of contrast sensitivity, resulting from SRI tracker stabilization of an objectively stationary grating, are included in both graphs. The subjects shown are Arend (top) and Kelly (bottom). In the authors's words, "The effect of pattern velocity and the overall shape of the curves agree with Kelly's. Under these stabilization conditions the 0-deg/s grating threshold was 50 times [1.7 log units] the 0.15-deg/s threshold at 1 cycle per degree (c/deg).* At higher spatial frequencies the elevation factor was smaller, decreasing to about 7 [0.84 log units] at 8.8 c/deg. As in Kelly's experiment, a drift velocity of only 0.012 deg/s (=43.2 sec of arc/s) increased sensitivity from the stabilized value by as much as 0.75 log unit" [a factor of 5.6] (p. 236). Arend and Timberlake go on to show that these impressive differences between stabilized and what they consider to be velocities similar to fixational drifts (0.15°/s) were, to no small degree, the result of their particular psychophysical threshold procedure, which was similar to the procedure Kelly had used 7 years before. Both experiments used the traditional Method of Adjustment, which exposes the test display continuously while the subject adjusts contrast during 'descending', as well as during 'ascending', trials. This means that half the trials began with contrast set to a high level and that contrast remained, more or less, above threshold until the subject decided that he had reached contrast threshold. Such continual exposure to relatively high contrasts will produce afterimages whenever the grating is relatively stationary on the retina (see Kelly's treatment of the 'sensitivity mask' in section 9.3). Such afterimages would have the effect of exaggerating the apparent loss of contrast sensitivity when a grating is stabilized as compared to contrast sensitivity measured when a grating was moving on the retina. This would be true regardless of the means by which the grating was moved, both when the stabilized grating was moved on the retina by experimentally introduced drifts and by natural fix-

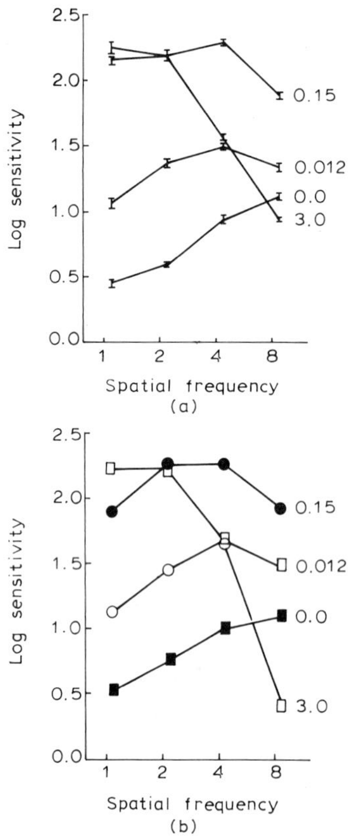

Fig. 21. Mean log sensitivity for stabilized gratings with superimposed constant-velocity drifts. Top panel shows data for subject LA and the bottom panel shows data for Kelly (1979b). Drift velocity is given as degrees/second on the right side of each graph. Bars in the top graph = 1 standard error of the mean. (From Arend and Timberlake, 1986)

* Note that this factor is larger than Kelly's (1979a) factor of 20 for the same condition. This difference probably reflects the improvement in tracker noise from Stage III to Stage IV. However, the fact that Arend and Timberlake confined all of their observations to spatial frequencies below 10 cycles/° might imply differences between the noise spectra of Stages III and IV, as well as differences in the noise properties of the various subjects' eyes.

ational drift eye movements when the display was not stabilized.

Burbeck and Kelly (1984) considered this problem and reduced the potential contribution of the 'sensitivity mask' to contrast sensitivity threshold measurements by using a 'reduced-exposure technique'. This psychophysical threshold procedure reduces the exposure to high contrast stimuli by employing only ascending tests and by only allowing contrast in the display during specific test intervals (a homogeneous display of the same space-average luminance was presented in the intervals between the tests). In effect, the contribution of the 'sensitivity mask' was reduced by using the traditional Ascending Method of Limits in which discrete test stimuli are used and the sequence of discrete tests always begins well below the expected threshold value. Arend and Timberlake (1986) used this reduced-exposure technique to compare the contrast sensitivity under stabilized and normal viewing (fixation with the head supported) and obtained much smaller effects of stabilization with a Stage IV SRI tracker than Kelly had reported for his noisier Stage III instrument. Arend and Timberlake's largest difference between stabilized (0.0°/s) and unstabilized (about 0.15°/s) contrast sensitivity thresholds was observed with a 1 cycle/° grating. The difference in stabilized and unstabilized viewing thresholds was now only 0.8 log unit (a factor of about 6 rather than the factor of 50 illustrated in Fig. 21). This means that the sensitivity mask reduced the contrast sensitivity of the Arend and Timberlake stabilized display by a factor of more than 8 (0.9 log unit). This suggests that Kelly's (1979a) reduction of contrast sensitivity with the stabilized image, if measured *without the sensitivity mask*, would have been less than a factor of 3 (0.4 log unit) rather than the factor of 20 (1.3 log unit) described in his original paper.* The difference between stabilized and unstabilized thresholds fell to about 0.3 log unit (a factor of 2) at 8 cycles/°, near the highest spatial frequency studied by Arend and Timberlake, using the reduced-exposure technique. This restricted spatial frequency range suggests that Arend's eye in the Stage IV tracker, like M. Clark's eye in Kelly's (1979a) earlier report with a Stage III tracker, contributed more noise to tracker performance than Kelly's eye in his Stage III tracker. Remember, Kelly could use his eye to study much finer spatial frequency displays, as fine as 12 cycles/°.

Arend and Timberlake's demonstration that stabilization with the SRI tracker is far less deleterious to contrast sensitivity when the contribution of the 'sensitivity mask' is reduced by using the reduced exposure technique was assumed (above) to apply to Kelly's (1979a) earlier report as well. This would bring tracker stabilization very much in line with previous reports based on contact lens optical lever stabilization. Kelly's claims of superiority over this method rest on a comparison with two experiments (see Kelly, 1979a, Fig. 9). The first, Tulunay-Keesey and Jones (1976), is not a fair comparison because the particular optical lever arrangements employed did not make provision for mounting the contact lens mirror to be normal to a line parallel to the visual axis, which means that eye torsions and translations would be confounded with eye rotations. Stabilization would have to be relatively incomplete and it is not surprising, therefore, that only modest differences between stabilized and normal viewing would be observed. The other comparison was with Gilbert and Fender (1969), whose stabilizing technique was not subject to this problem. These authors also did not keep their gratings in view continuously, as Kelly had, which means

* Burbeck and Kelly (1984) observed just this kind of reduction in the effectiveness of Stage IV SRI tracker stabilization when they used their 'reduced-exposure technique' to study local adaptation effects (0.16 log units for DK's eye at 3 cycles/°, a factor of 1.4, rather less than the factor of 20 reported for this spatial frequency and his eye when he used his noisier Stage III tracker). Note, however, that Burbeck and Kelly did not report the CSF during normal unstabilized viewing when they used their reduced exposure technique. It seems likely, on the basis of results obtained by Arend and Timberlake with the reduced-exposure technique, that the reduction in sensitivity produced by stabilization would be somewhat greater, perhaps 2.4, when local adaptation effects are prevented by an appropriate psychophysical procedure as well as by the drifts which occur during normal fixation.

that Gilbert and Fender's estimates of reductions in contrast sensitivity after stabilization were probably exaggerated less by the presence of a 'sensitivity mask' than Kelly's estimate. Arend and Timberlake (1986) found this to be quite important when estimating stabilization effectiveness from reductions of contrast sensitivity (see above). There are additional problems with Kelly's comparison of his with Gilbert and Fender's results. Kelly chose to describe the superiority of his over their results by comparing contrast sensitivity at only 3 cycles/°, a comparison most favorable for the conclusion he preferred. Gilbert and Fender's greatest loss of sensitivity was, as would be expected from Van Nes's (1968) and Arend's (1976) prior work (see Figs. 11 and 15), at lower spatial frequencies. In Gilbert and Fender's experiment, contrast sensitivity was reduced by a factor of about 6 (0.78 log unit) at 0.3 cycles/°, which is the same as Arend and Timberlake's factor when they used the reduced-exposure technique, and by a factor of about 4 (0.62 log units) at 1.2 cycles/°. At 3 cycles/°, the spatial frequency Kelly chose to compare, it was down to a factor slightly less than 2 (0.25 log units), but this factor is hardly representative of maximum loss of contrast sensitivity reported by Gilbert and Fender. Once it is assumed that Kelly's (1979a) reported reduction of contrast sensitivity with SRI tracker stabilization is exaggerated because over 90% of the reduction arises from the psychophysical procedure employed, as Arend and Timberlake showed was the case for their data, Kelly's maximum reduction due to stabilization falls from a factor of 20 to a factor of 2.4. This is less than half the maximum reduction in contrast sensitivity observed by Gilbert and Fender (1969).

It seems reasonable, then, to claim that Stage IV SRI tracker stabilization may be as good as, but not really better than, a properly designed contact lens optical lever stabilizing technique and that Stage III SRI tracker stabilization is worse. It is important to realize, moreover, that Gilbert and Fender were able to study spatial frequency gratings as fine as 30 cycles/°, almost 3 times as fine as could be studied with Kelly's best tracker subject (himself) and almost 4 times as fine as the other tracker subjects whose performance he and Arend and Timberlake (1986) described. Stage IV SRI tracker stabilization seems to be as good as optical lever stabilization with respect to the maximum possible reduction in contrast sensitivity, but the tracker restricts study to the lower part of the spatial frequency range the human eye is capable of resolving (at best only up to 12 cycles/° in the normal 60 cycle/° range). This spatial frequency restriction arises primarily from the noise of the stabilizing instrument, a fact that Arend and Timberlake (1986) go on to treat theoretically.

9.5. Calculation of stabilization accuracy required for disappearance

Arend and Timberlake point out that "if one's best-stabilized, 100% contrast gratings are detectable, there are two possible explanations: Either patterns are being detected by static pattern-detecting mechanisms [sustained or tonic neural elements] or one has not succeeded in eliminating all psychophysically important temporal change. To argue logically that static pattern-detecting mechanisms exist, one must (1) assume as a hypothesis that only dynamic mechanisms [transient or phasic neural elements] exist and then (2) somehow determine whether sufficient temporal change occurred to allow detection by dynamic mechanisms. Only if such change has not occurred is there need to postulate static mechanisms. The experimental problem is to determine how much temporal change is too much and whether one's stabilization technique produced that much. With any technique there is a formidable array of potential sources of stabilization failure. Whereas other sources of destabilization are potentially larger . . . [e.g., blinks, saccades, instrumentation delays], we have chosen to focus our argument conservatively on electronic noise in eyetracker position signals . . . One can directly measure the psychophysical consequences of small pattern movements only if the stabilization errors during measurements are small relative to the movements being evaluated. To evaluate directly movements as small as Purkinje image eyetracker noise (approximately 1 min of arc rms) one must be able to stabilize substantially better than that. To our knowledge no measurements meeting this requirement exist" (p. 238).

Arend and Timberlake (1986) pointed out that despite the fact that direct measurements were not available, with two simple assumptions it became possible to calculate the sensitivity of the visual system to small movements (imposed experimentally or by tracker noise) on the retinal image of a stabilized grating display. In other words, they proposed that it was possible to use available SRI tracker data obtained with counterphase flickering, stabilized gratings to evaluate Kelly's (or other) speculations about the neurological underpinnings of visual processing that had been inferred from a stabilization experiment with the tracker (or any other technique). This was possible because "a grating oscillating over a distance that is small relative to one grating period is closely approximated by the sum of two perfectly stabilized gratings" (p. 238). This can be accomplished by having one stabilized, relatively high contrast, grating remain invariant in time while a relatively much lower contrast, superimposed, as well as stabilized, grating undergoes counterphase-modulation. This kind of stimulus manipulation produces the same changes in the temporal variations of the illumination on a local retinal region as is produced when a relatively low spatial frequency grating wiggles with some temporal frequency (i.e., translates sinusoidally) through an amplitude small relative to the period of the spatial frequency of the moving grating. This can be visualized by imagining the very shallow slope of a low spatial frequency grating moving, ever so slightly, back and forth (try 1 cycle/° or shallower), over a very small portion of the retinal surface (perhaps 3 minutes of arc, which would contain a row of at most 9 cones at the center of the foveal bouquet). Readers with poor visual imagery might look at Fig. 5. Illumination varies very little over small distances in the situation illustrated in this figure.

The demonstration that there is a counterphase-modulated grating stimulus, which will have similar time-varying local illumination properties, required two equations and two assumptions, namely:

$$L(x,t) \approx L_M[1 + C_s \sin 2\pi fx + (C_s 2\pi fa)(\cos 2\pi vt)(\cos 2\pi fx)]$$

Here $L(x,t)$ is the luminance in space and time, L_M is the mean luminance, C_s is the contrast of the grating, a is the amplitude, f is the spatial frequency of the grating and v is the temporal frequency of the oscillatory movements of the grating. The left-hand term in the equation represents the stabilized, high-contrast, time-invariant grating and the right-hand expression represents the relatively low contrast, stabilized grating undergoing counterphase-modulation with contrast equal to $C_s 2\pi fa$. (See Appendix A in Arend and Timberlake, 1986, for the derivation of this equation.)

The two assumptions required to proceed are (a) dynamic (transient) variations of luminance are required to drive neural elements, i.e., there are no static (sustained) neural elements and the time-invariant high-contrast grating is not represented in any way in neural activity and cannot, therefore, be detected, and (b) the neural signals produced by this time-invariant high-contrast grating are not only imperceptible, they also do not affect the neural signals produced by temporal variations of the lower-contrast, counterphase-modulated, grating which can be detected, providing some threshold illumination change is exceeded. Accepting these assumptions allows us to ignore the time-invariant, high-contrast grating on the right-hand side of Equation 1 and the contrast required for threshold of the stabilized, low-contrast, counterphase-modulated grating is, therefore, represented by Equation 2, which assumes perfect, that is, noise-free, stabilization:

$$C_v f = C_s 2\pi fa$$

where C_v is the threshold for the counterphase-modulated grating of spatial frequency f, temporal frequency v. C_s is, as in Equation 1, the contrast of the counterphase-modulated grating. Equation 2 only works for perfectly stabilized gratings. So, how can we proceed from here?

Arend and Timberlake (1986) point out that "visual sensitivity to perfectly stabilized counterphase-modulated gratings will be closely approximated by actual eyetracker-stabilized sensitivity when the grating spatial period is large relative to eyetracker noise. Under this condition the temporal changes produced by the small oscillations of eyetracker noise are small relative to the temporal changes that are due to the counterphase modulation" (p. 239). This allowed them to use Equation 2 to estimate the threshold amplitude of grating displacement (a in Equation 2) that would produce a local variation of illuminance sufficient to just excite the dynamic neural elements. Their calculation was based on an extrapolation from existing measurements of contrast sensitivity thresholds to a sinusoidally flickered spatial frequency display, whose spatial frequency was sufficiently low to satisfy the requirement described just above. They calculated the hypothetical threshold displacement for a 4 Hz oscillatory sinusoidal movement of a perfectly stabilized, 100% contrast, 2 cycle/° grating. Their hypothetical displacement threshold calculation took contrast threshold data from Kelly's (1979b) measurements made with the same spatial and temporal frequencies. They extrapolated the peak-to-peak displacement threshold amplitude (2a) for a *hypothetical 100%* contrast, 2 cycle/° spatial frequency grating and found it to be only 0.0011° – only 8″! Arend and Timberlake (1986) suggested on the basis of their calculations that Kelly's assumed action of sustained neural elements at and below the noise level of his tracker was unwarranted. In their words, tracker "noise alone . . . prevents conclusions about dynamic detectors on the basis of data from electromechanical trackers" (p. 239).

Arend and Timberlake next attempted to test the equivalence of a moving and a flickering grating, whose parameters were chosen along the lines set forth in Equation 1. This led them to do 'a preliminary experiment' described, in their words, as "allowing direct comparison of thresholds for wiggling and counterphase-modulated gratings . . . In order to measure meaningful thresholds for sinusoidally translated [wiggling] gratings, the amplitude of movement must be small relative to one cycle of the grating and large relative to the noise of the stabilizing system. Both conditions can be met for a small range of spatial frequencies and movement amplitudes" (p. 240). A 1 cycle/° spatial frequency grating, oscillating through a peak-to-peak distance of 3.33′, was considered to meet this constraint sufficiently well to permit a direct comparison of the temporal CSF obtained by varying the temporal frequency of this stimulus (the contrast required to see the grating when it wiggled at various frequencies) with the temporal CSF obtained by counterphase-modulating a relatively low contrast grating of the same spatial frequency, superimposed on a similar, temporally invariant grating of much higher contrast. This second experimental condition is an example of the stimulating conditions, assumed to be equivalent to the stimulating conditions produced by a wiggling grating, in the calculations (described above) of the displacement threshold of the dynamic neural elements. In other words, the assumption that local temporal variation produced either by actually moving a grating (motion) or by counterphase modulation (flicker) has the same visual consequences was tested empirically. Temporal frequency was varied in octave-steps from 1.1 to 17.6 Hz. In the wiggle condition, these 5 frequencies moved the grating at average speeds ranging from 7.3′/s to 116′/s. The results of this experiment are summarized in Fig. 22.

Four of the 5 data points for flicker show greater sensitivity for counterphase modulation than for actual movement of the grating. In 3 of these 4 cases the standard deviations do not overlap, suggesting to us, at least, that Arend and Timberlake's description of "excellent agreement through 4.4. Hz" may be over-stated. Other features of potential significance in these results are the large and disorderly relationships at 8.8 and 17.6 Hz, which the authors suggest call into question their assumption that the time-invariant high-contrast grating is both undetectable and not interactive with the lower-contrast, counterphase-modulating grating. There is another disquieting feature in Fig. 22 that can be seen when it is compared with Fig. 21 (top), which reproduces the same subject's data for a drifting grating motion as a function of spatial frequency. Note that increasing the retinal image motion of the relatively low spatial frequency grating studied in Fig. 22 (1 cycle/°) led to a *reduction* in contrast sensitivity by a factor of almost 2 (0.3 log unit) whereas increasing retinal image speed with the same spatial frequency in Fig. 21 led to a modest *increase* in contrast sensitivity.* Furthermore, recall that when this subject's CSF was measured with the 'reduced-exposure technique' (described above), the difference between his SRI-tracker-stabilized contrast sensitivity and his contrast sensitivity when 'natural' biteboard fixational eye movements were permitted was as large as 0.8 log units (a factor of more than 6) with the same spatial frequency (his natural biteboard fixational drift eye movement speed, had it been recorded, would probably average about 9′/s). Ever since Van Nes's report (1968) we have come to expect an improvement in contrast sensitivity when motion is imposed on low spatial frequency gratings (see Fig. 11 for Van Nes's data, Fig. 15 for Arend's data and Fig. 20 for Steinman et al.'s data). The Arend and Timberlake (1986) result for a wiggling grating, which is reproduced in Fig. 22, is hard to understand when viewed in this historical perspective. Perhaps SRI tracker noise, which would have an average speed of 26′/s if it is assumed to be a 4 Hz sinusoid (a speed near the middle of the range shown in Fig. 22), had

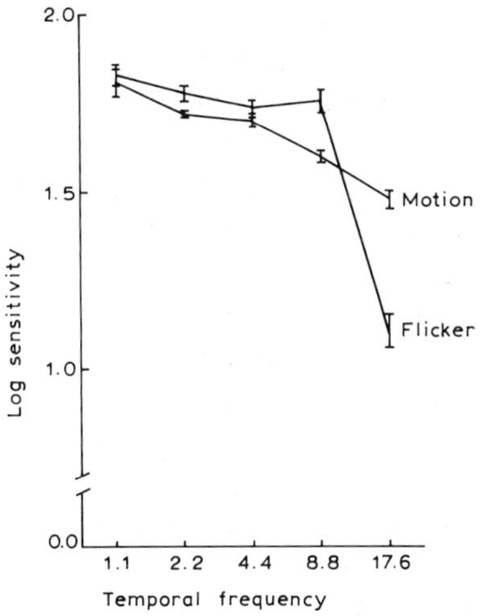

Fig. 22. Mean log sensitivities for stabilized 1 cycle/° gratings temporally modulated by two methods, i.e., by counterphase flicker (Flicker) or by moving the 1 cycle/° grating sinusoidally through 3.33 minutes of arc peak to peak (Motion). See the text for a discussion of the significance of this figure. (From Arend and Timberlake, 1986)

adverse effects on contrast sensitivity, adverse effects which would not be prominent with unidirectional drifting gratings or when tracker stabilization is not used.

We believe that the role of retinal image motion in the detection of contrast has not yet been worked out. Studies during the past decade in which the SRI tracker has been used to impose motion on stabilized gratings are less than completely satisfying in a number of respects. In addition to the uncertainties described above, we are disappointed by the fact that this technique has, because of its noise, confined study of the effects of retinal image motion on contrast sensitivity to the lower portion of the spatial frequency range to which the human visual system responds. Furthermore, the shape of the CSFs measured below the 7–12 cycle/° 'high' frequency spatial cutoffs reported for eyes of different subjects, may not be free from important distortion as has been assumed (e.g., Kelly, 1979b). If the spectrum of tracker noise is not actually known because no artificial eye can actually reproduce the characteristics of an individual's natural eye, it will not be possible to correct the shape of

* We are assuming that the data point plotted for 3°/s motion at 1 cycle/° lies above the value for 0.15°/s motion in Fig. 21 (top) entirely on the basis of the fact that Arend and Timberlake described their functions as similar to Kelly's (bottom) in Fig. 21 where different plotting symbols were used and one can be sure the the sensitivity was greater when the grating moved faster. If we are wrong, the results summarized by Arend and Timberlake in Fig. 21 are as mysterious as the results summarized in Fig. 22 in the light of previous observations by Arend and others.

an individual's stabilized CSF for artifacts introduced by stabilization. Tracker noise may well, as has been assumed, become less important with lower spatial frequency gratings but its actual contribution below 12, or 8.8 or 7 cycles/° probably should not simply be ignored – the common current practice. The situation above 12 cycles/° is even more troublesome. There are no meaningful tracker-stabilized data, whatsoever, in this region. The spatio-temporal surface modeled by Kelly (1979b) only covers a restricted range of spatial frequencies. The effects of retinal image motion on spatial frequencies falling in the range that was the domain called 'visual acuity' (30–60 or more cycles/°), throughout the century of pre-Fourier Optics, has not been and cannot be explored with this methodology in its current stage of development.

In our opinion, the most valuable, and possibly lasting, contribution of contemporary SRI tracker research with motion imposed on stabilized images can be found in the Arend and Timberlake (1986) paper. Specifically, their attempt to provide a quantitative technique for working out the potential contribution of instrumentation noise to threshold measurements of contrast sensitivity is intriguing and seems to be theoretically sound as well. Even if their estimates of displacement threshold, which were based on a *hypothetical* 100% grating contrast, prove to be in error by a large factor, their insistence on the need to estimate these thresholds and a technique for doing so provided a refreshing approach in a very old, much studied and technically very difficult problem area. Anyone considering working further in this area would probably benefit by thinking hard about their concluding remarks.

They concluded their provocative paper by calling attention to the fact that their "calculation focussed on noise in the eye-position signal, there are much larger potential sources of destabilization. No practical ramping of onset and offset can eliminate important stimulus transients... Eyeblinks produce large illuminance changes over the entire retina, often more frequently than the 15–20 s required for the effects of smaller transients to subside [see Burbeck and Kelly, 1982, for effects of transient stimulation]. The time delay between eye motion and the tracker signal also produces substantial retinal-illuminance transients at edges in the image during saccades or high-velocity smooth movements... Even if these large sources could be eliminated, there are smaller destabilization sources that are difficult or impossible to remove. Small shifts of the natural pupil relative to the artificial pupil [in the stabilizing device] could be significant because of the Stiles-Crawford effect. At the high threshold contrasts in Fig. 21 the just detectable grating appeared and disappeared in synchrony with the subject's heartbeat... Given the extreme sensitivity indicated by the observations and slow-drift calculations, the remarkable observation is not that we failed to get full disappearance but that Yarbus and Gerrits et al. did" (pp. 240–241).

In this section, we have seen that research on retinal image motion, imposed on a stabilized display, is incomplete, in large part because of technical limitations of instrumentation available for stabilizing images. These limitations arise more from the exquisite sensitivity of the human visual system to moving contrasts than from any lack of sophistication on the part of contemporary instrument builders. Stabilizing instruments, used with grating targets whose retinal contrast is physically realizable (i.e., well under the 100% assumed in Arend and Timberlake's calculations), need position accuracy better than 20″ and velocity accuracy better than 40″/s to be better than the visual system under study. Even such accuracy is very difficult to achieve in intact living organisms. Our current knowledge is incomplete at both ends of the spatial frequency spectrum. At the low end, we have not yet determined, after almost 40 years of stabilized image research, whether there are functionally significant sustained neural elements (called 'static' elements by Arend and Timberlake) which could provide vague visual outlines of patterned stimulation (the kind of percepts Barlow, 1963, reported), if prolonged, functionally 'perfect' stabilization could be achieved. It remains quite plausible to continue to subscribe to Yarbus's, Gerrits's,

Arend's and their coworkers's claim that transient stimulation is a *necessary* condition for vision. The upper part of the normal spatial frequency range (the region traditionally studied under the rubric 'visual acuity') has also been inaccessible to the best current non-invasive stabilizing instrumentation. We have no direct, meaningful, measurements made with an SRI tracker of the effects of motion imposed on sinusoidal gratings whose spatial frequencies are greater than 7–12 cycles/° (depending on the subject). Available data only cover a rather modest portion of the range of discriminable spatial frequencies – a range which extends as high as 60 cycles/° in normal observers.

We also still do not know whether unidirectional drifts imposed on stabilized gratings have the same effects on contrast sensitivity as imposed sinusoidal oscillations. This is important because a sinusoidal oscillation, rather than a unidirectional drift, is more like the image motion produced by the natural fixational eye movement pattern of a human being who is sitting without artificial head supports, standing or moving about. Arend and Timberlake (1986) have taken a small step towards answering this question. They have shown that very small amplitude sinusoidal oscillations (3.3′ p-p) and unidirectional drifts of a 1 cycle/° grating which have about the same average speed have somewhat similar effects on contrast sensitivity. Larger-amplitude oscillations (the kind observed when the head is not supported artificially) and higher spatial frequencies have not yet been compared.

In summary, detrimental effects of image motion on contrast sensitivity in the upper, 'acuity' range of discriminable spatial frequencies, and beneficial effects of image motion at the lower end of this range, have not been described adequately in the currently available literature which has studied effects of motion imposed on a 'stabilized' grating display. The most recent work by Arend and Timberlake (1986) on the significance of instrumentation noise and local retinal adaptation in stabilized image experiments suggests that it will be exceedingly difficult, perhaps even impossible, to use this kind of technique to eliminate all influences, other than image motion introduced by the experimenter, on measurements of contrast sensitivity across the entire functional range of the human visual system.

Is there an alternative way to find out how retinal image motion affects contrast sensitivity? Could it be that CSFs measured in experiments done with what we have called 'natural retinal image motion' (i.e., retinal image motion resulting from incomplete oculomotor compensation during oscillations of the head) provide a useful beginning of a description of the effects of retinal image motion on contrast sensitivity? These CSFs could provide the initial basis for developing models of visual information processing in the presence of image motion (and also suggest a technique for future work) if we could be sure that a subject making contrast threshold judgements while he shook his head actually followed instructions and made all of his observations near the center of his head trajectory, where retinal image speed would be close to its highest average value. In other words, the CSFs described in section 8.2.3 and illustrated in Fig. 20 might provide a valid, albeit very approximate, description of human contrast sensitivity across almost the entire range of discriminable spatial frequencies if we could be sure that the subjects made all of their threshold settings on the basis of information obtained when the image of the grating display was moving rapidly on their retinas. Said more succinctly, it would be easier to take the 'natural' CSFs, shown in Fig. 20, seriously if we could be sure that the subject did not sneak a peek when he turned about. In the next section, we will show that similar CSFs can be obtained when sneaking a peek is impossible.*

* We thank Dr. Z. Pizlo for making valuable suggestions about how we might treat the material reviewed in this and previous sections on research with the SRI tracker. Dr. Pizlo brought high-level engineering skills to an unfamiliar problem area and was prepared, therefore, to raise very cogent questions and demand justifications for assumptions and analyses that might be ignored or overlooked by visual scientists, such as ourselves, who have been measuring visual CSFs for many years.

10. Effect of motion on the CSF when natural image speed controls contrast

10.1. Instrumentation for monitoring head and retinal image speed

We used the revolving magnetic cube-surface field-sensor coil technique to monitor the absolute horizontal position of the head or eye in space while psychophysical measurements of contrast sensitivity were made, both while the subject (RMS) sat still and while he oscillated his head. The principle of this technique for measuring the orientation of the head or eyes in space was described originally by Collewijn (1977), who used it for the first time in his study of the eye movements of freely moving rabbits. The development of this type of instrumentation for use with human beings (first reported by Steinman and Collewijn, 1980), was described recently by Steinman (1986). The properties of the particular revolving field monitor (RFM) developed at the University of Maryland and used for the new research on contrast sensitivity, which will be reported for the first time in subsequent sections, were first described in Collewijn et al. (1981). Examples of its effectiveness in studying the full range of human binocular eye and head movement with exceptional accuracy and precision can be found in Steinman (1982) and, most recently, in Collewijn et al. (1988a,b) and Erkelens et al. (1989a,b).

Here, we will only describe the main features of the Maryland RFM and then describe a few specific elaborations of this instrumentation, which made it impossible for the subject to 'sneak-a-peek' while his thresholds were measured as he oscillated his head (the reader should consult the references cited above for additional details). A sensor coil, mounted either on a head-band or on a silicone annulus which was sucked on to the eye, was located in a large (3.6 m diameter) homogeneous magnetic field generated around the subject. This homogeneous magnetic field was rotating in the horizontal plane at 976 Hz. The phase of the alternating electric potential, which is induced by the rotating magnetic field in a sensor coil located within it, is linearly related to the angular orientation of the rotating magnetic field. It follows that the phase of the signal induced in the sensor coil indicates the orientation of the sensor coil with respect to an earth-fixed coordinate system (the coordinates are provided by the large stationary field coils that generate the revolving magnetic field).

In the Maryland RFM, the generation of the rotating magnetic field and the measurement of the phase of the signal induced in the sensor coil is accomplished primarily with digital instrumentation. This allows the measurement of very small changes in the angular orientation of the sensor coil within a very large range of possible orientations. Specifically, RFM rms noise with output at 488 Hz (the output sample rate used in the experiment described in the following sections) is less than 40″ and the linearity of RFM output is better than 0.01% within the instrument's 360° range of operation. The angular position output of the Maryland RFM is digital (16 bits) and its slewing speed is equivalent to angular velocities of 12000°/s. Drift (measured from a stationary sensor coil) is less than 6 seconds of arc for periods ranging from 1 second up to 24 hours. Measures of angular position (orientation) are not measurably sensitive to translations (linear displacements) of the sensor coil within a region of about 50 cm near the center of the rotating magnetic field where the subject sits. The stability of the self-adhering silicone annulus sensor coil, when it is inserted properly, was demonstrated by its inventors for saccadic eye movements as large as 20° (Collewijn et al., 1975) and reconfirmed in the Maryland RFM for much larger eye and head movements (Collewijn et al., 1981), and also during blinks and prolonged closures of the eyelids (Collewijn et al., 1985).

Digital indications of the orientation of the sensor coil (position output in angular units) were fed to a dedicated microprocessor running at 12 MHz, which stored them in a FIFO buffer (first in, first out), and did a running calculation of velocity as they passed through a programmable digital filter. These digital velocities were converted to speeds (absolute velocities) and then fed to a digital thresholding device, which permitted the output to be limited to some maximum value selected by the experimenter. The digital output of the thresholding device was then converted to a voltage analogue of speed, which was fed to the Z-axis of a CRT display, located 6 meters from the subject, where the display subtended 1.5° horizontally and 1.2° vertically (a Tektronix Model 604 display with a P-4 phosphor was used). The noise (rms) in the voltage proportional to speed was 0.15°/s (9′/s) with the parameters employed (viz., position signals fed at 488 Hz into a sliding window, whose width was 33 ms). This measurement of noise in the speed voltage output was made when the input to the microprocessor was provided by a stationary sensor coil.

Sinusoidal spatial frequency displays were generated and varied by conventional analogue techniques, which meant that, when the voltage derived from the rotational speed of the sensor coil was fed to the Z-axis of the display, the contrast of the grating was proportional to the speed with which the sensor coil was oscillating. The maximum contrast available to the subject was limited to a value chosen by the experimenter. This limit, coupled with the control of contrast by the speed of the sensor coil, made it possible to measure thresholds in, and always in, the presence of motion of a subject's head or eye, depending on the placement of the sensor coil. This was possible because when the coil was not moving, contrast was zero. In other words, there was no grating pattern – the display was homogeneous. A grating pattern was present in the stimulus when, and only when, the coil was moving. The contrast produced by motion might, or might not, allow the grating pattern to be above threshold. Exceeding the psychophysical contrast threshold required that the coil was moving fast enough, and also that the experimenter had set the maximum permissible contrast level above the threshold value needed for the particular spatial frequency under study. The Z-axis amplifier was adjusted so that a voltage proportional to a speed of either 50 or 5°/s produced a contrast of about 75%, depending on whether the sensor coil was mounted on the head or on the eye, respectively (these values were determined empirically in pilot work).

*10.2. Procedures in the 'sneak-a-peek' control experiments**

Two experiments were performed with this new instrumentation. Both were controls for the earlier work (see section 8 and Steinman et al., 1985), which had reported rather modest detrimental effects of natural retinal image motion on high spatial frequencies (that is, frequencies above 8 cycles/°) as compared with the detrimental effects of motion that had been imposed on stabilized displays (Kelly, 1979a,b; Arend and Timberlake, 1986). The previous experiments with natural retinal image motion had also shown beneficial effects of image motion on a wider range of 'low' spatial frequencies (up to about 6 cycles/°), whereas benefits of image motion were not observed for spatial frequencies above 2 cycles/° when motion was imposed on a stabilized display.

The sensor coil was mounted on the head in the first experiment. This permitted long psychophysical sessions in which contrast thresholds could be measured, and replicated carefully, both when the subject (RMS) sat still and when he oscillated his head. When he sat still, the contrast available depended entirely on the value set by the experimenter (JZL) before each trial. When he oscillated his head, the contrast available depended *both* on the speed of the head and on the value set by the experimenter before each trial. In this condition, contrast varied appreciably throughout the trial, depending on how fast the subject moved his head. The maximum available contrast, which had been set by the experimenter before the trial, was only available while the head was moving fast. Contrast was reduced by the microprocessor as the head slowed down and dropped to zero whenever the head stopped moving. This technique made it difficult, probably impossible, for the subject to set contrast

* We thank Dr. T. Park for his help in running these experiments.

thresholds during head movement to be similar to the contrast thresholds set when he sat still simply by basing his judgements on what could be seen when his head slowed down.

In both conditions, monocular contrast thresholds were measured with a double staircase procedure (Cornsweet's, 1962, method, which uses two randomly interleaved staircases). In both conditions, the subject continued on the pair of staircases until the experimenter was satisfied that steady-state performance had been achieved (see Nachmias and Steinman, 1965, for a comparison of the Double Random Staircase Procedure with the Method of Limits). A single spatial frequency grating was studied in each experimental session. Threshold measurements, made when the subject sat still or when he oscillated his head, were interleaved in alternating blocks of 10 trials each. The CRT display was surrounded by a homogeneous 'white' baffle which subtended about 8° horizontally and about 5° vertically. The light reflected from this baffle was adjusted to the same space average luminance as the CRT display, which could be seen through a rectangular cut-out at the center of the baffle. Trials, in both conditions, began with the subject fixating a black cross located 1.5° to the left of the center of the grating display (the cross was drawn on the left side of the baffle).

The subject started each 8-s trial when he felt ready after the experimenter had indicated that the contrast that would be available on the next trial had been prepared. When the subject started a trial during which he would keep his head still, he made a single saccade to the center of the display and continued to fixate at this position until either he reported that he could see the grating pattern or the trial ended, which was recorded as a failure to see the pattern. The test contrast was switched-on during the time the saccade was made to the center of the CRT display. This strategy was used to prevent the subject from basing his judgements either (1) on the appearance of the contrast in the eccentric display before the trial had started, or (2) on switching-transients in the CRT display, occurring after he had shifted fixation from the eccentric pre-trial fixation cross to the center of the CRT. In the second condition, the subject also began each 8-s trial when the experimenter indicated that contrast had been set but, in this condition, contrast in the display was only available while the head was oscillating. Its maximum was limited to a value selected by the experimenter on the basis of the report made by the subject on the preceding trial on the same staircase (the response on the preceding trial on the same staircase also determined the test contrast presented when the subject sat still – it is in this sense that staircase procedures are described as 'interactive'). The subject began to oscillate his head as he started the trial and shifted fixation to the center of the display while his head was in motion. The frequency and amplitude of his head oscillations were self-selected on the basis of what had been helpful during previous trials for obtaining the contrast required to see the grating (both the frequency and the amplitude of head oscillations were influenced by the particular spatial frequency under test). Here, as in the condition during which the subject sat still while his CSF was measured, either the subject reported seeing the grating pattern at some time during the trial or the trial was counted as below threshold, which meant that the next test on the same staircase would be made with a higher level of maximum contrast.

10.3. Results when head speed controlled contrast

Fig. 23 summarizes the psychophysical results obtained. The functions plotted in this figure should be compared with the functions for the same subject (RMS) in Fig. 20. The earlier data were obtained when this subject *could have* sneaked peeks near head-turnabouts as he judged high spatial frequency gratings and *could have* made threshold judgements near the center of head swings as he judged low spatial frequencies. The results of the new control experiment do not support these suggestions, particularly at the high spatial frequency end (above 8 cycles/° where the functions cross). Here, the detrimental effects of motion on contrast sensitivity are modest throughout the range of higher spatial frequencies (about 25% at and above 12 cycles/°). The extrapolated high-frequency cutoffs of both functions are also not very different, both falling well above 30 cycles/°. The beneficial effects of motion on low spatial frequency gratings were observed in a smaller range of spatial frequencies in the new control experiment than they were originally. In the original experiment, which is summarized in Fig. 20, this subject showed beneficial effects of motion at and below 8 cycles/°, whereas in the new experiment the benefits of motion only appeared at and below 4 cycles/°. The magnitude of the maximum beneficial effect of motion at the low frequency end was, however, quite comparable, namely a factor of about 2.5 at 2 cycles/°. The functions for both 'moving' and 'sitting still' were indistinguishable between 3 and 8 cycles/°, where they cross over as motion began to reduce contrast sensitivity.

It does not seem useful to try to explain the differences between the original and the sneak-a-peek control experiments, which are summarized in Figs. 20 and 23, because the new control experiment utilized a novel and very strange coupling of head motion and grating contrast, a coupling that could never occur under normal viewing. In other words, shaking the head to obtain contrast and shaking it faster to increase contrast precluded sneaking peeks but it does not provide a useful method for studying the normal relationship of head-movement-produced retinal-image slip to contrast sensitivity. We believe that the technique used in this control experiment seems no more likely to produce useful information about this relationship than imposing a unidirectional drift on a more-or-less stabilized grating display. The sneak-a-peek experiment did, however, serve its purpose inasmuch as it showed that the modest deleterious effects of image motion on high spatial frequencies observed in the previous experiment were not caused by the subject's carelessness, dereliction of duty or dishonesty.

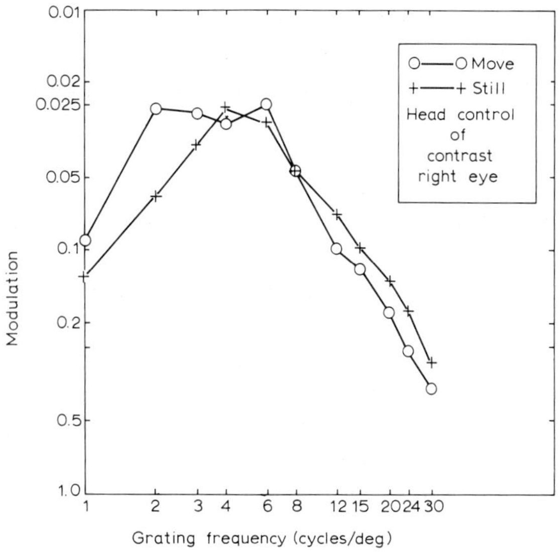

Fig. 23. Threshold grating contrast-modulation settings as fractions of 100% contrast at eleven spatial frequencies. These contrast sensitivity functions were obtained either while the subject (author RMS) sat still (Still), shown by the filled circles, or while he oscillated his head about its vertical axis (Move), shown by the open circles. When he oscillated his head, the speed with which the head was moving determined the maximum available contrast. See the text for a discussion of these functions.

10.4. Results when eye speed controlled contrast

The basic experiment was repeated with the sensor coil mounted on the eye, rather than on the head; a change which guaranteed that contrast sufficient to cause the perception of a grating would never be presented when the display was stationary on the retina. This change in the placement of the sensor coil only allowed a partial replication of the sneak-a-peek experiment because only relatively short psychophysical sessions were possible. Wearing the silicone annulus sensor coil restricted psychophysical sessions to 20 minutes.* Two-hour sessions had

* RMS is only comfortable for about 20 min when he wears the silicone annulus. Many other subjects are comfortable for much longer periods, up to 50 minutes, which is considered by many users to be the upper limit for the safe use of this kind of attachment to the eye (this limit is imposed by intraocular pressure, which increases slowly as the annulus is worn for prolonged periods).

been possible when the sensor coil was mounted on the head. This limitation made it relatively difficult to collect even the very modest set of threshold data that will be described below because it was deemed prudent to skip at least one day between sessions in addition to keeping the sessions very short. This restriction was partially overcome by using both of the eyes for making observations, one eye at a time in a single session and alternating eyes in successive sessions. The experiment was also simplified by reducing the number of spatial frequencies studied from 11 to 8 and by using a very modest number of reversals on the staircases to estimate thresholds, rather than continuing measurements until completely satisfied that the best possible estimate had been obtained in a given session. To sum up, using a silicone annulus sensor coil sucked on to the eye precluded the careful, well-replicated psychophysical measurements that were possible when the sensor coil was attached to the head.

The results of this control experiment are summarized in Fig. 24. The functions plotted are based on contrast sensitivity thresholds measured in 18 short sessions spread out over a period of more than 2 months (the data points are the means of RMS's right and left eye thresholds; his eyes had similar sensitivities). Measurements could not be extended above 20 cycles/° because the variability associated with contrast threshold measurements on the rapidly falling upper limb of the CSF precluded reasonable estimates with spatial frequencies above this value. In other words, sessions were too short to permit an acceptable estimate of sensitivity with the double random staircase we employed. Nevertheless, the, admittedly noisy, data summarized in Fig. 24 are, in our opinion, sufficiently clear to allow us to suggest that the main effects of motion on contrast sensitivity, which were measured when contrast was controlled by the speed of the head, can also be found in measurements made when contrast was controlled by the speed of retinal image (eye speed in space and retinal image speed are almost the same with distant targets; see Steinman et al., 1982; or Ferman et al., 1987). That is, the visibility of spatial frequency gratings below 3 cycles/° was enhanced by retinal image motion and retinal image motion had only relatively modest adverse effects on contrast sensitivity with higher spatial frequencies (above 6 cycles/° these modest effects of motion on contrast sensitivity were obscured by the noise of the psychophysical measurements). The basis upon which the visual system maintains contrast sensitivity in the presence of appreciable retinal image motion must still be worked out (see section 8.2.3 for our speculations about the way in which signals from the vestibular system might aid vision in the presence of retinal image motion).

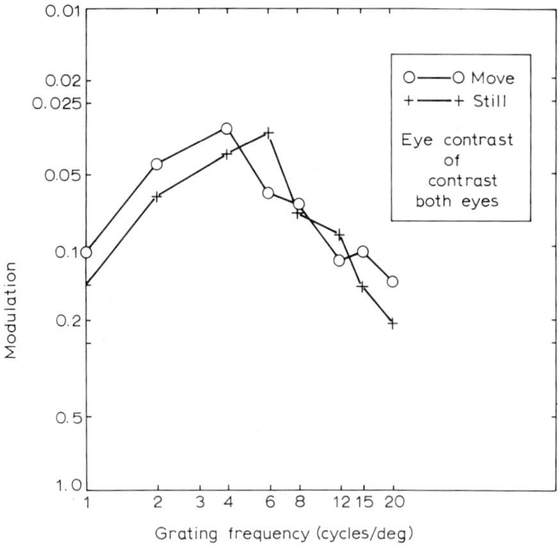

Fig. 24. Threshold grating contrast-modulation settings as fractions of 100% contrast at eight spatial frequencies. These contrast sensitivity functions were obtained either while the subject (author RMS) sat still (Still), shown by the filled circles, or while he oscillated his head about its vertical axis (Move), shown by the open circles. When he oscillated his head, the speed with which the retinal image was moving in either the right or the left eye determined the maximum available contrast. The functions during movement are the means of the threshold settings made with each eye at a separate session. See the text for a discussion of the significance of these functions and details about how these observations were made.

11. Conclusions

We began this chapter claiming that the role of eye

movements in basic visual information processing has a long history. Their role has varied from virtually complete neglect in 'static' theories to fundamental significance in 'dynamic' theories. A variety of intermediate roles have also been proposed. The reader will probably agree that we have justified this claim. We also began by claiming that current emphasis favors an important role for eye movement in basic visual information processing. At this time it is generally accepted that transient stimulation, which may be produced by movements of the eye as well as by movements of objects in the visual field, can drive visual neurons whose consequent action allows us to see. Exactly what would be seen with high-contrast targets in the central fovea if all retinal image motion were to be eliminated is still unknown and alternative expectations are plausible, i.e., either a completely homogeneous visual field or a low-contrast visual field with only low or medium spatial frequency content. It looks as though it may be exceedingly difficult, probably actually impossible, to resolve this issue because of the exquisite sensitivity of the visual neurons to motion of any appreciable extent across the retinal surface and the incessant motion of visual neurons embedded in pulsating retinal tissues.

Fortunately, it has also become clear in recent years that the unsuccessful attempt to resolve this classical question during the past 40 years may represent an unnecessary and misdirected effort. The retinal image is in no danger, whatsoever, of even approaching the level of stability observed when the head is artificially supported once the subject gets off the biteboard. The head resting only on its natural biological platform moves quite a bit and this motion is not compensated completely by eye movements. Natural retinal image motion, arising from incomplete oculomotor compensation of bodily motions, guarantees appreciable transient stimulation of visual neurons (several orders of magnitude greater than the minimum retinal image displacement required to provide effective transient stimulation). This is true even in the limiting case in which the human being attempts to sit or stand as still as possible while fixating a stationary target located at optical infinity. Here, only about 50% of the movements of his head are compensated by eye movements, and retinal image motions are 2–4 times faster than retinal image motions present when the head is on a biteboard. Once the subject relaxes or looks at near targets, retinal image motion more than doubles. As soon as he talks or moves or chews or does anything at all, the problem for the visual scientist changes the traditional question of how eye movements are used to provide transient stimulation into a complementary question. Namely, how do we see a clear and stable world in the presence of such turbulence. Actually, the oculomotor system does its job very well; on average, about 97.5% of bodily motion is likely to be compensated for by eye movements when the head is free and the subject makes rather natural movements. But 2.5% of uncompensated bodily motion allows the retinal image to move through several degrees of visual angle at velocities of several degrees per second during most non-violent natural activities. Also, remember that the motions in each of the eyes are different. This allows vergence (and absolute retinal disparity) to vary continually by like amounts whenever natural bodily motion is permitted.

Some of this turbulence has been shown to be beneficial for vision. In essence, the incomplete nature of oculomotor compensation is an inescapable but useful characteristic. Furthermore, there are suggestions that the degree of oculomotor compensation seems to be tuned at both ends of its effective functional range so as to facilitate some properties of visual information processing. Specifically, oculomotor compensation of bodily motion is far from complete when the subject sits or stands still. This allows effective transient stimulation. Also, even when compensation increases as the subject starts to move enough turbulence remains to facilitate perception of the global features of visual forms because the low spatial frequency content of the visual world benefits from increasing motion of the visual scene on the retina. Even the relatively high spatial frequency content required to make out fine details has been found to suffer only moderately when images move as a consequence of incomplete oculomotor compensation of bodily motion. How vision of high spatial frequencies manages to resist degradation in the presence of these natural retinal image motions is the major problem remaining.

It seems likely that the relationship between characteristics of oculomotor compensation and requirements for the detection of contrast and spatial detail is built-in and is maintained automatically without any voluntary oculomotor acts. It would be very awkward if the human being had to intentionally move her eyes so as to generate transient neural signals required to detect contrast or to achieve resolution of fine details. Simply living without artificial bodily restraint guarantees retinal image motion sufficient to activate all basic visual processing mechanisms. In essence, living and seeing go together naturally. It is only when stimuli are very faint or when contrast is extemely low that active looking for seeing comes into play. These conditions are likely to be encountered at night, in dense fog, with objects far in the periphery or in the visual science laboratory. In other situations, the interplay of oculomotor control and the processing of basic visual information are tuned to each other reflexively and voluntary oculomotor actions are unnecessary. This arrangement, from a teleological perspective, is a simple and useful way for the visual and oculomotor systems to cooperate. Significant features of visual stimuli appear effortlessly. Voluntary action is required only when we wish to search the visual array to find or to contemplate conspicuous features contained within it. More basic visual processing works well without explicit, willful oculomotor intervention.

Acknowledgement

The preparation of this chapter was supported, in part, by Grant EY 04647 from the National Eye Institute of the National Institutes of Health (U.S.A.).

References

Adler, F.H. and Fliegelman, M. (1934) Influence of fixation on the visual acuity. Arch. Ophthalmol. 12, 475–483.

Arend, L.E. (1973) Spatial differential and integral operations in human vision: implications of stabilized image fading. Psychol. Rev. 80, 374–395.

Arend, L.E. (1976) Temporal determinants of the form of the spatial contrast threshold MTF. Vision Res. 16, 1035–1042.

Arend, L.E. and Timberlake, G.T. (1986) What is perfect stabilization? Do perfectly stabilized images always disappear? J. Opt. Soc. Am. A 3, 235–241.

Attneave, F. (1957) Physical determinants of the judged complexity of shapes. J. Exp. Psychol. 53, 221–227.

Averill, H.L. and Weymouth, F.W. (1925) Visual perception and the retinal mosaic. II. The influence of eye movements on the displacement threshold. J. Comp. Psychol. 5, 147–176.

Barlow, H.B. (1952) Eye movements during fixation. J. Physiol. 116, 290–306.

Barlow, H.B. (1963) Slippage of contact lenses and other artefacts in relation to fading and regeneration of supposedly stabilized images. Q. J. Exp. Psychol. 15, 36–51.

Barlow, H.B., Fitzhugh, R. and Kuffler, S.W. (1957) Change in organization in the cat's retina during dark adaptation. J. Physiol. 137, 338–354.

Blakemore, C. and Campbell, F.W. (1969) On the existence of neurones in the human visual system selectively sensitive to the orientation and size of retinal images. J. Physiol. 203, 237–260.

Brindley, G.S. (1960) Physiology of the Retina and the Visual Pathway, Edward Arnold, London.

Brown, C.R. and Forsyth, D.M. (1959) Fusion contour for intermittent photic stimuli of alternating duration. Science 129, 390–391.

Bryngdahl, O. (1961) Effect of retinal image motion on visual acuity. Optica Acta 8, 1–16.

Burbeck, C.A. and Kelly, D.H. (1982) Eliminating transient artifacts in stabilized-image contrast thresholds. J. Opt. Soc. Am. 72, 1238–1243.

Burbeck, C.A. and Kelly, D.H. (1984) Role of local adaptation in the fading of stabilized images. J. Opt. Soc. Am. A 1, 216–220.

Byram, G.M. (1944) The physical and photochemical basis of visual resolving power. I. The distribution of illumination in retinal images. J. Opt. Soc. Am. 34, 571–591.

Campbell, F.W. and Robson, J. (1964) Application of Fourier analysis to the modulation response of the eye. J. Opt. Soc. Am. 54, 581.

Campbell, F.W., Kulikowski, J.J. and Levinson, J.Z. (1966) The effect of orientation on the visual resolution of gratings. J. Physiol. 187, 427–436.

Campbell, F.W., Carpenter, R.H.S., Levinson, J.Z. (1968) Visibility of aperiodic patterns compared with that of sinusoidal gratings. J. Physiol. 204, 283–298.

Clowes, M.B. (1962) A note on colour discrimination under conditions of retinal image constraint. Optica Acta 9, 65–68.

Collewijn, H. (1977) Eye and head movements in freely-moving rabbits. J. Physiol. 266, 471–498.

Collewijn, H. (1989) The vestibulo-ocular reflex: an outdated concept? In: J.H.J. Allum and M. Hulliger (Eds.), Afferent Control of Posture and Locomotion, Progress in Brain Research, Vol. 80, Elsevier, Amsterdam, pp. 197–209.

Collewijn, H. and Tamminga, E.P. (1984) Human smooth and saccadic eye movements during voluntary pursuit of different targets on different backgrounds. J. Physiol. 351, 21–250.

Collewijn, H., van der Mark, F. and Jansen, T.C. (1975) Precise recording of human eye movements. Vision Res. 15, 447–450.

Collewijn, H., Martins, A.J. and Steinman, R.M. (1981) Natural retinal image motion: origin and change. Ann. N. Y. Acad. Sci. 374, 312–329.

Collewijn, H., Martins, A.J. and Steinman, R.M. (1983) Compensatory eye movements during active and passive head movements: fast adaptation to changes in visual magnification. J. Physiol. 259–286.

Collewijn, H., Van der Steen, J. and Steinman, R.M. (1985) Human eye movements associated with blinks and prolonged eye-lid closures. J. Neurophysiol. 54, 11–27.

Collewijn, H., Erkelens, C.E. and Steinman, R.M. (1988) Binocular co-ordination of human vertical eye movements. J. Physiol. 404, 183–197.

Collewijn, H., Steinman, R.M., Erkelens, C.E., Pizlo, Z. and Van der Steen (1990a) The effect of freeing the head on eye movement characteristics during 3-D shifts of gaze. In: A. Berthoz, W. Graf and P.P. Vidal (Eds), The Head-Neck Sensory-Motor System, Oxford University Press, Wiley, New York, in press.

Collewijn, H., Steinman, R.M., Erkelens, C.E. and Regan, D. (1990b) Binocular fusion, steropsis and stereoacuity with a moving head. In: D. Regan (Ed.), Binocular Vision and Visual Dysfunction, Vol. 10A, Macmillan, London, in press.

Cornsweet, T.N. (1956) Determination of stimuli for involuntary drifts and saccadic eye movements. J. Opt. Soc. Am. 46, 987–993.

Cornsweet, T.N. (1962) The staircase method in psychophysics. Am. J. Psychol. 75, 485–491.

Cornsweet, T.N. and Crane, H.D. (1973) An accurate eye tracker using first and fourth Purkinje images. J. Opt. Soc. Am. 63, 921–928.

Craik, K.J.W. (1938) The effect of adaptation on differential brightness discrimination. J. Physiol. 92, 406–421.

Craik, K.J.W. (1939) The effect of adaptation upon visual acuity. Br. J. Psychol. 29, 252–266.

Crane, H.D. and Steele, C.M. (1978) Accurate three-dimensional eyetracker. Appl. Opt. 17, 691–705.

Crook, M.N. (1937) Visual discrimination of movement. J. Psychol. 3, 541–588.

Crozier, W.J., Wolf, E. and Zerrahn-Wolf, G. (1937) Critical illumination and critical flicker frequency for response to flickered light in dragonfly larvae. J. Gen. Physiol. 20, 363–392.

Cushman, W.B., Tangney, J.F., Steinman, R.M. and Ferguson, J.L. (1984) Characteristics of smooth eye movements with stabilized targets. Vision Res. 24, 1003–1009.

de Lange Dzn., H. (1957) Attenuation characteristics and phase-shift characteristics of the human fovea – cortex systems in relation to flicker-fusion phenomena. Thesis, Technical University, Delft.

de Lange Dzn., H. (1958) Research into the dynamic nature of the human fovea – cortex systems with intermittent and modulated light. J. Opt. Soc. Am. 48, 777–784.

Ditchburn, R.W. (1957) Report of N.P.L. symposium on colour vision. p. 415.

Ditchburn, R.W. (1973) Eye-Movements and Visual Perception, Clarendon Press, Oxford.

Ditchburn, R.W. (1980) The function of small saccades. Vision Res. 20, 271–272.

Ditchburn, R.W. and Drysdale, A.E. (1977a) The effect of retinal image motion on vision: I. Step-movements and pulse-movements. Proc. R. Soc. Lond. B 197, 131–144.

Ditchburn, R.W. and Drysdale, A.E. (1977b) The effect of retinal image motion on vision: II. Oscillatory movements. Pr. Roy. Soc. Lond. B 197, 385–406.

Ditchburn, R.W. and Ginsborg, B.L. (1953) Involuntary eye movements during fixation. J. Physiol. 119, 1–17.

Ditchburn, R.W. and Pritchard, R.M. (1956) Stabilized interference fringes on the retina. Nature 177, 434.

Dodge, R. (1903) Five types of eye movement in the horizontal meridian plane of the field of regard. Am. J. Physiol. 8, 307–329.

Dodge, R. and Cline, T.S. (1901) The angle velocity of eye movements. Psychol. Rev. 8, 145–157.

Duwaer, A.L. (1982) Assessment of retinal image displacement during head movement using an afterimage method. Vision Res. 22, 1379–1388.

Ercoles, A.M. and Zoli, M.T. (1968) Contrast thresholds for moving Landolt rings. Atti. Fond. G. Ronchi 23, 515–525.

Erkelens, C.E., Van der Steen, J., Steinman, R.M. and Collewijn, H. (1989a) Ocular vergence under natural conditions. I. Continuous changes of target distance along the median plane. Proc. R. Soc. Lond. B 236, 417–440.

Erkelens, C.E., Steinman, R.M. and Collewijn, H. (1989b) Ocular vergence undcr natural conditions. II. Gaze-shifts between real targets differing in distance and direction. Proc. R. Soc. Lond. B 236, 441–465.

Erkelens, C.E., Collewijn, H. and Steinman, R.M. (1989c) Asymmetrical adaptation of human saccades to to anisometropic spectacles. Invest. Ophthalmol. Vis. Sci. 30, 110–123.

Estevez, O. and Cavonius, C.R. (1976) Low-frequency attentuation in the detection of gratings: sorting out the artefacts.

Vision Res. 16, 497–500.

Falk, J.L. (1956) Theories of visual acuity and their physiological bases. Psychol. Bull. 53, 109–133.

Fechner, G.T. (1860) Elemente der Psychophysik, Breitkopf and Harterl, Leipzig.

Ferman, L., Collewijn, H., Jansen, T.C. and Van der Berg, A.V. (1987) Human gaze stability in horizontal, vertical and torsional direction during voluntary head movements, evaluated with a three-dimensional scleral induction coil technique. Vision Res. 27, 811–828.

Festinger, L. (1971) Eye movements and perception. In: P. Bach-y-Rita and C.C. Collins (Eds.), The Control of Eye Movements, Academic Press, New York.

Fiorentini, A. (1961) Dynamic characteristics of visual processes. In: E. Wolf (Ed.), Progress in Optics, North-Holland Press, Amsterdam.

Fiorentini, A. and Ercoles, A.H. (1957) Vision of oscillating non-uniform fields. Optica Acta 4, 150–157.

Graham, N. (1972) Spatial frequency channels in the human visual system: effects of luminance and pattern drift rate. Vision Res. 12, 53–69.

Gerrits, H.J.M. (1978) Differences in foveal and peripheral effects observed in stabilized vision. Exp. Brain Res. 32, 225–244.

Gerrits, H.J.M. and Vendrik, A.J.H. (1970) Artificial movements of a stabilized image. Vision Res. 10, 1443–1456.

Gerrits, H.J.M. and Vendrik, A.J.H. (1972) Eye movements necessary for continuous perception during stabilization of retinal images. Bibl. Ophthalmol. 82, 339–347.

Gerrits, H.J.M. and Vendrik, A.J.H. (1974) The influence of stimulus movements on perception in parafoveal stabilized vision. Vision Res. 14, 175–180.

Gerrits, H.J.M., Haan, B. de, Vendrik, A.J.H. (1966) Experiments with retinal stabilized images. Relations between the observations and neural data. Vision Res. 6, 427–440.

Gerrits, H.J.M., Stassen, H.P.W. and Erning, L.J. (1984) The role of drifts and saccades for the preservation of brightness perception. In: L. Spillmann and B.R. Wooten (Eds.), Sensory Experience, Adaptation, and Perception, Lawrence Erlbaum Associates, Hillsdale, NJ, pp. 439–459.

Gilbert, D.S. and Fender, D.H. (1969) Contrast thresholds measured with stabilized and non-stabilized sine-wave gratings. Optica Acta 16, 191–204.

Hartline, H.K. (1938) The response of single optic nerve fibers of the vertebrate eye to illumination of the retina. Am. J. Physiol. 121, 400–415.

Hartline, H.K. (1940) The receptive field of the optic nerve fibers. Am. J. Physiol. 130, 690–699.

Hartridge, H. (1922) Visual acuity and the resolving power of the eye. J. Physiol. 57, 52–67.

Hebb, D.O. (1949) The Organization of Behavior, John Wiley and Sons, New York.

Hecht, S. (1927) A quantitative basis for the relation between visual acuity and illumination. Proc. Nat. Acad. Sci. USA 13, 569–574.

Hecht, S. (1928) The relation between visual acuity and illumination. J. Gen. Physiol. 11, 255–281.

Hecht, S. and Mintz, E. (1939) The visibility of single lines at various illuminations and the retinal basis of visual resolution. J. Gen. Physiol. 22, 593–612.

Hecht, S., Shlaer, S. and Pirenne, M.H. (1942) Energy, quanta, and vision. J. Gen. Physiol. 25, 819–840.

Heckenmueller, E.G. (1965) Stabilization of the retinal image: a review of method, effects, and theory. Psychol. Bull. 63, 157–169.

Helmholtz, H.L.F. von (1863) Die Lehre von den Tonempfindungen ais physiologische Grundlage fur die Theorie der Musik, First Edition, Braunschweig.

Helmholtz, H.L.F. von (1866) Handbuch der Physiologischen Optik, Vol. 2, Voss, Hamburg-Leipzig.

Hering, E. (1899) Über die Grenzen der Schschärfe. Ber. d. math.-phys. Kl. d. Königl. Geo. d. Wissensch. zu Leipzig, 16–24.

Hering, E. (1920) Grundzuge der Lehre vom Lichtsinn, Springer, Berlin.

Hirsch, J. and Hylton, R. (1984) Quality of the primate photoreceptor lattice and limits of spatial vision. Vision Res. 24, 347–355.

Hofmann, F.B. (1920) Die Lehre vom Raumsinn des Auges, Springer, Berlin.

Jones, L.A. and Higgins, G.C. (1947) Photographic granularity and graininess III. Some characteristics of the visual system of some importance in the evaluation of graininess and granularity. J. Opt. Soc. Am. 37, 217–263.

Keesey, U.T. (1960) Effects of involuntary eye movements on visual acuity. J. Opt. Soc. Am. 50, 769–774.

Kelly, D.H. (1979a) Motion and vision I. Stabilized images of stationary targets. J. Opt. Soc. Am. 69, 1266–1274.

Kelly, D.H. (1979b) Motion and vision II. Stabilized spatio-temporal transfer surface. J. Opt. Soc. Am. 69, 1340–1349.

Köhler, W. and Wallach, H. (1944) Figural after-effects: an investigation of visual processes. Proc. Am. Philos. Soc. 88, 269–357.

Khurana, B. and Kowler, E. (1987) Shared attentional control of smooth eye movement and perception. Vision Res. 27, 1603–1618.

Kowler, E. and Steinman, R.M. (1979) The effect of expectations on slow oculomotor control: I. Periodic target steps. Vision Res. 19, 619–632.

Kowler, E. and Steinman, R.M. (1980) Small saccades serve no useful purpose: reply to a letter by R.W. Ditchburn. Vision Res. 20, 273–276.

Kowler, E., Martins, A.J. and Pavel, M. (1984a) The effect of expectations on slow oculomotor control – IV. Anticipatory smooth eye movements depend on prior target motions. Vision Res. 24, 197–210.

Kowler, E., Van der Steen, J. and Collewijn, H. (1984b) Voluntary selection of the target for smooth eye movement in the presence of superimposed, full-field stationary and moving stimuli. Vision Res. 24, 1789–198.

Krauskopf, J. (1957) Effect of image motion on contrast thresholds for maintained vision. J. Opt. Soc. Am. 47, 740–745.

Krauskopf, J. (1962) Effect of target oscillation on contrast resolution. J. Opt. Soc. Am. 52, 1306.

Krauskopf, J. (1963) Effect of retinal image stabilization on the appearance of heterochromatic targets. J. Opt. Soc. Am. 53, 741–744.

Kuffler, S.W. (1953) Discharge patterns and functional organization of the mammalian retina. J. Neurophysiol. 16, 37–68.

Le Grand, Y. (1967) Form and Space Vision. Revised Edition translated by M. Millodot and G. Heath, Indiana University Press, Bloomington and London.

Levinson, J.Z. (1959) Fusion of complex flicker. Science 130, 919–921.

Levinson, J.Z. (1960) Fusion of complex flicker. II. Science 131, 1438.

Levinson, J.Z. (1966) One-stage model for visual temporal integration. J. Opt. Soc. Am. 56, 95–97.

Levinson, J.Z. (1968) Flicker fusion phenomena. Science 160, 21–28.

Lit, A. (1968) Visual acuity. Annu. Rev. Psychol. 19, 27–54.

Ludvigh, E. (1948) The visibility of moving objects. Science 108, 63–64.

McCree, K.J. (1960) Colour confusion produced by voluntary fixation. Optica Acta 7, 281–290.

Marshall, W.H. and Talbot, S.A. (1942) Recent evidence for neural mechanisms in vision leading to a general theory of sensory acuity. Biol. Symp. 7, 117–164.

Matin, E. (1974) Saccadic suppression: a review and an analysis. Psychol. Bull. 81, 451–461.

Müller, J. (1826) Zur vergleichenden Physiologie der Geisichtssinnes der Menchen und Thiere, Leipzig.

Murphy, B.J. (1978) Pattern thresholds for moving and stationary gratings during smooth eye movements. Vision Res. 18, 521–530.

Murphy, B.J., Kowler, E. and Steinman, R.M. (1975) Slow oculomotor control in the presence of moving backgrounds. Vision. Res. 15, 1263–1268.

Nachmias, J. (1958) Brightness and visual acuity with intermittent illumination. J. Opt. Soc. Am. 48, 726–730.

Nachmias, J. (1959) Two-dimensional motion of the retinal image during monocular fixation. J. Opt. Soc. Am. 49, 901–908.

Nachmias, J. (1961) Determiners of drift of the eye during monocular fixation. J. Opt. Soc. Am. 51, 761–766.

Nachmias, J. and Steinman, R.M. (1965) An experimental comparison of the method of limits and the double-staircase method. Am. J. Psychol. 78, 112–115.

Osgood, C.E. (1953) Method and Theory in Experimental Psychology, Oxford University Press, New York.

Osgood, C.E. and Hyer, A.W. (1952) A new interpretation of figural aftereffects. Psychol. Rev. 59, 98–118.

Penner, M.J. (1978) Psychophysical methods and the minicomputer. In: M. Mayzner and T. Dolan (Eds.), Minicomputers in Sensory and Information Processing Research, Lawrence Erlbaum Associates, Hillsdale, NJ.

Polyak, S.L. (1941) The Retina, University of Chicago Press, Chicago.

Puckett, J. De W. and Steinman, R.M. (1969) Tracking eye movements with and without saccadic correction. Vision Res. 9, 695–703.

Ratliff, F. (1952) The role of physiological nystagmus in monocular acuity. J. Exp. Psychol., 43, 163–172.

Ratliff, F. (1965) Mach Bands: Quantitative Studies on Neural Networks in the Retina, Holden-Day, San Francisco.

Ratliff, F. (1984) Why Mach bands are not seen at the edges of a step. Vision Res. 24, 163–166.

Ratliff, F. and Riggs, L.A. (1950) Involuntary motions of the eye during monocular fixation. J. Exp. Psychol. 40, 687–701.

Riggs, L.A. (1965) Visual acuity. In: C.H. Graham (Ed.), Vision and Visual Perception, John Wiley and Sons, New York, pp. 321–349.

Riggs, L.A. and Armington, J.C. (1952) Angular displacements of the eye during prolonged fixation. Am. Psychol. 7, 252.

Riggs, L.A. and Ratliff, L.A. (1951) Visual acuity and the normal tremor of the eye. Science 106, 107–108.

Riggs, L.A. and Schick, A.M.L. (1968) Accuracy of retinal image stabilization achieved with a plane mirror on a tightly fitting contact lens. Vision Res. 8, 159–169.

Riggs, L.A., Ratliff, F., Cornsweet, J.C. and Cornsweet, T.N. (1953) The disappearance of steadily fixated visual test objects. J. Opt. Soc. Am. 43, 495–501.

Riggs, L.A., Armington, J.C. and Ratliff, F. (1954) Motions of the retinal image during fixation. J. Opt. Soc. Am. 44, 315–321.

Sachs, M., Nachmias, J. and Robson, J. (1971) Spatial frequency channels in human vision. J. Opt. Soc. Am. 61, 1176–1186.

Schade, O.H. (1956) Optical and photoelectric analog of the eye. J. Opt. Soc. Am. 46, 721–739.

Senders, V.L. (1948) The physiological basis of visual acuity. Psychol. Bull. 45, 465–490.

Senders, V.L. (1949) Visual resolution with periodically interrupted light. J. Exp. Psychol. 40, 453–465.

Shannon, C.E. (1948) A mathematical theory of communication. Bell System Tech. J. 27, 379–423; 623–656.

Skavenski, A.A., Hansen, R., Steinman, R.M. and Winterson, B.J. (1979) Quality of retinal image stabilization during small natural and artificial body rotations in man. Vision Res. 19, 365–375.

Stark, L. (1983) Normal and abnormal vergence. In: C.M. Schor and K.J. Ciuffreda (Eds.), Vergence Eye Movements: Basic and Clinical Aspects, Butterworths, Boston, pp. 3–13.

St.-Cyr, G.J. and Fender, D.H. (1969) Nonlinearities of the human oculomotor system: gain. Vision Res. 9, 135–1246.

Steinman, R.M. (1975) Oculomotor effects on vision. In: P. Bach-y-Rita and G. Lennerstrand (Eds.), Basic Mechanisms of Ocular Motility and Their Clinical Implications, Pergamon Press, Oxford, pp. 395–416.

Steinman, R.M. (1976) Role of eye movements in maintaining a phenomenally clear and stable world. In: R.A. Monty and J.W. Senders (Eds.), Eye Movements and Psychological Processes, Lawrence Erlbaum Associates, Hillsdale, NJ, pp. 121–149.

Steinman, R.M. (1986a) The need for an eclectic, rather than a systems, approach to the study of the primate oculomotor system. Vision Res. 26, 101–112.

Steinman, R.M. (1986b) Eye movement. Vision Res. 26, 1389–1400.

Steinman, R.M. and Collewijn, H. (1978) How our two eyes are held steady. J. Opt. Soc. Am. 68, 1359.

Steinman, R.M. and Collewijn, H. (1980) Binocular retinal image motion during natural active head rotation. Vision Res. 20, 415–429.

Steinman, R.M., Cunitz, R.J., Timberlake, G.T. and Herman, M. (1967) Voluntary control of microsaccades during maintained monocular fixation. Science 155, 1577–1579.

Steinman, R.M., Haddad, G.M., Skavenski, A.A. and Wyman, D. (1973) Miniature eye movement. Science 181, 810–819.

Steinman, R.M., Cushman, W.B. and Martins, A.J. (1982) The precision of gaze. Hum. Neurobiol. 1, 97–109.

Steinman, R.M., Levinson, J.Z., Collewijn, H. and Van der Steen, J. (1983) Vision in the presence of known natural retinal image motion. J. Opt. Soc. Am. 73, 1856.

Steinman, R.M., Levinson, J.Z., Collewijn, H. and Van der Steen, J. (1985) Vision in the presence of known natural retinal image motion. J. Opt. Soc. Am. A 2, 226–233.

Stork, D.G., Falk, D.S. and Levinson, J.Z. (1985) Receptive field asymmetry probed using converging gratings. J. Opt. Soc. Am. A 2, 275–279.

Talbot, S.A. and Marshall, W.H. (1941) Physiological studies of neural mechanisms of visual localization and discrimination. Am. J. Ophthal. 24, 1255–1264.

Tulunay-Keesey, U. and Jones, R.M. (1976) The effect of micromovements of the eye and exposure duration on contrast sensitivity. Vision Res. 16, 481–488.

Van Nes, F.L. (1968) Enhanced visibility by regular motion of the retinal image. Am. J. Psychol. 81, 367–374.

Van Nes, F.L. and Bouman, M.A. (1967) Spatial modulation transfer of the human eye. J. Opt. Soc. Am. 57, 401–406.

Van Nes, F.L., Koenderink, J.J., Nas, H. and Bouman, M.A. (1967) Spatiotemporal modulation transfer in the human eye. J. Opt. Soc. Am. 57, 1082–1088.

Volkmann, A.W. (1863) Physiologische Untersuchungen im Gebiete der Optik, Breitkopt and Hartel, Leipzig.

Volkmann, P.C. (1986) Human visual suppression. Vision Res. 26, 1401–1416.

Wald, G. (1948) Selig Hecht (1892–1947). J. Gen. Physiol. 32, 1–16.

Walls, G.L. (1943) Factors in human visual resolution. J. Opt. Soc. Am. 33, 487–505.

Walls, G.L. (1962) The evolutionary history of eye movements. Vision Res. 2, 69–80.

Westheimer, G. (1960) Modulation thresholds for sinusoidal light distributions on the retina. J. Physiol. 152, 67–74.

Westheimer, G. (1965) Visual acuity. Annu. Rev. Psychol. 16, 359–380.

Westheimer, G. (1981) Visual hyperacuity. Prog. Sensory Physiol. 1, 1–30.

Westheimer, G. and McKee, S. (1975) Visual acuity in the presence of retinal image motion. J. Opt. Soc. Am. 65, 847–850.

Weymouth, F.W., Andersen, E.E. and Averill, H.L. (1923) Retinal mean local sign; a new view of the relation of the retinal mosaic to visual perception. A.J. Physiol. 63, 410–411.

Wilcox, W.W. and Purdy, D. McL. (1933) Visual acuity and its physiological basis. Br. J. Psychol. 23, 233–261.

Williams, D.R. (1985) Aliasing in human foveal vision. Vision Res. 25, 195–206.

Wilson, V.J. and Melvill Jones, G. (1979) Mammalian Vestibular Physiology, Plenum Press, New York.

Winterson, B.J. and Collewijn, B.J. (1976) Microsaccades during finely-guided visuomotor tasks. Vision Res. 16, 1387–1390.

Woodworth, R.S. (1938) Experimental Psychology, Holt, New York.

Wülfing, E.A. (1892) Über den kleinsten Gesichtwinkel. Z. Biol. 29, 199–202.

Yarbus, A.L. (1957a) A new method for studying the activity of various parts of the retina. Biophysics 2, 165–167.

Yarbus, A.L. (1957b) The perception of an image fixed with respect to the retina. Biophysics 2, 683–690.

Yarbus, A.L. (1967) Eye Movements and Vision. Translated by B. Haigh and L.A. Riggs, Plenum Press, New York.

Yellott, J.I. Jr. (1983) Spectral consequences of photoreceptor sampling in the rhesus retina. Science 221, 382–385.

Eye movements and their role in visual and cognitive processes
E. Kowler, Editor

CHAPTER 4

Binocular eye movements and the perception of depth

Han Collewijn and Casper J. Erkelens

Department of Physiology I, Faculty of Medicine, Erasmus University Rotterdam, P.O. Box 1738, 3000 DR Rotterdam, The Netherlands

1. Introduction

Binocular viewing adds much to our appreciation of distance and depth. The use of two simultaneous viewpoints provides the main cue of binocular parallax, leading to retinal disparity and to vergence eye movement. Both retinal disparity and vergence eye movements relate to the topography of the projections of the world on the two retinae and therefore interact directly: eye movements change retinal image positions and, on the other hand, changes in retinal image position can elicit eye movements. Although this strong interaction seems fairly obvious, it has rarely been studied in a direct way. Studies in which reliable measurements of binocular eye movements have been combined with the evaluation of depth-perception are rare. Most studies of depth-perception have either neglected eye movements or tried to minimize them by providing fixation points or frames. On the other hand, studies of binocular eye movements have mostly concentrated on the control of vergence in extremely impoverished visual environments. In this chapter we shall review the relationship between binocular vision of a world with depth, and the control of the movements of the two eyes. We shall not deal with intraocular motor phenomena related to depth such as accommodation and pupillary responses, nor with monocular estimation of distance. Our approach will primarily follow the perspective of oculomotor researchers. For more comprehensive reviews of depth-vision including psychophysics, neurophysiology and computational aspects, we refer to a number of excellent reviews (Bishop and Henry, 1971; Bishop and Pettigrew, 1986; Foley, 1978, 1980; Graham, 1951, 1965; Julesz, 1978; Poggio and Poggio, 1984; Marr and Poggio, 1979; Nelson, 1975; Tyler and Scott, 1979).

A brief outline of the structure and the main problems discussed in this chapter follows here.

In section 2 we deal with the contribution of vergence as an isolated cue to the perception of distance. We start with a discussion of the geometrical relationships between target distances and ocular vergence angles, including consideration of vertical eye movements and the proper definition of vergence in distinct coordinate systems. Then we turn to discussing classical studies of the estimation of distance (absolute and relative) based on vergence cues; most of these relate to static conditions and assume more or less perfect binocular fixation. We shall point out that this assumption has not been verified in any of the extensive studies of this kind; as a result a strict attribution of any depth perception to either vergence or absolute disparity cannot be made.

In section 3 we discuss the role of disparity in depth perception. We start again with the pertinent geometrical relationships; the most fundamental point here is the distinction between absolute and relative disparities. The first parameter is defined by the difference in absolute angular retinal positions (relative to the fovea) of the images of a target. Absolute disparity is directly affected by ocular vergence, and in fact is the dominant signal used to control vergence. Relative disparity between two targets is defined as the difference between their absolute disparities; this difference is unaffected by eye movements. It will be argued that depth perception is almost exclusively based on relative, and not on absolute, disparity. The great functional advantage of this arrangement is that relative disparity detection can operate at threshold levels of a few seconds of arc, despite the fact that the precision of oculomotor control is considerably lower.

In section 4 we shall examine the control of vergence by disparity. The dynamics of this process will be examined extensively, and a number of concepts current in the literature will be critically evaluated. A new approach to the modelling of disparity-controlled vergence will be proposed, which may resolve a long-standing inconsistency between the responses to sinusoidal and step stimuli. We shall also discuss the imperfections of ocular vergence under various conditions.

Section 5 will deal with dynamic conditions, i.e., binocular vision of moving objects with moving eyes. The main topics will be the function of stereopsis under the constraints of imperfect control of vergence, and the perception of motion in depth. Again, it will be shown that perception of motion in depth is almost exclusively based on relative disparity, whereas changes in absolute disparity and/or vergence are perceptually only of secondary importance.

Finally, a number of conclusions will be summarized in section 6.

2. Vergence as a distance cue under static conditions

2.1. Geometric basis

2.1.1. The relationship between vergence and distance

An important parameter in binocular vision and a potential cue to distance is the angle of vergence. We shall first consider a simple case (Fig. 1A). Both eyes fixate a point P located in the median plane (symmetric vergence). The left and right eyes each contain a fovea (F_L and F_R), a center of rotation (C_L and C_R) and a nodal point (N_L and N_R). The baseline (b) connects C_L and C_R; the distance between C_L and C_R is the interocular distance.

We assume that the head is in the upright position and that the plane of regard (containing the line b and point P) is horizontal; in this case vergence is effected by purely horizontal eye movements.

The angle subtended between the two visual axes is the angle of ocular vergence, γ_O. The angle subtended by the two nodal points at P is the binocular parallax γ_P of P. In the case of binocular foveation (as in Fig. 1A), the visual axes intersect at P and $\gamma_O = \gamma_P$ (ocular vergence = binocular parallax).

The distance d of P to the subject is sometimes defined as the perpendicular distance of P to the baseline b or its extension (Graham, 1951, 1965). In the symmetric case this is equal to the distance between P and M, the midpoint of b. A more popular definition of the distance of an object is the length of PM (e.g. Foley; 1978, 1980). M is then considered to be the egocentric center.

For the angle of vergence γ_O we can write:

$$\tan \gamma_O/2 = b/2d \qquad (1)$$

For relatively small angles, tan γ_O is approximately equal to γ_O measured in radians; therefore

$$\gamma_O = b/d \qquad (2)$$

or, if γ_O is measured in degrees:

$$\gamma_O = 57.3\ b/d \qquad (3)$$

Logarithmic transformation leads to a linear relation with a slope of −1, since

$$\log \gamma_O = -\log d + \log 57.3\ b \qquad (4)$$

This relationship is shown in Fig. 2 for $b = 64$ mm,

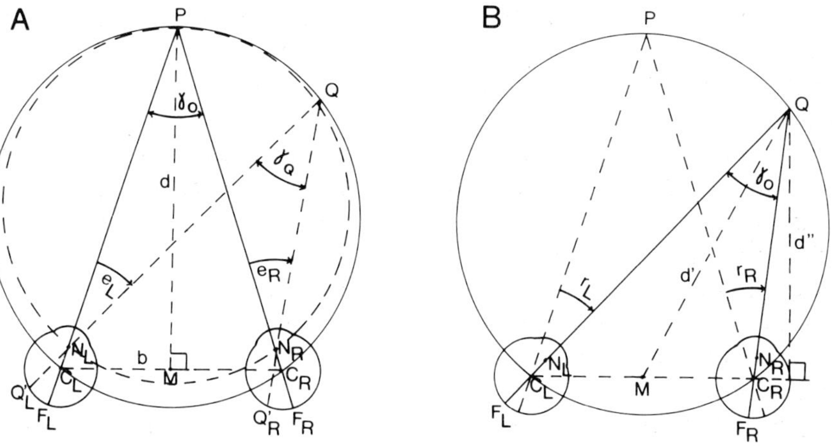

Fig. 1. Angles of vergence (γ) and distances (d) in the cases of symmetrical (A) and asymmetrical (B) convergence, with binocular fixation of target P or Q. Solid circles: locus of equal vergence = *isovergence circles*. Interrupted circle: Vieth-Müller circle. For further explanation, see text.

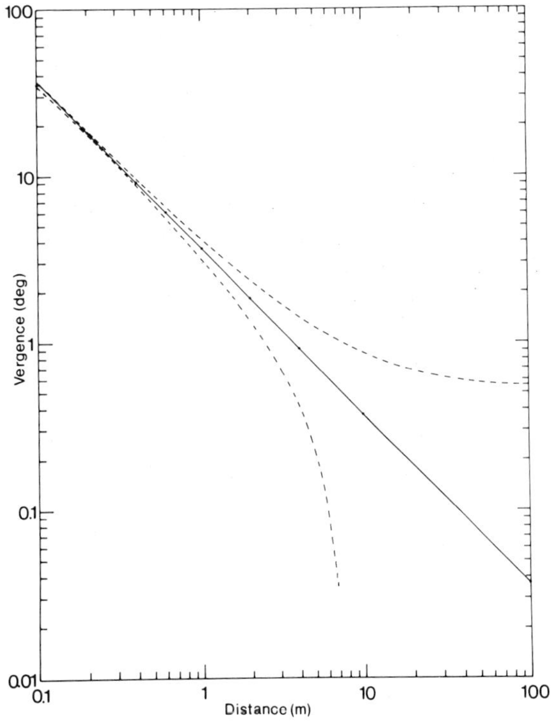

Fig. 2. The relationship between target distance (in meters) and required convergence angle (in degrees) for binocular fixation, for an interocular distance (b) of 64 mm, plotted on double logarithmic scales. The dotted lines mark the equivalent distances for errors in convergence of ± 1 degree; they show that at larger distances slight changes in convergence correspond to larger changes in distance.

together with some data points calculated exactly from Eqn. 1. The approximation in Eqns. 3 and 4 leads to a slight overestimation of d on the basis of γ_O, increasing with the shortening of target distance but not exceeding about 3% at distances of 10 cm. At this distance γ_O is of the order of 36 deg, close to the maximum obtainable for most subjects. Fig. 2 suggests that estimation of distance on the basis of vergence, if at all used, is most feasible at short distances, because this is where vergence varies steeply as a function of distance. About 90% of the vergence range is used for distances less than 1 m. At a distance of 2 m, a difference of ± 0.5 deg in vergence corresponds to a range in distance of more than 1 m, and at larger distances the sensitivity of any calculation of distance to minute errors of vergence or its estimated value becomes prohibitive.

There are at least two potential sources of error in using a vergence signal to estimate distance of a static target: (a) imprecision of binocular fixation; (b) errors in the estimation of the vergence angle.

(a) Imprecision of binocular fixation is common. For static conditions, fixation disparities have been extensively described (Ogle et al., 1967). With a moving head, fluctuations of vergence with amplitudes of the order of 0.5 – 1 deg have been recorded (Steinman and Collewijn, 1980). These imprecisions will be discussed in detail in section 4.9.

(b) The accuracy of the signal representing vergence angle (which should be independent of the conjugated version angle) is unknown; likewise its source (proprioceptive = inflow or efference-copy = outflow) remains undetermined. A reasonable assumption might be for the accuracy of the sensing of vergence to be comparable to the accuracy of the sense of versional eye position, which under certain experimental conditions may be considerably better than 1 deg (see Skavenski and Steinman, 1970; Hansen and Skavenski, 1977, 1985; and Skavenski's chapter in this volume).

A considerable further drawback of vergence as a cue to distance is that vergence has only a single value at any time and therefore can only signal the distance of one particular object at a time. It cannot, therefore, act as a substitute for visual, relative cues.

The considerations mentioned above make it unlikely that vergence is used as a major cue for distance. At best it may provide a rough indicator at close range (within manual grasping distance). As discussed later in this section, this expectation is largely borne out by psychophysical experiments. Before going into these, it is useful to explore the geometry of vergence a little further.

2.1.2. Relationship between visual and oculomotor angles

At relatively short target distances, the general relationship between the binocular parallax of a non-fixated target and the ocular vergence required for bifoveation of this target is complicated by the non-coincidence of the nodal point and the center of rotation. The center of rotation is commonly assumed to lie 13.5 mm behind the corneal surface, whereas the nodal point lies 6.2 mm more anteriorly (Alpern, 1962; Bennett and Francis, 1962). As a consequence, when the eye rotates through an angle α, the angular displacement β of the retinal image of a target P is larger by an angle $\Delta\alpha$:

$$\beta = \alpha + \Delta\alpha \tag{5}$$

For $\Delta\alpha$, the following relation can be derived:

$$\Delta\alpha = \tan^{-1} \frac{\sin \alpha}{CP/CN - \cos \alpha} \tag{6}$$

This equation, given by Steinman et al. (1982) with a slightly ambiguous notation, can be reasonably approximated by:

$$\Delta\alpha = (CN/CP) \cdot \alpha \tag{7}$$

which immediately shows that at target distances of 10 cm, $\Delta\alpha$ is of the order of 6% of α and therefore not negligible*. At optical infinity, $\Delta\alpha$ obviously reduces to zero.

Because the location of the centers of rotation in the head is independent of eye movements, in contrast to the location of the nodal points, target distances (*d*) and interocular distance (*b*) are best defined with C_L and C_R as references. In Fig. 1, a circle (continuous line) has been drawn through C_L, C_R and P, which represents the locus of equal vergence angles γ. Although this iso-vergence circle resembles the classic Vieth-Müller circle (dotted circle in Fig. 1A), it is slightly different because the latter passes through the nodal points, and represents the locus of (at least geometrically) equal angles of horizontal retinal eccentricity for both eyes.

Thus, there is a certain discrepancy between *visual* angles (eccentricity, binocular parallax, etc.), which are measured around the nodal point, and oculomotor angles, which are measured around the center of rotation. In order to deal with visual and oculomotor units that are equivalent, it is helpful to use the parameter *target vergence* (Rashbass and Westheimer, 1961) instead of binocular parallax.

---

* Any simple geometric description of visual optic relations remains an approximation. Strictly speaking, the assumption of C and N as single, fixed points in the eye is fictitious, and the visual axis does not pass through C, because the foveal center is located 4–5 deg temporal to the intersection of the optical axis with the retina. This constant difference between the orientations of the optical and visual axes does not affect Eqn. 5. Another consequence of this relation is the disappearance of targets in the extreme nasal visual field behind the nose when monocular gaze is directed at them (Mapp and Ono, 1986).

Target vergence is the angle subtended by the *centers of rotation* of the two eyes at the target, binocular parallax the angle subtended by the nodal points.

For targets outside the median plane the relations are more complex. During symmetric vergence (Fig. 1A), when a target Q is presented eccentrically, but on the isovergence circle, the programming of correct eye movements to achieve bifoveation of Q has to overcome several problems. Since Q lies outside the Vieth-Müller circle, it has a larger eccentricity on the right retina than on the left retina ($e_R > e_L$); furthermore its binocular parallax (γ_Q) is smaller than that of P ($\gamma_Q < \gamma_O$). Nevertheless, to achieve bifoveation both eyes have to rotate through a similar angle $r_L = r_R$, while $r_L < e_L$ and $r_R < e_R$. The final situation is shown in Fig. 1B; after bifoveation of Q the vergence angle γ_O is the same as during fixation of P (Fig. 1A), but the binocular parallax of Q has increased from γ_Q to γ_O. Thus, the binocular parallax of a target varies slightly with vergence as a result of Eqn. 6. Furthermore, the equal vergence required for fixation of either P or Q is not paralleled by equal distances of P and Q to the subject, irrespective of the definition of this distance. It is clear that in Fig. 1B the distance d' of Q to the midpoint of b (M) is different from the perpendicular distance d'' of Q to the extension of b, and that both are smaller than d in Fig. 1A. Thus, a locus of iso-vergence does not represent a locus of iso-distance, and vice versa; nor is this the case for a Vieth-Müller circle. (Theoretically, distance could still be calculated correctly by triangulation using the positions of each eye separately, or some combination of vergence and version.)

2.1.3. The generalized case: extension to the vertical dimension, and the need to define coordinate systems

We have so far restricted the discussion of vergence to movements of the visual axes in a single, horizontal plane of regard. In this case both visual axes always intersect in a single point of fixation, the eye movements are horizontal, and vergence equals the difference between the horizontal positions of the left and right eyes.

It is clear that a more realistic treatment has to include the vertical dimension. This cannot be done properly without careful consideration of the coordinate systems used to describe the eye movements, and their relation to the signals furnished by instruments used to measure eye positions. Although it is customary in oculomotor research to refer to 'horizontal' and 'vertical' in a loose way, usually in relation to a flat, cartesian coordinate system on a tangent screen, this is far from correct. Eye movements are rotations of a rigid body around a center of rotation and require a spherical coordinate system for proper description. All possible rotations can be described by a system using three axes, expressing eye position in three angular coordinates. The hierarchy of these axes has to be clearly defined; in this respect different conventions are in existence.

In the system designed by Fick, horizontal rotation (longitude, φ) is measured around a steady, vertical axis. Vertical rotation (latitude, θ) is measured around a horizontal axis. This coincides with the baseline when the eyes look straight ahead (horizontal zero position) and rotates in the horizontal plane along with horizontal eye movements. Finally, the eye can cyclorotate (torsion) around its visual axis (which moves along with horizontal as well as vertical eye movements).

A different hierarchy was chosen in Helmholtz's system: vertical rotation (elevation, λ) is measured around the steady baseline. Horizontal rotation (azimuth, μ) is subsequently measured around an axis which is vertical when the eyes look straight ahead (vertical zero) and rotates in a parasagittal plane with the vertical rotation. Torsion is measured around the visual axis.

Finally, Listing's system excludes torsion as an independent parameter and describes eye positions as being reached from the primary position by rotation through an angle of eccentricity around an axis in the equatorial (Listing's) plane with a specific meridional orientation. For details on coordinate systems we refer to Alpern (1962), Von Helmholtz (1962), Westheimer (1957) and Southall (1961).

Once we consider movements outside the horizontal plane, we have to include the possibility of vergence in the vertical direction. As long as both visual axes and the baseline are contained in a single flat plane of regard, the visual axes intersect in a fixation point and the vertical vergence equals zero. In this case we can retain the definition of vergence as the angle between the visual axes, measured in the plane of regard. The expression of this angle is most straightforward in Helmholtz's coordinate system: horizontal vergence is the difference between the azimuths of the left and right eye. For a single plane of regard, the elevations of both eyes are always equal.

If the two visual axes do not lie in a single plane and do not intersect, two components of vergence have to be distinguished. Vertical vergence is equal to the difference in the elevations of the eyes, horizontal vergence remains equal to the difference between left and right eye's azimuths. For true binocular fixation, the locus of fixation points with equal vergence is a toroid surface, formed by the rotation of an isovergence circle (as defined previously) around the interocular baseline.

Thus, the description of binocular eye movements is most elegantly done in Helmholtz coordinates. Unfortunately, no practical eye movement recorders furnish either Helmholtz or Fick coordinates directly. Of existing apparatus, only the magnetic scleral search coil system is capable of measuring binocular horizontal and vertical eye movements over large angles with great accuracy and precision. The formal relations between the horizontal and vertical electrical output signals of such a system – operated in the phase-locked amplitude detection mode – and the Fick coordinates have been worked out (Robinson, 1963; Ferman et al., 1987) and are reasonably simple*.

2.2. *Vergence as a distance cue: psychophysical evidence*

2.2.1. *Difficulty of isolating vergence as a cue*

The experimental evidence for ocular vergence acting as a distance cue has been highly controversial for more than a century. Early positive assertions in this respect (Wundt, 1862) were later denied (Hillebrand, 1893; Bappert, 1923) or supported (Bourdon, 1902; Swenson, 1932; Grant, 1942) but on balance the evidence appeared to be against a significant role of vergence in the estimation of distance (Ogle, 1962a). However, renewed interest in the problem has generated a series of contemporary experiments beginning in the early 1960s.

A serious problem in experiments on the relationship between ocular vergence and perceived distance has always been the elimination of all other cues to distance such as perceived size, brightness. accommodation cues and disparity. Although many of these additional cues can be minimized by proper manipulation of the target's optical

---

* To obtain the correct horizontal and vertical coordinates in the different systems, and to transform one system into the other one, the following relations may be used:

Definitions:

Fick's system: φ = longitude (horizontal); rightward positive
θ = latitude (vertical); upward positive

Helmholtz's system: μ = azimuth (horizontal); rightward positive
λ = elevation (vertical); upward positive

In Robinson's (1963) configuration, the following relations apply to the 'horizontal' and 'vertical' d.c. signals:

In Fick coordinates: longitude $e_\varphi \propto \sin\varphi\cos\theta$
latitude $e_\theta \propto \sin\varphi$ (8)

In Helmholtz coordinates: azimuth $e_\mu \propto \sin\mu$
elevation $e_\lambda \propto \sin\lambda\cos\mu$ (9)

Transformations

From Fick to Helmholtz:

$$\tan\lambda = \frac{\tan\theta}{\cos\varphi} \quad (10)$$

$$\sin\mu = \cos\theta\sin\varphi \quad (11)$$

From Helmholtz to Fick:

$$\tan\varphi = \frac{\tan\mu}{\cos\lambda} \quad (12)$$

$$\sin\theta = \cos\mu\sin\lambda \quad (13)$$

We thank our colleague H.G. Lemij for the derivation of these relations.

qualities, complete elimination is very difficult to achieve. The dissociation between ocular vergence and disparity is especially hard to establish since eye movements have not been recorded in any of the major psychophysical studies on the role of vergence in the perception of distance. The conclusions rest entirely on the assumption of accurate binocular fixation. In view of the common incidence of substantial fixation disparities (Ogle et al., 1967) this assumption will often be incorrect.

The best chances of achieving accurate binocular fixation occur when successive stimuli are presented with a sufficient time interval and a sufficient duration to eliminate any existing absolute disparities, although a transient disparity before vergence has been completed remains unavoidable. Thus, the distinction between vergence and disparity cues remains somewhat problematic. Probably the best isolation of vergence cues was reached in experiments of the old-fashioned type using real stimuli in large rooms with elaborate mechanical devices, requiring much time for rearrangement of a stimulus.

2.2.2. Estimation of relatively long distances

Relatively few studies have been devoted to the relationship between vergence and perception of distances beyond 1–2 m. Bourdon (1902) found in his subjects a fairly good ability to estimate the order of relative distances of successively presented point targets. Targets at about 6–7 m distance could be reliably recognized as closer than a target at 25 m; under favorable circumstances (repeated observation) even the difference between 10 and 25 m distance could be perceived. However, any estimate of the absolute magnitude of distances was extremely unreliable for all targets beyond a few meters. A more recent study is that of Crannell and Peters (1970), who used small light-targets viewed at distances of between 2 and 100 feet, and inexperienced subjects who had no information about the real dimensions of the stimulus space. Targets were exposed for 2–4 s, and subjects verbally reported the estimated distance. When all targets had the same objective size and luminance, subjects could use the relative change in apparent size and brightness to judge the relative distances of the targets in about the correct order, with a clear tendency to underestimate distances, especially the larger ones. When the cue of relative brightness was eliminated, subjects could still detect the relative distances of the targets, but variability between subjects increased greatly. Finally, when the cue of relative size was also removed, leaving only accommodation and vergence, the estimate became totally unreliable, with even a tendency for distances to be reported in reversed order. Under none of these three conditions was there any significant difference between monocular and binocular viewing. In control experiments with simultaneous presentation of several targets, subjects could easily discriminate relative distances with binocular viewing, but again performed below chance level with monocular vision. These results of Crannel and Peters (1970) strongly suggest that vergence alone, in the absence of cues of brightness, size or relative disparity, is an inadequate cue to distance.

These authors were apparently not aware of the elaborate studies by Gogel (1961a,b, 1962), published a decade earlier in the same journal. Using somewhat more artificial stimulus arrangements in an ingenious visual alley experiment, Gogel tested the successive discrimination of distances on the exclusive basis of convergence. Vergence varied between 0 and 4 deg, corresponding to object distances between infinity and 90 cm. This is about the same (relatively large) range as studied by Crannel and Peters, which a priori (see section 2.1.1) would be expected to yield weak cues of oculomotor nature. Instead of verbal reports, Gogel used a matching technique in which subjects adjusted a monocularly seen reference target (including cues of perspective and size) to the same distance as perceived for the test target. For successive presentations at intervals of about 1 min, only 3 out of 12 subjects showed a systematic tendency to associate increased convergence with a decreased perceived distance. The same three subjects, who happened to be experienced observers in laboratory experiments on binocular vision, were still able to make the same distance discriminations based on vergence when the interstimulus interval was increased to 20 min. However, the changes in perceived distance were small compared to the physical equivalent range of 90 cm to infinity; they did not exceed 8 feet in the most sensitive subject. These results were obtained with the accommodative distance of the target at infinity; a control experiment in which accommodative distance was appropriately covaried with binocular parallax revealed an improvement of distance discrimination in 6 out of 12 subjects. Finally, a continuous change of binocular parallax *during* the observation, rather than a successive viewing of discrete settings, enabled 9 out of 12 subjects to make correct judgements about the *direction* of change in distance; the perceived change amounted to about 2.5 feet (76 cm) for changes in the convergence angle between 1 and 3 deg (still a considerable underestimate of the equivalent physical distance change of 244 cm). Gogel (1961a) concluded that at the relatively long distances tested, vergence is not an effective determiner of perceived distance.

In a further study, Gogel (1961b) explored the effect of using multiple binocular target configurations. Again, for most subjects changing the absolute convergence to an otherwise unchanged binocular configuration had little if any effect upon either the apparent position of the configuration or the perceived distances between objects within the configuration. Some subjects, however, showed a definite but limited change in apparent distance with a change in vergence. In these subjects, the apparent distances between the objects within the configuration covaried with the perceived distance of the configuration as a whole.

However, it seems possible that at relatively short (virtual) distances of targets, vergence signals are more effective as a distance cue. Indeed, experimenters using shorter target distances in general have found more positive evidence for a role of vergence in perception of distance.

2.2.3. Estimation of relatively short distances

The outcome of experiments covering this nearer range (roughly within arm's length) has been quite varied. Bourdon (1902) found moderately good discrimination of relative distances at a close range. At 1 m distance, differences of about 20 cm could be reliably discriminated between successive presentations. A target at 3 m was discriminated as farther than one at 2 m. In general, the difference threshold corresponded to a change in binocular parallax, and presumably vergence, of about 40 min arc. Bourdon (1902) also found that within reaching distance absolute estimates of distance of single targets were possible, although this point was not tested very rigorously. Bappert's (1923) entirely negative findings are of limited value as they were based on monocular viewing. Distance could thus only be estimated on the basis of accommodative cues and accommodative vergence. Surprisingly accurate distance estimates in the range 25–40 cm were reported by Swenson (1932), using a haploscope with adjustable binocular parallax and a manual pointing technique by which subjects indicated the perceived distance of a luminous disc. Size and luminance were kept constant. Swenson's (1932) attempts to dissociate accommodative from vergence cues, and his conclusion that vergence was about three times as powerful as accommodation in signalling distance, were clearly fallacious. The construction of his apparatus would almost certainly induce accommodation to the plane of a size-limiting aperture at a constant distance, rather than to the plane of the more distant homogeneous light source.

Grant (1942) recognized this limitation and achieved better control of accommodation, but used a rather dubious indicator of perceived distance (the setting of a monocularly viewed coin of known size at the estimated depth). His results were much less positive than Swenson's (1932). Even with accommodation and vergence appropriately covaried, subjects were only able to report target distances of 25, 33 and 50 cm in the correct order but with erroneous values, compressed into a narrow range (34–41 cm). Grant (1942) estimated that vergence and accommodation were about equally potent in determining distance judgments.

Gogel (1962) extended his studies to the range of

convergence up to 12 deg, using the same general methods as before (Gogel, 1961a,b). Even at this closer range, less than half of Gogel's subjects showed any relation reflecting smaller perceived distances at greater angles of convergence. Even when present, such a relation had a small slope.

Richards and Miller (1969) further investigated this problem, introducing mismatches between accommodative and vergence cues. Observers had to change the distance of a reference point target, seen with normal binocular viewing, until it matched the perceived distance of a test target, seen through various combinations of prisms and lenses, but never at the same time as the reference target. It was found that responses were distributed bimodally. Two-thirds of subjects followed vergence cues in setting distances, with little effect of accommodative stimuli, while the remaining one-third of subjects tended not to use vergence but to base their settings on other cues such as size and brightness.

The accuracy of (unseen) manual pointing to a distance appropriate to vergence was investigated again by Foley and Held (1972). Using point targets of which only the binocular parallax was varied, they found that subjects could indicate the distances in the right order but with great errors of absolute values. Cued distances of 15–36 cm were consistently overreached, with a median error of about 25 cm.

Komoda and Ono (1974), using stimuli of constant retinal size and artificial small pupils to prevent secondary effects of accommodation, confirmed that increased convergence leads to decreased perceived distance. But, once more, the perceived distances were only correctly ordered and lacked veridicality. The range was strongly compressed. A special effort was made to study the possible effects of assumptions by the subject on identity or non-identity of the successive stimulus objects. Such effects were weak, but a small trend was demonstrated for perceived changes in distance to be larger for discrete vergence steps between successive stimulus presentations than for continuously viewed, gradual changes in binocular parallax.

Finally, Von Hofsten (1976), using point targets (oscilloscope spots) displayed with different binocular parallax (range 1–6 deg convergence) with relatively short inter-stimulus intervals (1.5 s), obtained surprisingly good verbal distance estimates. A majority of his subjects not only consistently perceived the fused dot as farther away in the position with the smaller convergence angle, but also estimated the egocentric distance with remarkable accuracy. However, the results were affected by slight changes in the procedure (making the subject close his eyes before and between stimulus presentations); this may indicate the use of extraneous cues. Furthermore, the distinction between the use of either vergence or disparity or both is impossible in Von Hofsten's experiment.

A direct comparison between the use of manual pointing and of verbal reports (Foley, 1977, 1978) showed that slopes of perceived distance as a function of binocular parallax were substantially flatter for pointing than for verbal estimates. (In both cases there was a substantial underestimation of the objective distance range.) Thus, there is no basis for supposing that the motor-related vergence signal would be better expressed in a motor activity such as pointing than in a verbal report, although such a preference has been found for spatial localization in connection with saccades (Hansen and Skavenski, 1977, 1985).

At this point it should be mentioned that a visual stimulus without any distance information (a luminous point in darkness, viewed monocularly through a small artificial pupil) is perceived at a relatively short distance (about 0.7–2 m; Gogel and Sturm, 1972; Foley, 1978). Also accommodation and vergence under such deprived conditions take on values corresponding to relatively small target distances (for references see Foley, 1978). Gogel and Sturm (1972) have called this default distance the 'specific distance' and proposed that with limited distance information available, perceived distance will tend toward this specific distance.

2.2.4. Effects of vergence on perceived size

For all targets of some perceptible size (i.e., all except point targets) the estimation of distance may be complicated by the fact that the perceived size of a target subtending a constant visual angle decreases with increasing convergence. This effect was first noted by Wheatstone (1852) when he changed the binocular parallax of images in his stereoscope. It was confirmed in careful studies by Heinemann et al. (1959), Komoda and Ono (1974) and many others (see Foley, 1978, p. 190, for further references). The effect seems to be due to vergence alone and not to accommodative and pupillary changes (Heinemann et al., 1959) and would normally work in the direction of size-constancy. A rigid object observed at a smaller distance will subtend a larger visual angle, but still be perceived as having the same size. Part of this size-constancy may be due to the vergence associated with nearness of the target, although its contribution appears to be relatively small (Heinemann et al., 1959). This effect demonstrates the availability of a vergence-related signal to the perceptual process. However, its direction is such that it detracts from the use of vergence as a distance cue: decreasing size would suggest increase rather than decrease in distance. This conflict may be the basis of the tendency, found in several laboratory experiments (Bappert, 1923; Crannel and Peters, 1970; Heinemann et al., 1959), to report distances in reversed order as appropriate for the associated convergence.

2.2.5. Conclusions

Strictly speaking, the relative contribution of vergence and absolute disparity is unknown for any of the psychophysical experiments discussed so far, because vergence was not measured. The experiments discussed above (a representative but by no means complete survey), taken together, suggest that it is likely that extraretinal signals, related to the vergence of the eyes, mediate some perception of distance, in agreement with Foley's (1980) conclusion. This signal is relatively weak and virtually useless at distances beyond about 2 m. Even within arm's range, some subjects cannot use vergence cues at all. The signal appears to be barely reliable enough to detect relative differences in distance (i.e., correct order). The magnitude of perceived distances is usually erroneous, with large mistakes in mean value and range. The estimated values are easily influenced by experimental conditions (manner of presentation, additional cues) and cognitive factors (the subject's assumptions about or knowledge of the dimensions and properties of targets and experimental apparatus).

3. Disparity as a distance cue

3.1. Geometric basis

3.1.1. Disparity

Implicit in the discussion in section 2 on the use of vergence in estimating distance is the requisite that the eyes achieve bifoveation first, in the same manner in which the two images have to be brought into correspondence by the observer in an optical range-finder. The ultimate criterion for perfect vergence is the absence of retinal disparity for the foveated target. Disparity, an important stimulus for vergence, is illustrated in Fig. 3A for the simple symmetric case. The eyes are converged on P, the point of fixation. Ocular vergence (γ_O) is equal to the angle between the visual axes. The targets A and B have binocular parallaxes γ_A and γ_B, the angles subtended by the nodal points of the two eyes at A and B. The absolute disparities of A and B are:

$$\delta_A = \gamma_A - \gamma_O \text{ and } \delta_B = \gamma_B - \gamma_O \qquad (14)$$

Thus, the absolute disparity of a target is equal to the difference between its binocular parallax and the ocular vergence. For targets closer than the fixation point, the disparity is positive and is usually called 'crossed'; for targets farther than the fixation point, the disparity is negative, and is usually called 'uncrossed'. The terms 'crossed' and 'uncrossed' refer to the eye–image relationship when A and B are seen in diplopia: for A ('crossed') the left of the two images is seen by the right eye, whereas for B ('uncrossed') the right one of the pair of images is seen by the right eye. Crossed and uncrossed images are not to be equated with the projection on the

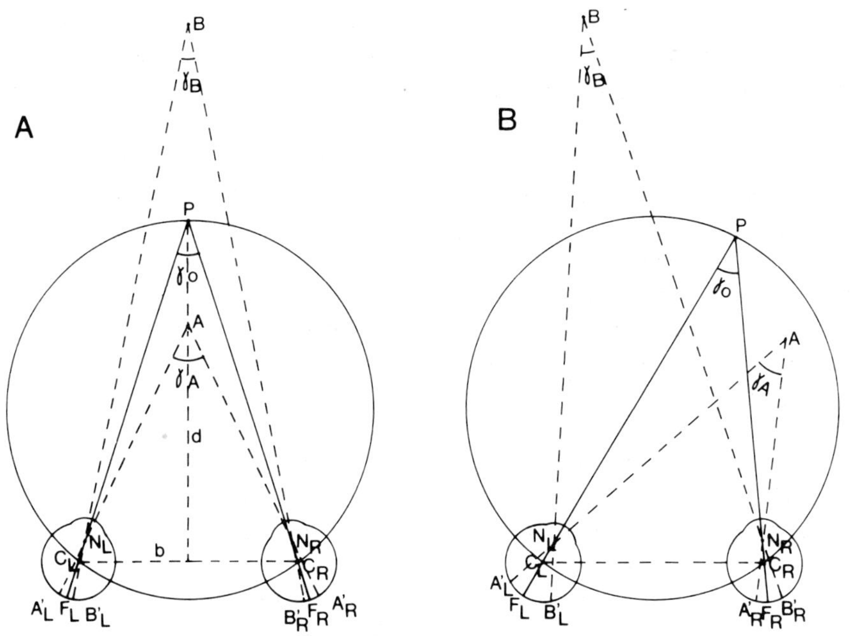

Fig. 3. Angles of ocular vergence (γ_0) and of binocular parallax ($\gamma_{A,B}$) with symmetric (A) and asymmetric (B) convergence. See text for further explanation.

temporal and the nasal halves of the retina, as is made clear by the more general asymmetric case sketched in Fig. 3B, with P moved laterally on the iso-vergence circle (γ_O unchanged) and A and B on either side of it. δ_A and δ_B are called absolute disparities, because they are scaled with respect to γ_O, which depends directly on the orientations of the lines of sight with the foveae as fixed reference points.

Crossed disparities evoke convergence; uncrossed disparities evoke divergence. These vergence movements will tend to diminish the absolute disparity of the target. No natural targets have a target vergence smaller than zero (corresponding to optical infinity); accordingly there is no natural need for divergence beyond parallelity of the lines of sight and in fact most subjects can overdiverge only a few degrees, although yoked eye movements can reach temporal deviations of 40–50 deg. The geometrical relations described do not, by themselves, initiate or control vergence, any more than retinal coordinates initiate or control other types of eye movement such as smooth pursuit and saccades. For instance, in the situation of Fig. 3, a decision will have to be made first whether A or B should become the fixated target. In the real world a multitude of targets at different distances may be present within the visual field and compete for visual attention. It is clear that higher-level, cognitive decisions must be involved in this selection process.

For the decision to fixate A or B and to induce the correct vergence it is not necessary for a target to be present in P, the intersection of the lines of sight. Actually, Fig. 3B is much simplified as it deals only with horizontal disparities. The lines of sight may also deviate vertically, in which case they do not intersect and technically there is no binocular point of fixation. However, we may assume that vertical disparities induce vertical vergence similar to the horizontal case, at least over a limited range.

For any given angle γ_O, there will be a collection of points in space (including P) that have disparity zero and require no vergence. In principle, this absence of a stimulus for vergence is one way of defining the horopter (Ogle, 1964), although no empirical determinations of the horopter have been made using this oculomotor criterion, as far as we know. Geometrical point horopters, representing the locus of zero geometrical disparity, can be constructed for several locations of the fixation point P. When P is in the horizontal visual plane passing through the two nodal points and the two foveae (with the head upright, torsion and optical aberrations being considered absent) the geometrical horopter consists of a circle (known as the Vieth-Müller circle) through P and the two nodal points, and in addition a vertical line through the intersection of the Vieth-Müller circle with the median plane. For the generalized case of asymmetric fixation outside the horizontal plane, the point horopter becomes a curve of the third degree, forming a single-loop spiral passing through P and the nodal points of the two eyes, and approaching the vertical line described before asymptotically (see Tyler and Scott, 1979; Graham, 1951; Von Helmholtz, 1962).

Empirical horopters deviate from these theoretical constructions due to a variety of factors which are not completely understood. A detailed discussion of this subject is beyond the scope of this chapter and we refer to Ogle (1964), Graham (1965) and Tyler and Scott (1979). It should be emphasized, though, that no such ambiguities arise with respect to the isovergence locus, which is a valid description of the locus of fixation points requiring equal vergence, and perfectly yoked eye movements (measured in Helmholtz's coordinates) to change binocular gaze between any two points on the same isovergence locus.

3.1.2. Absolute and relative disparity

In the configuration sketched in Fig. 3, we have defined the absolute disparities of A and B, δ_A and δ_B as $\gamma_A - \gamma_O$ and $\gamma_B - \gamma_O$. These relations are valid irrespective of whether a target is actually present at P. When P is a real target, B will be seen farther away than P, and A nearer than P through the mechanism of stereopsis. A and B will be perceived as single objects (with fusion of the two disparate retinal images) as long as the absolute disparities of A and B are not too large: the range of disparities allowing fusion and stereopsis is known as Panum's area. The points A and B have a relative disparity with respect to each other:

$$\delta_{AB} = \delta_A - \delta_B = \gamma_A - \gamma_B \tag{15}$$

In the latter expression, neither ocular vergence nor conjugate eye position is involved; thus relative disparity is independent of absolute retinal coordinates and of eye movements. In experiments on stereopsis absolute and relative disparities are often confused. In nearly all psychophysical research, subjects have to decide whether a variable target is nearer or farther away than a reference target. The latter usually also serves as a fixation point, or otherwise some additional frame of reference is used to keep the eyes appropriately directed and converged. The conclusions from many studies apply to relative disparities, but are typically stated as if they applied to absolute disparities.

Although the significance of disparity in stereopsis has been firmly established since Wheatstone's (1838, 1852) invention of the stereoscope, the history of research on disparity and its role in depth vision is a rather tangled one. This is so because in many investigations absolute and relative disparities have not been recognized (or at least have not been clearly described) as separate entities.

The distinction between absolute and relative disparity was clearly described by Blakemore (1969). Yet the importance of this distinction has been generally overlooked. In particular, most investigators have failed to realize that the presence of fixation points or any other visual frame of reference makes the absolute disparity of any test target become a relative disparity in relation to the fixation target. As we shall emphasize throughout this chapter, this has grave consequences for the interpretation of many experiments, since absolute and relative disparities have entirely different significances in binocular visual processes.

3.1.3. Corresponding points and the horopter

A major line of research on binocular vision has been the determination of corresponding retinal points and the horopter. One of the strictest criteria for corresponding points (Tschermak, 1930) is that of identical *primary* subjective visual directions of the images formed in the two eyes (Ogle, 1964), 'Primary' is used here in the sense of the perceived direction of the monocular, unfused images. The reference for these directions is the point of fixation in object space, and the fovea at the retinal level. Since this criterion is difficult to use experimentally if accurate and precise results are desired, it has often been replaced by the criterion that corresponding retinal points are represented by targets in an 'apparent fronto-parallel plane' (Hering, 1879)*. In this case, stereopsis is used to establish the absence of a perceived depth difference between the point of fixation and other points on the horopter. This paradigm may be the origin of the erroneous association of stereopsis with absolute retinal coordinates. As Ogle (1964, p.18) formulated it: "... the sensation of depth appears to arise from a psychic appreciation of the number of subjective direction units corresponding to the number of retinal elements between the fovea and the image in one eye compared to that in the other eye". In another passage, Ogle (1964, p.137) stated: "... the disparity of images in the two eyes provides stimuli not only for a stereoscopic sensation of depth, but also for fusional movements which, if made, would eliminate that disparity". A similar strong association between disparity, perception of depth and control of vergence is found in many text books. The formulation above does not distinguish between absolute and relative disparity and is therefore confusing. The fact that a fixation target is often present near the point of convergence should not lead to the misinterpretation that it is the retinal disparity with respect to the *fovea* (absolute disparity) which encodes depth: stereopsis is based on the relative disparity between one target and another target, irrespective of whether either (or none) of them is precisely fixated. If this were not the case, eye movements would have to be controlled with a precision matching that of stereoacuity (of the order of 10 seconds of arc), which is clearly not the case. Absolute disparity is changed by disjunctive eye movements and is used to control the latter; relative disparity is unaffected by eye movements (see section 3.1.2, Eqn. 15). This is of course only true if two targets A and B are presented simultaneously, or at least close enough in time for some sort of visual integration. When two targets are presented successively, in the absence of any other visible features which could act as a reference, judgements on the relative distance of these targets could be made only by comparing the successive absolute disparities of these targets. Although this could be called a relative disparity in time, it is clear that this would be an entirely different process, requiring some sort of memory and being affected by eye movements. A comparable point can be made for the discrimination of differences in lateral position (direction) of two successively presented targets. The superiority of stereoacuity for simultaneously, compared to successively, presented targets was first demonstrated by Westheimer (1979a), who also discussed the consequent increased tolerance of stereoacuity for ocular instabilities (see also Poggio and Poggio, 1984).

It should be emphasized that 'simultaneity' in the discussion above refers to targets, not to eyes. Interocular delays between the presentation of the right and left half-images of a stereogram disrupt stereopsis too, but in a different way. In this case the effect is not on the correlation between the near and far target, but on the correlation between the right and left eye views of these two targets. Ogle (1962a,b), within the limitations of the techniques of his time, found that true depth could not be demonstrated without temporal overlap of successive images presented to the left and right eyes. Ross and Hogben (1974) used an elegant display technique for dot stereograms on oscilloscopes with a decay to 1% luminosity in 10 μs. They demonstrated that stereopsis started to degrade with inter-

* As pointed out by Ogle (1964, p.19), the fundamental logic of this criterion is somewhat obscure, since the points in such a plane are obviously *not* equidistant to the subjective center of the individual. Maybe this is a reason why some investigators defined distance as the perpendicular distance of an object to the interocular base line or its extension (e.g., Graham, 1965).

ocular delays longer than about 36 ms, and decayed to chance performance for delays of about 150 ms.

3.1.4. Binocular correlation, fusion and stereopsis
A fundamental problem in binocular vision and control of vergence is the correlation between the images on the right and left retinas. Once the proper correspondence between the left and right images has been detected, the two images can be integrated.

At very large absolute disparities between the two retinal images, it must be still possible to initiate vergence. The values on the ordinate of Fig. 1 also represent the absolute disparities of targets at the distances on the abscissa of Fig. 1 when the visual axes are parallel (focussed at infinity). As we are able to converge from targets at infinity to very close ones and vice versa, it seems likely that sensory correlation of sufficient quality to initiate vergence in the proper direction must be possible throughout the vergence range, including disparities of 30 deg and more (crossed as well as uncrossed), at least for real-world targets. The purpose of vergence, which will be treated in detail in section 4, is to bring the two retinal images into sufficient register for binocular information to be correlated at a high level of resolution. Thus, there is a range of large disparities which does not allow binocularly integrated perception, but from which vergence in the right direction can be initiated.

In a smaller disparity range, binocular viewing has the important qualities of fusion and the various grades of stereopsis. A number of zones were clearly shown by Ogle (1962a) and later by Richards (1971); for a summary see Fig. 4. When the eyes are converged at a fixation target and a simple, monocularly recognizable target such as a vertical line or bar is seen in stereopsis, three different ranges of relative disparity can be distinguished. Around zero disparity there is a region where *perceived depth increases monotonically as a function of disparity.* This is called the region of *quantitative or patent stereopsis.* In a narrower subdivision within this region the target is also seen single or fused; this area is called *Panum's fusional zone.* Outside Panum's zone the line target is seen double. When

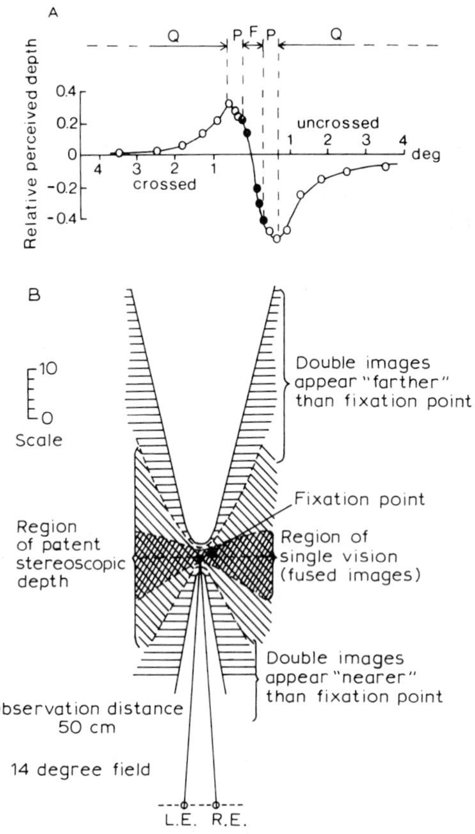

Fig. 4. The different zones of binocular vision. A. Relative perceived depth as a function of crossed or uncrossed disparity (after data of Richards, 1971); F, zone of single, fused vision; P, zone of patent or quantitative stereopsis (perceived depth increasing with disparity); Q, zone of qualitative stereopsis; B. The same zones as defined by Ogle, drawn in the horizontal plane of regard. Scale in cm. (B reproduced from Ogle, 1962)

disparity exceeds the zone of patent stereopsis, the target is still perceived at some depth, but the magnitude of depth decreases as a function of disparity until it disappears. This outer zone is the region of *qualitative stereopsis.*

The actual size of these zones is not a fixed property even for a given retinal region, but depends upon the spatial spectral composition and extent of a visual stimulus. For instance, measurements by Richards and Kaye (1974) have shown that a 3 min arc wide vertical bar (height 0.5 deg) yields a limit of patent stereopsis of about 0.5 deg and a limit for qualitative stereopsis of about 2 deg. For a bar 0.8

deg wide these limits are 2 deg and 8 deg, respectively. The maximal range of qualitative stereopsis allowing a reasonably reliable discrimination 'near' and 'far' is about 10 deg of relative disparity between target and reference (fixation point), as measured by Westheimer and Tanzman (1956) and Blakemore (1970).

Some other classifications of stereopsis are used, but not always consistently. Bishop and Henry (1971) used the terms 'fine' and 'coarse' stereopsis in relation to small (maybe up to 2 deg) and large (up to about 10 deg) disparities. In contrast, Julesz (1978) defined the stereopsis of narrow bars (i.e., *high spatial frequencies*) as *fine stereopsis,* and stereopsis of wide bars (*low spatial frequencies*) as *coarse stereopsis.* A further distinction, introduced in relation to random-dot stereograms by Julesz, is between local and global stereopsis. *Local stereopsis* refers to depth localization (on the basis of disparity) of elements whose correspondence (and thus disparity) can be unambiguously established, such as in classical stereograms, with non-camouflaged features that can be seen both monocularly and binocularly in isolated regions of the visual field without reference to the disparities present in other regions or even at the same location (Julesz, 1978; Schor et al., 1984a; Tyler, 1983). In random-dot stereograms with many potential correspondences between elements at the local level, a higher-order process called *global stereopsis* is assumed to select a preferred set of local depth localizations, which form a dense surface (Julesz, 1978). 'Local' and 'global' should not be confused with 'fine' and 'coarse'.

3.2. Disparity and perception of depth: psychophysics

3.2.1. Traditional estimates of Panum's area

In the traditional description, non-corresponding points on the two retinae, when stimulated separately, lead to different perceived visual directions. Simultaneous stimulation of such points by the disparate images of an object leads to perception of a single object in a fused visual direction. The maximum disparity beyond which diplopia occurs is conventionally represented by considering that a point on one retina corresponds not to a single point on the other, but to a 'Panum's area' of finite size (Panum, 1858; Ogle, 1964; Mitchell, 1966a,b). When defined in this way, Panum's area relates to *absolute,* overall disparities of the two retinal images; one of its main virtues would be to induce a tolerance for imperfect binocular alignment. Panum's area would allow single vision despite instabilities or constant errors (fixation disparity) of vergence. In practice, however, Panum's area is usually determined as the disparity range allowing single vision around a fixation target. Although the fixation point may closely correspond to the foveal center, this means that most practical determinations of Panum's area are actually estimates of the maximal *relative* disparity between fixation target and test object allowing single vision. There are suggestions in the literature that the maximal absolute and retinal disparities compatible with single fusion are indeed different entities. Classical, static determinations of Panum's area in the fovea have yielded values of about 14 min arc peak-to-peak for the total crossed to uncrossed range (Ogle, 1964; for review see Mitchell, 1966a). However, values as large as about 20 min arc (Palmer, 1961; Mitchell, 1966b) and as small as 2–4 min arc (Woo, 1974) have been found. Duwaer and Van den Brink (1981) found that diplopia thresholds for horizontal disparities in the fovea could vary over two orders of magnitude (0.25 – 22.2 min arc) depending on subjects, amount of training, the criteria used for diplopia, and surrounding stimuli. Schor and Tyler (1981) found that the static value of 8 min arc for a line stereogram could be extended by spatio-temporal modulation of the disparity to maximally about 20 min arc. When instead of lines bars are used, which had been spatially filtered with a narrow band, much larger relative disparities can be fused, as shown by Schor et al. (1984b). Peak-to-peak values of Panum's area as large as 400 min arc (centered on the fovea) were found for stimuli with spatial frequencies of 0.075 cycles/deg, in horizontal as well as vertical directions. At these low frequencies the sensory fusion limit equalled the upper limit for stereoscopic depth perception. When conventional bars of varying width were used instead of spatially filtered bars, a much more limited extension of Panum's area was found as a function of bar width. The high spatial frequencies contained in the edges of the bars caused diplopia at relatively small disparities (Schor et al., 1984b).

It is well known that the depth of Panum's fusional zone increases as a function of eccentricity. Ogle's data (see Ogle, 1962a, Figs. 33 and 34) suggest that the peak-to-peak depth of Panum's zone increased from about 14 min arc at 1 deg eccentricity to about 17 min arc at 4 deg eccentricity. Beyond 4 deg eccentricity, the total width of Panum's zone was estimated at about 6% of the angle of eccentricity. Ogle's typical result for the extent of the fusional zone in the horizontal plane is shown in Fig. 5A. Attempts to extend these measurements into three-dimensional space have apparently been rare; an impression of the shape of the three-dimensional fusional volume was given by Tyler and Scott (1979). Fig. 5B,C shows this shape and its probable change due to eccentric gaze positions.

Traditional investigations have not dealt with the limits of fusion at very small eccentricities. Burt and Julesz (1980a,b) introduced the concept of a disparity-gradient limit. Using two-dot stereograms in a wallpaper configuration, they showed that diplopia occurred whenever the ratio of the binocular relative disparity to the binocular dot separation exceeded a critical value, which turned out to be close to unity. For example, at the low end of the scale, fusion was lost for a disparity of 2 min arc at a binocular inter-dot distance of 2 min arc. Elaborating on these findings, Burt and Julesz (1980a,b) have suggested extensive modifications of the classical concept of Panum's zone. They claimed that Panum's zone (see Figs. 4 and 5) represents the fusional volume for a *single* object, whereas interactions would occur between multiple objects. Each object would create a cone-shaped 'forbidden zone' around itself, within which no fusion with a new object would be possible.

A number of problems with the arguments of

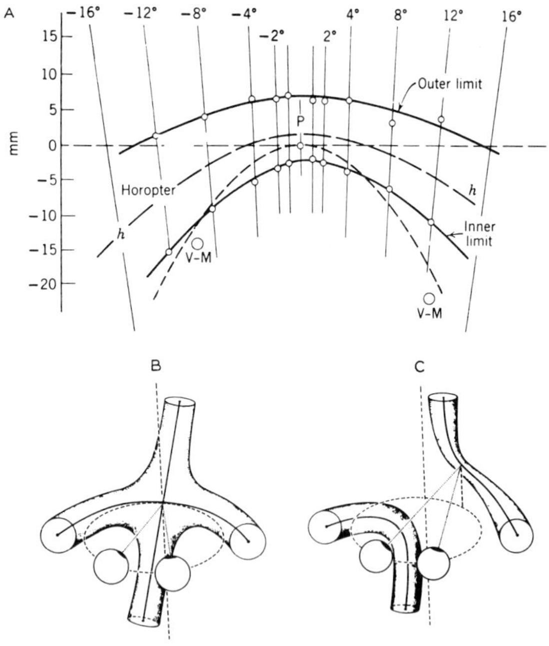

Fig. 5. The spatial extent of the fusional zone. A. Region of binocular single vision in the horizontal plane of regard, as determined by Ogle. The observation distance to the fixation point (F) was 40 cm. Ordinates are magnified 2-fold. (From Ogle, 1964) B,C. Sketches of three-dimensional fusional space around the horopter (solid lines) in the case of symmetric (B) and asymmetric (C) convergence. (Reproduced from Tyler and Scott, 1979)

Burt and Julesz have been pointed out by Krol and Van de Grind (1982). In the present context, a fundamental concern is that Burt and Julesz did not consider the fact that all traditional determinations of Panum's zone already involve two objects, viz. the fixation target and the test target. Thus, the classical diagrams may already contain the aspect of object interaction, and the introduction of extra forbidden zones (Burt and Julesz, 1980b, Fig. 5b) may be unnecessary. However, the interesting observations of Burt and Julesz may imply that the depth of the fusional zone becomes very small when the distance between the fixation point and test object is of the order of a few min arc, a range not explored in the classical experiments. On the other hand, Prazdny (1985) has reported that the disparity-gradient limit can be significantly raised (to values of 2 or 3) when the two interacting objects are not identical in size or contrast polarity.

The interpretation of many of the published observations of disparity tolerance is difficult because vergence was not measured. Although attempts were made to control vergence by fixation marks, it is not certain how effective this control was, and, moreover, fixation marks introduce relative disparity. Even the use of nonius lines has been discredited as unreliable, at least in the case of vertical vergence (Kertesz et al., 1983). We shall return to the important issue of the fusional zone in section 4, where we shall discuss the results of experiments in which vergence was recorded and absolute disparity was controlled.

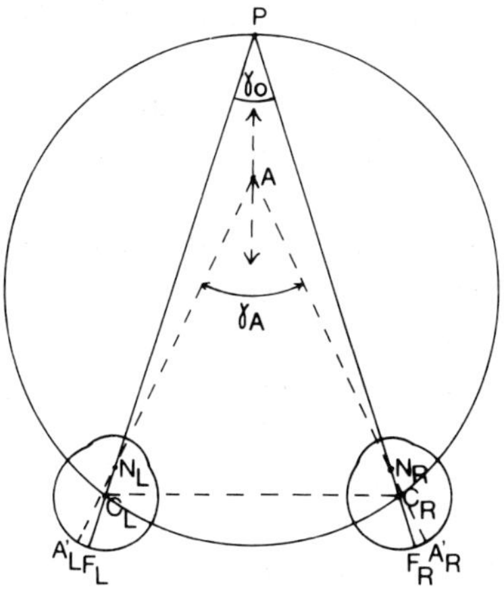

Fig. 6. Absolute disparity and depth perception: the eyes are converged at point P, where no target is present. Target A is seen in isolation, with an absolute disparity $\delta_A = \gamma_A - \gamma_O$. The question is whether δ_A conveys information on distance, and whether changes in δ_A lead to perception of motion in depth, in the absence of relative disparity information derived from reference targets, for instance a real target at P.

3.2.2. Absolute disparity and perception of depth

Now that the distinction between absolute and relative disparity has been made it is possible to determine whether absolute disparity of a single target provides a cue for depth. In Fig. 6 the eyes are converged at point P, where no target is present. A target A is presented at a different distance, with absolute disparity δ_A. Theoretically, a subject might correctly estimate the absolute distance of A even without making any eye movements by using information on the vergence angle γ_O as well as absolute disparity $\delta_A = \gamma_A - \gamma_O$. Alternatively, a subject might converge first on target A and then estimate the distance. As psychophysical tests of absolute estimates are difficult to perform, it is easier to investigate first the question whether a subject can discriminate relative changes in depth on the sole basis of the successive presentation of a single target at different absolute disparities, without any visual frame of reference, and with vergence preferably dissociated from disparity.

The literature on successive discrimination of absolute disparities, with vergence minimized, is quite limited. Foley (1976) did very careful experiments using lines presented on an oscilloscope, with the left and right eye stimulation separated by crossed polarizers. The first binocular line was shown for 2 s, and after an interval of 0–32 s a second line was shown for 100 ms at a different disparity (stereo condition) or in a different direction (vernier condition). A forced-choice technique was used, with the subjects receiving feedback about their performance. No fixation point was used and presumably no other visual frame of reference was available. Thresholds for discrimination increased as a function of the interstimulus time interval. They were as low as 1 min arc for intervals of 0–0.1 s, and rose to 20–30 min arc for intervals of 3.2–32 s. Thresholds for direction (successive vernier discrimination) were slightly lower than for disparity discrimination. Foley (1976) interpreted these results in the context of an earlier model of Kinchla and associates (Kinchla and Smyzer, 1967: Kinchla and Allan, 1969) in which error accumulates over time as a result of uncompensated eye movements and loss of memory for the first target position. A longer presentation of the second target (1 s), permitting more accurate control of vergence, reduced the thresholds very slightly. A point of caution in the interpretation of this and other experiments using oscilloscope images is the possibility of image persistence on the screen. Foley (1976) gave no details of the type of phosphor used in his oscilloscopes, but it is important to stress that even so-called fast phosphor compounds such as P31 contain slower components resulting in prolonged visibility of a weak residual image after the beam has been turned off. This would of course change the absolute into relative disparities.

Westheimer (1979a) compared stereoscopic thresholds for ordinary, simultaneously presented line pair stereograms with those for successively presented lines at different absolute disparities. A single binocular line executed a step in disparity and therefore acted as a self-reference. No effective comparison stimulus was available within several degrees of visual angle. Thresholds for discrimination of distance of the steps of this 'successive' presentation were of the order of 1 min arc, in accordance with Foley (1976). These thresholds were at least 10-fold larger than a subject's best stereo threshold for stimuli presented simultaneously. Westheimer (1979a,b) was probably the first to express clearly the idea that good stereoacuity requires the simultaneous presence of the targets which have to be distinguished in depth, and the operation of some differentiating mechanism, which would extract relative disparities, independent of eye movements. (Notice that no interocular delays were involved in Westheimer's experiments; see section 3.1.3.)

Jones (1977) studied the detection of disparity by successive presentation as well as vergence responses to large steps in disparity (0.6–4.6 deg), created by the sudden, brief replacement of a fixation point by a target with a given disparity. Although these experiments were presented as a follow-up of Richards' (1970, 1971) work on stereoanomalies for crossed or uncrossed disparities, an essential difference is that in the experiments of Richards a fixation point was continuously present. Thus, Richards studied discrimination of relative disparity, whereas Jones studied absolute disparities. This may be the reason for the surprisingly high proportion of stereo-anomalous subjects (18 out of 30) identified in the experiments by Jones (1977). Only one third of the 'stereo-anomalous' subjects showed some form of anomaly in the vergence responses, and all subjects had normal fine stereoacuity (better than 20 sec arc) in a standard stereoscopic test. Although Jones (1977) interprets his large number of 'anomalous' subjects as indicating a commonly occurring specific defect of coarse stereopsis, the successive presentation he used in his task is a more likely contribution to the poor performance.

3.2.3. Relative disparity and perception of depth

In marked contrast to absolute disparity as a cue to depth, relative disparity is an extremely powerful cue for the perception of relative depths, or stereopsis. Only some aspects of the prolific literature on stereopsis can be reviewed here. The lowest thresholds for relative differences in depth have been found for conventional, monocularly recognizable, fine line stereograms; they are of the order of 10 sec arc or better (e.g. Howard, 1919; Ogle, 1964; Westheimer, 1979a). This acuity is found only in the fovea; thresholds rise rapidly as a function of eccentricity and stereopsis becomes very poor beyond 20 deg in the periphery (Ogle and Ellerbrock, 1945; Tyler, 1977). This is also true for motion in depth (Beverley and Regan, 1973, 1975).

Richards and Kaye (1974) proposed that fine and coarse stereopsis (local and global, in their terms) formed a continuous range. Marr and Poggio's (1979) computational theory of stereopsis follows this concept and predicts that the disparity range over which depth is processed is proportional to the receptive field size of disparity coding neurons. In order for coarse and fine stereopsis to be part of this continuum, both upper and lower limits of stereopsis should increase with stimulus size. Accordingly, depth would not be stimulated by fine disparities subtended by large targets, or by coarse disparities subtended by small targets (Schor and Wood, 1983). Investigations using local narrow-band spatially filtered stimuli have indeed shown such a continuum. Lower disparity limits for the perception of depth were about 0.25 min arc for narrow stimuli (up to 0.42 deg) and increased proportionally with stimulus width for wider stimuli. Similarly, upper disparity limits for stereopsis also increased from a lowest value of 40 min arc for stimuli up to 0.42 deg wide to 2 deg at the broadest stimulus width used (13.6 deg) but at a lower rate, i.e. proportionally to the square root of the stimulus diameter (Schor and Wood, 1983). A similar square-root relationship between upper disparity limit and stimulus diameter was observed for bars by Richards and Kaye (1974) and also for dynamic random-dot stereograms by Tyler and Julesz (1980). The maximal relative disparities in random-dot stereograms which could still be perceived as depth, called by Tyler and Julesz (1980) the depth of the cyclopean retina, was about 2 deg of crossed or uncrossed disparity, reached for a width of the disparate region of 10 deg. Clearly, this range is lower than that found for monocularly recognizable stimuli, which show a *maximum* depth at 2 deg disparity (Richards and Kaye, 1974).

A further spatial limitation of stereopsis is the bandwidth of the variations in relative disparity across the visual field. Using wavy-line stereograms, Tyler (1973, 1975) described the area of depth perception contained between the threshold values and the upper limits of disparity. Tyler found a linear relationship between the upper limit of disparity and the period length (reciprocal of spatial frequency) of the disparity modulation. This effect was called disparity scaling, as it implies a constant ratio between the maximal disparity still perceived as depth and the spatial period of disparity. An absolute upper frequency limit for the perception of spatial variation of disparity as modulation of depth is about 4 cycles/deg for wavy-line stereograms (Tyler, 1973, 1975) as well as random-dot stereograms (Tyler, 1974).

In conclusion, we know that relative disparity is an effective cue to depth, whereas absolute disparity is probably not, or only marginally effective. However, serious attempts to relate purported retinal conditions to percepts via neural mechanisms must rely on *known* retinal conditions. Therefore, we have to discuss the control of vergence. Also, vergence and perception of depth may rely on either similar or different binocular visual mechanisms, and understanding one may help in understanding the other.

4. Control of vergence by disparity

4.1. Introduction

As discussed in the preceding sections, humans are able to synthesize a single, binocular percept from the retinal images in the two eyes. A stimulus in one retina can be physiologically fused with a range of similar stimuli around the point of precise correspondence in the other retina. Eye movements provide the conditions under which the sensory process of fusion can succesfully operate to obtain or maintain a single percept. They bring or keep the binocular retinal stimuli within the area of tolerance permitted by the fusional process. In this section we will discuss vergence performed in response to absolute retinal disparity, and evaluate conclusions which have been drawn from experimental observations in the literature. We will show that the problem of describing vergence responses to stepwise and sinusoidal stimuli by a single model, which has been discussed many times in the literature, may be solved by a better interpretation of experimental results with regard to the latency and the dynamics of vergence responses. We will also discuss the accuracy and precision of ocular vergence.

4.2. Stimuli for vergence

Westheimer and Mitchell (1956) were the first to show that absolute disparity is an effective stimulus for ocular vergence in the absence of other cues. The vergence response reduced the amount of disparity. Thus, vergence responds to sensory feedback (absolute disparity) in a way typical of a negative feedback system.

Vergence is also stimulated by cues other than retinal disparity. For example, blur of the retinal image, which is the effective stimulus for accommodation, also produces a vergence response (Allen, 1953; Troelstra et al., 1964). This vergence response (called ‘accommodative vergence’) was objectively recorded first by Alpern and Ellen (1956). Another cue is the size of the image in the two eyes. Alpern (1958) discovered that static differences in size produce vergence responses. More recently, Erkelens and Regan (1986) found that dynamic changes in retinal image size induce small, but consistent, vergence responses.

The cues 'blur' and 'change in size', unlike 'disparity', induce vergence responses in a feed-forward way, because the vergence response does not affect the stimulus. Another way that blur and change in size are different from binocular disparity is that they induce vergence responses during monocular stimulation. Change in size, however, is more effective during binocular than during monocular stimulation (Erkelens and Regan, 1986). Binocular accommodative vergence has been reported to be weaker than monocular accommodative vergence (Semmlow and Venkiteswaran, 1976). This result could be questioned because the authors recorded movements of the right eye only and they did not open the disparity-loop to avoid interference with induced disparity.

Of the three cues discussed above, i.e., disparity, blur and change in size, disparity has been shown to be the strongest in human (Semmlow and Wetzel, 1979; Erkelens and Regan, 1986) and in monkey (Cumming and Judge, 1986). As was mentioned previously, we will discuss only one type of vergence, i.e., horizontal vergence induced by retinal disparity, because it is most directly related to the perception of depth and to the maintenance of binocular fusion. Knowledge about the dynamics of ocular vergence may lead to conclusions about how much absolute retinal disparity is tolerated by the fusional process under dynamic viewing conditions. To introduce this discussion, it will be necessary to describe and evaluate the experimental technique of disparity stabilization, which has been central to investigations of the dynamics of vergence.

4.3. Interpretation of vergence derived from monocular recordings

In order to study the dynamics of vergence properly, it is necessary to record the positions of both eyes accurately and simultaneously. This may seem an obvious demand, but, until fairly recently, accurate and precise binocular eye-movement recording systems were practically unavailable. As a consequence, many experiments on binocular eye movements have been carried out with inferior techniques, such as electrooculography (EOG), or with accurate, monocular, and therefore incomplete, recording systems. Data from such experiments have led to confusing results. For example, Zuber and Stark (1968) measured ocular vergence elicited by small changes in target vergence (up to 1.7°) under closed-loop conditions with a monocular eye-movement recording system. They found that gains were considerably larger than unity for frequencies below 0.4 Hz, and phase lags were larger than 180° for frequencies larger than 2.0 Hz. Gains larger than unity and phase lags larger than 180° seem puzzling, because such responses do not eliminate retinal disparity. Also, phase lags larger than 180° may lead to instabilities so that even no vergence response at all to such small stimulus disparities would result in smaller retinal disparity. The results of Zuber and Stark (1968) were not confirmed by others who measured vergence responses to sinusoidally changing disparity under closed-loop conditions with binocular eye-movement recording systems. Erkelens and Collewijn (1985b), using large stereograms as stimuli, measured vergence responses under closed-loop conditions and found gains lower than unity and phase lags less than 120° for frequencies up to 1.5 Hz and amplitudes up to 5°.

The gain–phase relationships reported by Zuber and Stark (1968) may be related to the fact that these authors measured the horizontal movements of the left eye only, and assumed mirror-symmetrical vergence movements of the other eye. This procedure is inappropriate because vergence responses to small disparities are not distributed equally between the two eyes (Erkelens, 1987). Examples of unequal vergence movements in the two eyes are shown in Fig. 7.

The inequality of vergence movements in the two eyes is particularly striking at high stimulus frequencies (> 1 Hz), when fusion is lost. Under such

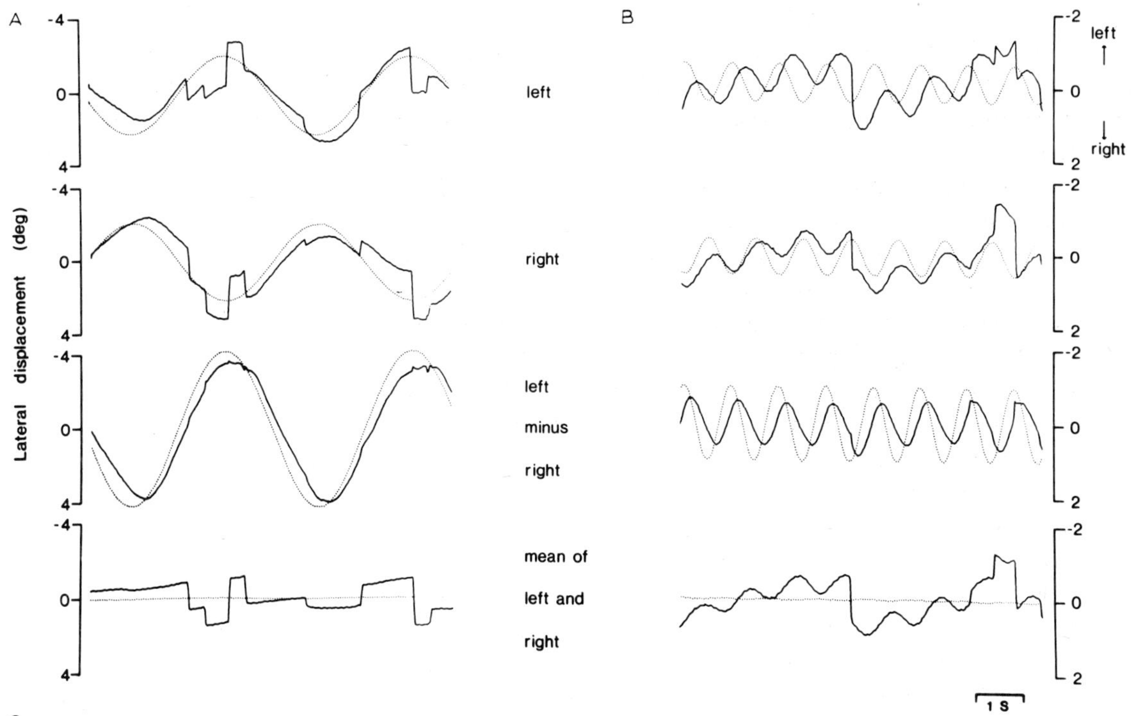

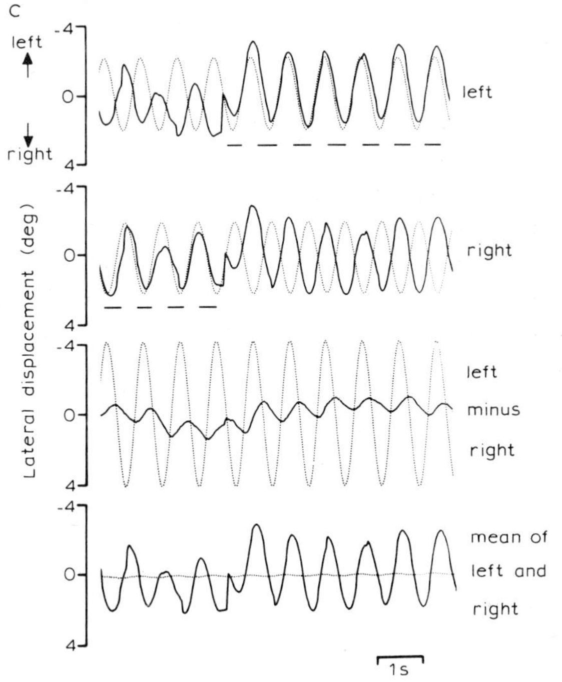

Fig. 7. Vergence responses (continuous lines) to symmetric stimulation with sinusoidal changes in target vergence (dotted lines). The inequality of the vergence responses of the two eyes is best demonstrated by the oscillations in the version traces (bottom figures). The target was viewed in binocular fusion in A and B, but in binocular rivalry in C. The dashed lines (in panel C) indicate the time during which the eye tracked the monocular stimulus. (From Erkelens and Collewijn, 1985b)

conditions one eye starts to track its stimulus monocularly. Little – if any – vergence is left under such viewing conditions and the other eye is pulled along conjugately with the eye dominating the response (Erkelens and Collewijn, 1985b). In this light, it seems likely that the claim by Zuber and Stark (1968) of a continued presence of vergence movements up to at least 4 Hz was based on the version movements of the measured eye misinterpreted as vergence. In the literature on ocular vergence we found several reports in which the authors recorded the movements of only one eye (Zuber and Stark, 1968; Krishnan et al., 1973; Semmlow and Venkiteswaran, 1976; Krishnan and Stark, 1977, 1983; Semmlow and Wetzel, 1979; Semmlow and Heerema, 1979). Conclusions with respect to vergence in these reports have to be viewed with great caution.

4.4. Stabilization of retinal disparity

The study of the relationship between disparity and vergence requires opening of the feedback loop by which disparity is processed. This so-called open-loop condition for disparity can be created by the experimental stabilization of disparity, which prevents the vergence movements from changing disparity. This stabilization can be achieved by superimposing the ocular vergence signal upon the signal controlling the target vergence. Additionally, disparity with a specific time function can be imposed on the stimulus. As a result the disparity of the stimulus is under complete experimental control. In practice, half of the vergence signal is added to the signal controlling the position of each of the half-images. This technique allows the experimental control of retinal disparity without the disadvantage of image-fading or ocular instability which may occur with complete image stabilization in each eye. A minor disadvantage of the technique is that ocular vergence is imposed symmetrically upon the positions of each of the images presented to the two eyes. This means that the binocularly fixated targets are driven off the foveae when the two eyes respond unequally to the disparity stimulus. The drift of the fixation point, however, can easily be corrected by a non-stabilized versional eye movement, which has no consequences for the disparity of the target.

The technique of stabilization of retinal disparity gives interpretable information about the normal behavior of vergence only when results from such experiments are compatible with those from experiments done under normal, closed-loop conditions. Smooth-pursuit versional eye movements under open-loop conditions do not meet this criterion. Smooth pursuit under the open-loop conditions has been hard to interpret because of the emergence of idiosyncratic smooth eye-movement patterns (Cushman et al., 1984; Collewijn and Tamminga, 1986) and because in some cases subjects exercise some, albeit limited (Cushman et al., 1984), voluntary control (Van den Berg and Collewijn, 1987). We have tested whether vergence responses to retinal disparity under closed- and open-loop conditions are compatible (Pobuda and Erkelens, in preparation). Vergence responses to stimulation with sinusoidally changing target vergence were recorded under closed-loop conditions. Retinal disparity was computed from the recordings of target and ocular vergence. Subsequently, these disparities were presented as a stimulus under open-loop conditions. As shown in Fig. 8, the vergence responses under both conditions were very similar most of the time. This result justifies using the technique of stabilization of retinal disparity for studying the vergence response to controlled changes in disparity.

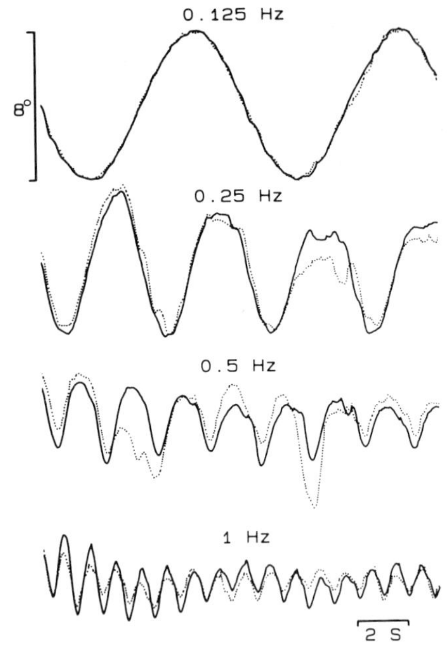

Fig. 8. Vergence responses to oscillating changes in disparity. The effective changes in stimulus disparity were the same under closed-loop (continuous lines) and under open-loop (dotted lines) viewing conditions. (From Pobuda and Erkelens, in preparation)

Stabilization of retinal disparity can be succesfully applied only if the movements of both eyes are precisely recorded without any drift in the recording system. Rashbass and Westheimer (1961), who were the first to implement this technique, developed an elaborate recording technique based on the relationship between angular differences in the directions of light beams reflected from the limbus and the cornea, and the angular position of the eye. This system, which recorded horizontal positions of both eyes with a noise level below 5 min arc, allowed them to achieve a substantially drift-free ocular vergence during stabilization with zero disparity.

4.5. Vergence responses to controlled changes in disparity

In their landmark paper Rashbass and Westheimer (1961) used the technique of stabilization of retinal disparity to study vergence responses to small step or sinusoidal changes in disparity. They found that a step change in disparity induced an ocular vergence movement with a uniform velocity after a latency of about 160 ms. The velocity of vergence was linearly related to the amplitude of the disparity step for disparities up to 0.5°. Rashbass and Westheimer (1961) also showed that the velocity of vergence responses started to saturate for disparity steps larger than 0.5° (Fig. 9A). Very similar results have recently been obtained in monkeys (Cumming and Judge, 1986; Fig. 9C).

Rashbass and Westheimer (1961) concluded from the vergence responses to disparity steps that the velocity of vergence movements is proportional to the disparity existing one reaction time earlier. They wrote this statement in the form of the following simple equation:

$$\dot{V} = k\, d(t - \tau_v) \tag{16}$$

where $\dot{V}$ is the velocity of vergence, k is a constant of proportionality, $d(t)$ is disparity as a function of time, and τ_v is the latency or reaction time of the response. Rashbass and Westheimer (1961) tested the general validity of this relationship between vergence velocity and disparity by probing the vergence system with sinusoidal disparities. Such disparities can be written as:

$$d(t) = A \cos(\omega t) \tag{17}$$

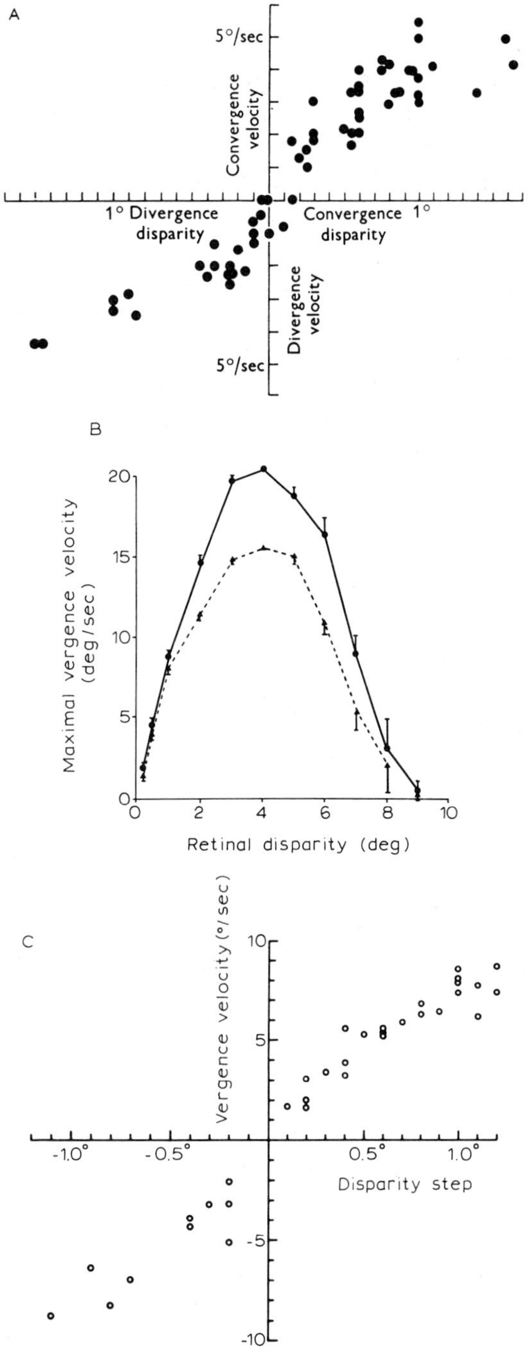

Fig. 9. Velocity of vergence as a function of the disparity step. A. Data of Rashbass and Westheimer (1961). B. Data of Erkelens (1987) for crossed steps of disparity between the half-images of a random-dot stereogram (continuous line) and a single-line stereogram (dashed line). C. Data of Cumming and Judge (1986) for monkeys.

where A is the amplitude (in deg) and ω is the frequency (in rad/s) of stimulation. Time integration of $\dot{V}$ after substitution of Eqn. 17 into Eqn. 16 gives:

$$V(t) = \frac{kA}{\omega}\cos\{\omega(t-\tau_v) - \frac{\pi}{2}\} \quad (18)$$

The gain of vergence, which is defined as the ratio between the amplitudes of vergence and disparity, and the phase lag of the vergence response with regard to the disparity stimulus, follow directly from Eqns. 17 and 18.

$$\text{Gain: } G(\omega) = \frac{k}{\omega}$$

$$\text{Phase lag: } \varphi(\omega) = \tau_v\omega + \frac{\pi}{2} \quad (19)$$

Eqn. 19 predicts that the gain of vergence is inversely proportional to the frequency of disparity stimulation, and that the phase lag is a linear function of frequency with a minimum of 90° for frequencies approaching 0 Hz. Rashbass and Westheimer (1961) found that there was good agreement between the experimental and predicted results for gain as a function of stimulus frequency, but not for phase. For sinusoidal disparities at frequencies below 1 Hz the phase lags were smaller than 90°. In general, the phase lags were much smaller than was predicted by the phase relationship between vergence and disparity in Eqn. 19. These short phase lags of vergence in response to sinusoidal stimulation seemed to suggest some kind of prediction or anticipation of the change in disparity. However, Rashbass and Westheimer (1961) rejected this possibility because responses to stepwise alternation of crossed and uncrossed disparity showed no evidence of anticipation; responses occurred invariably after one reaction time. They concluded that the short phase lags of vergence in response to sinusoidally modulated disparity were not caused by genuine anticipation. They favored the hypothesis that vergence was sensitive to higher time derivatives of disparity, i.e., rate of change in disparity.

In a late study, Krishnan et al. (1973) claimed to have evidence for anticipation of repetitive square-wave changes of target vergence based on their finding that reaction times were short – close to 0 ms at 0.5 Hz and about 80 ms at 0.2 and 0.8 Hz in two subjects. Reaction times were longer than 132 ms for all frequencies in a third subject. But this would not account for Rashbass and Westheimer's result, because even with reaction times of about 0 ms, Eqn. 19 would still predict phase lags of 90° for all frequencies of sinusoidal stimulation. Thus, the effect of anticipation, such as that reported by Krishnan et al. (1973), was too small to explain the short phase lags of vergence in response to sinusoidally modulated disparity. Moreover, the conclusions of Krishnan et al. (1973) are questionable because these authors only recorded the horizontal movements of one eye and assumed symmetrical eye movements. This procedure leaves the possibility open that versional eye movements were misinterpreted as vergence movements. This point was addressed in more detail in section 4.3.

As noted above, Rashbass and Westheimer (1961) suggested that higher time derivatives of disparity might be responsible for the short phase lags. Sensitivity of vergence to the rate of change in disparity would predict that anticipation would not occur to step changes of disparity because steps do not have a finite velocity. Thus, sensitivity to higher time derivatives would give additional terms in Eqn. 18 (the response to sinusoids), but not in Eqn. 16 (the response to steps). But Rashbass and Westheimer (1961) did not consider the implication of adding terms to one equation and not to the other. The main implication is that the gain of vergence for sinusoidal disparities should also be inconsistent with the gain of vergence to steps, i.e. the gain of vergence to sinusoidal changes in disparity would be different from that predicted by Eqn. 19. Gains, however, were neatly predicted by this equation. This implies that either the gain or the phase lags, but not both, can be predicted correctly by Rashbass and Westheimer's model. One resolution to this inconsistency is that responses to step and sinusoidal changes of disparity cannot be simulated by a single model, in contrast to Rashbass and Westheimer's model.

The attempt to reconcile the responses to sinusoidal and step changes in disparity has attracted the attention of many investigators. In the next subsection we will show that the differences in vergence responses to step and sinusoidal disparities are probably only apparent, and due to misinterpretations of the experimental results.

4.6. The time delay of disparity processing

Rashbass and Westheimer (1961) showed that a step in disparity induced an ocular vergence movement with a uniform velocity, after a latency of about 160 ms. The usual interpretation of this observation (e.g., Rashbass and Westheimer, 1961; Zuber and Stark, 1968; Cumming and Judge, 1986) can be questioned. The usual interpretation, to use engineering terminology, is illustrated in Cumming and Judge (1986). They stated that the vergence system responds to step changes in disparity as if it has an open-loop transfer function of an integrator plus a delay. This delay was assumed to be equal to the latency of a vergence response to a step in disparity. However, this interpretation can be questioned because it neglected the contribution of the orbital plant to the vergence response. This neglect is justified only for the late (> 500 ms) phase of the vergence response to a step in disparity because the time constant of the plant is short (about 150 ms in a first-order approximation; Robinson, 1973) relative to the time constant of the vergence controller, which was assumed to be infinitely large (see Eqn. 16).

The dynamics of the plant have to be taken into account in the computation of the time delay of the vergence loop because the time constant of the plant (about 150 ms) is of the same order as the latency of the vergence response (about 160 ms). Using a first-order approximation of the plant dynamics, the transfer function of vergence induced by a step in disparity can be written as:

$$H(s) = \frac{G\, e^{-\tau_v s}}{(\tau_1 s+1)\,(\tau_2 s+1)} \qquad (20)$$

where τ_v is the time delay in the loop, G and τ_1 are gain and time constant of the disparity integrator, and τ_2 is the time constant of the plant. *H* is the transfer function in the Laplace domain of a second-order system with delay, for which it holds that τ_v and τ_2 are of the same order and τ_1 is much larger. A feature of such a system is that its latency to a step input is not equal to τ_v, but approximately equal to $\tau_v+\tau_2$. Latencies of vergence induced by steps in disparity, computed according to the method shown in Fig. 10, had a mean value of 195 ms (Pobuda and Erkelens, in preparation). Taking 150 ms as an approximation for τ_2, it follows that the time delay, τ_v, is approximately 45 ms instead of 160 ms as is generally assumed.

In addition to the interpretation of the time delay, the validity of assuming an infinite time constant of the vergence controller for disparity integration can be questioned. Conclusions about the

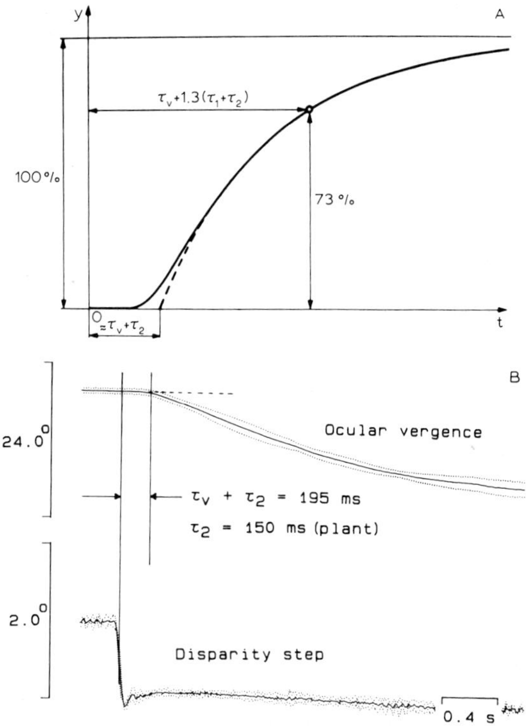

Fig. 10. A. Theoretical response of a second-order system with a delay to a step stimulus. The dashed line represents the response of a first-order system to a step stimulus. B. Mean vergence responses to step changes in disparity. The dotted lines indicate the response and the stimulus ± 1 SD.

time constant of the vergence controller were based on the early portion of the vergence response, as the imposed steps of disparity had durations of at most 2 s (Rashbass and Westheimer, 1961; Cumming and Judge, 1986). Thus, the apparent perfect integration of disparity might well be accounted for by a leaky integration with a time constant longer than a few seconds. In fact, vergence responses to small disparity steps lasting about 8 s show that 4 s is a more realistic value for the time constant of integration (Erkelens, 1987).

The short time delay, in combination with the finite time constant of disparity integration, may close the gap which apparently existed between vergence responses to sinusoidal and step changes in disparity. A shorter time delay than previously assumed does not affect the gain of vergence to sinusoidally changing disparity predicted by vergence responses to disparity steps. However, it strongly reduces the predicted phase lags. A finite time constant further reduces the predicted phase lags but it also changes the gain. Taken together, the short time delay and the finite time constant of disparity integration bring the predicted and the actual vergence response to sinusoidally changing disparity closer together. That predicted and actual vergence responses can be brought into complete agreement with each other will be shown in section 4.9.

4.7. Dependence of vergence on the frequency and amplitude of disparity changes

Until now we have treated vergence as a linear system with the transfer function shown in Eqn. 20. There is evidence from different types of experiment that vergence induced by disparity shows strongly non-linear behavior. For example, Rashbass and Westheimer (1961) showed that the vergence response to sinusoidally changing disparity under open-loop conditions is dependent on amplitude. Similar results were obtained under closed-loop conditions in which target vergence was changed sinusoidally (Erkelens and Collewijn, 1985b; Cumming and Judge, 1986). These studies showed that the gain of vergence, but not the phase, depended strongly on amplitude. The gain also showed considerable individual differences, while the phase did not. Erkelens and Collewijn (1985b) found that the gain of vergence could be well described as a uniform function of the maximum velocity of target vergence, independently of amplitude (Fig. 11). Gain decreased progressively with the increase of velocity of target vergence. Gain did not fall to zero even for velocities of almost 50°/s. Convergence and divergence are often unequal. Either of the two may be faster, but one type of vergence has consistently faster dynamics in individual subjects (Mitchell, 1970; Jones, 1977).

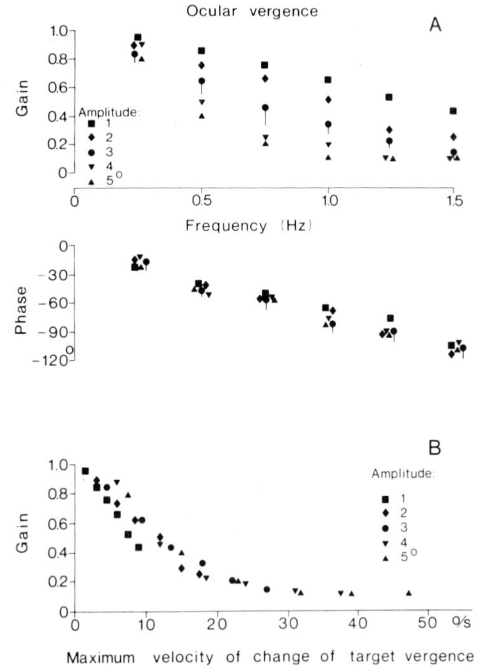

Fig. 11. A. Mean frequency responses of vergence for different amplitudes of modulation of target vergence. Standard deviations are plotted for one amplitude (3°). B. The same mean gain responses of vergence as in A, but now plotted as a function of the maximum rate of change of target vergence. (From Erkelens and Collewijn, 1985b)

Vergence responses to sinusoidally changing stimuli under either open- or closed-loop conditions may be adequate to demonstrate the non-linear behavior of vergence. Sinusoidal stimuli, however, are poorly suited for a quantitative analysis of the dependence on amplitude because disparity is not restricted to a specific amplitude but passes through a whole range of amplitudes during each cycle. The dependence of vergence on the amplitude of the disparity is, therefore, better estimated from responses to steps in disparity. Results from such experiments are shown in Fig. 9. The velocities of vergence induced by steps in disparity, found in three different studies, agree well for small disparities (< 1°) (Rashbass and Westheimer, 1961; Cumming and Judge, 1986; Erkelens, 1987).

An extensive description of the dependence of velocity of vergence on the amplitude of disparity is given by Erkelens (1987), who stimulated with disparities up to 10°. This study showed that the velocity of vergence increased in proportion to disparity for amplitudes up to about 1° (see Fig. 9B). The rate of increase in vergence velocity with stimulus amplitude then slowed, reaching a peak of 4°. Above this amplitude, the velocity of vergence decreased with increasing disparity.

Erkelens (1987) further discovered that vergence responses showed adaptation to large, sustained disparities. To study these effects, subjects were stimulated for periods of 15 s with constant disparities up to 10° under open-loop conditions (Fig. 12). Vergence responses to disparity steps up to 2° consisted of movements with a more or less uniform velocity over distances ranging between 15 and 25°. The responses saturated between 25 and 35° of convergence and were sustained for the duration of stimulation. Responses to disparities of 2° and larger were transient. After initial vergence responses which reached convergence angles up to 35°, the eyes drifted back to angles between phoria and 5° convergence. The amplitude as well as the duration of the transient response decreased with increasing disparity. The gradual decrease in convergence angle whenever a long-lasting, large disparity was imposed suggested that vergence adapts to disparities larger than 2°. The adaptation was selective for a band of disparities centered on the disparity which induced the adaptation, because vergence responses were still obtained to small, secondary steps in disparity after vergence had been adapted to the initially presented disparity (Fig. 12). These responses were stronger for larger secondary disparity steps. The selective adaptation suggests that the vergence subsystem processes disparities of different amplitudes through independent, parallel channels of varying coarseness.

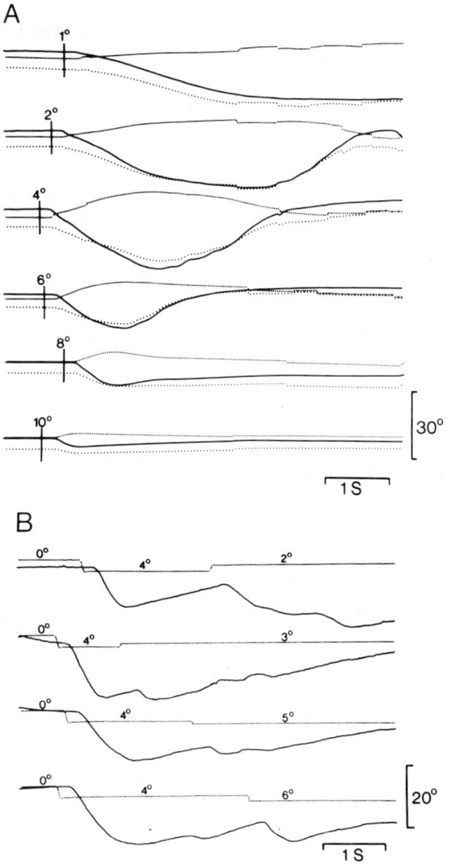

Fig. 12. Ocular vergence (continuous lines) and horizontal movements of the left (coarsely dotted lines) and right (fine dotted lines) eyes in response to disparity steps with amplitudes indicated by the numbers on top of the vertical bars which mark the onset of the disparity step. B. Ocular vergence responses (continuous lines) to two subsequent steps in disparity (dotted lines). The initial steps had an amplitude of 4° in the crossed direction and the secondary steps had amplitudes of 1° or 2° in the crossed or in the uncrossed direction. The numbers indicate the total amount of disparity. Rightward eye movements and convergence are represented by downward movement. All ocular vergence traces start at 5° of convergence. (From Erkelens, 1987)

No model of disparity-controlled vergence has been described in the literature which simulates vergence responses to long-lasting, large disparities.

In all models disparity is lumped together into a single input for the vergence controller. Very recently, we developed a vergence model, which will be discussed in subsection 4.9, that processes disparities of different amplitudes through independent, parallel channels (Pobuda and Erkelens, in preparation).

4.8. The time course of vergence responses

When a step stimulus is presented to a system with low-pass filter characteristics (Eqn. 20), one expects the response to be a ramp-like movement which saturates at a specific level. Time courses of vergence in response to steps in disparity do not show such behavior. Westheimer and Mitchell (1956) noticed that vergence responses to steps in target vergence larger than 1.5° were biphasic. After a fast initial response the vergence movement almost stopped for a period of about one reaction time, after which a fast secondary response completed the vergence movement. Rashbass and Westheimer (1961) observed sequences of fast and slow phases in the vergence responses to ramp and sinusoidal changes of target vergence. Semmlow et al. (1986) observed that slow ramps (1.4°/s) induced smooth vergence tracking, while faster ramps (2.7°/s) evoked a combination of smooth tracking and step-like dynamic behavior. Very different explanations have been proposed for the slow and fast phases in the time courses of vergence: (1) the vergence system contains two controllers, one having slow and the other having fast dynamics (Semmlow et al., 1986), and (2) a high gain of the vergence loop in combination with long latencies of vergence responses cause oscillatory behavior (Erkelens and Regan, 1986). To understand the mechanisms that underly vergence it is important to find the correct explanation. In this subsection we will discuss arguments from which we conclude that slow and fast phases in the time course of vergence responses are caused by the combination of high gains and long latencies.

Semmlow et al. (1986) and Hung et al. (1986) investigated slow and fast phases in vergence responses by studying ocular vergence responses to ramps of target vergence at various speeds. These authors suggested that the vergence system contains two modes of disparity control: a fast, transient component, activated at disparities larger than about 0.5° to 1°, and a slow, sustained component working at small disparities. The hypothesis of two modes of disparity control was inspired by a suggestion made by Jones (1980) that vergence acts as a two-stage process consisting of fusion-initiating and fusion-sustaining components. Several investigators showed that dissimilar targets presented to each eye could produce transient vergence responses (Westheimer and Mitchell, 1969; Mitchell, 1970; Jones and Kerr, 1971; Jones, 1980). Jones (1980) found that the transient response produced by a fusable stimulus (a pair of identical vertical lines), presented in a brief flash (200 ms), was identical to that produced by a long-duration, non-fusable target (a vertical line paired with a horizontal line). In the case of the non-fusable target the transient response was followed by a gradual return to the phoria position. Semmlow et al. (1986) and Hung et al. (1986) believed that the fusion-initiating and fusion-sustaining components were activated intermittently, resulting in alternating slow and fast phases in the time course of vergence responses. A crucial element in the view of Semmlow et al. (1986) and Hung et al. (1986) was that vergence should respond slowly to disparities below 1° and much faster to larger disparities. The velocities of vergence responses to steps in disparity (Fig. 8) show that this does not occur (Rashbass and Westheimer, 1961; Cumming and Judge, 1986; Erkelens, 1987). The opposite is the case: the velocity of vergence is linearly related to the size of the disparity step for disparities up to about 0.5°, but shows soft saturation for larger disparities. Another argument against the view of Semmlow et al. (1986) and Hung et al. (1986) is that slow and fast phases do not occur in the time course of vergence responses made under open-loop conditions. Rashbass and Westheimer (1961) did not find such phases in vergence responses to step, ramp and sinusoidal changes of disparity under open-loop viewing conditions. Inspection of Figs. 12, 15 and 21 in their paper shows that alternation of slow and fast phases did not occur. We can confirm from our own open-loop experiments that alternating fast and slow responses to step, ramp and sinusoidal changes in disparity are absent. This finding seems to be at odds with the experimental results of Semmlow et al. (1986), but it is not. Semmlow et al. (1986) claimed to have stimulated the vergence system with *disparity* ramps of constant velocity. In their experiments, however, they controlled only *target vergence*, which changed in a ramp-like way. They did not compute disparity as the difference between target vergence and ocular vergence. The vergence responses were irregular in their time course, whereas target vergence changed smoothly with a uniform velocity. It is evident that disparity did not change according to smooth ramps, but was as irregular as the vergence responses. In conclusion, we believe that slow and fast phases in the time courses of vergence are not caused by two modes of disparity control with different dynamics.

The absence of biphasic or oscillatory responses under open-loop conditions may indicate that the time delay in the disparity loop is the main cause of the oscillations under closed-loop conditions. The time delay has inevitable consequences for the dynamics of vergence under closed-loop conditions, but it is not relevant for the dynamics of vergence under open-loop conditions.

In a recent paper, Erkelens and Regan (1986) addressed the role of the time delay in a study of the phase lags of ocular vergence in response to sinusoidally changing target vergence and in response to sinusoidally changing target size. They found that phase lags in response to those two stimuli were quite similar for frequencies between 0.2 and 2.0 Hz. This result might create the false impression that neural processes underlying the two responses have the same processing time. However, a fundamental difference between vergence induced by disparity and by changing size is that processing of disparity occurs within a closed loop, whereas changing target size is an open-loop stimulus for vergence. Time delays for responses to changing size can be computed directly from the phase lags. Erkelens and Regan (1986) found time delays which did not depend on the stimulus frequency and had durations between 194 and 230 ms. Time delays for responses to changing target vergence cannot be directly computed from the phase lags. Suppose that the target vergence (V_t) changes as follows:

$$V_t(t) = A \sin(\omega t) \tag{21}$$

where A is the amplitude, ω is the frequency in rad/s and t is time. If it is assumed that the ocular vergence (V_o) follows the target vergence according to a sinusoidal wave form with amplitude B and phase shift φ, then V_o can be expressed as:

$$V_o(t) = B \sin(\omega t+\varphi) \tag{22}$$

This results in a disparity change (d) given by:

$$d(t) = V_t(t) - V_o(t) = A \sin(\omega t) - B \sin(\omega t+\varphi) \tag{23}$$

This equation can be rewritten as:

$$d(t) = A[\sin(\omega t) - G \sin(\omega t+\varphi)] = A\, C \sin(\omega t+\theta) \tag{24}$$

where G is the gain of ocular vergence in relation to target vergence, and C and θ are the amplitude and the phase of the disparity relative to the target vergence. Since G and φ are known from the gain–phase relationship of ocular vergence relative to target vergence, $C \sin(\omega t+\theta)$ can be computed by vectorial subtraction of $G \sin(\omega t+\theta)$ from $\sin(\omega t)$ in the vector field of which $\sin(\omega t)$ and $\cos(\omega t)$ are the orthogonal unit vectors. Erkelens and Regan (1986) computed the time delays of ocular vergence in response to disparity from the phase lags of ocular vergence in response to target vergence by this method. They found that the time delays decreased from 833 ms at 0.2 Hz to 265 ms at 2.0 Hz. Thus, latencies of vergence responses to the effective stimulus were found to be much longer for changes in disparity than for changes in size, in particular for low frequencies. It was also found that oscillations of the vergence responses to ramps of target ver-

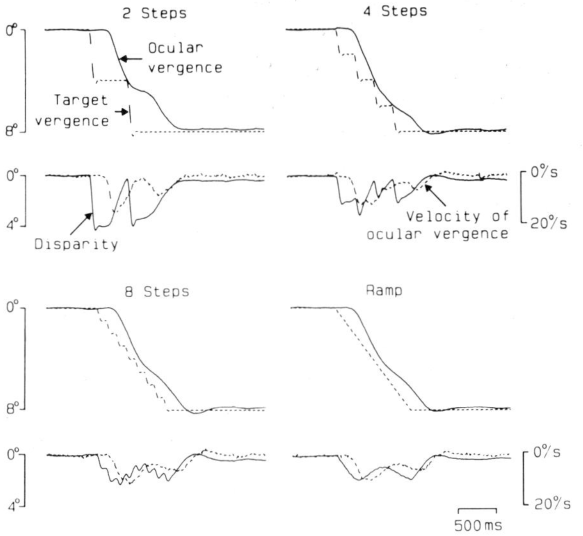

Fig. 13. The time course of vergence responses. Target vergence of a random-dot stereogram was changed by 8° in 2, 4 or 8 steps, or smoothly (as shown in the four panels). Average velocity of target vergence was 8°/s in all cases. The upper half of each panel shows target vergence and ocular vergence. The time course of ocular vergence was smooth, irrespective of the velocity profile of the change in ocular vergence. The lower half of each panel shows the effective disparity (target vergence minus ocular vergence), as well as the velocity of ocular vergence. Vergence velocity was roughly a low-pass filtered copy of effective disparity, lagging by one reaction time (about 160 ms). (From Pobuda and Erkelens, in preparation)

gence were reduced, when the changes in target vergence were accompanied by commensurate changes in target size. This shows a relationship between the long latencies in the disparity-vergence loop and the oscillatory vergence responses. Do the long latencies cause the oscillation? This is plausible because it is well known that latency is a major determinant of the dynamic stability of a feedback system.

If the oscillations are caused by the long latencies, this implies that the oscillations are predictable from the time course of disparity: fast phases in the time course of vergence occur about one reaction time after a maximum in disparity and slow phases occur about one reaction time after a minimum in disparity. This relationship between disparity and vergence is illustrated by the following example taken from Pobuda and Erkelens (in preparation) (Fig. 13). Target vergence was changed over 8° in 2, 4 or 8 steps, or smoothly with a ramp velocity of 8°/s. Ocular vergence showed fast and slow phases in response to the step, as well as to the ramp changes in target vergence. Comparison of the computed disparity traces with the computed velocity of ocular vergence traces showed that the velocity of ocular vergence was roughly a low-pass filtered copy of the disparity which lagged about one reaction time behind. Or in other words, fast phases in the time course of vergence occurred about one reaction time after a maximum in disparity and slow phases occurred about one reaction time after a minimum in disparity. Furthermore, the responses in Fig. 13 show that vergence was not sensitive to the velocity of disparity as such. The time course of vergence was very similar, irrespective of whether target vergence was changed in 8 steps or changed smoothly in a rampwise fashion. In the first case disparity changed very abruptly while in the latter case disparity changed smoothly. The time course of the velocity of vergence was very similar in both cases, while the velocity of disparity was very dissimilar.

From the discussion in this section we conclude that vergence in response to ramps of disparity has characteristics of a low-pass filter, similar to the relationship found between vergence and disparity steps as expressed by Eqn. 20. Consequently, the fast and slow phases in the time course of vergence responses are caused by the long latencies.

4.9. Descriptive models of disparity-controlled vergence

In the previous subsections we discussed specific aspects of the relationship between vergence and disparity and proposed new interpretations of previous experimental results. The following conclusions were proposed: (a) the vergence loop contains a pure delay of about 45 ms instead of about 160 ms as is generally assumed (section 4.6); (b) the vergence loop processes disparity through parallel, independent channels (section 4.7); (c) the channels have low-pass filter characteristics (sections 4.6 and

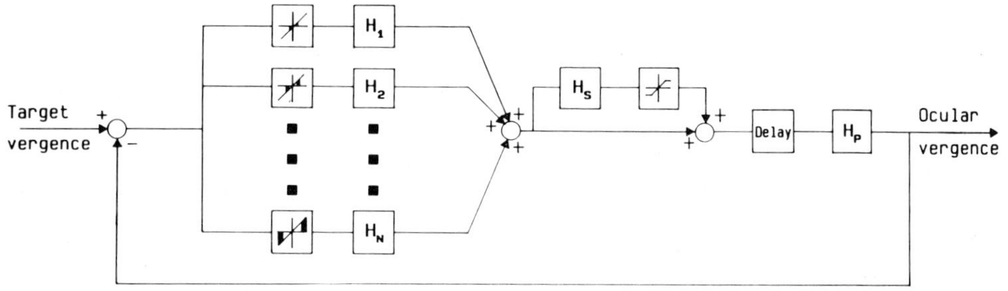

Fig. 14. Block diagram of the disparity-controlled vergence model proposed by Pobuda and Erkelens (in preparation). An essential feature of the model is the processing of disparity in several (here taken as five) parallel channels, each of which is sensitive to a specific disparity range and has its own low-pass filter characteristics. H_n represents the transfer function of a channel, and in the Laplace domain is given by: $H_n(s) = G_n/(\tau_n s+1)$

4.7); (d) the vergence loop is insensitive to the rate of disparity change (section 4.8). It seems likely that any model designed to describe disparity-controlled vergence successfully has to incorporate these features.

Four different models have been described in the literature on disparity-controlled vergence. In the oldest model (Rashbass and Westheimer, 1961), discussed in section 4.5, vergence control consisted of perfect time-integration of disparity delayed by a propagation time of 160 ms. This model was inadequate in describing vergence responses to sinusoidal disparities. In the model described by Krishnan and Stark (1977), the vergence controller consisted of an imperfect disparity-integrator parallel to an imperfect disparity-differentiator, both in combination with a pure delay of 160 ms. This model simulated vergence responses to sinusoidal disparities better than the model of Rashbass and Westheimer (1961), but it was sensitive to the rate of disparity change, and therefore would simulate different vergence responses to staircases and ramps of disparity with equal mean velocities. A model which is sensitive to the rate of disparity change seems not realistic, as was demonstrated in Fig. 13. In a third model (Schor, 1979b), the vergence controller consists of two imperfect disparity-integrators parallel to each other, in series with a pure delay of 160 ms. Basically, this model is similar to that described by Rashbass and Westheimer (1961), with the special feature of a second integrator, which was introduced to describe the reduction of fixation disparity with prolonged binocular fixation (Schor, 1979b, 1980). The fourth and most recent model of Hung et al. (1986) was based on the idea that vergence is controlled by disparity in two modes (Semmlow et al., 1986). This idea was discussed and criticized in section 4.8, and consequently a model based on this idea seems less attractive.

The foregoing models are all unsatisfactory in that they are not able to describe the dynamics of vergence in response to disparities with all kinds of different time functions. None of the models shows all of the four features, specified above, that were considered essential for adequate modelling of disparity-controlled vergence. Very recently, we developed a model which incorporates these features (Pobuda and Erkelens, in preparation). In this model, which is shown in Fig. 14, disparity is processed via several (here, taken as five) parallel, imperfect integrators with slightly different low-pass filter characteristics, each of them susceptible to a specific range of disparities. Gains and time constants of the individual integrators, each representing a channel, were determined from steady-states and maximum velocities of vergence responses to open-loop disparity steps falling within the working range of a specific channel. The model also contains a pure delay of 45 ms and a slow integrator (H_s) similar to that proposed by Schor (1979b) to simulate the reduction in fixation disparity with pro-

TABLE 1

Characteristics of the low-pass filters derived from vergence responses to open-loop constant disparities of one subject

Filter	Disparity range (deg)	Gain (G_n)	Time constant (τ_n) (s)
H_1	0 – 0.2	14.8	3.0
H_2	0.2 – 0.5	12.0	2.2
H_3	0.5 – 1.0	8.9	1.3
H_4	1.0 – 2.0	5.6	0.7
H_5	>2.0	2.9	0.5
H_s		20.0	33.0

longed binocular fixation. The plant has been modelled by a second-order low-pass filter with time constants of 8 and 150 ms. Optimal gains and time constants derived from the experimental data of one subject are shown in Table 1.

Gains as well as phase lags of vergence responses of the same subject to sinusoidal disparities are accurately simulated by this model (Fig. 15). The lower gains and the shorter time constants of the low-pass filters processing larger disparities mean that the gain of the response falls off rapidly for larger disparities and higher frequencies. For small, slowly changing disparities, the response is almost perfectly proportional to the time integration of the disparity input, owing to the characteristics of the slow integrator, H_s. For large disparities the response reaches the limits of the vergence range so rapidly that the influence of H_s is hardly felt. As a consequence of the different time constants of the low-pass filters, the model correctly simulates the alternation of fast and slow phases in response to steps and ramps of target vergence, which are characteristic of real vergence responses.

4.10. The accuracy and precision of ocular vergence

How accurate and stable is the control of vergence? An answer is needed, because theories of binocular vision will have to take into account whether fixated images fall on corresponding points. Several

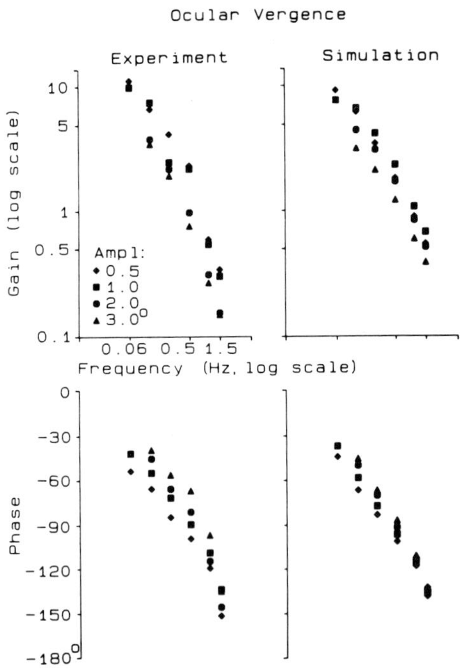

Fig. 15. Experimental gains and phase lags of vergence responses of one subject to open-loop sinusoidal disparity changes compared to values simulated by the model in Fig. 14. (From Pobuda and Erkelens, in preparation)

types of error contribute to the imperfection of vergence: (a) the dynamic limitation of vergence in response to changes in target vergence, as has been discussed earlier in this section; (b) steady-state errors (fixation disparity); (c) non-conjugated components of smooth and saccadic eye movements during maintained fixation of the target; (d) dynamic errors associated with saccadic eye movements; (e) imperfect yoking of compensatory eye movements associated with head movements. Because of the technical difficulties in obtaining veridical binocular eye movement recordings the number of objective measurements of vergence, i.e., not relying on psychophysical techniques such as afterimages or nonius lines, is limited. The number of studies in which objective recordings of eye movements were combined with psychophysical data on fusional limits is even more limited.

The characteristics of steady-state fixation disparity have been somewhat controversial in the literature. Forced duction techniques using prisms and nonius lines have strongly suggested the accumulation of vergence error as a function of demanded vergence, the eye movements being invariably too small (Ogle, 1964; Ogle et al., 1967; Crone and Hardjowijoto, 1979; Schor, 1979a,b). The errors increase at a low rate as long as vergence stimuli are small, and more rapidly as the limits of convergence and divergence are approached. Types I, II and III have been described (Ogle et al., 1967), in which error accumulates equally fast with convergence and divergence, more rapidly with divergence, or more rapidly with convergence, respectively. The slopes differ between subjects, and also depend on target configurations. Typical disparities for a 6 diopter base-out prism (requiring a convergence of about 3.4 deg) are about 5 min arc for type I and II subjects, but often more than 20 min arc for type III subjects (Schor, 1979a).

Early objective recordings of vergence had been provided by Westheimer and Mitchell (1956), Tani et al. (1956) and Alpern (1957). However, these observations have been subject to the criticism of technical shortcomings (sometimes by the authors themselves, who did not like their own results, e.g. Tani et al., 1956). In an influential study, Riggs and Niehl (1960), using an optical lever–scleral contact lens technique with photographic recording, discounted the occurrence of any substantial vergence errors. They claimed that vergence movements over a range of 3° were accurate to about 2 min arc. Such values are not incompatible with Ogle's findings for fixation disparity, but of course they represent only a small part of the vergence range.

Hebbard (1962) compared subjectively measured fixation disparity with objective eye position recordings (using scleral contact lenses) and found a good agreement. He measured about 0.60 min arc/prism diopter objectively and 0.44 min arc/prism diopter subjectively . He measured over a range of 20 prism diopters base-in and base-out, corresponding to 11.3° divergence and convergence. Hebbard's findings would predict a vergence error of 3 min arc for a convergence of 3 deg, which is compatible with Riggs and Niehl's (1960) results, except that fixation disparity is of course a systematic error, increasing as a function of the vergence angle. Recent objective recordings made by Kertesz and Lee (1988) confirm the existence of significant, systematic fixation disparities.

In addition, there are instabilities of vergence during maintained fixation. Krauskopf et al. (1960) analysed eye movements during monocular and binocular fixation using the contact lens optical lever. They found that the smooth movements of the two eyes were not correlated over short periods (2 s sample intervals). Microsaccades in one eye, however, were always accompanied by simultaneous saccades in the other eye, in the same direction and of about the same size. Later, Fender and Julesz (1967) noticed the imperfect correlation of binocular eye movements in normal vision and, puzzled by the fact that this fluctuation of (absolute) disparity does not affect stereopsis, quantitatively analysed this fluctuation using the scleral contact lens technique. They found disjunctive drift of the order of 1 min arc/s, but much larger errors due to imperfect yoking of microsaccades. The probability that any saccade changed the disparity by 3 min arc or more in 40 ms was 0.57 when a point target (a pinhole) was viewed and 0.89 for a random-dot pattern. Some saccades produced vergence changes greater than 20 min arc. A later investigation by St.-Cyr and Fender (1969) confirmed the occurrence of fluctuations in vergence of at least 10 min arc (see their Fig. 1) during binocular fixation. Hebbard (1962), also using scleral contact lens techniques, found a maximum range of vergence of about 10 min arc over a period of 75 s during steady binocular fixation.

Not much is known about conjugacy during voluntary gaze changes and, actually, perfect conjugacy would not be expected in a general case, because gaze changes require a combination of version and vergence, unless the targets between which gaze is changed happen to be located on a single iso-vergence plane (see section 2.1.2). Recently, Collewijn et al. (1988) recorded binocular saccades between targets on an iso-vergence locus and found systematic, transient deviations from conjugacy for horizontal saccades. The eye moving in the temporal direction showed consistently faster dynamics than the eye moving nasally, causing a transient divergence. For a 30° saccade this had a maximal value of 1–3 deg, with a total duration of about 300 ms. Whether such asymmetries occur during other types of eye movement is unknown, since no experiments have been done under the required iso-vergence stimulus conditions. Recent recordings in our laboratory suggest that during the slow phase of OKN in humans, the nasally moving eye has a higher velocity than the temporally moving eye, irrespective of whether monocular or binocular viewing is used (Van den Berg and Collewijn, 1988).

For compensatory eye movements during head movements there is compelling evidence that compensation is imperfect not only in the sense of a non-unity gain, but also in the sense of considerable non-conjugacy, increasing with the frequency of head motion. Objective recording of such gaze instability is possible only with search coil techniques using a large homogeneous magnetic field. The first evidence of this kind was gathered by Steinman and Collewijn (1980). Further experiments, in which potential sources of artefact are progressively ruled out, were described by Collewijn et al. (1981a,b, 1983), and Steinman et al. (1983, 1985). In these papers, and also in Steinman et al. (1982) and Ferman et al. (1987), the various technical pitfalls and their remedies are discussed in detail. Calculations of retinal image motion can become very complicated when targets at finite distances, subjects wearing corrective glasses, or recording systems sensitive to translation are used. The data most pertinent to stereopsis were published by Steinman et al. (1985). Vergence speeds in subjects with unrestrained heads, looking binocularly at a structured pattern, varied from about 20 min arc/s when the head was held still, to more than 1 deg/s when subjects made voluntary head oscillations at 1.33 Hz (amplitude about 10 deg). Peak-to-peak amplitudes of the fluctuations in vergence (which roughly followed a sinusoidal pattern in synchrony with the head movements) were about 0.5 – 1 deg. However, it should be noted that Duwaer (1982), using an afterimage technique, has reported considerably smaller vergence errors and gaze instability during voluntary head movements. For the most recent objective recordings of monocular gaze instability, which essentially confirm the earlier work of Steinman and Collewijn but also show considerable variation between subjects, see Ferman et al. (1987).

The balance of the evidence discussed above suggests that considerable inaccuracy of vergence occurs commonly during steady fixation, during changes in gaze, and particularly during natural head movements. None of these inaccuracies of vergence, however, appears to interfere with normal binocular vision and stereopsis; this point will be further treated in section 5.

4.11. Concluding remarks

Stabilization of retinal disparity is used extensively in the analysis of vergence. In this section we have shown the validity of this technique. Reproducible vergence responses, elicited by modulations of disparity in time by simple functions, have encouraged the use of engineering tools to analyse experimental results. In view of some misconceptions with regard to the time delay of disparity processing, the presence of predictive mechanisms, and the so-called dual mode of disparity control, this approach has not always been successful.

Reinterpretation of experimental results led to the formulation of four characteristic features of disparity-controlled vergence that were considered essential in the understanding of disparity processing. Vergence responses to disparities with different time functions could be adequately simulated by a model which incorporated these features.

An important observation made in this section is that vergence is far from perfect. This results in vergence errors occurring in different, natural conditions such as during binocular fixation of a target moving in depth, after saccadic eye movements, or during head movement.

5. Perception of depth under dynamic conditions

5.1. Introduction

In natural behavior, binocular vision will rarely operate under static conditions. Absolute disparities will frequently change owing to the imperfect control of vergence, particularly during head motion (see section 4.10). Relative disparities will change when objects move, relative to other objects, away from or towards an observer. In this section we will review the effects of such changes on binocular vision. Specifically, two main questions will be addressed: (1) what is the effect of disjunctive retinal image motion on binocular visual processes; (2) what is the relationship between changes in disparity and the perception of motion in depth?

5.2. Stereopsis in relation to retinal image motion

Early interest in the effects of retinal image motion on stereopsis goes back to 'dynamic' theories of stereopsis, which postulated an important role of the involuntary, miniature eye movements in stereopsis (e.g., Ogle and Weil, 1958). These were disproved by Shortess and Krauskopf (1961), who showed that stereoscopic thresholds – as a function of exposure time – were virtually identical under normal viewing and stabilized-image conditions. Thus, stereopsis thresholds are not increased by the elimination of retinal image motion.

The effect of retinal image motion on stereopsis was also investigated by Westheimer and McKee (1978). In a previous paper they had shown that Landolt C and vernier acuity were not adversely affected by retinal image speeds up to about 2 or 3 deg/s (Westheimer and McKee, 1975). In their experiments on stereopsis the target was a line stereogram consisting of two vertical lines, one above the other, presented in each trial for about 190 ms. In addition, four corner dots outlining a square around the line stereogram were continuously presented to both eyes. This square defined the plane of fixation and convergence. The line targets were moved together with respect to the fixation square,

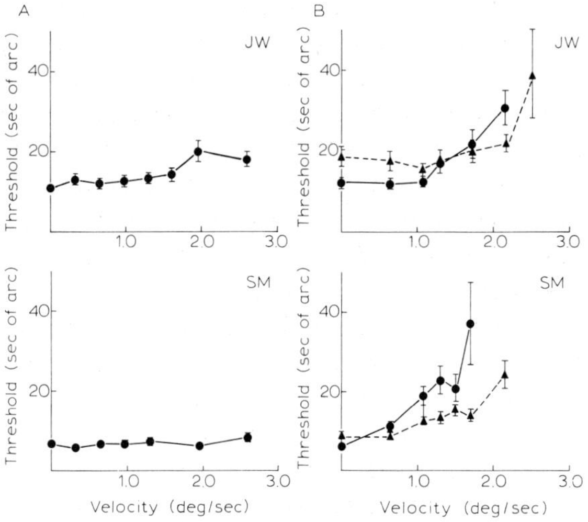

Fig. 16. Disparity threshold for stereoscopic depth resolution by two subjects (J.W. and S.M.) of two vertical lines, 15.5 min arc in length, one above the other, vertically separated by 3 min arc. A. Foveal stimulus presentation (duration 190 ms); thresholds as a function of *lateral* motion of both targets in the frontal fixation plane. B. Stimulus exposure times of 95 ms (triangles) or 190 ms (round dots); thresholds as a function of the velocity of change in *target vergence* that sweeps the stereogram in a convergent or divergent direction through the fixation plane. (From Westheimer and McKee, 1978)

while the relative disparity between the upper and the lower line was varied between trials in order to establish the threshold of stereopsis. In one experiment the upper and lower lines moved together laterally. Target velocities up to 2 deg/s had essentially no effect on the threshold of stereopsis, which remained at about 10 sec arc (Fig. 16). The result was similar when only the upper line moved, while a constant relative disparity with respect to the lower line was maintained; in this condition any uniocular cue was abolished. In view of the brief exposure times, retinal image speed was probably essentially similar to target speed. These results of Westheimer and McKee show the insensivity of stereopsis to lateral motion. In a second experiment, Westheimer and McKee (1978) oscillated the line stereogram in depth by moving its right and left eye half-images in opposite directions relative to the fixation square. In this case, stereopsis thresholds were significantly increased at target speeds of 2 deg/s, i.e., motion in depth was more detrimental to stereopsis than lateral motion (Fig. 16). An explanation was sought in the fact that at higher velocities of motion in depth, the targets were seen a greater part of the time with "disparity with respect to the fixation plane". Apparently, the authors alluded here to absolute disparity, and they proceeded with experiments in which the target line pair was statically presented at different absolute disparities, while the fixation plane was maintained by the continuously shown square. Thresholds for relative disparity between the two lines were found to rise significantly beyond 2–3 min arc away from the fixation plane. However, Westheimer and McKee's (1978) experiments do not necessarily show a high sensitivity of stereopsis to absolute disparity because relative disparity varied as well. Since the fixation target was continuously visible, the subjects actually viewed an array of targets with two ranges of relative disparity: 3 – 10 min arc between fixation square and line targets, and less than 1 min arc (the threshold) between the two lines. Thus, Westheimer and McKee's (1978) results could be interpreted as showing that the presence of a large relative disparity increases the threshold for the discrimination of a simultaneously seen small relative disparity.

A similar point applies to the experiments by Blakemore (1970), who investigated the threshold for relative disparity as a function of absolute disparity, which was varied over a larger range. Since all measurements were done with the eyes fixating a continuously present target, Blakemore's (1970) findings actually also show an increased threshold for the discrimination of one relative disparity in the presence of another (larger) one.

This effect was explicitly demonstrated in subsequent experiments by Westheimer (1979a), who found at least a doubling of the stereo-threshold by a 'standing disparity' as small as 1 min arc. Similarly, Schumer and Julesz (1984) found a systematic increase in stereo thresholds as a function of the height of 'depth pedestals'. Schumer and Julesz's (1984) attempt to account for certain asymmetries in their results for crossed and uncrossed disparities in terms of fixation disparity forms an example of a typical confusion between relative and absolute disparities.

If vergence or absolute disparity were to provide primary sensory cues underlying the perceived distance of a visual display, the display should appear to move toward and away from the observer whenever vergence changes. In the experiments of Steinman et al. (1985) vergence changes were produced by having subjects shake their heads. The resulting changes in vergence (Fig. 17A) and the high retinal image speeds in each eye did not affect perception. Stereopsis was tested and found to be functioning normally with bar stereograms as well as random-dot stereograms. The bar stereograms were presented for at most 3 s while subjects were oscillating their heads. Relative disparities between the parts of the stereogram as small as 11.4 sec arc (crossed or uncrossed in random order) were correctly identified by the subjects as 'near' or 'far' in more than 85% of the trials (Fig. 17B). Differences between data obtained while sitting still and while moving the head were not large or statistically reliable, nor were there reliable correlations between retinal image speed and incorrect responses. Similarly, a Julesz random-dot stereogram (relative disparity between central figure and background was 22.7 min arc) was seen continuously in stereopsis during head oscillation. It proved to be impossible to break fusion during the fastest voluntary head oscillations possible within a range of about 25 deg peak-to-peak, even though vergence speeds reached values up to 8.2 deg/s, with a standard deviation of the vergence angle of 0.38 deg (Fig. 17C). Not only was fusion easily maintained during such motion, but stereopsis was also acquired without difficulty within a second when the stereogram was suddenly presented while head oscillation was going on.

The psychophysical aspects of these experiments by Steinman et al. (1983, 1985) have been confirmed by Patterson and Fox (1984) without recording of the eye movements but with the use of dynamically generated random-dot stereograms (refreshed every 16 ms). During head oscillation at up to 2 Hz, the threshold for recognition of a target in

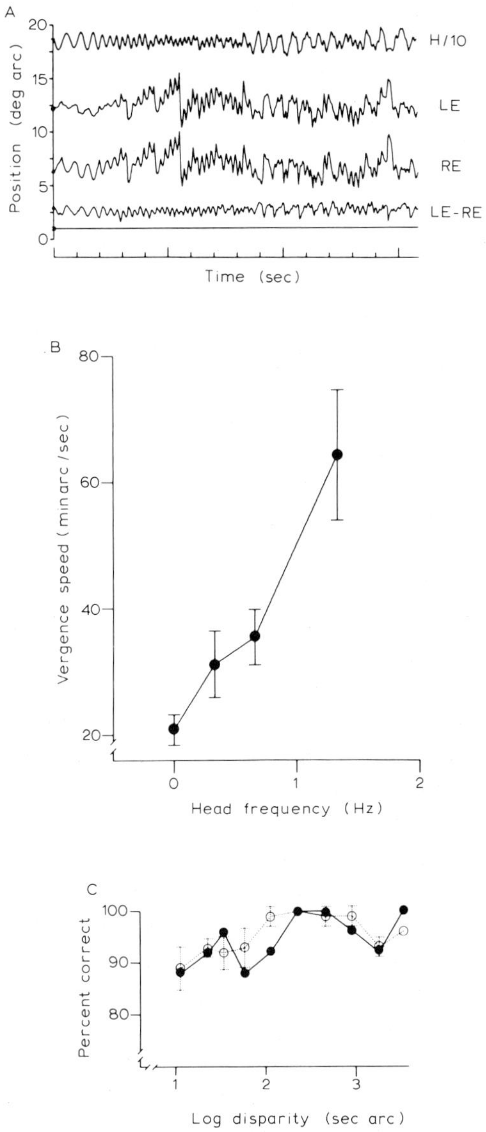

Fig. 17. A. Recordings of head and eye movements of subject R.S. with respect to an earth-fixed frame of reference during voluntary head oscillation (about 25° peak to peak), made at increasing frequency in an (unsuccessful) attempt to break fusion of a large random-dot stereogram. Head rotations are reduced in scale by 10. Eye rotations, RE and LE, show considerable, but certainly incomplete, and variable, compensation when the head moved. If compensation had been perfect, the eye traces would be horizontal straight lines, i.e., the target would not move on the retina. These residual eye rotations, then, represent retinal image motion in each of the eyes. The trace labeled LE–RE represents changes in vergence resulting from different degrees of compensation in each of the eyes. B. Mean vergence speed (absolute velocity) as a function of head frequency for three subjects. The error bars (standard deviations) show intersubject variability. C. Accuracy of psychophysical observation of target position in depth (percent correct) as a function of (relative) disparity of a large stereogram (a vertical bar on a random-dot background). Averaged data of three subjects. The closed circles show average performance when the subjects kept their heads still (0 Hz). The open circles show average performance when they moved their heads at 1/3, 2/3 and 4/3 Hz. The error bars (standard deviations) show the variability associated with moving the head at three different frequencies. (From Steinman et al., 1985)

the stereogram (relative disparity 11 min arc crossed) remained unchanged relative to the 75% correct baseline level with the head steady.

The considerable tolerance of binocular vision and stereopsis for vergence errors is further corroborated by experiments in which the head was stationary, and absolute disparity of the half-images of a stereogram was manipulated deliberately. Obviously, any potential recording artifacts related to the freedom of head movement are absent in such experiments. Fender and Julesz (1967), Erkelens and Collewijn (1985b) and Piantanida (1986) showed that fusion and stereopsis of random-dot stereograms was maintained despite the presence of absolute disparities up to between 1° and 2° between the half-images. Indications as to how much disparity of a small, isolated foveal target is tolerated by the fusional system come from the studies of Fender and Julesz (1967) and Piantanida (1986). These authors found that the fusional limits of a single-line target ranged between 42 and 77 min arc when disparity was changed very slowly (at a velocity of a few min arc/s).

The experiments discussed above show that the substantial fluctuations of vergence and, therefore, absolute retinal image disparity do not disturb stereo vision. The computation of relative disparities within the retinal images, which are of course invariant with vergence or version movements, may be the basis of the stable steropsis.

5.3. Motion in depth

Subjects have some ability to discriminate successively presented absolute disparities (section 3.2.2), although it is clearly inferior to the discrimination of simultaneous, relative disparity (3.2.3). Change in absolute disparity is effective in the control of vergence eye movements and may, therefore, be available for perception. For instance, it might not be surprising to find that subjects can discriminate between crossed and uncrossed disparities, since these categories also lead to opposite motor responses. A different question is whether such differences are truly perceived as differences in depth. If this were the case, then a continuous change in absolute disparity should induce a vivid perception of motion in depth (Fig. 6). Recent experiments have clearly shown that this is not the case.

Erkelens and Collewijn (1985a) provided significant observations in this respect. Their subjects viewed a Julesz-type random-dot stereogram (size 30 × 30 deg), which contained a central figure seen in front of the background. The depth difference was due to the relative disparity between the central figure and the background. The continuous perception of this relationship ensured that binocular fusion and global stereopsis were indeed engaged. The investigators were interested in the effects of motion of the entire half-images of the stereogram on the perception of a stereogram as a whole. The two half-images were moved in counterphase, following a triangular waveform at 0.125–0.5 Hz at amplitudes of 0.3–3 deg. The ratio of the amplitudes of the motion of the right and left eye image could be varied. No fixation point or other frame of reference was available. The most striking observation was made when both half-images moved at equal amplitudes in counterphase. In this condition the stereogram was continuously perceived as stationary, completely fused, and in normal depth. No motion in depth of the stereogram as a whole or any part of it was perceived, even though careful observation revealed modest changes in apparent size (smaller size being associated with crossed disparity). Movements of the half-images at unequal

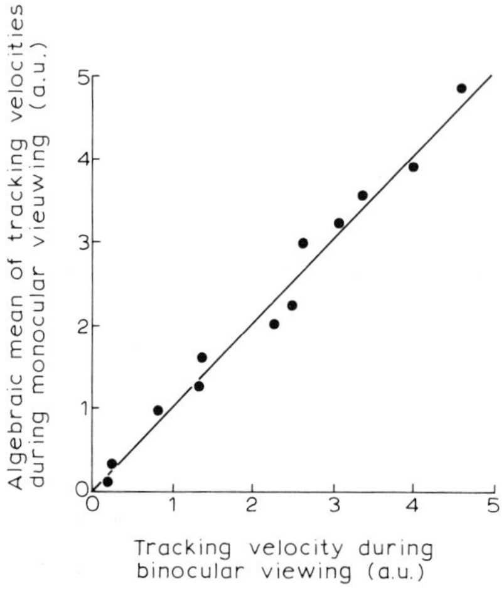

Fig. 18. Relation between the algebraic mean of the two average velocities of manual tracking during monocular viewing, and the average velocity of manual tracking during binocular viewing, showing that the binocularly perceived target velocity equals the algebraic mean of the two monocularly perceived target velocities. Both scales in (the same) arbitrary units. (From Erkelens and Collewijn, 1985a)

velocities induced perception of motion; however, this was always sideways, never in depth. By the use of manual tracking of the perceived motion it was quantitatively demonstrated that the binocularly perceived sideways motion was equal to the algebraic mean of the two separately observed monocular motions (Fig. 18). For equal but opposite velocities this mean is of course zero. Also more complex stimulus combinations (e.g., the half-images moving 90 deg out of phase) induced apparent motion reflecting the moment-to-moment mean of the two velocities. It had been previously shown (Ono et al., 1977; Sheedy and Fry, 1979) that during static convergence the oculocentric direction of a fused image is the mean of the oculocentric directions of the two monocular images. This is clearly also the case when the entire images on the left and right retina are moving: binocularly perceived motion is then the mean of the two monocularly perceived motions. These observations relate to absolute motion. The binocular perception of relative (sideways or in-depth) motion, in the presence of a frame of reference, follows different rules (see Regan and Beverley, 1973a,b). What is unusual about the Erkelens and Collewijn (1985a) result is that no sensation of motion-in-depth was produced despite the changes in disparity.

The stimuli used by Erkelens and Collewijn (1985a) induced vergence movements. The eyes did not track the moving targets with perfect accuracy, as discussed in section 4 (Fig. 11) and below. Substantial changes in disparity were taking place at the retinal level; nevertheless, neither this nor the vergence movements elicited any apparent motion in depth. This may seem in conflict with the many earlier demonstrations that changes in disparity are sufficient to induce perception of motion in depth (e.g., Wheatstone, 1852; Tyler, 1971; Richards, 1972; Beverley and Regan, 1973, 1975; Regan and Beverley, 1973a,b, 1979). However, in all this previous research motion was presented relative to a background or a fixation point. In the experimental conditions of Erkelens and Collewijn (1985a) a vivid perception of motion in depth was immediately induced in all subjects when any stationary reference was added to the stimulus. When the reference was small (e.g., a single bar), it was seen in motion against the stationary stereogram. A more extended stationary reference (e.g., a grating) was seen as stationary. Instead the stereogram appeared to move. Apparently relative motion is important. It can be distributed between different components of the viewed scene according to principles not yet worked out. A similar point has been made for sideways motion (Duncker, 1929; see also Wallach's chapter in this volume).

Erkelens and Collewijn (1985b) recorded binocular eye movements (with scleral search coils) in subjects observing random-dot stereograms, while the left and right eye half-images were moved in order to find the effects of controlled amounts of absolute disparity while the relative disparity between central figure (a diamond) and background in the stereogram remained constant. The size of the stereogram was 30 × 30 deg and it consisted of 100 × 100 pixels each subtending 18 × 18 min arc. The relative disparity in the stereogram was 36 min arc (2 pixels). The half-images were moved sinusoidally in counterphase at frequencies between 0.25 and 1.5 Hz and amplitudes of 0.5–2.5 deg, centered on an angle of 10 deg convergence. The positions of both eyes and half-images were continuously recorded, so that it was possible to correlate the motion perceived by the subject with changes in vergence as well as with changes in absolute disparity. Fusion and stereopsis were maintained as long as the velocity of the change in the angle between the half-images remained above a maximum, which varied between subjects (range 6–13.5 deg/s). Only observations below this limit will be discussed, Counterphase motion of the half-images at equal amplitude induced no perceived motion, as already mentioned above (Erkelens and Collewijn, 1985a). Subjects perceived a figure against a background in the stereogram, which did not seem to move as a whole. The typical relations between target and eye movements for this condition are shown in Fig. 19. Since there was no fixed plane of fixation (no fixation marks were present) considerable ocular vergence movements were elicited, tracking the changes in target vergence. In addition, both eyes made frequent saccades as the subject looked at various parts of the stereogram, but these were quite well yoked and did not affect vergence. Ocular vergence was clearly not perfect, but always smaller than target vergence. As a result there were large, sinusoidal fluctuations in absolute retinal disparity. As shown in Fig. 20, the maximal fluctuations of absolute disparity compatible with fusion were independent of the frequency of oscillation and amounted to a zone between 1–2 deg crossed and 1–2 deg uncrossed (the actual width varied between subjects). Interestingly, this is similar to the maximum extent of Panum's zone found for random-dot stereograms by Fender and Julesz (1967) in their experiments with stabilized viewing. The pertinent point here is that maximal fluctuations of absolute disparity within the fusional zone did not elicit the slightest perception of motion in depth; neither did the associated changes in vergence. However, these same stimuli combined with any non-moving visual reference induced very compelling perception of motion in depth (Erkelens and Collewijn, 1985a,b); this is apparently only medi-

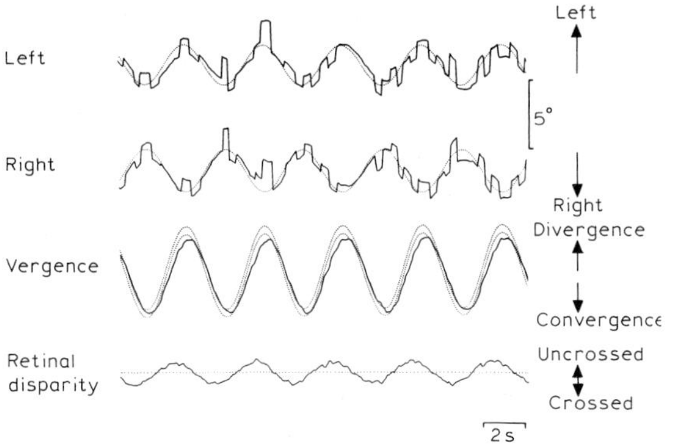

Fig. 19. Relations between eye movements and oscillations of half-images of random-dot stereogram. Upper two traces: position of left and right eye (solid lines) and half-image seen by that eye (dotted lines). Third trace: ocular vergence (solid line) and target vergence (dotted lines) of background (upper curve) and figure (lower curve). Bottom: absolute retinal disparity changes caused by vergence tracking error. (From Collewijn et al., 1986)

ated by changes in relative disparity. This is clearly different from the perception of sideways motion, which is elicited by absolute retinal image motions and/or the associated versional eye movements (see Erkelens and Collewijn, 1985a,b).

In a later collaboration, Regan et al. (1986a) confirmed and extended the observations of Erkelens and Collewijn (1985a,b). One important aspect of this investigation was the effect of target size. All of their six subjects reported that there was a range of stimulus oscillations of a single dot for which clear motion in depth was experienced when a stationary reference (a surrounding random-dot pattern) was present. But when the reference was removed, the dot's motion immediately ceased. Threshold determinations showed that for a single dot without a stationary reference this effect amounted to a substantial elevation of the threshold for detection or of motion-in-depth (by a factor of 2–7), rather than a complete abolition of stereomotion perception. Stereomotion perception was completely abolished, however, for extended multidot targets when absolute, unreferenced changes in disparity were shown. As will be discussed later, the results could not be accounted for by the reduction of effective retinal disparities due to vergence eye movements.

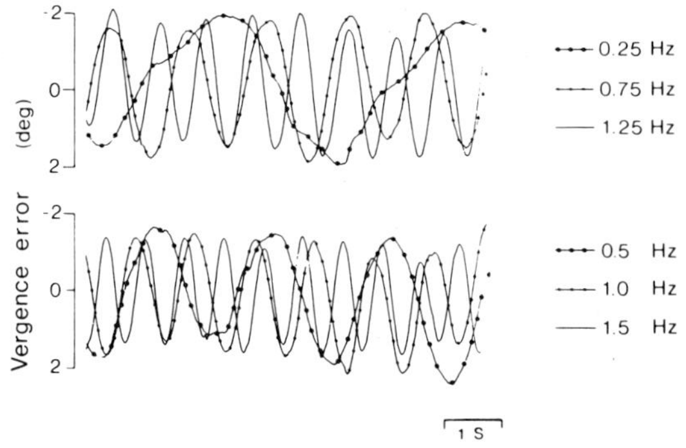

Fig. 20. Examples of variation of absolute binocular disparity as a function of time, obtained from one representative subject, for different frequencies of modulation of image vergence at the limit for fusion. (From Erkelens and Collewijn, 1985b)

These results suggested that absolute disparity changes did induce some motion in depth of a small, unreferenced target (which would be in agreement with Foley, 1976, and Westheimer, 1979a) but none for a multi-dot target. In principle, this difference might be due to a lateral interaction. In a further experiment, Regan et al. (1986a) attempted to resolve this point by using stimuli with intermediate configurations. In a multidot stimulus (diameter 28 deg) with randomly, but more or less evenly, spaced dots (each of diameter 0.3 deg) a blank annulus of variable width was introduced around a central dot, and two such (identical) images were oscillated as a whole in counterphase and viewed separately by the two eyes. The observers directed their attention to the central dot; no stationary reference was available. In the complete pattern, the central dot gave no impression of motion in depth for any amplitude of oscillation, nor was this the case when it was surrounded by a blank annulus with a radius of 0.6 deg. However, when the radius of the blank zone was increased beyond 1–2 deg and oscillation amplitude was raised to just below the point of fusional breakdown, the central dot appeared to move weakly in depth relative to the surrounding dots. (It should be emphasized that there was never any real relative displacement between the central and surrounding dots). In the limiting case, with only the central dot remaining, motion-in-depth threshold was approximately the same as with a blank annulus of 2 deg radius. This experiment produced evidence for a lateral interaction: any apparent motion of a single target, induced by modulation of absolute disparity, was suppressed by the presence of coherently moving targets within a distance of 1–2 deg. This lateral interaction may contribute to the suppression of apparent motion in depth induced by disjunctive eye movements, since any residual movement impression resulting from the unreferenced retinal disparity changes would be suppressed by the coherent motion of all adjacent targets.

Although we have been treating the perception of depth, based on either constant or changing relative disparities, as a continuum, some caution in this respect may be warranted. Certain differences between the perception of static depth and motion in depth are suggested by the rather common occurrence of different types of defect. Richards and Regan (1973) and Regan et al. (1986b) have described scotomata in the visual fields of many normal subjects which show specific defects for the perception of motion in depth on the basis of changes in disparity, although a static disparity was often perceived as depth at the same loci in the visual field. This difference between static and dynamic depth might be due to local bandwidth limitations in the dynamic processing of disparity. These limitations would not necessarily affect the perception of stereomotion in all cases, even though they may extend over a whole quadrant or hemifield. They are usually limited to either crossed or uncrossed disparities. Thus, in practical situations we may compensate for these limitations by (1) using unaffected parts of the visual field; (2) changing the fixation point in depth, thus inverting the sign of disparity; (3) making use of additional cues, such as changing size.

The bandwidth limitation discussed above relates to a 'single population' hypothesis (Regan et al., 1986b) in which the same neuronal pool detects static and dynamic disparities. An alternative is the 'two population' hypothesis, in which the defects in sensitivity to motion in depth would be due to the absence of a pool of neurons reacting to changes in disparity, with the preservation of a different pool of neurons exclusively responding to static disparities (i.e., d.c. up to a fraction of a Hz; Regan et al., 1986b). Strong evidence for the 'two population' hypothesis would be the independent occurrence of either static or dynamic disparity detection anomalies. There is good evidence for defects in dynamic disparity detection with maintained static stereopsis (Richards and Regan, 1973; Regan et al., 1986b). Evidence for the occurrence of the reversed case has been recently found by Hong and Regan (personal communication).

In a similar vein, Schor et al. (1984a) have described differences in spatial tuning of static and dynamic local stereopsis, using band-filtered luminance profiles (DOGs, differences of two Gaussian functions). Their results indicated the presence of sustained mechanisms, tuned to high spatial frequencies, that were equally sensitive to static and dynamic (modulated at 1 Hz) disparities. In addition, they found evidence for transient mechanisms, tuned to low spatial frequencies, that were more sensitive to dynamic than static disparities.

5.4. The perceived direction of motion in depth

Object motion has an arbitrary direction in three-dimensional space, and the perception of this direction of motion is of great practical importance. In an extensive series of investigations, Regan and Beverley have investigated the psychophysics of the discrimination of the direction of motion in depth (Beverley and Regan, 1973, 1975; for a recent review see Regan, 1986). This discrimination has a high acuity (about 0.2 deg) for directions not too far from a line directed close to the nose. It has been proposed that this high acuity can be explained in terms of sensitivity to relative motion, in this case a velocity ratio. Because of the horizontal distance between the eyes, the left and right eyes' images of a target moving in depth move with different velocities. There is a unique relationship between the ratio of these velocities and the direction of motion in depth. We are referring here to motions that are relative in two respects: (1) the left and right eye image velocities are referred to some other binocular target (e.g., a surrounding structure or fixation target); (2) relative velocities seen by the right eye are compared to those seen by the left eye. Such movements in general contain an in-phase component, representing a change in direction (or a sideways motion), and an out-of-phase component, representing a change in distance. On the basis of adaptation experiments (Beverley and Regan, 1973) eight channels tuned to different directions of motion have been proposed, each of which is fatiguable separately. These channels could be based on tuning to different retinal image velocity ratios, or on specific combinations of rates of change in disparity (depth component) with frontal plane velocity (lateral component). A realistic analysis of the perception of generalized three-dimensional motion also requires consideration of changes in apparent size, i.e., changes in visual angle subtended by the borders of an object. This introduces yet another kind of change in relative distances, this time within the moving object (for a discussion of the algorithms which can be used in the analysis of visual motion, see Regan et al., 1986a, and Regan, 1986). The main point to be stressed here is that the in-depth component of three-dimensional motion can be efficiently decoded using only angular changes that have a clear reference in object space, while absolute retinal coordinates are relatively unimportant.

5.5. Interaction between vergence and perception of motion in depth

Experiments in which psychophysical observations are combined with objective recordings of eye movements can be used to distinguish the contributions of disparity and vergence to the perception of depth. Regan et al. (1986a; see also Collewijn et al., 1986) did experiments addressing this point, using retinal image stabilization in the horizontal direction. With this technique, constant absolute disparities could be imposed, which were dissociated from the induced vergence movements. The stimuli consisted of large random-dot stereograms. Fig. 21

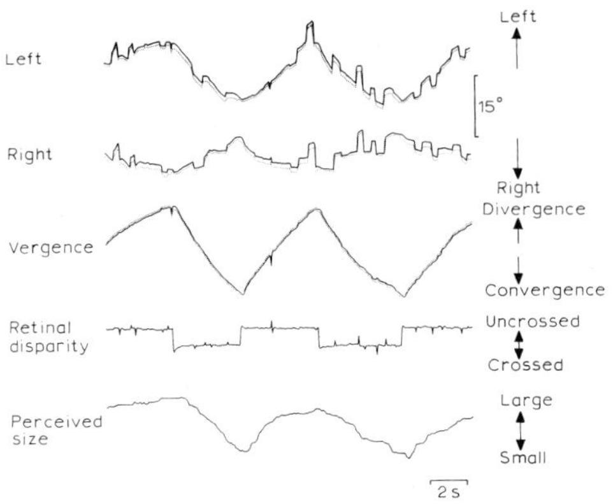

Fig. 21. Perceptual and oculomotor response to open-loop steps of stabilized half-images of random-dot stereogram. Upper two traces: position of left and right eye (solid lines) and (retinally stabilized) target, seen by that eye. Third trace: ocular vergence (solid line) and target vergence (dotted line). Fourth trace: imposed steps in absolute disparity; sensitivity 5× higher than in upper traces. Lower trace: perceived changes in size of stereogram. (From Collewijn et al., 1986)

shows the responses to steps in disparity between 0.5 deg crossed and uncrossed. These steps (made about every 5 s) elicited large (> 20 deg) vergence movements with a triangular wave form. The triangle was, roughly, the integral of the disparity steps. Thus, the time course of the changes in absolute disparity and changes in vergence was dissociated. The subjects did not perceive motion in depth, and fusion was maintained, similar to the results of Erkelens and Collewijn (1985a,b). The new aspect of the results was that the large vergence movements introduced a marked apparent change in size. Convergence was associated with apparent shrinkage by a factor of as much as about 3. Although the perceived size change was vivid and could be tracked by a joy-stick (Fig. 21, bottom trace), it was not associated with apparent motion in depth! This contrasts with the strong perception of motion in depth induced by objective changes in stimulus size, even when only one eye views the stimulus (Regan and Beverley, 1979). Size changes also induce vergence (Erkelens and Regan, 1986), but in this case convergence is associated with a large stimulus size. This suggests that the increased size is interpreted as decreased distance. These results may help to interpret the apparent shrinkage of a stimulus with constant retinal size during convergence observed by Regan et al. (1986a). With this stimulus the conflict between the convergence and maintenance of constant (rather than increased) retinal size seems to be interpreted as a result of object shrinking. This would suggest that the perception of size is a higher-order perceptual scaling effect resulting from the contribution of various cues to distance. Perception of motion in depth may be similar.

In a further experiment, done to determine the interaction between vergence and disparity in the perception of motion-in-depth, Regan et al. (1986a) used a random-dot stereogram in which the absolute disparity of center and surround could be controlled independently. When center and surround were stabilized horizontally on the retina and oscillations of absolute disparity (± 0.5 deg) were imposed, none of the subjects reported any sensation of motion in depth, as expected from the experiments above, although a large (20 deg peak-to-peak) oscillation of ocular vergence was induced. Subsequently, the gain of the stabilization of the surround was slightly displaced from unity, whereas the center remained exactly stabilized. This introduced changes in relative disparity, coherent with but smaller than the changes in absolute disparity, and much smaller than the vergence oscillations. It turned out that all subjects experienced the central figure as moving in depth with respect to the surround. It stood out most in front when the relative disparity of the center with respect to the surround was crossed. This was the case irrespective of whether the gain of the feedback controlling the stabilization of the surround was set slightly above or slightly below unity, although such a change inverted the polarity of the changes in relative disparity with respect to the oscillations of vergence. Formal determinations of thresholds of relative disparity changes for the viewing of vivid motion in depth showed that these were identical, whether the relative disparity change was in-phase or out-of-phase with the vergence. Thus, very clear motion in depth was perceived with relative disparity changes of 10–18 min arc, independently of simultaneous changes in absolute disparity over a range of 1 deg and vergence movements over a range of 20 deg in either direction. The conclusion seems inescapable that only relative disparity leads to percepts of depth.

5.6. The Pulfrich depth illusion

Several of the conclusions reached in the previous section are corroborated by recent investigations of the well-known Pulfrich illusion (Pulfrich, 1922). When a target is oscillated in a flat, fronto-parallel plane and is viewed binocularly with an attenuating filter in front of one eye, it will appear to swing in an elliptical path in the plane of regard. This depth illusion is traditionally explained by a delay of the signals produced by the filtered eye, producing an effective retinal disparity. This explanation is in principle plausible (see e.g. Williams and Lit, 1983; Julesz and White, 1969; Ross and Hogben, 1975), but disregards eye movements. When a stationary fixation point or background is provided, one might assume that tracking is suppressed and that the oscillating target moves sinusoidally across the retina, with the signal of one retina delayed and disparity as a result. Indeed, it was noticed long ago (Kahn, 1931) and has been confirmed several times (Ogle, 1962a; Enright, 1970; Rogers et al., 1974) that the depth illusion does not occur when the oscillating target is the only object in view. One theoretical explanation would be that both eyes will track the target perfectly, placing the target's image on the foveae of both eyes and thus abolishing any disparity. The other explanation, in line with the above considerations of relative disparity, is that in the absence of a reference, the nervous system does not interpret changes in absolute disparity of a single target as a change in depth. Rogers et al. (1974) showed that the depth illusion was preserved when subjects pursued the oscillating target in the presence of a stationary background. They accounted for this by the effects of the filtered background sweeping across the retinae and being delayed in one eye. The disparity change would thus occur in the background but rather than a moving background the subjects would see a moving target ('induced depth') analogous to the phenomenon of 'induced motion' as studied originally by Duncker (1929).

Adequate recordings of the eye movements while the target was pursued (with a background present) and the depth illusion was perceived have been published by Ono and Steinbach (1983) and Enright (1985). The outcome was that the eyes made conjugate pursuit movements of the physical target path; no vergence component in relation to the illusory, periodic displacement in depth was present, except during the initial phase (the first 100 ms) of pursuit. Although tracking was planar after this initial phase, Enright (1985) showed that the target was not bifoveated, as one would intuitively expect: constant divergent fixation disparities of 38–55 min arc relative to the target were recorded, compared to tracking in the unfiltered condition.

In the light of the preceding discussions, the best interpretation of such findings seems to be that the nature of the eye movements is immaterial for the illusion, which is due to the change in relative disparity between target and background. This change in relative disparity is the result of the delay of the observed relative velocity between target and background in the filtered eye. This would be another example of the discrimination of motion in depth on the basis of different relative (i.e., referenced) perceived velocities of a target on the right and left retinae (see Regan, 1986).

The actual relationships between the delays and the resulting relative disparities may be quite complex. Morgan (1975), Ross and Hogben (1975) and Burr and Ross (1979) have shown Pulfrich-like phenomena with stroboscopic targets presented with an interocular delay. In this case stereopsis appears to be based on 'virtual disparities', which are somehow extracted by binocular processes from interpolated monocular activities (see also Poggio and Poggio, 1984).

6. General conclusions

1. Although there is a strong interaction between binocular visual processes and binocular eye movements, investigations in which objective binocular eye movement recordings were combined with psychophysical study of binocular perception have rarely been done. As a result, effects of vergence and disparity cannot be clearly demarcated in most studies on the perception of distance.

2. The few existing studies make it clear that any role played by vergence-related signals in the estimation of distance is a weak one. Some subjects can probably use such a signal in estimating the correct order of distances among a number of objects within arm's range.

3. In the evaluation of the role of disparity in binocular processes, insufficient distinction has been made in the past between absolute and relative disparity. Many studies claiming to investigate absolute disparities do in fact deal with relative disparities, owing to the presence of fixation marks or other visual points of reference. As a consequence, many classic conclusions about the role of disparity in fusion and stereopsis are suspect.

4. Some more recent studies did distinguish absolute from relative disparity. They showed that for small, isolated, foveal targets some (successive) depth discrimination is possible on the basis of absolute disparity, with thresholds at least an order of magnitude above those for the discrimination of simultaneously present, relative disparities. However, such targets are untypical of any real-life stimulus condition because targets are usually embedded in rich visual surroundings.

5. For larger targets, or targets within a visual context, absolute disparity is used exclusively to control vergence, and does not lead to any sensation of depth. Modulation of absolute disparity drives vergence, but the residual modulation of retinal absolute disparity is not perceived as motion in depth. However, this latter sensation is invariably elicited by any modulation of relative disparities.

6. As a result, binocular perception is exquisitely sensitive to relative disparities, used in stereopsis, while at the same time considerable fluctuations in absolute disparity, originating, for example, from imperfections in oculomotor control, have no perceptual consequences.

7. The remarkable insensitivity of fusion and stereopsis to absolute disparities up to 1–2° is functionally very meaningful, as it turns out that the inaccuracy of the control of vergence is substantial. During natural head movements, vergence position errors up to 1–2° and vergence velocity errors up to 1°/s are easily generated. As a result, static as well as dynamic fixation disparities occur very commonly, without any noticeable deterioration of fusion or stereopsis.

8. In future studies of the relationships between disparity, vergence and the perception of depth it will be important to combine psychophysical techniques with high-quality eye movement recordings, in order to avoid ambiguities in the interpretation of the results.

Acknowledgements

We thank Suzanne Markestijn for secretarial assistance and Professor D. Regan for critical comments on an earlier draft of this chapter. Our research was in part supported by the Foundation for Medical Research MEDIGON, grant No. 900-550-92.

References

Allen, M.J. (1953) An investigation of the time characteristics of accommodation and convergence of the eyes. Am. J. Optom. 30, 393–402.

Alpern, M. (1957) The position of the eyes during prism vergence. A.M.A. Arch. Ophthalmol. 57, 345–353.

Alpern, M. (1958) Vergence and accommodation: can change in size induce vergence movements? A.M.A. Arch. Ophthalmol. 60, 355–357.

Alpern, M. (1962) Kinematics of the eye. In: H. Davson (Ed.), The Eye, Vol. 3, Academic Press, New York, pp. 15–27.

Alpern, M. and Ellen, P. (1956) A quantitative analysis of the horizontal movements of the eyes in the experiments of Johannes Muller. II. Effect of variation in target separation. Am. J. Ophthalmol. 42, 296–303.

Bappert, J. (1923) Neue Untersuchungen zum Problem des Verhaltnisses von Akkommodation und Konvergenz zur Wahrnehmung der Tiefe. Z. Psychologie 90, 167–203.

Bennett, A.G. and Francis, J.L. (1962) The eye as an optical system. In: H. Davson (Ed.), The Eye, Vol. 4, Academic Press, New York, pp. 101–131.

Beverley, K.I. and Regan, D. (1973) Evidence for the existence of neural mechanisms selectively sensitive to the direction of movement in space. J. Physiol. 235, 17–29.

Beverley, K.I. and Regan, D. (1975) The relation between discrimination and sensitivity in the perception of motion in depth. J. Physiol. 249, 387–398.

Bishop, P.O. and Henry, G.H. (1971) Spatial vision. Annu. Rev. Psychol. 22, 119–160.

Bishop, P.O. and Pettigrew, J.D. (1986) Neural mechanisms of binocular vision. Vision Res. 26, 1587–1600.

Blakemore, C. (1969) Binocular depth discrimination and the nasotemporal division. J. Physiol. 205, 471–497.

Blakemore, C. (1970) The range and scope of binocular depth discrimination in man. J. Physiol. 211, 599–622.

Bourdon, B. (1902) La Perception Visuelle de l'Espace, Schleicher Freres, Paris.

Burr, D.C. and Ross, J. (1979) How does binocular delay give information about depth? Vision Res. 19, 523–532.

Burt, P. and Julesz, B. (1980a) A disparity gradient limit for binocular fusion. Science 208, 615–617.

Burt, P. and Julesz, B. (1980b) Modifications of the classical notion of Panum's fusional area. Perception 9, 671–682.

Collewijn, H. and Tamminga, E.P. (1986) Human fixation and pursuit in normal and open-loop conditions: effects of central and peripheral retinal targets. J. Physiol. 379, 109–129.

Collewijn, H., Martins, A.J. and Steinman, R.M. (1981a) Natural retinal image motion: origin and change. Ann. N.Y. Acad. Sci. 374, 312–329.

Collewijn, H., Martins, A.J. and Steinman, R.M. (1981b) The time course of adaptation of human compensatory eye movement. Doc. Ophthalmol. Proc. 30, 123–133.

Collewijn, H., Martins, A.J. and Steinman, R.M. (1983) Compensatory eye movements during active and passive head movements: fast adaptation to changes in visual magnification. J. Physiol. 340, 259–286.

Collewijn, H., Erkelens, C.J. and Regan, D. (1986) Absolute and relative disparity: a re-evaluation of their significance in perception and oculomotor control. In: E.L. Keller and D.S. Zee (Eds.), Adaptive Processes in Visual and Oculomotor Systems, Pergamon, Oxford, pp. 177–184.

Collewijn, H., Erkelens, C.J. and Steinman, R.M. (1988) Binocular co-ordination of human horizontal saccadic eye movements. J. Physiol. 404, 157–182.

Crannell, C.W. and Peters, G. (1970) Monocular and binocular estimations of distance when knowledge of the relevant space is absent. J. Psychol. 76, 157–167.

Crone, R.A. and Hardjowijoto, S. (1979) What is normal binocular vision? Doc. Ophthalmol. 47, 163–169.

Cumming, B.G. and Judge, S.J. (1986) Disparity-induced and blur-induced convergence eye movement and accommodation in the monkey. J. Neurophysiol. 55, 896–914.

Cushman, W.B., Tangney, J.F., Steinman, R.M. and Ferguson, J.L. (1984) Characteristics of smooth eye movements with stabilized targets. Vision Res. 24, 1003–1009.

Duncker, K. (1929) Ueber induzierte Bewegung. Psychol. Forsch. 12, 180–259.

Duwaer, A.L. (1982) Assessment of retinal image displacement during head movement using an afterimage method. Vision Res. 22, 1379–1388.

Duwaer, A.L. and Van den Brink, G. (1981) What is the diplopia threshold? Percept. Psychophys. 29, 295–309.

Enright, J.T. (1970) Distortions of apparent velocity: a new optical illusion. Science 168, 464-467.

Enright, J.T. (1985) On Pulfrich-illusion eye movements and accommodation vergence during visual pursuit. Vision Res. 25, 1613–1622.

Erkelens, C.J. (1987) Adaptation of ocular vergence to stimulation with large disparities. Exp. Brain Res. 66, 507–516.

Erkelens, C.J. and Collewijn, H. (1985a) Motion perception during dichoptic viewing of moving random-dot stereograms. Vision Res. 25, 583–588.

Erkelens, C.J. and Collewijn, H. (1985b) Eye movements and stereopsis during dichoptic viewing of moving random-dot stereograms. Vision Res. 25, 1689–1700.

Erkelens, C.J. and Regan, D. (1986) Human ocular vergence movements induced by changing size and disparity. J. Physiol. 379, 145–169.

Fender, D. and Julesz, B. (1967) Extension of Panum's fusional area in binocularly stabilized vision. J. Opt. Soc. Am. 57, 819–830.

Ferman, L., Collewijn, H., Jansen, T.C. and Van den Berg, A.V. (1987) Human gaze stability in horizontal, vertical and torsional direction during voluntary head movements, evaluated with a three-dimensional scleral induction coil technique. Vision Res. 27, 811–828.

Foley, J.M. (1976) Successive stereo and vernier position discrimination as a function of dark interval duration. Vision Res. 16, 1269–1273.

Foley, J.M. (1977) Effect of distance information and range on two indices of visually perceived distance. Perception 6, 449–460.

Foley, J.M. (1978) Primary distance perception. In: R. Held, H. Leibowitz and H.L. Teuber (Eds.), Handbook of Sensory Physiology, Vol. VIII; Perception, Springer, Berlin, pp. 181–213.

Foley, J.M. (1980) Binocular distance perception. Psychol. Rev. 87, 411–433.

Foley, J. and Held, R. (1972) Visually directed pointing as a function of target distance, direction and available cues. Percept. Psychophys. 12, 263–268.

Gogel, W.C. (1961a) Convergence as a cue to absolute distance. J. Psychol. 52, 287–301.

Gogel, W.C. (1961b) Convergence as a cue to the perceived distance of objects in a binocular configuration. J. Psychol. 52, 303–315.

Gogel, W.C. (1962) The effect of convergence on perceived size and distance. J. Psychol. 53, 475–489.

Gogel, W.C. and Sturm, R.D. (1972) A comparison of accommodative and fusional convergence as cues to distance. Percept. Psychophys. 11, 166–168.

Graham, C.H. (1951) Visual perception. In: S.S. Stevens (Ed.), Handbook of Experimental Psychology, Wiley, New York, pp. 868–920.

Graham, C.H. (1965) Visual space perception. In: C.H. Graham (Ed.), Vision and Visual Perception, Wiley, New York, pp. 504–547.

Grant, V.W. (1942) Accommodation and convergence in visual space perception. J. Exp. Psychol. 31, 89–104.

Hansen, R.M. and Skavenski, A.A. (1977) Accuracy of eye position information for motor control. Vision Res. 17, 919–926.

Hansen, R.M. and Skavenski, A.A. (1985) Accuracy of spatical localizations near the time of saccadic eye movements. Vision Res. 25, 1077–1082.

Hebbard, F.W. (1962) Comparison of subjective and objective measurements of fixation disparity. J. Opt. Soc. Am. 52, 706–712.

Heinemann, E.G., Tulving, E. and Nachmias, J. (1959) The effect of oculomotor adjustments on apparent size. Am. J. Psychol. 72, 32–45.

Hering, E. (1879) Der Raumsinn und die Bewegungen des Auges. In: L. Hermann (Ed.), Handbuch der Physiologie, Vol. III, Teil 1, Vogel, Leipzig, pp. 343–601.

Hillebrand, F. (1893) Die Stabilitat der Raumwerte auf der Netzhaut. Z. Psychol. Physiol. Sinnesorgane 5, 1–60.

Howard, J.H. (1919) A test for the judgement of distance. Am. J. Ophthalmol. 2, 656–675.

Hung, G.K., Semmlow, J.L. and Ciuffreda, K.J. (1986) A dual mode dynamic model of the vergence eye movement system. IEEE Trans. Biomed. Eng. BME-33, 1021–1028.

Jones, R. (1977) Anomalies of disparity detection in the human visual system. J. Physiol. 264, 621–640.

Jones, R. (1980) Fusional vergence: sustained and transient. Am. J. Optom. Physiol. Opt. 57, 640–644.

Jones, R. and Kerr, K.E. (1971) Motor responses to conflicting asymmetrical vergence stimulus information. Am. J. Optom. 48, 989–1000.

Julesz, B. (1978) Global steropsis: cooperative phenomena in stereoscopic depth perception. In: R. Held, H. Leibowitz and H.L. Teuber (Eds.), Handbook of Sensory Physiology, Vol. VIII; Perception, Springer, Berlin, pp. 215–256.

Julesz, B. and White, B. (1969) Short term visual memory and the Pulfrich illusion. Nature 222, 639–641.

Kahn, R.H. (1931) Ueber den Stereoeffekt von Pulfrich. Pflugers Arch. 228, 213–224.

Kertesz, A.E. and Lee, H.J. (1988) The nature of sensory compensation during fusional response. Vision Res. 28, 313–322.

Kertesz, A.E., Hampton, D.R. and Sabrin, H.W. (1983) The unreliability of nonius line estimates of vertical fusional vergence performance. Vision Res. 23, 295–297.

Kinchla, R.A. and Allan, L.G. (1969) A theory of visual movement perception. Psychol. Rev. 76, 537–558.

Kinchla, R.A. and Smyzer, F. (1967) A diffusion model of perceptual memory. Percept. Psychophys. 2, 219–229.

Komoda, M.K. and Ono, H. (1974) Oculomotor adjustments and size-distance perception. Percept. Psychophys. 15, 353–360.

Krauskopf, J., Cornsweet, T.N. and Riggs, L.A. (1960) Analysis of eye movements during monocular and binocular fixation. J. Opt. Soc. Am. 50, 572–578.

Krishnan, V.V. and Stark, L. (1977) A heuristic model for the human vergence eye movement system. IEEE Trans. Biomed. Eng. BME-24, 44–49.

Krishnan, V.V. and Stark, L. (1983) Model of the disparity vergence system. In: C.M. Schor and K.J. Ciuffreda (Eds.), Vergence Eye Movements: Basic and Clinical Aspects, Butterworths, Boston, pp. 349–371.

Krishnan, V.V., Farazian, F. and Stark, L. (1973) An analysis of latencies and prediction in the fusional vergence system. Am. J. Optom. Physiol. Opt. 50, 933–939.

Krol, J.D. and Van de Grind, W.A. (1982) Rehabilitation of a classical notion of Panum's fusional area. Perception 11, 615–619.

Mapp, A.P. and Ono, H. (1986) The rhino-optical phenomenon: ocular parallax and the visible field beyond the nose. Vision Res. 26, 1163–1165.

Marr, D. and Poggio, T. (1979) A computational theory of human stereo vision. Proc. R. Soc. Lond. B 204, 301–328.

Mitchell, D.E. (1966a) A review of the concept of 'Panum's fusional areas'. Am. J. Optom. 43, 387–401.

Mitchell, D.E. (1966b) Retinal disparity and diplopia. Vision Res. 6, 441–451.

Mitchell, D.E. (1970) Properties of stimuli eliciting vergence eye movements and stereopsis. Vision Res. 10, 145–162.

Morgan, M.J. (1975) Stereo-illusion based on visual persistence. Nature 256, 639–640.

Nelson, J.I. (1975) Globality and stereoscopic fusion in binocular vision. J. Theor. Biol. 49, 1–88.

Ogle, K.N. (1962a) Spatial localization through binocular vision. In: H. Davson (Ed.), The Eye, Vol. 4, Academic Press, New York, pp. 271–324.

Ogle, K.N. (1962b) The visual space sense. Science 135, 763–771.

Ogle, K.N. (1964) Researches in Binocular Vision, Hafner, New York.

Ogle, K.N. and Ellerbrock, V.J. (1945) Stereoscopic sensitivity in the space eikonometer. Arch. Ophthalmol. 34, 303–310.

Ogle, K.N. and Weil, M.P. (1958) Stereoscopic vision and the duration of the stimulus. Arch. Ophthalmol. 59, 4–17.

Ogle, K.N., Martens, T.G. and Dyer, J.A. (1967) Oculomotor imbalance in binocular vision and fixation disparity, Lea and Febiger, Philadelphia.

Ono, H. and Steinbach, J. (1983) The Pulfrich phenomenon with eye movement. Vision Res. 23, 1735–1737.

Ono, H., Angus, R. and Gregor, P. (1977) Binocular single vision achieved by fusion and suppression. Percept. Psychophys. 21, 513–521.

Palmer, D.A. (1961) Measurement of the horizontal extent of Panum's area by a method of constant stimuli. Optica Acta 8, 151–159.

Panum, P.L. (1858) Physiologische Untersuchungen ueber das Sehen mit Zwei Augen, Schwerssche Buchhandlung, Kiel.

Patterson, R. and Fox, R. (1984) Stereopsis during continuous head motion. Vision Res. 24, 2001–2003.

Piantanida, T.P. (1986) Stereo hysteresis revisited. Vision Res. 26, 431–437.

Poggio, G.F. and Poggio, T. (1984) The analysis of stereopsis. Annu. Rev. Neurosci. 7, 379–412.

Prazdny, K. (1985) On the disparity gradient limit for binocular fusion. Percept. Psychophys. 37, 81–83.

Pulfrich, C. (1922) Die Stereoskopie im Dienste der isochromen und heterochromen Photometrie. Naturwissenschaften 10, 553–564.

Rashbass, C. and Westheimer, G. (1961) Disjunctive eye movements. J. Physiol. 159, 339–360.

Regan, D. (1986) Visual processing of four kinds of relative motion. Vision Res. 26, 127–145.

Regan, D. and Beverley, K.I. (1973a) Some dynamic features of depth perception. Vision Res. 13, 2369–2379.

Regan, D. and Beverley, K.I. (1973b) The dissociation of sideways movements from movements in depth: psychophysics. Vision Res. 13, 2403–2415.

Regan, D. and Beverley, K.I. (1979) Binocular and monocular stimuli for motion in depth: changing-disparity and changing-size feed the same motion-in depth stage. Vision Res. 19, 1331–1342.

Regan, D., Erkelens, C.J. and Collewijn, H. (1986a) Necessary conditions for the perception of motion in depth. Invest. Ophthalmol. Vis. Sci. 27, 584–598.

Regan, D., Erkelens, C.J. and Collewijn, H. (1986b) Visual field defects for vergence eye movements and for stereomotion perception. Invest. Ophthalmol. Vis. Sci. 27, 806–819.

Richards, W. (1970) Stereopsis and stereoblindness. Exp. Brain Res. 10, 380–388.

Richards, W. (1971) Anomalous stereoscopic depth perception. J. Opt. Soc. Am. 61, 410–414.

Richards, W. (1972) Response functions for sine- and square-wave modulations of disparity. J. Opt. Soc. Am. 62, 907–911.

Richards, W. and Kaye, M.G. (1974) Local versus global stereopsis: two mechanisms? Vision Res. 14, 1345–1347.

Richards, W. and Miller, J.F. (1969) Convergence as a cue to depth. Percept. Psychophys. 5, 317–320.

Richards, W. and Regan, D. (1973) A stereo field map with implications for disparity processing. Invest. Ophthalmol. Vis. Sci. 12, 904–909.

Riggs, L.A. and Niehl, E.W. (1960) Eye movements recorded during convergence and divergence. J. Opt. Soc. Am. 50, 913–920.

Robinson, D.A. (1963) A method of measuring eye movement using a scleral search coil in a magnetic field. IEEE Trans. Biomed. Electron. BME-10, 137–145.

Robinson, D.A. (1973) Models of the saccadic eye movement control system. Kybernetik 14, 71–83.

Rogers, B.J., Steinbach, M.J. and Ono, H. (1974) Eye movements and the Pulfrich phenomenon. Vision Res. 14, 181–185.

Ross, J. and Hogben, J.H. (1974) Short-term memory in stereopsis. Vision Res. 14, 1195–1201.

Ross, J. and Hogben, J.H. (1975) The Pulfrich effect and short-term memory in stereopsis. Vision Res. 15, 1289–1290.

Schor, C. (1980) Fixation disparity: a steady state error of disparity-induced vergence. Am. J. Optom. Physiol. Opt. 57, 618–631.

Schor, C.M. (1979a) The influence of rapid prism adaptation upon fixation disparity. Vision Res. 19, 757–765.

Schor, C.M. (1979b) The relationship between fusional vergence eye movements and fixation disparity. Vision Res. 19, 1359–1367.

Schor, C.M. and Tyler, C.W. (1981) Spatio-temporal properties of Panum's fusional area. Vision Res. 21, 683–692.

Schor, C.M. and Wood, I. (1983) Disparity range for local stereopsis as a function of luminance spatial frequency. Vision Res. 23, 1649–1654.

Schor, C.M., Wood, I.C. and Ogawa, J. (1984a) Spatial tuning of static and dynamic local stereopsis. Vision Res. 24, 573–578.

Schor, C., Wood, I. and Ogawa, J. (1984b) Binocular sensory fusion is limited by spatial resolution. Vision Res. 24, 661–665.

Schumer, R.A. and Julesz, B. (1984) Binocular disparity modulation sensitivity to disparities offset from the plane of fixation. Vision Res. 24, 533–542.

Semmlow, J. and Heerema, D. (1979) The synkinetic interaction of convergence accommodation and accommodative convergence. Vision Res. 19, 1237–1242.

Semmlow, J. and Venkiteswaran, N. (1976) Dynamic accommodative vergence components in binocular vision. Vision Res. 16, 403–410.

Semmlow, J. and Wetzel, P. (1979) Dynamic contributions of the components of binocular vergence. J. Opt. Soc. Am. 69, 639–645.

Semmlow, J.L., Hung, G.K. and Ciuffreda, K.J. (1986) Quantitative assessment of disparity vergence components. Invest. Ophthalmol. Vis. Sci. 27, 558–565.

Sheedy, J.E. and Fry, G.A. (1979) The perceived direction of the binocular image. Vision Res. 19, 201–211.

Shortess, G.K. and Krauskopf, J. (1961) Role of involuntary eye movements in stereoscopic acuity. J. Opt. Soc. Am. 51, 555–559.

Skavenski, A.A. and Steinman, R.M. (1970) Control of eye position in the dark. Vision Res. 10, 193–203.

Southall, J.P.C. (1961) Introduction to Physiological Optics, Dover, New York.

St.-Cyr, G.J. and Fender, D.H. (1969) The interplay of drifts and flicks in binocular fixation. Vision Res. 9, 245–265.

Steinman, R.M. and Collewijn, H. (1980) Binocular retinal image motion during active head rotation. Vision Res. 20, 415–429.

Steinman, R.M., Cushman, W.B. and Martins, A.J. (1982) The precision of gaze. Human Neurobiol. 1, 97–109.

Steinman, R.M., Levinson, J.Z., Collewijn, H. and Van der Steen, J. (1983) Vision in the presence of known natural retinal-image motion. J. Opt. Soc. Am. 73, 1856.

Steinman, R.M., Levinson, J.Z., Collewijn, H. and Van der Steen, J. (1985) Vision in the presence of known natural retinal image motion. J. Opt. Soc. Am. A 2, 226–233.

Swenson, H.A. (1932) The relative influence of accommodation and convergence in the judgment of distance. J. Gen. Psychol. 7, 360–380.

Tani, G.T., Ogle, K.N., Weaer, R.W. and Martens, T.G. (1956) On the precise objective determination of eye movements. A.M.A. Arch. Ophthalmol. 55, 174–185.

Troelstra, A., Zuber, B.L., Miller, D. and Stark, L. (1964) Accommodative tracking: a trial-and-error function. Vision Res. 4, 585–594.

Tschermak, A. (1930) Beitrage zur physiologischen Optik III, Raumsinn, Handbuch der normalen und pathologischen Physiologie, Vol. 12, Part 2, Springer, Berlin, pp. 833–1000.

Tyler, C.W. (1971) Stereoscopic depth movement: two eyes less sensitive than one. Science 174, 958–961.

Tyler, C.W. (1973) Stereoscopic vision: cortical limitations and a disparity scaling effect. Science 181, 276–278.

Tyler, C.W. (1974) Depth perception in disparity gratings. Nature 251, 140–142.

Tyler, C.W. (1975) Spatial organization of binocular disparity sensitivity. Vision Res. 15, 583–590.

Tyler, C.W. (1977) Spatial limitations of human stereoscopic vision. SPIE Report 120, 36–42.

Tyler, C.W. (1983) Sensory processing of binocular disparity. In: C.M. Schor and K. Ciuffreda (Eds.), Vergence Eye Movements: Basic and Clinical Aspects, Butterworths, Boston, pp. 199–295.

Tyler, C.W. and Julesz, B. (1980) On the depth of the cyclopean retina. Exp. Brain Res. 40, 196–202.

Tyler, C.W. and Scott, A.B. (1979) Binocular vision. In: R.E. Records (Ed.), Physiology of the Human Eye and Visual System, Harper and Row, Hagerstown, MD, pp. 643–671.

Van den Berg, A.V. and Collewijn, H. (1987) Voluntary smooth eye movements with foveally stabilized targets. Exp. Brain Res. 68, 195–204.

Van den Berg, A.V. and Collewijn, H. (1988) Directional asymmetries of human optokinetic nystagmus. Exp. Brain Res. 70, 597–604.

Von Helmholtz, H. (1962) Treatise on Physiological Optics, Vol. III. Translated from the Third German Edition. In: J.P.C. Southall (Ed.), Dover, New York.

Von Hofsten, C. (1976) The role of convergence in visual space perception. Vision Res. 16, 193–198.
Westheimer, G. (1957) Kinematics of the eye. J. Opt. Soc. Am. 47, 967–974.
Westheimer, G. (1979a) Cooperative neural processes involved in stereoscopic acuity. Exp. Brain Res. 36, 585–597.
Westheimer, G. (1979b) The spatial sense of the eye. Invest. Ophthalmol. Vis. Sci. 18, 893–912.
Westheimer, G. and McKee, S.P. (1975) Visual acuity in the presence of retinal-image motion. J. Opt. Soc. Am. 65, 847–850.
Westheimer, G. and McKee, S.P. (1978) Stereoscopic acuity for moving retinal images. J. Opt. Soc. Am. 68, 450–455.
Westheimer, G. and Mitchell, D.E. (1969) The sensory stimulus for disjunctive eye movements. Vision Res. 9, 749–755.
Westheimer, G. and Mitchell, G. (1956) Eye movement responses to convergence stimuli. A.M.A. Arch. Ophthalmol. 55, 848–856.
Westheimer, G. and Tanzman, I.J. (1956) Qualitative depth localization with diplopic images. J. Opt. Soc. Am. 46, 116–117.
Wheatstone, C. (1838) Contributions to the physiology of vision. Part the first. On some remarkable, and hitherto unobserved, phenomena of binocular vision. Phil. Trans. R. Soc. 128, 371–394.
Wheatstone, C. (1852) Contributions to the physiology of vision. Part the second. On some remarkable, and hitherto unobserved, phenomena of binocular vision. Phil. Trans. R. Soc. 142, 1–17.
Williams, J.M. and Lit, A. (1983) Luminance-dependent visual latency for the Hess effect, the Pulfrich effect and simple reaction time. Vision Res. 23, 171–179.
Woo, G.C.S. (1974) The effect of exposure time on the foveal size of Panum's area. Vision Res. 14, 473–480.
Wundt, W. (1862) Beitrage zur Theorie der Sinneswahrnehmung, Wintersche, Leipzig.
Zuber, B.L. and Stark, L. (1968) Dynamical characteristics of the fusional vergence eye-movement system. IEEE Trans. Syst. Sci. Cybern. SSC-4, 72–79.

Note added in proof

Recently, Erkelens et al. (1989a,b) found that "when ocular vergence was studied under relatively natural conditions in which there were many cues to the distance of [relatively nearby] targets, oculomotor vergence was both much faster and much more accurate than could have been anticipated from previous studies done under more restricted stimulating conditions" (p. 418). Furthermore, "asymmetric vergence was largely saccadic and... the generation of saccades of unequal sizes in each of the eyes is a normal feature of oculomotor performance whenever gaze is shifted between targets that differ in distance as well as direction" [the most common arrangement in everyday life] (p. 442).

References

Erkelens, C.J., Van der Steen, J., Steinman, R.M. and Collewijn, H. (1989a) Ocular vergence under natural conditions. I. Continuous changes of target distance along the median plane. Proc. R. Soc. Lond. B 236, 417–440.
Erkelens, C.J., Steinman, R.M. and Collewijn, H. (1989b) Ocular vergence under natural conditions. II. Gaze stifts between real targets differing in distance and direction. Proc. R. Soc. Lond. B 236, 441–465.

Eye movements and their role in visual and cognitive processes
E. Kowler, Editor

CHAPTER 5

Eye movement and visual localization of objects in space

Alexander A. Skavenski

Department of Psychology, Northeastern University, Boston, MA, U.S.A.

1. Introduction

Historically, there has been continuing interest in eye movement and visual localization because the eyes of many animals, including humans, move with respect to the head. These movements, as well as movements of the head with respect to the body and the body with respect to the environment, effectively decouple the position of images of objects in the environment on the receptor surface from the position of those objects with respect to the animal's body. As a result, the animal cannot tell where an object is located with respect to his body based only on the retinal image position because retinal image position is determined by the relative positions of the eye in the head and head on the body as well as the position of the body relative to the object. Of course knowing where objects are located is crucial if one is going to do anything more than simple passive observation. This review deals primarily with what is known about how we localize in the fronto-parallel plane.

Helmholtz (1925) proposed a solution to the localization problem in which he noted that both retinal and extraretinal signals accompanied motions of the eyes in the head. He also noted that the visual world appears to shift when the eyeball is passively pressed with the finger. This observation supports the idea that the signals used in compensating for eye movements relative to the head are derived from an extraretinal source, namely, the commands generated to move the eye. Grusser (1986a) noted that, in fact, Helmholtz's ideas were actually elaborations of earlier views proposed by Purkinje. There was a slow evolution of an understanding of the algebra needed to accomplish compensation for eye movements using extraretinal signals and there have been numerous formal statements of what is needed; for examples, see von Holst and Mittelstaedt (1950), Sperry (1950) and Hansen and Skavenski (1977). The essence of these models is that neurally coded analogues of the position of an object relative to the head may be obtained by adding a neural analogue of the retinal image position of an object to a neural analogue of eye position in the head, with all of these expressed in suitable coordinate systems. Similarly, the position of the object relative to the body, or to the outside world, may be obtained by adding the neural analogue of its position relative to the head to neural analogues of head position relative to the body or head position relative to the world, respectively. While such a schema is realizable with neural elements, a number of tests of the quality of the various signals that would be used in such a compensatory system have produced discrepant results, and this fact has raised doubt about whether such a mechanism is actually useful in localization and space perception in normal viewing (e.g., see reviews by Bridgeman, 1983; Howard, 1982; Matin, 1983).

2. Quality of the retinal signals

2.1. Acuity measures

Coding of the retinal image position is accepted as being of very high resolution. One measure of the upper limit (lowest quality) of this coding is given by various acuity indices, the minimum angle resolved being the lowest of these, with a foveal threshold of about 1 min arc (Westheimer, 1981). Other measures, such as those describing performance in several hyperacuity tasks, indicate that the spatial resolution of visual images (i.e. determining the relative position of two visual features) is an order of magnitude higher (Westheimer, 1981). Of course, these measures were for the central fovea and high-contrast, stationary test targets, conditions under which seeing was best. Presentation of test targets to the peripheral retina, reducing contrast, or imposing motion can increase thresholds and degrade acuity. Westheimer (1981) showed the minimum angle resolved to be about 5 min arc at 10 degrees retinal eccentricity and that it sharply rose as one tested more peripheral retina. Retinal image motion of up to about 2 deg arc/s had relatively small effects on the spatial resolving capacities (Westheimer and McKee, 1975; Steinman et al., 1985) although higher retinal image speeds do cause deterioration of resolution (Arend, 1976; Kelly, 1979). In sum, we can resolve detail to within about 5 min arc in the central 20 degrees of the retina when the detail is high-contrast and moving at less than 2 deg arc/s. This is good resolution (see Ch. 3 of this volume, by Steinman and Levinson, for further discussion of visual resolution with moving and stationary images).

However, acuity measures may not be the optimal indicator of the spatial resolving capacity of the eye in so far as spatial localization is concerned. Most acuity measurements are made with the critical detail included in visual features that are close to each other and, therefore, require local comparisons of the spatial positions of receptors stimulated, regardless of the place on the retina being tested. What is crucial for the mechanisms of localization described at the beginning of this chapter is whether or not this local sensitivity is also maintained when the comparison is made to some remote reference position on the retina, such as the fovea. For example, while it is clear that two places separated by about 5 min arc and located at 10 deg arc eccentricity provide sufficient spatial information for a subject to determine that two places are stimulated, it does not automatically follow that a single stimulus on one of these places would be seen as 5 min arc further from the fovea than a stimulus on the other when they are separated in time.

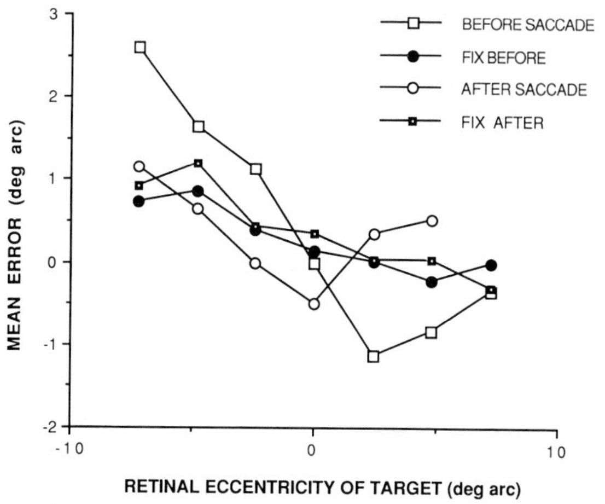

Fig. 1. Mean error, the distance between the subject's setting of a pointer indicating target position and physical location of that target, plotted as a function of the *retinal eccentricity* of that target for subject N.C. Open symbols show mean error on trials when targets were presented *before* the saccade started and *after* it had ended. Filled symbols show error on trials when the target was presented to the fixating eye 200 ms after fixation was established. Positive signs indicate target presentation in the right visual field and mean pointing errors to the right of target location. Data replotted from Fig. 6, O'Regan (1984), with permission.

2.2. Direct localization measures

There have been relatively few measures of the absolute position coding of the retina, but the few that were done indicated that the absolute position sensitivity of the retina may be much poorer than was indicated by measurements of acuity. For example, Bischof and Kramer (1968) concluded that mislocalization of flashes presented near and during saccades was due, in part, to retinal factors, in addition to extraretinal factors. O'Regan (1984) replicated and extended Bischof and Kramer's study (1968) by asking subjects to set a visible marker to the position of a flash they had seen at various times around the occurrence of a saccade or during steady fixation. Two fixation marks were always visible and the subjects either made saccades between them or fixated one of them under dim ambient room illumination. The retinal locus of the test flash and its time of presentation were systematically manipulated. The errors one of the subjects made in localizing flashes seen before and after the saccade and during fixation are shown as a function of the retinal locus of the test flash in Fig. 1. Although there was inconsistency across subjects, it was generally true that subjects were very accurate in localizing flashes presented to the fovea but made large errors in localizing flashes presented to the peripheral retina. O'Regan (1984) suggested that input about eye movement could be assumed to be constant during steady fixation so that accuracy of localization of flashes presented during fixation would reflect the accuracy of retinal coding of the target position only. O'Regan's results showed that the retinal coding of target position was subject to error. He found that peripheral targets were mislocalized toward the fovea for all subjects. Errors were as large as 1 deg arc for targets presented at 7.2 deg arc eccentricity during fixation. This error was at least a factor of 10 larger than might be expected based on acuity at the same eccentricity; viz., acuity limitations suggested that the largest error should have been less than 5 min arc. It is also important to note that the error was about the same whether the test flashes were presented to the fixating eye or very near the time of a saccadic eye movement. This was interpreted by O'Regan to mean that eye-movement-related extraretinal signals had very little to do with the error and that the error was based solely on retinal factors.

Subjective underestimates of the retinal eccentricity of peripherally presented targets have been noted before. For example, Osaka (1977) asked subjects to point to targets briefly presented in 10 deg arc increments over a range of ± 50 deg arc on both the horizontal and vertical meridians. Pointing error was about 1.5 deg arc at 10 deg arc eccentricity and increased to about 6.5 deg arc at 50 deg arc eccentricity. Osaka (1977) hypothesized that refraction by the optics of the eye for images off the visual axis led to these localization errors; however, no quantitative analysis to compare refractive errors with obtained errors was reported. In addition, Osaka's (1977) account seems implausible for the following reason. Distortion due to refractive error is a product of the optics of the eye and is relatively invariant over one's life. Central compensation for imperfections of the optics of the eye is known to occur for color fringes, for example. Also, there is both perceptual and oculomotor compensation when lenses of differing power are prescribed for the two eyes (see Erkelens et al., 1989, for discussion of short- and long-term adaptation to anisometropic spectacles). So it would be odd if compensation for refractive error in eccentric targets did not take place.

It is interesting to note that superficially the pointing errors which Osaka (1977) measured appear to be of the same order of magnitude as the error in primary saccades made to targets presented more than 10 deg arc in the periphery (Optican, 1985). Ordinarily, such distant targets are acquired with two saccades: a primary saccade covers about 90% of the distance and a secondary saccade positions the fovea on target (Becker and Fuchs, 1969). Although the reason for programming such movements in two steps remains unclear (Optican, 1985), it does not seem to be due to error in the retinal signals of target location, because a corrective second saccade is still generated even when the goal is removed from view before the first saccade ends (Becker and Fuchs, 1969). It should be noted that thorough quantitative studies on the accuracy of eye movements made to targets at large eccentricities and in a variety of directions from the fovea are rare (however, for recent papers concerned with the accuracy and dynamic properties of large saccades, see Collewijn et al., 1988a,b). The problem has been that, until fairly recently, high-resolution, linear, eye movement recording systems have not been available for large movements. Also, the idea of using eye movements to characterize position coding of the retina is novel to eye movement research.

Any inhomogeneity or inaccuracy in the quality of coding of eccentric retinal position signals which was not corrected or compensated for by the viewer would not necessarily preclude accurate localization under normal viewing conditions, because the person could quickly rotate the eye to view the object to be localized with their fovea. In virtually all reports of localization with foveal targets, errors were of the order of a few minutes of arc (e.g., Hansen and Skavenski, 1977; O'Regan, 1984; Osaka, 1977). However, O'Regan has correctly noted that foveal versus peripheral differences in localization accuracy of the retinal image could have contributed to misinterpretations in a number of studies whose intent was to describe accuracy of extraretinal signals. Most of the previous work assumed that the retina was homogeneous with respect to position coding, and therefore no attempt was made to control or factor out effects due to retinal eccentricity. O'Regan noted particularly the work of Bischof and Kramer (1968), Matin and Pearce (1965), Matin et al. (1969, 1970b), Monahan (1972) and Mateeff (1978), who all found relatively large mislocalizations of targets presented around the time of saccades, which O'Regan attributed to purely retinal factors. Certainly, future work will need to carefully control the eccentricity at which test targets are presented to determine how much localization error may be attributed to retinal, in contrast to extraretinal, factors. The relative contribution of retinal and extraretinal factors to localization will be discussed further under subsequent headings.

3. Quality of extraretinal signals

3.1. Control of eye position using extraretinal eye position signals

A number of approaches have been taken to assess the quality of nonretinal eye position information. The key problem in making these measurements is that the subject must provide a response which indicates the seen position of a target under conditions which prevent the subject from making that judgement solely on the basis of retinal information. The most direct approaches have involved attempts to hold the line of sight in place in darkness or return it to the position of a previously seen fixation target when the subject is in complete darkness. The rationale behind these studies is that we know the eye can be positioned quite accurately on visible targets, so that errors in establishing or maintaining eye position in darkness should provide a sensitive measure of the quality of extraretinal signals of eye position with respect to the head. Measurements of a subject's ability to maintain the line of sight in the position of a previously visible fixation target showed that the eye moved slowly away from that position until the subject was about 2 deg arc from the starting position (Skavenski and Steinman, 1970). There were no further drifts of any consequence. Statistical analysis of the eye movement patterns indicated deviations from the predictions of a random-walk model and provided evidence that the subjects were attempting to hold the position of the target (Matin et al., 1970a; Skavenski, 1971). This would indicate use of at least some extraretinal information for effective control of eye position.

Further evidence for use of extraretinal information comes from demonstrations that subjects were able to return their eyes to within about 2–4 deg arc of a reference position after different types of eye movement (saccades, smooth pursuit, or the slow phase of vestibular nystagmus) had driven the eye out of the reference position in total darkness (Merton, 1961; Skavenski and Steinman, 1970; Hansen and Skavenski, 1977; Miller, 1980). Miller

(1980) used a paradigm similar to Hansen and Skavenski (1977) in which either saccades or smooth pursuit drove the eye from the starting position. In addition to a saccade back on some trials, Miller (1980) asked his subjects to set a pointer to the start position without making an eye movement to that position. Miller (1980) found errors to be just under 2 deg arc in both the psychophysical and the two eye movement tasks, errors very similar to those obtained by Hansen and Skavenski (1977). Errors of 2 deg arc, however, are too large to be able to account for the accurate visual localization we observe in normal viewing. This has been noted by several investigators (e.g., see Matin, 1972; Hansen and Skavenski, 1977; Howard, 1982). Indeed, if the error reflected only the accuracy of the extraretinal eye position signal, and, therefore, the quality of target localization with respect to the head, then that signal was too poor to account for much of visual localization. However, in the tasks studied by the investigators cited above, subjects were attempting to keep their eyes in a remembered position and it was unlikely that memory for absolute spatial position was perfect. The exact contribution of poor spatial memory to the large errors observed in the control of eye position in the dark could not be directly determined because memory for the target position and the sensitivity with which extraretinal signals were compared to remembered position were confounded in the previous work. Indirect methods of separating memory from the process of comparing extraretinal eye position signals to remembered position include Skavenski and Steinman's (1970) comparison of short-term mean error and variability over the course of a long attempt to hold a constant eye position in the dark. Short-term variability was uniform, with SDs less than 20 min arc over 7.5-s intervals, while mean error steadily grew. This suggested that subjects were using extraretinal signals to compare eye position to remembered position with good sensitivity, but that memory slowly decayed over time to lead to errors of a few degrees.

Interestingly, the decay in spatial memory for target position was influenced little by the pattern of eye movement required of the subjects. Mean error was about the same (about 2 deg arc) whether the subjects used their preferred pattern of eye movement to stay in the remembered position for 30 s or were asked to make 30 large saccades in randomly chosen directions over a 30-s time interval (Skavenski and Steinman, 1970). Nemire and Bridgeman (1987) recently performed a variation of this procedure in which they asked subjects to make a saccade or to point the hand to a peripherally presented target either (1) immediately after it disappeared, (2) after a 20-s wait in the dark, or (3) after making 40 trained saccades in the dark. When manual pointing data had been corrected for pointing bias, (determined by pointing to a continuously visible peripheral target without fixating on it) manual error and oculomotor pointing error were identical within conditions (their Fig. 3). Error after the wait (3.5 deg arc) was somewhat larger than error when pointing immediately after target disappearance. However, error after executing a pattern of saccades was nearly twice as large. Why did they see such a big difference when Skavenski and Steinman (1970) did not? A key difference was that in Skavenski and Steinman's study the subject had to return to the position the eye was in before executing the saccade pattern. In Nemire et al.'s (1987) study the subject had to look at a target that was in a different position after executing the sequence of saccades. So, it may be that the process of going to a location seen originally by peripheral retina was more disrupted by intervening saccades than was returning to the place where the subject started. Nemire et al. (1987) concluded that since both manual and eye pointing errors were affected equally by the eye movement patterns required of the subjects, then both share the same mapping of visual space. It was also clear that the performance in the tasks used to measure the mapping (tasks in which subjects look at or point to remembered positions) must be subject to memory decay. As a result, the numerical data from control in the dark (Skavenski and Steinman, 1970; Hansen and Skavenski, 1977) must be taken as the lower limit (worst case) of the quality of the extraretinal indicators of eye position. The estimate of the quality of the extraretinal signal would be better in tasks less sensitive to visual spatial memory.

3.2. Visual psychophysical judgement of location using extraretinal signals

Other methods of assessing the quality of extraretinal signals have apparently avoided the memory problem but have introduced other difficulties in interpretation. To illustrate, several investigators have asked subjects to judge the seen location of a briefly flashed target relative to the location of a continuously visible scale (Bischof and Kramer, 1968; Mateeff, 1978; O'Regan, 1984) or to a previously seen reference mark (Matin et al., 1969, 1970b; Monahan, 1972). The primary objective of these experiments was to characterize the accuracy of visual localization during and around the time of saccadic eye movements and to infer the temporal course of the change in the extraretinal signals that accompanied the saccades.* In general, the finding was that localization of test targets was quite good, with errors of the order of a few tens of min arc or less, when flashes were presented several hundred milliseconds before or after the saccade, but that localization was very poor for targets flashed temporally near or during the saccade (e.g., see Mateeff, 1978; Matin, 1972). Localization accuracy generally recovered much more quickly following the saccade when judgements were made in the presence of a continuously visible marker or scale than when judgements were made with reference to a previously seen marker. The presence of visual markers at the time the test target was flashed permitted the judgement to be based on retinal factors alone, so those studies which used continuously visible markers will not be considered further here. Location judgements made with reference to a previously visible marker require an extraretinal signal. An example of the temporal course of errors made in this paradigm may be seen in Fig. 2. Also shown is a model which Hansen and Skavenski (1977) found would simulate the data obtained

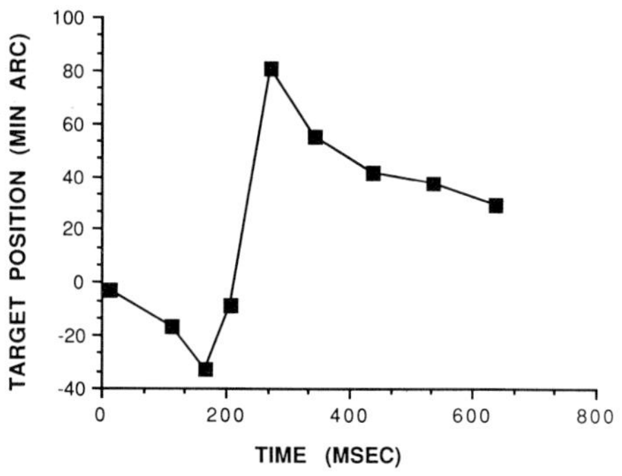

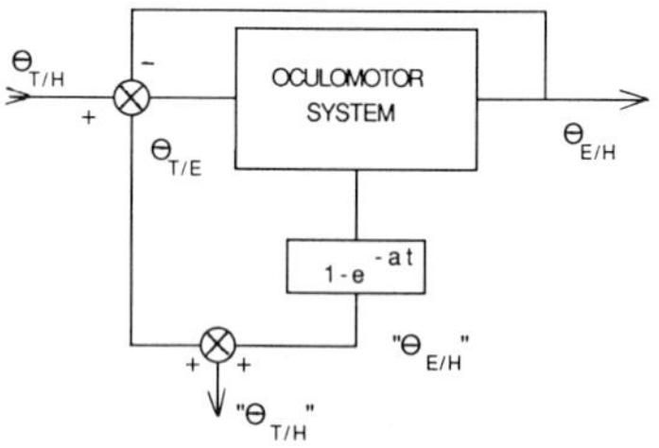

Fig. 2. Graph shows *target position* that a representative subject could not discriminate as being to the left or right of a previously visible fixation point when the target was briefly exposed at various *times* during or around a saccade. The saccades were about 2 deg arc amplitude and began at 200 ms. The data points show physical positions required for the subject to perceive the target as being in a single locus. Data were taken from Matin (1972). The model below was adapted from von Holst et al. (1950) by inserting a filter in the path of the efference copy signal ('$\theta_{E/H}$') that causes it to follow eye position ($\theta_{E/H}$) exponentially. When the time constant of the filter is made long (between 200 and 500 ms) the model very closely simulates the data shown in the graph above. That is, the perceived location of the target ('$\theta_{T/H}$') is constant when its physical location ($\theta_{T/H}$) is changed as shown in the graph above and it is presented around the time of saccades. The model does not show a pure delay needed to account for changes in target position that began before the saccade. Additional details of this model may be found in Skavenski and Hansen (1978).

* Some authors have the mistaken impression that the investigators, using the paradigm of presenting targets during saccades to study localization, have a secondary aim which is to demonstrate that vision is useful during the saccade. This secondary aim is distinctly not the issue in studies of localization regardless of its merit for other issues in visual processing. Rather, we use the saccade to produce an abrupt, natural shift in eye position (to approximate the step response in engineering analysis) and localization performance is measured. If extraretinal signals were to be responsible for good localization during brief intersaccadic intervals, then such signals would follow the eye closely during the saccades (Hansen and Skavenski, 1977).

using this general paradigm. The model is an adaptation of the von Holst and Mittelstaedt (1950) mechanism in which the extraretinal eye position signal is made to follow eye position through a filter and with some asynchrony. As an example, we were able to get good fits to Matin's (1972) localization data using time constants for the filter of between 200 and 450 ms. The data of other workers may be fit with somewhat shorter time constants (e.g., see Grusser, 1986b). Nevertheless, all of these time constants were so long that they led ultimately to the inference that the extraretinal eye position signal was so poorly matched in time to the actual changes in eye position as to be of little use in normal localization (Matin, 1972; Hansen and Skavenski, 1977). Alternatively, investigators have been turning to mechanisms of localization based solely on information contained within the retinal image (e.g., see Matin, 1982, 1983).

There is another possible interpretation of the results obtained using the previously visible marker paradigm (after Matin et al., 1972) which closely links it to the task of comparing the seen location of the test flash with a continuously visible reference mark, which can be done on the basis of retinal information alone (Skavenski and Hansen, 1978; Howard, 1982; O'Regan, 1984). O'Regan (1984) adopted this view and claimed that extraretinal eye position was not needed in the task. He assumed that the extraretinal signal remained constant and tried to account for performance based on retinal information alone. Recall that O'Regan's analysis described above (section 2.2) showed that localization error was about the same during steady fixation or near the time of saccade onset and offset. O'Regan (1984) argued that the errors could be accounted for by retinal factors and that a sloppy extraretinal signal need not be invoked at all. He applied his analysis to the paradigm of Matin and co-workers (1970) and Monahan (1972) in which the reference mark was removed from view before the test flash was presented. O'Regan assumed only that the subject had an obscure notion of the time of saccade occurrence and made the judgement on the basis of the retinal information available after the saccade was over. He reasoned that the subject had an afterimage or some persisting visual memory image of the flash which decays fairly rapidly. If that image was faint, it would tell the subject that the flash occurred at the beginning of the saccade. In this case the subject would respond that the flash was to the left of the reference mark if the image was to the left of the fovea or to the right of the reference if the image was to the right of the fovea. If the memory image was strong, then the subject would conclude that the flash occurred late in the saccade and its image would be near its veridical position. The subject could base his judgement of the flash location relative to the reference mark on some internal estimate of the size of the saccade he made. Errors in localization (which might appear to be due to a sluggish extraretinal signal) would be expected using this strategy because the subject would not know the exact time of the saccade and therefore could mistakenly believe that the flash occurred earlier with respect to the onset of the saccade than it actually had. Lest O'Regan's rationale seem somewhat strained here, it should be recalled that the subjects in the previous work were highly experienced, there were large numbers of trials, and the saccades in a particular experiment were all of the same size and direction, all conditions that might foster the making of judgements solely on the basis of the intensity of retinal signals, as O'Regan claimed. At the very least his ideas reinforce the notion that unless the conditions force the subjects to make judgements in the head-centric frame of reference, there is no reason to assume they will automatically do that (Howard, 1982). At most, the errors seen when visually localizing brief flashes presented during saccades might be explained by retinal factors without recourse to time-varying extraretinal signals at all (O'Regan, 1984).

3.3. Location judgements made by pointing with the eye or hand

Hallett and Lightstone (1976a,b) used a similar display but with a task that forced the subjects to make spatial judgements relative to the position of the head by requiring them to saccade to the target. The most revealing of their conditions was the situation in which a target abruptly shifted position in a totally dark environment and then disappeared. The subject initiated a saccade toward the shifted position and during this saccade the target again briefly appeared in a new location. It was seen against a totally dark background. Individual records of eye movements indicate that subjects made secondary saccades of size and direction appropriate to the physical location of these targets relative to the head, rather than appropriate to the retinal location of the target. A regression analysis confirmed that the size of the corrective saccade was predicted better by the error that existed between eye position and the physical location of the target than by the retinal eccentricity at which the test flash was presented. It was most likely that subjects were using an extraretinal eye position signal to determine where the target was presented in the framework of the head. This is an important and oft-cited result which has one potential problem. The target steps were shown on an oscilloscope equipped with a P15 phosphor which decays to 10% starting output in under 0.01 ms and there was a chance that there was enough persistence for the spots to remain visible when the eye had come to rest after the first saccade. The force of the Hallett and Lightstone (1976a,b) argument depends critically on the targets for the second saccade only being seen by an eye that was rapidly changing position. This was most likely the case, but it would be useful to see the results replicated using a visual display less subject to persistence.

Another way to encourage subjects to use extraretinal eye position signals in target localization is to require them to point to target location with the unseen hand. This task, however, requires an additional computation over localization in the head-centric frame of reference. Namely, the position of the head relative to the body must be added to the position of the target relative to the head to reconstruct the position of the target with respect to the body. This computation allows the limb to be directed to the target location and would, of course, be expected to introduce a bit more noise in the responses. Nevertheless, ballistic pointing responses can be very accurate and have a relatively small variance. To illustrate, Hansen and Skavenski (1977) found that the mean position of hammer blows was less than 5 min arc from the target when four subjects attempted to strike small targets seen against a totally dark background. Standard deviations of the position of the blows relative to the target ranged from 0.5 to 1.0 deg arc.* Next, they used this response to determine how well subjects could localize targets which were flashed-on briefly at various times before, during and after the making of saccadic eye movements by the subjects (Hansen and Skavenski, 1985). Specifically, subjects attempted to strike a black line centered horizontally on a 3×4 deg arc transilluminated panel. Subjects could not see any part of their bodies or anything else in the totally darkened room. Auditory cues were eliminated with loud white noise. Subjects were not given feedback about their performance. The 2-ms flash, which allowed the target to be seen, was timed to a large spontaneous saccade subjects made in total darkness. Saccade amplitude was, of course, somewhat variable and had a mean amplitude of 5 deg arc for one subject and 8 deg arc for the other. Surprisingly, there was relatively little variation in the mean position of the hammer blows as a function of the time of target exposure relative to the saccade, as can be seen in Fig. 3. There was variation in the position of the blows, of the order of 0.5 deg arc, for targets exposed during and just after the saccades, but this variation was more than an order of magnitude less than would have been ex-

* These small mean errors and variability often draw skepticism when, in fact, they are common requisites in a variety of manual tasks and in many sports. For example, the head on an ordinary carpenter's hammer subtends about 1.7 deg arc diameter at the distance I use it when I start nails (holding the nail in the other hand). At the accuracy cited here, I could expect to miss about 5% of the time. Heavy driving is usually done at a greater distance and would require smaller variability. We (with Lynne Kiorpes) first made measurements of the accuracy of ballistic pointing movements using the NU Varsity Women's Basketball Team. Their mean error was about 3 min arc and standard deviations were less than 0.5 deg arc for their foul shots.

pected from previous observations (e.g., Matin et al., 1970). Such performance could be accounted for only if the subjects had a very accurate extraretinal eye position signal which was very closely time-locked to actual changes in eye position during their saccades.* In fact, a good fit to the data shown in Fig. 3 was obtained using the model shown in Fig. 2 with time constants of 9 milliseconds for R.H. and 12 milliseconds for A.S. for the coupling between the extraretinal signal and actual eye position during the saccade. Recall that time constants of 200–450 milliseconds were needed to fit the Matin (1972) data. Clearly, the results of Hansen and Skavenski (1985) show that the coupling can be tight. With a time constant of 12 milliseconds, the model in Fig. 2 will produce a stable output when the visual world is stable and the input is a pattern of large saccades such as a person might make in looking around the room (Skavenski and Hansen, 1978). There were some small displacements at the instants of the saccades but they were of such short duration that saccadic suppression and or metacontrast mechanisms might be sufficient to blank vision during the saccades and prevent perception of the brief displacement (Matin, 1974). Saccadic

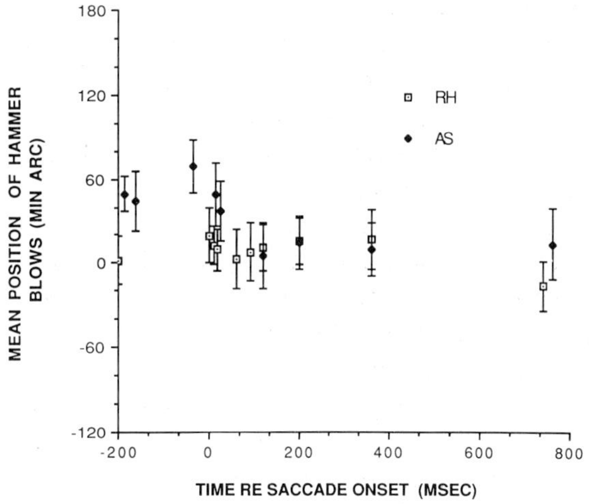

Fig. 3. Mean position of hammer blows struck at small targets briefly flashed on at variouis *times relative to saccade onset* for subjects R.H. and A.S. Zero position indicates blows directly on target and positive numbers signify position to the right and time after saccade onset. Each point is the mean of 45 blows and error bars show + 2SEM. Mean saccade amplitude was 5 deg arc for R.H. and 8 deg arc for A.S. Data redrawn from Hansen and Skavenski (1985). There was a modest shift in the position of the blows during the saccades but it was only a small percentage of that seen in Fig. 3.

suppression or metacontrast would not be sufficient to suppress perceptual displacements if the extraretinal signal did not keep up with the saccade (if the coupling had a 200-millisecond time constant) because a slow extraretinal signal would produce localization error for several hundred milliseconds after the saccade. If these errors were suppressed, then vision in general would be seriously degraded during intersaccadic intervals (Skavenski and Hansen, 1978). Of course, vision is not seriously degraded during intersaccadic intervals because, for example, we know that people ordinarily make 3 or 4 saccades per second when they read.

3.4. Comparison of visual psychophysical and pointing measures

There have been several studies which showed large differences in localization accuracy when localization was done by pointing the eye or arm to the target as compared to verbal judgement of the per-

* In this series of experiments biteboards were not used to restrain the subjects' heads and they sat on an ordinary wood chair, as found in many offices. This means that their bodies, as well as their heads, were allowed to move during the course of an experimental run. These arrangements add to other measures we employed to preclude the possibility of the subject memorizing a finite set of ballistic movements in space and then using crude localization to determine which member of the finite set was to be performed. In this case, body motions on the chair would have introduced enormous errors. These arrangements also contribute to a reduction in mean errors. We noted larger mean errors (pointing biases) when subjects' head movements were restrained by a biting board in other experiments. Biguer et al. (1984) also observed reduction in the constant error in a pointing task when their subjects' heads were free to move. These authors explained that coding of eye position was accurate only up to some small limiting eccentricity in the head. Beyond this limit, error became large. When the head was free, subjects moved it to bring the eye into the range where coding was accurate. Whatever the reason, the ballistic pointing response became more accurate when subjects could make a coordinated orienting motion of head and eyes to the target position even when the target wasn't there.

ceived location of the test target. For example, Bridgeman et al. (1979) examined whether subjects could detect a 2 deg arc shift in the position of the test target. The shift occurred during a 20 deg arc saccade. They also asked the subject to point to the target in its final location. Subjects reported seeing the shifts on approximately one-half of the trials, but pointing was accurate regardless of whether subjects reported detecting the shift. In a control experiment, Bridgeman (1983) showed that subjects could reliably report this 2 deg arc shift, as well as shifts down to 0.25 deg arc, when they were fixating and the shift was applied to a target moved by 18 deg arc to simulate target motion during a saccade. The subjects' task here was to indicate which of two target displacements was the larger when they were temporally separated by about 1 s. Certainly the extraretinal information about eye position was good enough to allow accurate pointing. However, the fact that displacements which were easily detected by the fixating eye were missed when seen during saccades led Bridgeman (1983) to argue that the extraretinal signals were degrading the subject's sensitivity to stimulus position when assessed by a more cognitive task than pointing (as in verbal reports).

Howard (1982) argued that the control condition does not duplicate exactly the saccade condition in the Bridgeman work. One difficulty was that the subject's task appeared very different in the saccade and control conditions. The control condition required the subject to make a judgement about the difference between two target jumps separated by a short time interval, while the saccade condition required an absolute judgement of the size of the eye movement and position of the target (an absolute position judgement). Absolute judgements are notoriously less accurate than relative judgements. Another complicating factor in Bridgeman's saccade condition is that it closely parallels conditions used to study saccadic dysmetria (see Optican, 1985). To study dysmetria, experimenters displace the goal target by a small amount during the saccade to simulate over- or under-shooting and mimic a problem in the peripheral oculomotor system. The paradigm produces rapid adjustment of saccade metrics. This finding leads to the suggestion that subjects failed to detect small displacements in the Bridgeman paradigm because the brain assumed that something had gone wrong in the execution of the motor program. For example, during a 20 deg arc saccade, the target was stepped 2 deg arc further in the direction of the saccade, so that at saccade offset it was 2 deg arc in peripheral retina rather than on the fovea. This could as well be interpreted as the eye only having moved 18 deg arc while the target remained stationary. It was an ambiguous situation in which the final target position on the retina could have resulted from a saccade that was too short or from an abrupt movement of the target. Which to prefer? The rapid adaptation of saccades to dysmetria (Optican, 1985) would suggest that dysmetria was the default assumption the brain made, unless the difference between the target step and the saccade was so large that some sort of proprioceptor signal indicated that dysmetria was unlikely. It is, therefore, not so clear that when subjects fail to notice a disparity between the size of their eye movements and the final position of the targets, it is necessarily due to insensitivity of the extraretinal signals.

In an alternative approach made to reconcile the discrepancy in localization accuracy measured with verbal reports and manual pointing, several investigators have proposed a kind of dualism in visual processing with a cognitive branch that has poor extraretinal information about eye position and a visuo-motor branch with good extraretinal information (Trevarthen, 1968; Skavenski and Hansen, 1978; Bridgeman et al., 1979). In fact, it can be shown that this speculation may be premature. I will return to it in a subsequent section since it has also been offered to explain differences in localization by pointing or verbal reports in studies of the quality of extraretinal signals during smooth pursuit eye movements.

4. Quality of extraretinal signals during smooth pursuit eye movements

A substantial number of experiments, beginning with Fleischl (1882), Aubert (1887) and Dodge (1904), have documented that humans regularly misperceive the path of motion of objects seen when their eyes are smoothly pursuing a different target (Festinger and Easton, 1974; Festinger et al., 1976; Mack and Herman, 1972; Sedgwick and Festinger, 1976; Stoper, 1973). Although a variety of stimulus configurations have been used, the pattern used by Dodge (1904) had much in common with many of them. Specifically, the subject tracked a stimulus light moving sinusoidally. A second moving stimulus was presented and it was moving through the same amplitude but 180 degrees out of phase with the tracked target. If both targets were the only objects visible to the subjects, then they described the path of motion of the untracked target as being much greater than that of the tracked target ('the pendular whiplash illusion'; Carr, 1907).

4.1. Visual psychophysical judgement of object motion

More recent quantitative measurements (e.g. see Mack and Herman, 1972, 1973, 1978) showed that there was consistent under-registration of the actual eye motion during pursuit. To illustrate, Mack and Herman (1972) found that subjects underestimated both the speed and the extent of motion of objects by 10–25% when subjects viewed them while generating smooth pursuit. These errors were much larger than errors in judging the speed or extent of motion of targets seen when subjects fixated or made a saccade (Festinger and Canon, 1965). The large errors observed during smooth pursuit is known as the Aubert-Fleischl paradox. Using an anchored magnitude estimation procedure, Dichgans et al. (1975) found that the magnitude of this paradox depended on the pattern subjects viewed. Specifically, grating patterns of 30 cycles/deg produced the largest difference in apparent speed when tracked or viewed during fixation, while a single edge produced no difference.

A quantitatively similar loss of position constancy was obtained when subjects viewed a stationary background while they made smooth-pursuit eye movements (Mack and Herman, 1973). Specifically, on about 2/3 of the trials, subjects perceived stationary objects as moving in the opposite direction to the smoothly moving eye. Subjects required the object to be moved at about 20% of eye velocity to perceive the object as being stationary (Mack and Herman, 1978). This is called the Filehne illusion. These observations led to the suggestion that the extraretinal eye position signals under-represent eye motion during pursuit by approximately 20% (Mack and Herman, 1978).

All the preceding studies found only a partial loss of eye position information. There were, however, instances where the loss was total and perception completely neglected the fact that the eye was moving smoothly. Among the first of these was the report of Stoper (1973) that stimuli flashed sequentially from the same physical location to the smoothly pursuing eye resulted in the perception of motion. No motion was perceived when the flashes originted from different physical locations causing the same retinal locus to receive the flash. This result was just the opposite of that obtained by Rock and Ebenholtz (1962), who did an analogous experiment with saccadic eye movements. Taken together, these results would indicate good compensation for eye motion due to saccades and almost no compensation for smooth eye motion.

A dramatic and direct demonstration of the failure of the viewer to account for the position of the pursuing eye was obtained by Festinger et al. (1976), who used a version of Dodge's original stimulus configuration which is shown in Fig. 4. The special case shown in the figure was for horizontal sinusoidal motion of the tracked target. The untracked target moved in-phase with the tracked target and its physical path was vertical. However, when seen against a totally dark background, the untracked target was perceived to move at approximately a 45 deg angle to the path of the tracked target. In other words, it was perceived to move

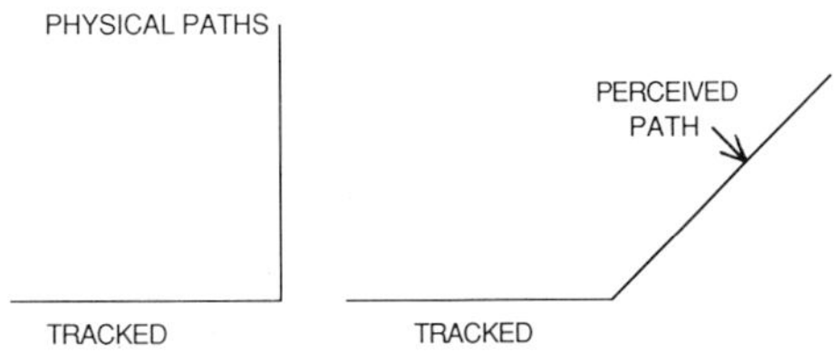

Fig. 4. Schematic drawing of the paths of two targets used to measure localization accuracy during smooth pursuit. On the left the *physical paths* of two moving targets are shown. The horizontally moving stimulus was tracked by the subject, who then judged the direction of motion of the vertically moving target. On the right is shown the most frequent verbal description subjects give for the *perceived path* of motion of the untracked target.

along a path very close to the path of its image on the retina. Festinger et al. (1976) found that this was true for many paths other than the one illustrated. Thus, visual perception of the motion path appeared to incorporate very little information about the movement of the eye (Festinger et al., 1976).

Much the same conclusion was reached by Becklen et al. (1984) when they replicated portions of the Festinger et al. experiment. Becklen et al. (1984) asked their subjects to adjust the orientation of a rod to match the perceived path of a vertically moving, untracked target. The tracked target consisted of a point or a field a vertical lines moving horizontally. Perceived paths were always much closer to the path of the retinal image than to the objective path of the untracked target. This illusion of perceived tilt disappeared when the subjects tracked the target whose path they were to judge. However, when the display was changed so that both the tracked and untracked targets moved vertically in the presence of horizontally moving lines, Wallach et al. (1985) found very good compensation for the smooth-pursuit eye movements. Here the horizontal motion of the grating induced a constant horizontal component in the paths of the vertically moving targets so they were seen as moving on an oblique path. The perceived obliqueness of the path did not vary when subjects tracked the target whose path they were judging or tracked the other target. This means that there was very good compensation for the pursuit because the perceived tilt did not vary when pursuit made the retinal image motion of the untracked target greater or less than its objective motion. Wallach et al. (1985) offered no explanation about why components of image motion caused by pursuit can be subtracted out when the target is moving colinearly with eye motion but not for targets moving in other diretions. Earlier, Bacon et al. (1982) had shown that the shift in the perceived location of a dot, in the presence of an inducing stimulus, depended on the inducing pattern shifting its center relative to the test target. When the same pattern was moved behind a target-centered window, it also induced perceived motion in the target, but subjects' performance, assessed by a pointing task, showed that they continued to perceive the target's location veridically (Bacon et al., 1982). Wallach and his coworkers used the center-aligned display for experiments with moving gratings, and it was possible that it lacked effectiveness in generating shifts in perceived location because compensation is easier when the stimulus pattern is simple. But there were other questions as well.

Recently, Swanston and Wade (1988) repeated the 2-moving-dot version of the foregoing experiments using a much more extensive set of motion paths. They compared the accuracy in setting a rod to the path of target motion when subjects fixated or tracked a second target with smooth-pursuit eye or with translatory head motions. Subjects were very accurate in setting the rod to the objective path of the untracked target in most of the smooth-pursuit conditions, including those of Festinger et al. (1976) and Becklen et al. (1984). Their results show an average of about 95% compensation for the smooth pursuit. Swanston et al. (1988) claimed that they found more compensation for the pursuing eye than previous investigators did because their tracking target moved through an amplitude 3 times that of the judged target. In fact, when they reduced the amplitude of tracked to judged motion to 1:1, the compensation for the pursuit dropped to about 70%. Nevertheless, the result was clearly in conflict with that of Festinger et al. (1976) and Becklen et al. (1984).

Unfortunately, there are two unresolved concerns about the recent work of Becklen, Wallach, Bacon, Swanston and their coworkers. One is that eye movements were not recorded in any of these experiments. Mostly naive subjects were tested and it was not known whether they performed the tracking as well as they could have. Subjects in the Swanston et al. (1988) study may not have smoothly pursued the tracking target at all, and therefore would have no eye movement component in the retinal image motion. Becklen et al. (1984), on the other hand, may have obtained good tracking in their more experienced subjects. This could account for the discrepancy in the results of the two studies. There is another possibility. Namely, all subjects pursued very well but were operating under different implied instructions about how to make the psychophysical judgements. None of the reports contained details about how the subjects were instructed to make their judgements. This is important because it is well known that the subjects' set can influence how they perform complex perceptual tasks. In the present case, Becklen et al.'s (1984) subjects could have assumed that they were to describe retinal image motion since that was easy to do. Swanston and Wade's (1988) subjects might have assumed that they were to make judgements relative to their bodies. Combined, these two issues preclude any firm conclusions, except that potentially complex methodological issues need to be resolved.

4.2. Pointing judgement of moving object location

Instructions to subjects were probably less ambiguous in an experiment by Hansen (1979) because a motor, rather than a perceptual, task was used to measure perceived location of targets. The motor task would encourage judgements to be made relative to the body rather than to other parts of the retinal image. Hansen asked subjects to try to strike moving targets with a hammer. The targets were exposed only when the subjects were smoothly pursuing another target. Eye movements were recorded with the magnetic-field search-coil technique hav-

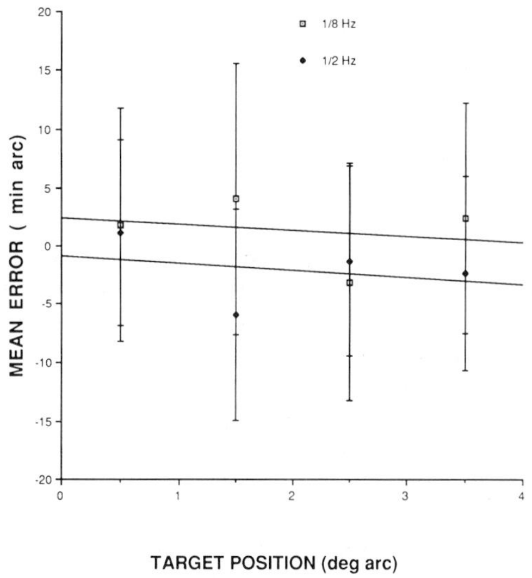

Fig. 5. Mean Error, the distance of the mean position of hammer blows struck at stimuli flashed on at various *Target Positions* along the vertical path shown on the left in Fig. 4. Subject J.C. tracked the horizontally moving stimulus at 1/8 and 1/2 Hz. Each mean was based on 8 hammer blows and error bars show + 1 SEM. Linear regression lines fitted to each frequency of tracking have nearly zero slope. It should be noted that these lines would be expected to have +1 slope if the ballistic pointing had matched the subject's verbal description from other reports. Other features as in Fig. 3.

ing a sensitivity of 5 min arc. Targets for hammer blows were shown either superimposed over the tracking target for 10 ms, or continuously under viewing conditions duplicating those of Festinger et al. (1976) (see Fig. 4). In both conditions, hammer blows landed within about 15 minutes of arc of the target position. Fig. 5 shows representative data obtained from one subject when the target to be struck moved orthogonally to the tracked target. A tone sounded when the subject was to hit the untracked target. Responses were sorted according to physical target position at the time the tone sounded and mean errors were calculated for each target position. As can be seen, the data were best fit by a horizontal line, rather than the oblique that would have been expected if localization was based solely on the retinal image position of the untracked target. Using these data, Hansen (1979) estimated that compensation for the position of the smoothly moving eye was good to 95–97% in this localization task. In a demonstration, Hansen (1979) also tested perceived location using a psychophysical task. He provided subjects with control over the path of motion of the untracked target using the viewing conditions of Fig. 4. The untracked target was exposed only when subjects were tracking the horizontal target. Hansen (1979) required subjects to adjust the path of the untracked target so that it appeared parallel to their midsaggital planes. He found that they were very accurate in doing so, in spite of the fact that they were experiencing the illusion that it was moving at an oblique angle to the tracked target.

In a recent report, Bedell and Klopfenstein (ARVO, 1988) found that subjects could accurately point to targets that were flashed briefly in total darkness when subjects were undergoing the primary phase of optokinetic afternystagmus. Optokinetic afternystagmus is a smooth movement, but it is more primitive, phylogenetically older and more 'reflexive' than smooth pursuit.

The findings of Hansen (1979) and Bedell and Klopfenstein (1988) dealing with localization during smooth eye movements, like those for saccades in section 3.3, point to a difference in localization accuracy depending on the kind of response required of the subject. Motor responses yield much better compensation for eye position than do visual judgements of perceived direction or position. In fact, Honda (1985) compared visual judgements and pointing responses to targets which were stepped to elicit a saccade or moved smoothly to elicit smooth pursuit. There were large, idiosyncratic response biases in the pointing responses which prevented comparison of the accuracy of the responses. Nevertheless, subjects showed few differences in pointing to the final position of a target whether they acquired it with a saccade or tracked it there with pursuit. There were, however, consistent differences between the saccade and pursuit eye movement conditions when subjects set the separation of two LEDs to match the extent of visually perceived motion. The extent of the displacement was always judged larger when seen on a saccade trial than when it was pursued.

One potential difficulty with comparing motor responses with perceptual reports and performance during saccades with smooth pursuit might be that the decay of spatial memory may again be intruding. During pursuit, subjects must integrate motion that continues for several seconds to estimate the final position or extent of motion of the target. During saccades, on the other hand, changes in position are abrupt so temporal integration of motion signals may not be needed. Perhaps the reduced demands on spatial memory, resulting from the reduced need for temporal integration of retinal displacements during saccades, accounts for why perceived location during saccades is reported to be more accurate than perceived location during pursuit. Pointing judgements require only that the subject indicates where the target is at the instant the response is made. Pointing does not require the subject to judge the extent of motion, which requires the subject to know where the target has been. Thus, it appears that the pointing response may not rely on spatial memory and, for this reason, may yield more accurate localization responses than does verbal report or target motion seen with the smoothly pursuing eye.

To complicate matters a bit further, there is at least one report in which findings were obtained that were opposite to those described above. Mitrani et al. (1979) asked subjects to track a stimulus moving at constant velocity. Arrangements were made for the stimulus to disappear at a randomly chosen place along its path and subjects attempted to report the location of the disappearance on a clearly visible ruler. Subjects also consistently made saccades back towards the place of target disappearance without explicit instruction to do so. The offset position of corrective saccades showed a consistent 2 deg arc error in the direction of the smooth movement. This would imply insufficient compensation for the smooth eye movements. In contrast, reported position of disappearance was displaced by 2 deg arc, also in direction of target movement, only for targets that disappeared early in the ramp. Error in reporting the position of disappearance systematically decreased to zero for targets that disappeared near the end of the ramp. Mitrani et al. (1979) argued that this resulted from a dissociation of motor and perceptual localization of the tracked target, with the former being determined by a 'primitive' motor programmer, and the latter by higher centers which are subject to 'set and expectation'. Alternatively, the corrective saccades may not imply different localization mechanisms, but may simply have reflected the tendency to undershoot targets for saccades (Becker and Fuchs, 1969, noted in section 2).

Post and Leibowitz (1985) have offered a model which is quite specific regarding the way the 'cognitive' and motor localization systems make use of the efference copy that contributes to motion perception. The model is summarized here because it has been applied to visual localization (e.g. see Bridgeman, 1986) and it deals explicitly with the source of efference copy signals. Post and Leibowitz (1985) hypothesized that the efference copy signal used for perception is derived from the oculomotor commands to generate smooth-pursuit eye movements. Moreover, they proposed that the signals used to generate compensatory vestibular and optokinetic nystagmus do not contribute. They argue that the phylogenetically older compensatory systems were designed to stabilize the eyes in space during body motion (after Walls, 1961; Robinson, 1981). Post et al. (1985) argued that if these signals contributed to the perception of motion, then observers would see the stationary world as moving whenever they moved so as to produce compensatory eye movements. The phylogenetically newer pursuit system is different. It was designed to maintain fixation of moving objects, and, consequently, it was essential that the movement commands issued by this system contribute to motion perception. Post et al. (1985) indicate that such a system accounts for a large number of illusory motion phenomena. They described a number of examples, one of which is reviewed here.

In the Duncker illusion (induced motion), a small stationary object, seen on a moving background or surrounded by a moving frame, will be seen as moving while the frame will be seen as stationary. Post et al. (1985) claimed that the larger moving image generated optokinetic nystagmus which was not signalled at a perceptual level, but which was cancelled by an opposite-going pursuit movement. The efferent copy signals accompanying the pursuit commands do affect perception. Therefore, the smaller object, which was 'pursued', was seen as moving. If indeed the system works this way, then the Post et al. (1985) reasoning raises a set of dilemmas. Specifically, the model deals only with motion perception relative to the head. As noted in the introduction, a complete system to process motion and position must also incorporate signals indicating how the head and body move relative to each other and in space. It would seem counterproductive for nature to have evolved good oculomotor compensation for head/body movement via OKN and VOR, and not have provided a means of knowing where the objects were located or how they were moving. There are also data on this subject.

One straightforward prediction made by the Post et al. (1985) model is that a textured drum moving about the subject would not be perceived as moving when subjects track it with OKN. In fact, motion is perceived, and quite often the perception is that it is the self moving relative to the stationary environment (Dichgans and Brandt, 1978). So, obviously, subjects are perceiving some sort of motion, and an internal motion signal must be generated by the stimulus that supposedly produces the optokinetic response. Visual information is needed to help the organism organize its relationship to the environment because the vestibular system is poor at signalling sustained constant motions (see Simpson and Graf, 1985, and Young, 1985, for reviews of this topic). With this in mind, one could view the Duncker illusion as arising because movements of the frame contributed information that the head/body was moving relative to the environment. Since the dot was continuously fixated with the same part of the retina without eye motion it must have been moving with the subject. Such an interpretation is as plausible as the Post et al. (1985) explanation and it seems to take more of the facts into account.

5. Source of extraretinal signals

The work described in previous sections makes it clear that some extraretinal information was available for visual localization under impoverished viewing conditions in which visual cues alone would be insufficient to judge object location. Several investigations (beginning with Helmholtz, 1925) have been aimed at revealing what kind of nonretinal cues to eye position were involved. Helmholtz noted that when one passively deviated the eye, or restrained the eye and attempted to make an eye movement, the visual world was perceived to move. The reader can readily verify the latter by pressing the outer canthus of one eye while observing the environment with the other eye closed. Helmholtz argued that objects changed position during passive deviations because there was a shift in the position of the retinal image without an accompanying signal to indicate eye rotation, i.e., there was no sensory (proprioceptive) registration of eye rotation (i.e. 'inflow'). Recently, Bridgeman (1985) questioned Helmholtz's interpretation. He found that during an eye press, the subject maintains fixation of a single point by changing the innervation to the extraocular muscles to overcome the eye press. The change in innervation made the eye press very similar to the condition in which the subject attempted to move a restrained eye in that there was a change in the motor program to the eye muscles without an accompanying change in the position of the retinal image.

5.1. Location judgements with inflow and outflow decoupled by loads

Helmholtz's observations were replicated in qualitative form using different paradigms (Brindley and Merton, 1960; Irvine and Ludvigh, 1936) and led to the consensus that the extraretinal signal for the perception of direction was derived from the commands sent to the muscles (i.e. 'outflow'). These early experiments, however, did not provide quantitative comparisons of the relationship between shifts in perceived direction and the changes in the commands sent to the eye muscles and, consequently, left open the possibility that there was partial compensation by an inflowing sensory signal. That possibility was eliminated in an experiment by Skavenski et al. (1972), who applied known loads to an eye by means of a suction contact lens. Perceived direction of a target was measured when the eye was passively deviated by the load, or when the innervation was changed to compensate for the load and keep the eye in the same position. Under both circumstances, perceived direction varied directly with the loads and, consequently, the commands sent to the eye muscles. There was no evidence for partial compensation by an inflowing signal. The result further strengthened the conclusion that the extraretinal signal for the visual perception of direction was based on the commands sent to the eye muscles.

5.2. Pharmacological decoupling of inflow and outflow

One difficulty with the monocular loading experiments (Skavenski et al., 1972; Stark and Bridgeman, 1983; to be described below) is that it places inflow signals from the loaded eye in conflict with inflow from the other eye and outflow to both eyes. It is conceivable that the brain ignores these contradictory inflowing signals entirely. Systemic pharmacological blocking of neuromuscular junctions is probably the only technique which will separate inflow from outflow while maintaining interocular consistency within the two signals. The procedure has been performed in several labs, and most recently by Matin et al. (1982). In their experiment, subjects were partially curarized while they attempted to fixate targets placed at various horizontal and vertical positions relative to the head. A second target was adjusted so that its perceived location fell on the subject's median plane at horizontal eye level. Results shown in Fig. 6 indicate that subjects perceived the fixation target to be displaced linearly as a function of the eccentricity of the fixation target relative to head position, and the magnitude of perceived displacement was much

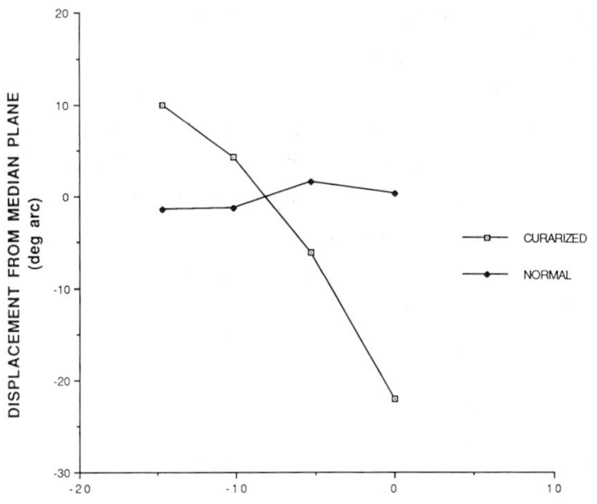

Fig. 6. Positions of a target subject L.M. had adjusted to coincide with his median plane (plotted as *displacement from median plane*) when he looked at a lamp in various *fixation positions* while *curarized* or *normal* (drug-free). The nearly horizontal arrangement of the data under normal viewing indicates veridical perception of the location of the fixation targets. The marked negative slope obtained under curare indicated that the increased innervation to the eye muscles to overcome the neuromuscular block caused the subject to see the fixation lamp as being further displaced from the median plane than it actually was. Data redrawn from Matin et al. (1982).

larger than the actual physical displacement. This result was obtained only when the paralysed subject was in the dark, and not when the room was normally illuminated. It was not obtained with unparalysed subjects in the light or in the dark. Subjects were also asked to match the location of a sound source to the perceived location of the fixation targets. Auditory-visual matches indicated that when the subjects were curarized, they perceived the visual targets to be displaced by much more than their physical eccentricity relative to the head in both dark and light. Among the conclusions Matin et al. (1982) drew was that the data were inconsistent with inflow (proprioception) as the sole source of the eye position signals because the localizations performed in the dark indicated that the eye was perceived to be rotated further than it actually was in the curarized state. In other words, when curarized, subjects had to change oculomotor innervation by a much larger amount than they would ordinarily require to fixate an eccentric target, and, consequently, localized the target at a much larger eccentricity. One limitation of this paradigm is that it does not provide a quantitative measure of the magnitude of the change in oculomotor innervation (outflow). As a result, partial compensation by an inflow signal could not be ruled out (Matin et al., 1982). At this juncture it seems clear that inflow plays a modest role, if any, in visual localization.

Matin and co-workers also drew additional conclusions from their results with curarized subjects that deal with the contribution of retinal and extraretinal signals to localization. Specifically, they tried to explain the paradox that curarized subjects mislocalize only in the dark or when making auditory-visual matches by assuming that extraretinal eye position signals were used for these judgements but were superseded by visual signals when the full visual field was present (Matin et al., 1982, 1983). These authors extended their hypothesis to suggest that under normal viewing conditions people make their visual localizations solely on the basis of retinal information and that extraretinal signals are not involved (Matin et al., 1983b, p244), a phenomenon some have labelled 'visual capture' (Stark and Bridgeman, 1983).

This last conclusion of Matin et al. (1983) was not supported by an experiment by Stark and Bridgeman (1983), who used a finger press on one eye to dissociate its inflow and outflow signals. The magnitude of the dissociation was estimated from an independent experiment in which they measured the displacement of the nonpressed and nonseeing yoked eye to estimate the change in innervation to the seeing and pressed eye, a procedure which leaves uncertain the actual change in outflow at the time judgements of direction were made. It was also a procedure that produced very modest changes in the outflow signals (about 2 deg arc). Nevertheless, outflow signals did influence judgements of visual direction both in the dark, and when the room was normally illuminated, while the eye was pressed and subjects pointed with the unseen hand to the fixation target or matched the position of an unseen sound source to the target. Eye press also biased setting of a target to the subjective 'straight-ahead' in the dark, but not in the normally illuminated room. Stark et al. (1983) concluded that only in the latter condition has visual capture superseded the offset produced by corollary discharge signals.

Seen from a somewhat different perspective, these experiments also allow suggestions about the nature of 'visual capture'. As noted above, several authors (e.g. Howard, 1982) have cited the difficulties in using localization data in normal illumination because subjects could simply align the target and pointer images visually in spite of what they actually perceive to be the position of the target relative to themselves. In setting the straight-ahead position, subjects could note some visible feature of the scene that was straight ahead before the press and then align the marker to that feature while pressing. In fact, when Bridgeman (1986) used an illuminated environment made up of similar bars, the perceived straight-ahead position shifted as the eye was pressed just as it did in the dark. In all situations where direct vision of the pointing arm was prevented (e.g. Stark and Bridgeman, 1983), or an unseen auditory stimulus was used as a marker, perceived location was seen to closely follow the extraretinal signals. The point of this discussion is that most localization experiments have been done in the dark to prevent subjects from using cues in the retinal images to align targets and pointers. One could argue that accurate pointing in the light in the paralysed state was the illusory situation, and not the mislocalizations seen in the dark as Matin and co-workers (1982) have argued. Put together, the foregoing arguments show that 'visual capture' during paralysis may not necessarily mean that extraretinal eye position signals are ignored or neglected during localization in a lighted environment by unparalysed viewers.

5.3. Location judgements after surgical realignment of eye muscles

Returning to the main issue of this section, which is concerned with the source of the extraretinal signals used in localization, Steinbach and Smith (1981) were perhaps the only investigators to report that inflow signals influence the visual perception of direction. In their experiment, 14 patients, who had undergone strabismus surgery with large monocular shifts of eye position relative to extraocular muscle coordinates, were tested for accuracy of pointing with the unseen hand to 3 visible target positions. Measurements were made before surgery, and from 7 to 48 hours after surgery, when the bandages were first removed from the operated eye. In 8 out of 9 patients having their first strabismus surgery, postoperative pointing error for targets seen by the operated eye was only about 25% of the angle the eye had been physically rotated on the muscles (Steinbach and Smith, 1981). The remaining 5 patients who were tested had one or more previous strabismus surgeries on the tested eye. In these patients post-operative pointing errors coincided with the amount the eye had been rotated by repositioning the insertions of the extraocular muscles. The authors account for these results by suggesting that the patients with no prior surgical experience must have used an inflow signal as the extraretinal signal for visual localization, or at least that the inflow was used to recalibrate the relation between ouflow and actual eye position under the bandage because the patients had no visual experience between surgery and testing. Recovery from prior surgery prevented the remaining patient group from having access to the inflow information, and, consequently, their pointing errors were consistent with outflow and the preoperative relation between muscles and eye position (Steinbach and Smith, 1981).

The Steinbach and Smith (1981) result refuted previous anecdotal evidence of 'past pointing' (mislocalization) that was consistent with the use of outflow signals (Ambrose and von Noorden, 1976). Steinbach's result was surprising to many, including the investigators. There was no clear means by which an inflow signal from receptors located in the muscle could provide quantitative information about the magnitude of the eye rotation relative to the muscles (Boch and Kommerell, 1986) because the surgery has only minor effects on muscle stretch. To resolve this issue, Steinbach (1987) argued that there was a high degree of cooperation between the three pairs of extraocular muscles, and that information from the 4 or 5 untouched muscles could provide the information needed to determine how much the operated muscle was changed. However, he offered no quantitative demonstration of how this could take place. Miller and Robinson (1984) also noted that extraocular muscle surgery could result in changes in mechanoreceptor activity which could ultimately influence oculomotor innervation. In fact, Robinson's (1975) simulation of the changes in muscle length with globe position supports Steinbach's (1987) contention because there were rather substantial changes in the lengths of all of the muscles when the eye moved primarily in the plane of one of the rectus muscle pairs. For example, Robinson's (1975) Table 1 shows that the superior oblique muscle changes length compared with its length at primary position by 9.4%, 18.6% and 25.1% when the eye is elevated by 30 deg arc and is either adducted 30 deg, straight ahead horizontally, or abducted 30 deg arc, respectively. With the same eye movement on the horizon, Miller and Robinson's (1984) Squint computer model showed that both superior and inferior recti increased length by about 3 mm in going from 30 deg nasal to 30 deg temporal on the horizontal meridian (Miller, personal communication). The model also showed an increase in force of 5.5 *g* in the inferior rectus and 3.5 *g* in the superior rectus during the same movement. These were systematic changes, and the question arose whether there could be a unique mapping of the lengths of the 4 or 5 untouched eye muscles onto all possible eye positions. The Miller et al. (1984) model could provide the simulation data, but unfortunately it did not include some very recent findings on orbital mechanics which Miller (personal communication) believes could alter the simulation. In addition, there were no published reports showing contour maps of muscle length versus eye position. This all means that there is some support for Steinbach's (1987) contention that eye position can be determined from the intact muscles following surgery, but a great deal more work with models and muscle measurements would be needed to answer the question quantitatively.

An alternative source for the inflow signal which would detect how far the eye was rotated on the muscles would be some orbital mechanoreceptor that sensed a feature on the globe (e.g. the corneal bulge) and used that feature to establish the new relationship between eye position and muscle innervation. In the absence of direct evidence, it is difficult to conceive of tactual receptors with sufficient resolution to achieve that objective.

Gauthier et al. (1986) and Boch and Kommerell (1986) repeated the Steinbach and Smith (1981) experiment independently and obtained past pointing error that was consistent with the use of outflow rather than with inflow. Their patients required several days of visual experience after the operation for pointing accuracy to return to normal. Boch and Kommerell (1986) stated that the main difference in their procedure was that they used many more test target positions, which made it less likely that the subjects memorized the test positions during the preoperative evaluation. Nevertheless, one out of 14 subjects in Boch and Kommerell's pool did point accurately in spite of a 16 deg arc eye rotation from the surgery. Boch and Kommerell (1986) explained that egocentric localization tended to be quite variable in strabismic patients, and, also, that some patients admitted to memorizing the 9 positions used in the preoperative testing. Although not explicitly admitted by the patient, it was suggested that the patient with accurate pointing used spatial memory from before the operation to make postoperative judgements (Boch and Kommerell, 1986).

More recently, Steinbach (1987) noted that there was a difference in the anesthesia used in the different experiments which could account for these discrepant results. The Steinbach and Smith (1981) patients were given a general anesthetic while the Boch and Kommerell (1986) patients received retrobulbar blocks. The retrobulbar block could have disrupted inflowing stretch receptor signals completely, according to Steinbach (1987).

The main point to be drawn from this analysis is that there is some evidence, albeit controversial, supporting the notion that inflow signals may contribute to the calibration of extraretinal eye position signals (Steinbach, 1987). However, the evidence also indicates that the extraretinal signal used in localization in real time is derived from outflow (efference copy). Perhaps the only study in which it was suggested that inflow influenced spatial localization directly was Fiorentini et al.'s (1985) demonstration that cats with sections of the ophthalmic branch of the trigeminal nerve (to block inflow) were unable to use binocular cues to judge depth. When the nerve was cut, either bilaterally or unilaterally, binocular thresholds for detecting depth overlapped monocular thresholds when cats were tested on a jumping stand (Fiorentini et al., 1985). Certainly, depth is important in making localization responses to the body. However, the role of inflow in the present case was unclear. It may be involved in establishing or maintaining vergence position or in the neural processing of binocular disparity information (Fiorentini et al., 1985). In the latter case, the signals could provide information on vergence position to evaluate retinal disparity, but this remains speculative.

6. Deriving egocentric localization from visual field flow

This section is concerned with recent evidence on the localization information contained in the flow of the visual image over the retina. Long ago Gibson (1950) realized there was rich information contained in the retinal image flow produced by an animal as it moves in its environment. He argued that this information could be used by an organism to determine its relative location and motion relative to the environment and the objects within it. An enormous body of data has been compiled on motion processing since then (see Nakayama, 1985, for a review of this literature). Is there, in fact, quantitative information which would support the contention that animals, and people, determine the direction of objects relative to their bodies on the basis of retinal image flow information (as in visual capture) under normal viewing conditions?

Several investigators have extended Gibson's work by offering quantitative accounts of how the visual system could, in principle, extract both rotational and translational components of eye motion from the information based on the flow of the retinal image of a rigid environment (for examples see Lee, 1980; Longuet-Higgins and Prazdny, 1980). Lee's analysis included details about how the retinal image movement field could be scaled to body dimensions (such as the height of the eye from the ground) to permit precise visual navigation in the environment. These were theoretical accounts. In empirical tests, Regan and Beverly (1982) noted that the center of origin of the optic flow pattern during forward body motion varies substantially when the subject changes eye position and, consequently, would not serve as a reliable cue to the subject's destination. They asked whether the location of the maximum rate of change of magnification within the retinal imge could be judged accurately, since this variable is invariant with changes in gaze position. When rate of magnification was made uniform over the whole field so that the only cue was the center of origin of the flow pattern, subjects were unable to judge the direction of self motion (Regan and Beverly, 1982). This showed that the center of the flow pattern was ineffective. However, when the rate of magnification of the expanding pattern was made much greater at one place compared with the rest of the field, subjects became very accurate at judging that location (Regan and Beverley, 1982). Interestingly, threshold measurements published by Regan and Beverley (1983) indicate that an object the size of a refrigerator would be above threshold for detecting both changing size and changing disparity when it was approached at a speed of 0.5 mph, a speed well within the 'physiological range'. Clearly, these cues can and do provide important information about the depth of objects (or relative distance from the observer) in normal viewing. Depth is crucial for accurate localization of objects, even in the fronto-parallel plane, when the response requires a limb movement. This need arises because visual localization and the limb movement originate from different spatial locations. To note the obvious, the subject's hand would intersect the plane of the target with a very large error on both the horizontal and vertical meridians if the subject misjudged the depth of the target plane.

From everyday experience we all know that motion of a large portion of the visual field can lead to a profound sense that our body is moving. In the laboratory, there have been numerous demonstrations that people show compensatory body postural responses to large-field optic flow patterns presented to peripheral retina (e.g., see Dichgans and Brandt, 1978; Lee and Aronson, 1974; Stoffregen et al., 1987). In eye movement control, where the characteristics of compensation are well established with high-resolution recording, it is also well known that visual information about head motion is used in conjunction with vestibular signals to generate both compensatory eye movements and the perception of self motion (e.g., see review by Dichgans and Brandt, 1978). The need for this synergy arises because the labyrinths are useful in providing only the higher-frequency components of head motion (Fernandez and Goldberg, 1971) and visual signals are needed to signal the sustained DC components of head motion. There is also evidence that these two signals share many of the paths that drive the eye (Keller and Precht, 1979; Waespe and Henn, 1977). Robinson (1977) and Raphan et al. (1977) have proposed a mechanism for combining visual and vestibular signals to provide the oculomotor system with the best estimate of the velocity of the head in space and, thereby, improve the quality of ocular compensation for this movement. Although there is no direct experimental proof that these signals are combined in that fashion, the model does account for a great deal of the physiology. An efficient way to compute the velocity of an object in space would be to add the best estimate of head velocity in space to a signal indicating velocity of the object relative to the head, obtained by adding eye velocity in the head (an extraretinal signal) to retinal image velocity of the object. This is efficient because all of these signals are present and are used by the nervous system (e.g., see review by Nakayama, 1985; and by Robinson, 1977, on oculomotor control systems).

Current understanding suggests that cues about relative location and depth can be extracted from the environment best when the observer is moving. There appear to be no theoretical accounts that permit extracting location from the stationary visual field. Investigators who emphasize the importance of the optic flow field in the perception of visual space often note that animals are constantly in motion. They overlook the fact that there are times when the body is relatively motionless and yet localization must be good. One well documented example was the paralysed subjects in the Matin et al. (1982) study who were able to accurately localize targets when the room lights were on and when they were motionless on a stretcher. There were no apparent visual cues that allowed them to do this other than the fact that they were simply aligning the pointer and the target with each other or with a common feature in the room. Certainly there was insufficient optic flow to provide reliable cues to position. Another is a case reported by Zihl et al. (1983) of a patient with bilateral brain damage and an accompanying almost pure loss of movement vision in all three dimensions. In detailed psychophysical tests, the patient showed normal performance in a variety of tasks, including localization in depth, as long as the targets were not moving. When they did move smoothly at more than a few deg arc/s, she could not follow them or predict where they would be. She would see moving objects as frozen at points along the movement path. The example indicates that the ability to completely process motion in the flow field is not essential to veridical localization of static objects no matter how disabling the disorder may be to navigation in the normal environment.

7. Conclusions

This chapter has reviewed several experiments on manual pointing which supported the existence of an extraretinal signal that remains quite faithful to eye position, even during rapid eye motions, and is, therefore, of value in accurate localization of objects. On the other hand, much psychophysical evidence has characterized the extraretinal eye position signal as so sloppy and sluggish that it would have a minimal role in normal visual localization. In some respects this latter outcome seems unlikely given the high degree of accuracy and precision of oculomotor control, which could, in principle, mean that accurate and precise copies of the commands are available within the nervous system. Another observation which might inspire confidence that extraretinal (outflow) signals are important for localization comes from Helmholtz's classical demonstration summarized earlier. Readers are now invited to try it for themselves if they have not already done so. Close one eye and fixate an object in the field with the other. Note the position of that object. Then press the outer canthus of the open eye with your finger. You should notice that you can maintain fixation on the object, but it, as well as the whole visual field, has shifted position. Bridgeman (1985) has shown that fixation of the object is maintained by changing the innervation pattern sent to the eye being pressed so as to overcome the external rotational force applied to the eye by the finger. The eye does not change position in the head, except for a small amount of translation. The image does not shift position on the retina. The only change is in the commands sent to the eye, and, presumably, efferent copies of these commands. The fact that we perceive a shift in position of a normal visual scene implies that the efference copy has a profound influence on the perception of visual direction. The observation, of course, is quite old! It has been cited by many authors.

The root of the controversy about the role of the extraretinal signals in visual localization may be the differences in the way the subjects approach the localization task. Knowing the subject's approach to the task may be critical in interpreting the experimental results because different localization tasks place different kinds of demands on the subject. For example, setting a visible marker to the perceived location of a test target may encourage subjects to localize solely in a retinal frame of reference. On the other hand, pointing to or hitting a target, which requires localization relative to the head and body, may encourage localization in a head or body frame of reference. It would now be of interest to begin to test this 'frame-of-reference' hypothesis. If we are to understand spatial localization, we must understand precisely which factors control and limit the subject's ability to shift from one to another frame of reference, and to discover what makes a retinal frame of reference valuable in some cases and detrimental in others.

References

Ambrose, P.S. and von Noorden, G.K. (1976) Past pointing in comitant strabismus. Arch. Ophthalmol. 94, 1896–1898.

Arend, L. (1976) Temporal determinants of the form of the spatial contrast threshold MTF. Vision Res. 16, 1035–1042.

Aubert, H. (1887) Die Bewegungsempfindungen. Pflugers Arch. Ges. Physiol. 40, 459–480.

Bacon, J.H., Gordon, A. and Schulman, P.H. (1982) The effect of two types of induced-motion displays on perceived location of the induced target. Percept. Psychophys. 32, 353–359.

Becker, W. and Fuchs, A. (1969) Further properties of the human saccadic system: Eye movement and correction saccades with and without visual fixation points. Vision Res. 9, 1247–1257.

Becklen, R., Wallach, H. and Nitzberg, D. (1984) A limitation of position constancy. J. Exp. Psychol. Hum. Percept. Performance 10, 713–723.

Bedell, H. and Klopfenstein, J. (1988) Eye position information for involuntary eye movement: optokinetic afternystagmus. Invest. Ophthalmol. Vis. Sc. 29, 133.

Biguer, B., Prablanc, C. and Jeannerod, M. (1984) The contribution of coordinated eye and head movements in hand pointing accuracy. Exp. Brain res. 55, 462–469.

Bischof, N. and Kramer, E. (1968) Untersuchungen und Uberlegungen zur Richtungswahrnehmung bei Willkurlichen sakkadischen Augenbewegungen. Psychol. Forsch. 32, 185–218.

Bock, O. (1986) Contribution of retinal versus extraretinal signals towards visual localization in goal-directed movements. Exp. Brain Res. 64, 476–482.

Bock, O. and Kommerell, G. (1986) Visual localization after

strabismus surgery is compatible with 'outflow' theory. Vision Res. 26; 1825–1829.
Bridgeman, B. (1983) Mechanisms of space constancy. In: A. Hein and J. Jeannerod (Eds.), Spatially Oriented Behavior. Springer-Verlag, New York, Berlin, pp. 263–279.
Bridgeman, B. (1986) Multiple sources of outflow in processing spatial information. Acta Psychol. 63, 35–48.
Bridgeman, B. and Fishman, R. (1985) Dissociation of corollary discharge for gaze position does not induce a straight-ahead shift. Percept. Psychophys. 37, 523–528.
Bridgeman, B., Hendry, D. and Stark, L. (1975) Failure to detect displacement of the visual world during saccadic eye movements. Vision Res. 15, 719–722.
Bridgeman, B., Lewis, S., Heit, G. and Nagle, M. (1979) Relation between cognitive and motor oriented systems of visual position perception. J. Exp. Psychol. Hum. Percept. Performance 5, 692–700.
Brindley, G. and Merton, P. (1960): The absence of position sense in the human eye. J. Physiol. Lond. 153, 127–130.
Bruce, V. and Green, P.R. (1985) Visual Perception Physiology. Psychology and Ecology. L. Erlbaum Associates, London.
Carr, H. (1907) The pendular whiplash illusion. Psychol. Rev. 14, 169–180.
Collewijn, H., Erkelens, C. and Steinman, R. (1988a) Binocular coordination of human horizontal saccadic eye movements. J. Physiol. Lond. 404, 157–182.
Collewijn, H., Erkelens, C. and Steinman, R. (1988b) Binocular coordination of human vertical saccadic eye movements. J. Physiol. Lond. 404, 183–197.
Dichgans, J. and Brandt, T. (1978) Visual-vestibular interaction: Effects on self-motion perception and postural control. In: R. Held, H. Leibowitz and H. Teuber (Eds.), Handbook of Sensory Physiology. Springer, New York, pp. 755–804.
Dichgans, J., Wist, E., Diener, H.C. and Brandt, T. (1975) The Aubert-Fleischl Phenomenon: a temporal frequency effect on perceived velocity in afferent motion perception. Exp. Brain Res. 23, 529–533.
Dodge, R. (1904) The participation of eye movements in the visual perception of motion. Psychol. Rev. 11, 1–14.
Erkelens, C., Collewijn, H. and Steinman, R.M. (1989) Asymmetrical adaptation of human saccades to anisometropic spectacles. Invest. Ophthalmol. Vis. Sci. 30, 1132–1145.
Fernandez, C. and Goldberg, J.M. (1971) Physiology of the peripheral neurons innervating semicircular canals of the squirrel monkey. II. Responses to sinusoidal stimulation and dynamics of peripheral vestibular system. J. Neurophysiol. 34, 661–675.
Festinger, L. and Canon, L.K. (1965) Information about spatial location based on knowledge about efference. Psychol. Rev. 72, 373–384.
Festinger, L. and Easton, A.M. (1974) Inferences about the efferent system based on a perceptual illusion produced by eye movements. Psychol. Rev. 81, 44–58.
Festinger, L., Sedgwick, A. and Holtzman, J.D. (1976) Visual perception during smooth pursuit eye movements. Vision Res. 16, 1377–1386.
Fiorentini, A., Maffei, L., Cenni, M. and Tacchi, A. (1985) Deafferentation of oculomotor proprioception affects depth discrimination in adult cats. Exp. Brain Res. 59, 296–301.
Fleischl, E.V. (1882) Physioloisch-optische Notizen. Akad. Wiss. Wien. Abs. 3, 86, 17–25.
Gauthier, G., Berard, P., Deransard, J., Semmlow, J. and Vercher, J. (1986) Adaptation processes resulting from surgical correction of strabismus. In: E. Keller and D. Zee (Eds.), Adaptive Processes in Visual and Oculomotor Systems. Pergamon Press, Oxford, pp. 185–189.
Gibson, J.J. (1950) The perception of the visual world. Houghton-Mifflin, Boston.
Grusser, O.J. (1986a) Interaction of efferent and afferent signals in visual perception. A history of ideas and experimental paradigms. Acta Psychol. 63, 3–21.
Grusser, O.J. (1986b) Some recent studies on the quantitative analysis of efference copy mechanisms in visual perception. Acta Psychol. 63, 49–62.
Hallett, P.E. and Lightstone, A.D. (1976a) Saccadic eye movements towards stimuli triggered by prior saccades. Vision Res. 16, 99–106.
Hallett, P.E. and Lightstone, A.D. (1976b) Saccadic eye movements to flashed targets. Vision Res. 16, 107–114.
Hansen, R.M. (1979) Spatial localization during pursuit eye movements. Vision Res. 19, 1213–1221.
Hansen, R.H. and Skavenski, A.A. (1977) Accuracy of eye position information for motor control. Vision Res. 17, 919–926.
Hansen, R.M. and Skavenski, A.A. (1985) Accuracy of spatial localizations near the time of saccadic eye movements. Vision Res. 25, 1077–1082.
Helmholtz, H. (1925) Treatise on Physiological Optics; Translation by J.P. Southall. Dover, New York.
Honda, H. (1984) Eye-position signals in successive saccades. Percept. Psychophys. 36, 15–20.
Honda, H. (1985) Spatial localization in saccade and pursuit eye movement conditions: a comparison of perceptual and motor measures. Percept. Psychophys. 38, 41–46.
Howard, I. (1982) Human Visual Orientation. Wiley, New York.
Irvine, S. and Ludvigh, E. (1936) Is ocular proprioceptive sense concerned in vision? Arch. Ophthalmol. 15, 1037–1049.
Jeannerod, M., Kennedy, H. and Magnin, M. (1979) Corollary discharge: its possible implications in visual and oculomotor interactions. Neuropsychologia 17, 241–258.
Keller, E. and Precht, W. (1979) Adaptive modification of central vestibular neurons in response to visual stimulation through reversing prisms. J. Neurophysiol. 42, 896–911.
Kelley, D.H. (1979) Motion and vision. II. Stabilized spatio-temporal transfer surface. J. Opt. Soc. Am. 69, 1340–1349.
Koenderink, J.J. and van Doorn, A.J. (1981) Exterospecific component of the motion parallax field. J. Opt. Soc. Am. 71, 953–957.

Lee, D.N. (1980) The optic flow field: the foundation of vision. Phil. Trans. R. Soc. Lond. B 290, 169–179.

Lee, D.N. and Aronson, E. (1974) Visual proprioceptive control of standing in human infants. Percept. Psychophys. 15, 529–532.

Longuet-Higgins, H.C. and Prazdny, K. (1980) The interpretation of a moving retinal image. Proc. R. Soc. Lond. B 208, 385–397.

Mack, A. and Herman, E. (1972) A new illusion: the underestimation of distance during pursuit eye movements. Percept. Psychophys. 12, 471–473.

Mack, A. and Herman, E. (1973) Position constancy during pursuit eye movement: an investigation of the Filehne Illusion. Q. J. Exp. Psychol. 25, 71–84.

Mack, A. and Herman, E. (1978) The loss of position constancy during pursuit eye movements. Vision Res. 18, 55–62.

Mateeff, S. (1978) Saccadic eye movements and localization of visual stimuli. Percept. Psychophysics 24, 215–224.

Matin, E. (1974) Saccadic suppression: a review and an analysis. Psychol. Bull. 81, 899–917.

Matin, L. (1972) Eye movements and perceived visual direction. In: D. Jameson and L.M. Hurvich (Eds.). Handbook of Sensory Physiology: Visual Psychophysics. Springer Verlag, Berlin, pp. 331–380.

Matin, L. and Pearce, D.G. (1965) Visual perception of direction for stimuli flashed during voluntary saccadic eye movements. Science 148, 1485–1488.

Matin, L., Matin, E. and Pearce, D. (1969) Visual perception of direction when voluntary saccades occur. I. Relation of visual direction of a fixation target extinguished before a saccade to a flash presented during the saccade. Percept. Psychophys. 5, 65–80.

Matin, L., Matin, E. and Pearce, D. (1970a) Eye movements in the dark during the attempt to maintain a prior fixation position. Vision Res. 10, 837–857.

Matin, L., Matin, E. and Pola, J. (1970b) Visual perception of direction when voluntary saccades occur. II. Relation of visual direction of a fixation target extinguished before a saccade to a subsequent test flash presented after the saccade. Percept. Psychophys. 8, 9–14.

Matin, L., Picoult, E., Stevens, J., Edwards, M. and MacArthur, R. (1982) Oculoparalytic illusion: visual-field dependent spatial mislocalizations by humans partially paralyzed with curare. Science 216, 198–201.

Matin, L., Stevens, J. and Picoult, E. (1983) Perceptual consequences of experimental extraocular muscle paralysis. In: A. Hein and M. Jeannerod (Eds.), Spatially Oriented Behavior. Springer-Verlag, New York, Berlin, pp. 243–262.

Merton, P.A. (1961) Accuracy of directing the eyes and the hand in the dark. J. Physiol. Lond. 156, 555–557.

Miller, J. (1980) Information used by the perceptual and oculomotor systems regarding the amplitude of saccadic and pursuit eye movements. Vision Res. 20, 59–68.

Miller, J. and Robinson, D.A. (1984) A model of the mechanics of binocular alignment. Comput. Biomed. Res. 17, 436–470.

Mitrani, L., Dimitrov, G., Yakimoff and Mateeff, S. (1979) Oculomotor and perceptual localization during smooth eye movements. Vision Res. 19, 609–612.

Monahan, J.S. (1972) Extraretinal feedback and visual localization. Percept. Psychophys. 12, 349–353.

Morgan, C.L. (1978) Constancy of egocentric visual direction. Percept. Psychophys. 23, 61–68.

Nakayama, K. (1985) Biological image motion processing: a review. Vision Res. 25, 625–660.

Nemire, K. and Bridgeman, B. (1987) Oculomotor and skeletal motor systems share one map of visual space. Vision Res. 27, 393–400.

O'Regan, J.K. (1984) Retinal vesus extraretinal influences in flash localization during saccadic eye movements in the presence of a visible background. Percept. Psychophys. 36, 1–14.

Optican, L.M. (1985) Adaptive properties of the saccadic system. In: A. Berthoz and G. Melvill Jones (Eds.), Reviews of Oculomotor Research: Adaptive Mechanisms in Gaze Control. Elsevier, Amsterdam, pp. 71–79.

Osaka, N. (1977) Effect of refraction on perceived locus of a target in the peripheral visual field. J. Psychol. 95, 59–62.

Post, R.B. and Leibowitz, H. (1982) The effect of convergence on the vestibulo-ocular reflex and implications for perceived movement. Vision Res. 22, 461–465.

Post, R.B. and Leibowitz, H.W. (1985) A revised analysis of the role of efference in motion perception. Perception 14, 631–643.

Raphan, T., Cohen, B. and Matsuo, V. (1977) A velocity storage mechanism responsible for optokinetic nystagmus (OKN), optokinetic afternystagmus (OKAN) and vestibular nystagmus. In: R. Baker and A. Berthoz (Eds.), Control of Gaze By Brain Stem Neurons. Elsevier, Amsterdam, pp. 37–47.

Regan, D. and Beverley, K.I. (1982) How do we avoid confounding the direction we are looking and the direction we are moving? Science 215, 194–196.

Regan, D. and Beverley, K.I. (1983) Visual fields for frontal plane motion and for changing size. Vision Res. 23, 673–676.

Robinson, D.A. (1975): A quantitative analysis of extraocular muscle cooperation and squint. Invest. Ophthalmol. 14, 801–825.

Robinson, D.A. (1977) Vestibular and optokinetic symbiosis: an example of explaining by modelling. In: R. Baker and A. Berthoz (Eds.), Control of Gaze by Brain Stem Neurons. Elsevier, Amsterdam, pp. 49–58.

Rock, I. and Ebenholtz, S. (1962) Stroboscopic movement based on change of phenomenal location rather than retinal location. Am. J. Psychol. 75, 193–207.

Sedgwick, H.A. and Festingr, L. (1976) Eye movements, efference and visual perception. In: R. Monty and J. Senders (Eds.), Eye Movements and Psychological Processes, L. Erlbaum Assoc., Hillsdale, NJ, pp. 221–230.

Shebilske, W.L. (1987) An ecological efference mediation theory of natural event perception. In: H. Heuer and A.F. Sanders

(Eds.), Perspectives on Perception and Action, L. Erlbaum Assoc., Hillsdale, NJ, pp. 195–213.

Simpson, J. and Graf, W. (1985) The selection of reference frames by nature and its investigators. In: A. Berthoz and G. Melvill Jones (Eds.), Reviews of Oculomotor Research: Adaptive Mechanisms in Gaze Control. Elsevier, Amsterdam, pp. 3–16.

Skavenski, A.A. (1971) Extraretinal correction and memory for target position. Vision Res. 11, 743–746.

Skavenski, A.A. (1972) Inflow as a source of extraretinal eye position information. Vision Res. 12, 221–229.

Skavenski, A.A. (1976) The nature and role of extraretinal eye position information in visual localization. In: R.A. Monty and J.W. Senders (Eds.), Eye Movement and Psychological Processes. L. Erlbaum Assoc., Hillsdale, NJ, pp. 277–287.

Skavenski, A.A. and Hansen, R.M. (1978) Role of eye position information in visual space perception. In: J.W. Senders, D.F. Fisher and R.A. Monty (Eds.), Eye Movements and the Higher Psychological Functions. L. Erlbaum Assoc., Hillsdale, NJ, pp. 15–34.

Skavenski, A.A. and Steinman, R.M. (1970) Control of eye position in the dark. Vision Res. 10, 193–203.

Skavenski, A.A., Haddad, G. and Steinman, R.M. (1972) The extraretinal signal for the visual perception of direction. Percept. Psychophys. 11, 287–290.

Sperry, R.W. (1950) Neural basis of the spontaneous optokinetic response produced by visual inversion. J. Comp. Physiol. Psychol. 43, 482–489.

Stark, L. (1985) Space constancy and corollary discharge. Percept. Psychophys. 37, 272–273.

Stark, L. and Bridgeman, B. (1983) Role of corollary discharge in space constancy. Percept. Psychophys. 34, 371–380.

Steinbach, M. (1987) Proprioceptive knowledge of eye position. Vision Res. 27, 1737–1744.

Steinbach, M. and Smith, D. (1981) Spatial localization after strabismus surgery: evidence for inflow. Science 213, 1407–1409.

Steinbach, M.J. (1986) Inflow as a long-term calibrator of eye position in humans. Acta Psychol. 63, 297–306.

Steinman, R.M., Levinson, J., Collewijn, H. and van der Steen, J. (1985) Vision in the presence of known natural retinal image motion. J. Opt. Soc. Am. A 2, 226–233.

Stoffregen, T.A., Schmuckler, M.A. and Gibson, E. (1987) Use of central and peripheral optical flow in stance and locomotion in young walkers. Perception 16, 113–119.

Stoper, A. (1973) Apparent motion of stimuli presented stroboscopically during pursuit movement of the eye. Percept. Psychophys. 13, 201–211.

Swanston, M. and Wade, N. (1988) The perception of visual motion during movements of the eyes and of the head. Percept. Psychophys. 43, 559–566.

Trevarthen, C.B. (1968) Two mechanisms of vision in primates. Psychol. Forsch. 31, 299–337.

Von Holst, E. and Mittelstaedt, H. (1950) Das reafferenzprinzip. Wechselwirkungen zurischen Zentralnervensystem und Peripherie. Naturwissenschaften 37, 464–476.

Waespe, W. and Henn, V. (1977) Neuronal activity in the vestibular nuclei of the alert monkey during vestibular and optokinetic stimulation. Exp. Brain Res. 27, 523–538.

Wallach, H. (1985) The perception of motion during colinear eye movements. Percept. Psychophys. 38, 18–22.

Westheimer, G. (1981) Visual hyperacuity. In: Progress in Sensory Physiology 1. Springer-Verlag, Berlin, New York, pp. 1–30.

Westheimer, G. and McKee, S. (1975) Visual acuity in the presence of retinal image motion. J. Opt. Soc. Am. 65, 847–850.

Young, L. (1985) Adaptation to modified otolith input. In: A. Berthoz and G. Melvill Jones (Eds.), Reviews of Oculomotor Research: Adaptive Mechanisms in Gaze Control. Elsevier, Amsterdam, pp. 155–162.

Zihl, J., von Cramon, D. and Mai, N. (1983) Selective disturbance of movement vision after bilateral brain damage. Brain 106, 313–340.

Eye movements and their role in visual and cognitive processes
E. Kowler, Editor

CHAPTER 6

The role of eye movements in the perception of motion and shape

Hans Wallach

Department of Psychology, Swarthmore College, Swarthmore, PA 19081, U.S.A.

1. Motion perception

Smooth eye movement is one of several kinds of stimulation that play an important role in the perception of visual motion. But, because it is rarely the only stimulation condition in operation at a given time, assessing its importance requires consideration of smooth-pursuit eye movement along with the two other conditions of stimulation.

Duncker (1929) distinguishes two kinds of distal stimulation which are evoked by the motion of an object in our visual environment. One is a change in the direction in which the moving object lies. Duncker called this change subject-relative displacement. The other is a change in the location of the moving object relative to stationary items in the object's surround, or with respect to its background, which may be either stationary or moving.

The first of these two distal conditions of stimulation, subject-relative displacement, results in two proximal stimulus conditions. First, the motion of the object relative to the observer can evoke pursuit eye movements, which may operate as stimuli for the percept of the object's motion. Second, the displacement of the moving object's image on the retina serves as stimulation, provided the eyes are fixed on a stationary point. Object-relative displacement, the second of the distal conditions of stimulation, results in a proximal stimulus which consists of a change in the configuration of the retinal pattern in the region in which the moving object is located. (A fourth stimulation condition, orientation change (Wallach and O'Leary, 1985), will not be considered.)

When an object moves in a homogeneous surround, its motion can be mediated by subject-relative displacement only and, since there is no stationary point visible on which the eye can fasten, the motion is given by ocular pursuit. But in patterned (non-homogeneous) environments, subject-relative and object-relative displacement take place simultaneously and provide redundant stimulation conditions. We thus do not know which of the two causes the perceived motion. In fact, how do we know that, all in all, both operate in motion perception? There is evidence that both do. Consider the evidence for the role of configurational change in determining perceived motion. Configurational change can sometimes result in perceived motion of a stationary object, which, on the grounds of subject-relative stimulation, would be correctly perceived as stationary. We owe to Duncker (1929) the explanation of how this can happen: configurational change represents only the displacement of different objects with respect to one another. Which object is really moving, and which is stationary, is not transmitted by this stimulus condition. This ambiguity, however, is not reflected in perceptual experience. Experienced motion is an absolute, a temporary property of the moving object, and that is the case even when configurational change mediates only relative displacement between an object and its surround. Configurational change tends to cause the percept that the object is moving and that the surround is stationary. This makes configurational change, under most circumstances, a veridical cue. That configurational change results in perceived motion of the surrounded object is now called Duncker's rule.

It is because configurational change transmits only relative displacement between object and surround, and because what is perceived to move is determined by a perceptual rule (i.e., Duncker's rule) rather than by stimulation, that configurational change sometimes results in the perceived motion of a stationary object. When a stationary object is seen in a surround that is in translatory motion, the object is perceived to move in the direction opposite to the motion of the surround. The non-veridical motion of the surrounded object is called induced motion. The apparent motion of the moon when it is seen among drifting clouds is a familiar example. Induced motion occurs even when the motion of the surround is also perceived, because the motion of the surround may be represented by one or the other subject-relative conditions of stimulation.

1.1. The effectiveness of three conditions of stimulation is compared

Induced motion demonstrates that configurational change is a stimulus for motion perception. Induced motion is also a valuable tool in research on visual motion. Under ordinary circumstances the motion of an object represented by configurational change and by one of the subject-relative conditions of stimulation is the same. In induced motion, on the other hand, motion or rest represented by subject-relative conditions of stimulation and that represented by configurational change are in conflict with each other. For example, when the observer looks at a stationary object whose surround or background is moving, both of the subject-relative conditions of stimulation (image displacement and ocular pursuit) indicate that the object is stationary. If induced motion of the object is perceived in this situation, then configurational change emerges as more potent than the subject-relative conditions of stimulation.

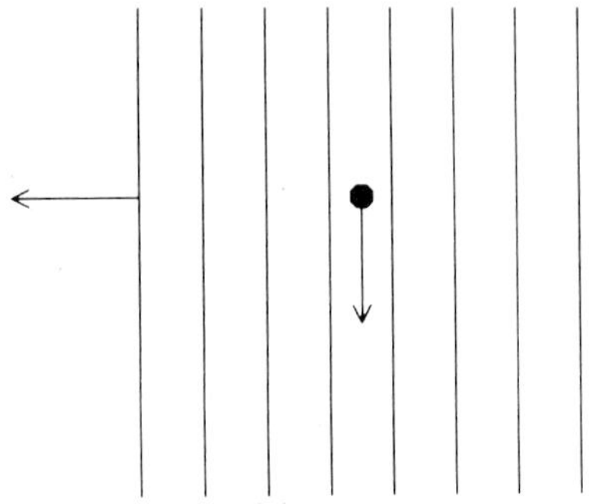

Fig. 1. A pattern of very long vertical lines was in reciprocating horizontal motion while a dot moved up and down, changing motion direction simultaneously with the line pattern. The extents of the two motions were equal.

In experiments by Wallach et al. (1982) configurational change was made to conflict with one of the two subject-relative stimulation conditions, either ocular pursuit or image displacement. This was achieved by giving the surrounded object a motion of its own while subjecting it to induced motion in a different direction. A dot seen against a background of evenly spaced parallel vertical lines moved vertically up and down as the line pattern moved left and right, at the same rate and in phase with the motion of the dot (Fig. 1). The vertical motion of the dot encountered virtually no landmarks and was not given by configurational change because the surrounding pattern consisted of only vertical lines that were quite long. Also, the displacement between the dot and the lines defined only a horizontal component of motion rather than a motion in a purely horizontal direction. Straight lines whose ends are not visible cannot transmit their specific direction of motion when they are being displaced (Fig. 2) (Wallach, 1935; see also p. 202 in Wallach, 1976). Therefore the relative displacement between a dot and lines that reach into the periphery of vision defines no definite direction for the displacement of the dot, and the relative displacement between the dot and the line pattern is compatible with any perceived motion of the dot that has a horizontal component opposite to the line

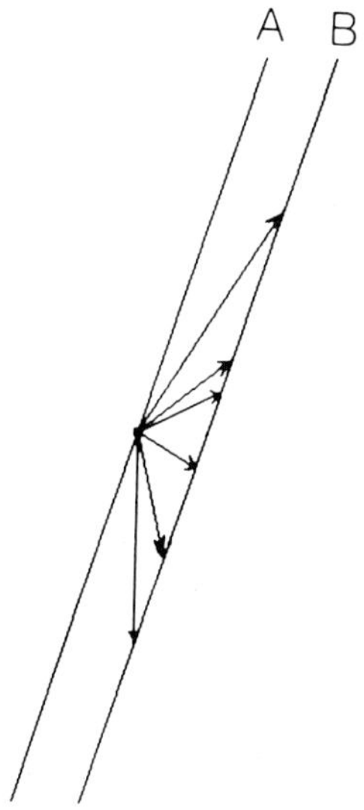

Fig. 2. Two locations of a smooth, long moving line. As long as its ends are not visible, the line could have reached location B by moving in any direction within nearly 180 deg. No specific motion direction is transmitted to the eye.

motion. If the horizontally moving pattern did not consist of endless vertical lines but was, say, a pattern of dots, the vertical motion of the dot would be given as a relative displacement between the dot and the pattern. That relative displacement would be oblique, the result of the vertical motion of the dot and the horizontal motion of the dot pattern. This relative displacement of the dot would be given to the eyes as an oblique configurational change, and it would partially represent the vertical motion of the dot. As the background pattern consisted of vertical lines, this oblique configurational change was avoided. The vertical dot motion was given only subject-relatively and the dot's object-relative motion was horizontal. Under these conditions, the perceived vertical motion of the dot, which resulted from either one of the subject-relative conditions of stimulation, was combined with the horizontal induced motion of the dot, and the dot was seen to move on an oblique path. This would, of course, not happen unless the two perceptual motion processes, one based on configurational change and the other on one of the subject-relative stimuli, were able to combine. This combining took place although the processes evoked by the different conditions of stimulation were quite different. The vertical motion was produced by a process that registered eye movements or evaluated changes in retinal location. The horizontal induced motion was produced by a form-perception process. The slope of the oblique motion path depended on the relative effectiveness of the two kinds of stimulation responsible for its vertical and horizontal components. Earlier, Wallach et al. (1978) had used this stimulus arrangement to measure diminished induced motion that resulted from adaptation. Wallach et al. (1982) used it to measure the relative effectiveness of configurational change that caused the horizontal induced motion, and of the subject-relative cues (either ocular pursuit or image displacement) that mediated the vertical motion of the dot.

The perceived angle of the motion of the dot depended on whether the subjects tracked the dot or maintained a stationary line of sight. It also depended, of course, on the extents of the dot and line motions, which in these experiments were equal. When subjects tracked the vertical motion of the dot, so that the vertical motion of the dot was given by ocular pursuit, the mean estimate of the slope angle was 45.4 deg when the vertical is assigned a slope angle of 0 deg (12 subjects). Earlier, Wallach et al. (1978) had obtained under the same conditions a mean estimate of 43.9 deg, with 25 subjects participating. In kinematics, a horizontal and a vertical displacement of the same extent combine to form a path with a slope of 45 deg. That the mean slope estimates in these experiments were very close to 45 deg means that the induced motion and the perceived vertical motion of the dot were equal, just as the real vertical motion of the dot and the horizontal motion of the lines were of the same extent. (If, as the authors assumed, the vertical dot motion was correctly transmitted, the conditions causing induced motion were fully effective, but these considerations played no role in the conclusions drawn from the results.) That the combined motion path was close to 45 deg demonstrates that configurational change which is responsible for induced motion fully prevailed over the ocular pursuit by which the dot's vertical motion was given. In contrast to the horizontal component of the perceived motion path, the vertical component represented a motion with definite direction, and the fact that the perceived motion path was sloping means that ocular pursuit yielded to configurational change. This was not the case when the experiment was performed with subjects fixating a stationary point, so that the vertical motion of the dot was given by image displacement. Here, the mean slope estimate was only 23.2 deg (n=12) from the vertical. The horizontal component of this perceived motion path amounted to only 0.43 of the extent of the motion of the line pattern, and the difference between the direction of the perceived motion path and the direction of the image path was a bit less than half of what it would have been had configurational change been fully effective. It was concluded that configurational change and image displacement were about equally effective. The relative contribution of the vertical, subject-relative motion was greater when the subject-relative cue was given by image displacement than when it was given by smooth-pursuit eye movement.

Becklen and Wallach (1985, experiment 3) investigated the effect of speed on induced motion. They obtained at their lowest speed (0.26 cycles per second) results very similar to those just described, although they used a slightly different stimulus. The two motion components were not in phase. Instead the vertical motion of the dot and the horizontal motion of the line pattern were combined with a 90 deg phase shift. An oval or circular motion path resulted, whose shape represented the relative effectiveness of the conflicting stimulation conditions. The height of the oval path represented the subject-relative stimulation and its width the configurational change. Estimates of the height and the width of the perceived path were, therefore, measures of the relative effectiveness of the two conditions of stimulation. When the subjects tracked the vertical motion of the dot, so that the vertical motion was given by ocular pursuit, the mean of the ratios of the width estimate to the height estimates obtained from 8 subjects was exactly the same as the ratio of the real extent of the line motion and the real extent of the dot motion. This result corresponded to the mean estimates of 45 deg for the sloping linear motion path obtained by Wallach et al. (1982). Again, it demonstrated the dominance of configurational change over ocular pursuit. When, on the other hand, the eye was stationary so that the vertical motion of the dot was given by its image displacement, the mean ratio of the width to height estimates was one half of what it was in the combination of configurational change with ocular pursuit. Again, configurational change and image displacement appeared to be equally effective, while ocular pursuit was the least effective of the three conditions of stimulation under comparison.

That these stimulus arrangements yield well-shaped motion paths, straight lines or ovals, is in itself a remarkable fact, since the horizontal and vertical dimensions of these paths are given by different kinds of stimulation. Ocular pursuit and configurational change evoke different processes in the nervous system before they yield components of a unified path. There does not seem to be an analogue to these stimulus arrangements in ordinary experience; that is, instances in which the results of different processes combine to provide a single motion experience different from either of the motions that would result from each stimulus alone. When under ordinary conditions ocular pursuit and configurational change represent the motion of a single object the different stimuli are not in conflict. So, in terms of the underlying functions, perceiving such combined motions may have been novel events for our subjects. The interesting question is whether such a combination of two motion processes also takes place when, under ordinary conditions, ocular pursuit and configurational change represent the same motion. An alternative possibility is that some people may habitually use one stimulus condition and some the other. But an argument will be presented below that the two processes operate in concert, nevertheless. If that is the case, the cooperation of motion processes of different origins is not so singular.

In physics, simultaneous motions of an object, of

course, also combine. When simple harmonic reciprocating motions combine, the resultant motion paths are called Lissajous figures. Had the objective vertical and the induced horizontal motion, which in the experiment of Wallach et al. (1982) combined to form a straight motion path, both been objectively given, the straight motion path would have been a Lissajous figure. The same would have been true of the oval paths that Becklen and Wallach (1985) obtained, when they combined an objective vertical and an induced horizontal motion with a 90 deg phase shift. If both motions had been objective, the resultant motion path could have served as a distal stimulus. But since the horizontal components in these experiments were produced by the motions of the line patterns, the straight or oval motions existed only in experience and were the perceptual equivalent of Lissajous figures.

Linear and oval paths result when the periods of the reciprocating motions are of equal duration. When two periods of vertical motion combine with one period of horizontal motion, or when the two motions are combined with frequency ratios of 3 to 2, the resultant motion paths are more complex. O'Leary et al. (1988) produced the perceptual counterparts of these more complex Lissajous paths using objective vertical and induced horizontal motion. When their subjects reproduced these perceived paths, there were large individual differences between subjects' ability to reproduce such complex motion paths, but the reproductions of psychological Lissajous paths were not worse than the reproductions obtained when subjects observed a dot move on the corresponding real Lissajous paths and when ocular pursuit was the condition of stimulation. There was a further condition in which real Lissajous paths were given as configurational change only, that is, where the path of the moving dot was entirely given as induced motion. A stationary dot was seen against a background consisting of vertical and horizontal lines forming a square pattern. This pattern was given both the horizontal and the vertical motions that resulted in the Lissajous path, and the motions of the pattern induced the Lissajous motion path in the dot. Reproductions of the dot's induced motion were as good as those obtained when real dot motion was given by ocular pursuit. The complex induced motions that were perceived were another instance of configurational change prevailing over subject-relative stimulation conditions which represented the dot as stationary. However, what is important in the present discussion is the results for the psychological Lissajous paths. There was no striking loss of accuracy of the reproductions, which would have been expected if the combining of different perceptual processes that takes place when these paths are perceived had never occurred before. It seemed unlikely that the combinations of the two processes which result from different conditions of stimulation were altogether novel events. This suggests that, in ordinary motion perception, the different processes which result simultaneously from configurational change and from ocular pursuit operate at the same time to produce the percepts.

1.2. Other consequences of redundant stimulation

The experiments described in the previous section show that an objective motion can be simultaneously represented by two conditions of stimulation. This phenomenon may serve as an explanation of a type of motion event that for many years has been regarded as an instance of perception performing a vector analysis which causes two motions to be seen where a single motion is given. Johansson (1950) discovered a number of motion displays in which each of two or more moving dots are perceived to move simultaneously in two directions. Wallach et al. (1985) proposed that this happens because the objective motions are simultaneously represented by different conditions of stimulation.

The reciprocating motion represented by the arrows in Fig. 3, panel A, is one of the best-known examples. As one dot moves vertically and the other horizontally, they are perceived to move toward and then away from each other, as shown by the solid arrows in panel B. In addition to this colinear motion, some subjects also report a motion perpendicular to the colinear motion, a motion repre-

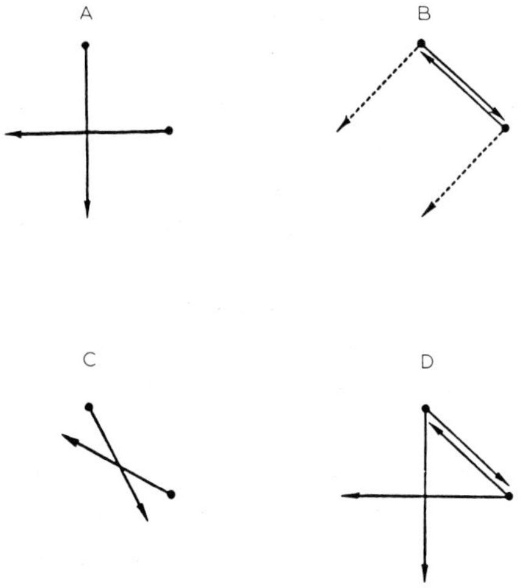

Fig. 3. The arrows in these panels represent reciprocating motions. Panel A shows the actual motions of Johansson's crossing paths display and panel B the perceived motions described by Johansson. The motions shown in panel C are perceived when the processes resulting from the stimulation shown in panel D are combined.

sented by the dotted arrows in panel B. These motions are kinematic components of the objective motions shown in panel A, and were attributed to a perceptual process that resolved the given motion into two components (Johansson, 1950). Wallach et al. (1985) proposed an alternative, namely, that the two perpendicular motions are perceived because the objective motions are represented by two different stimulation conditions operating at the same time. Configurational change represents the colinear components of the dots' motions, and one of the kinds of subject-relative stimulation (image displacement or smooth pursuit) represents the component perpendicular to the colinear motion of the dots. Because configurational change registers only the displacement that the dots undergo relative to each other, that is, their changing distance from each other, it represents only the colinear components of the dots' motions. Why subject-relative stimulation represents those components of the dot's motion which are perpendicular to the colinear motions will be explained below. When the perceptual processes evoked by the two stimulation conditions do not combine, the motions described by Johansson (1950) are perceived. This explanation recognizes that the component motions represented by the different conditions of stimulation are physical properties of the objective vertical and horizontal motions. In the physical world, the component motions are just as real as the resultant motion. So, the stimulation could just as readily be caused by the component motions as by the objective motions. There is no need for psychological processes to explain events that can be attributed to physical characteristics of the stimuli.

Wallach et al.'s (1985) explanation of the perceived motions is supported by their finding that half their subjects saw paths which crossed each other at an angle of 30 or 40 deg as shown in Fig. 3, panel C. These crossed paths were explained as the combination of two motion processes that resulted from the two stimulation conditions shown in panel D. One was configurational change representing the colinear motion components, and the second was one or the other of the subject-relative stimuli representing the objective vertical and horizontal motions of the dots. Why did only half of the subjects report the crossing motion that resulted from process combination and why did the other half report the colinear motions that resulted from configurational change only? Wallach et al. (1985) proposed that the latter happens when the two dots form a group and when their individual motions are not available for process combination.

Group formation is also responsible for the parallel motion path represented by the dotted arrows in panel B. Wallach et al. supported this explanation with two experiments employing another of Johansson's displays which could be altered to favor group formation. It consisted of two dots moving next to each other. One dot moved straight up and down in reciprocating simple harmonic motion, and the other performed a circular motion of which the vertical component was in phase with the motion of the other dot (Fig. 4A). Configurational change between the two dots represented the horizontal distance change between them and resulted in horizontal motion of the circling dot. This horizontal motion could combine with the circular motion of the dot given by subject-relative stimulation

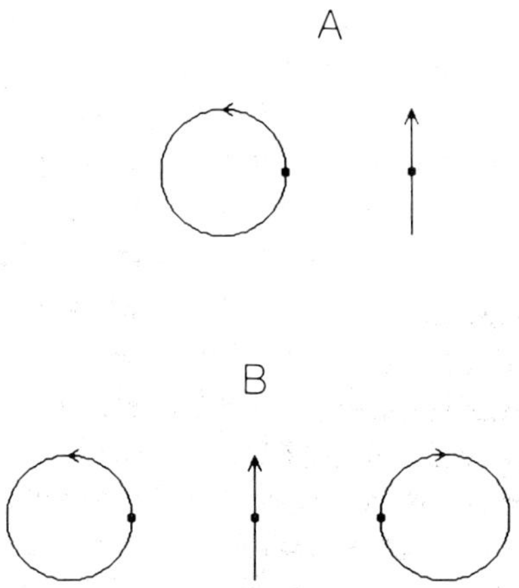

Fig. 4. Panel A shows one dot on a circular and another on a reciprocating vertical motion path. The motions are so arranged that the vertical component of the circular motion and the vertical motion of the other dot go together up and down. Configurational change representing the changing distance between the dots causes the dot on the left to move horizontally. If grouping of the dots causes the vertical component of the motion of the circling dot to be perceived, that dot also appears to move vertically, together with the other dot. The simultaneous horizontal and vertical motion of the circling dot described by Johansson (1950) results. When the dots do not form a group, the horizontal motion of the circling dot combines with its circular motion to form an elliptic motion path. If grouping is strengthened by adding another circling dot (panel B), more subjects see simultaneous horizontal and vertical motion.

and form an elliptic motion path. This combination of the two processes corresponded to the crossing motion in the previous experiment. When the dots moved as a group and the vertical component of the circular motion and the vertical motion of the other dot went together, the process combination was prevented, as happened in the previous experiment. The circularly moving dot was, in addition to its vertical motion, also seen to move horizontally. But these two motions were reported only 7 times, while 16 subjects reported elliptical motion. In a second experiment grouping was favored by adding a third moving dot (Fig. 4B). That raised the number of subjects who reported simultaneous vertical and horizontal motion of the circling dots to 21, while only 8 saw elliptical motions of the circling dots. Increasing grouping strength tended to prevent process combination.

1.3. Adaptation in motion perception

Earlier it had been pointed out that perceived motion may be thought of as a temporary property of the moving object. This manner of describing motion perception is in agreement with the subject-relative condition of stimulation which represents the displacement of the moving object provided the observer is at rest. But it is not consistent with configurational change, which represents only the relative displacement between the moving object and its surround and provides no information which of the two is really moving. That is an argument for proposing that configurational change is either a learned condition of stimulation or a late phylogenetic development. Moving objects are very frequently seen while surrounded by stationary objects or by a stationary patterned background. In such situations two kinds of motion cue are present, configurational change and subject-relative displacement. Simple stimulus substitution may result in configurational change coming to evoke the perceived motion of the object. If such are the occasions when configurational change becomes a stimulation condition for motion, Duncker's rule will also be learned or developed, because on these occasions it is always the surrounded object that is displaced relative to the observer and is, therefore, perceived to move.

When a percept depends on more than one kind of stimulation, as is the case with motion, it is often possible to alter the effect of one of the stimuli by means of perceptual adaptation. By interposing a device which alters one of the redundant stimuli, a cue conflict is created where the outcomes of the processes which the two stimuli evoke are no longer in agreement. During prolonged exposure to such cue conflict one of the processes may change so that the difference between their outcomes is diminished. When that happens we speak of perceptual adaptation (e.g., Wallach and Frey, 1972, where the relationship of ocular convergence and perceived distance was altered). In motion perception, no interposed device was needed to obtain a cue conflict. Inherent in the stimulation conditions that result in induced motion is a conflict between configurational change and subject-relative stimulation, as has been stated above. Making use of this natural cue discrepancy, Wallach et al. (1978) produced an alteration of the relationship between configurational change and the extent of the perceived motion it evoked.

A natural pairing of ocular pursuit with image displacement also made it possible to change the relationship between ocular pursuit and the motion it evokes. Such an adaptation was obtained by Bacon and Wallach (1982) on the basis of the following considerations. When an object starts to move, the eyes remain still for a brief time before they begin to smoothly track the moving object. Thus, pursuit is typically preceded by image displacement. In the case of linear motion, image displacement and subsequent pursuit have the same direction. Instances of this sequence may provide the occasions on which a connection between ocular pursuit and perceived motion becomes established and pursuit comes to evoke the perceived motion caused by the preceding image displacement. This possibility prompted Bacon and Wallach (1982) to perform an adaptation experiment involving image displacement and ocular pursuit. Their experiment was different from the traditional adaptation experiment in that the two stimulation conditions occurred sequentially instead of simultaneously. In their experiment, adaptation altered the direction of the perceived motion which is the result of ocular pursuit. A cue conflict between image displacement and subsequent ocular pursuit was created by altering the objective direction of the target motion at the moment when ocular pursuit began. Repeated exposure to such a motion sequence altered the perceived direction resulting from the pursuit phase of the motion sequences.

During the adaptation period the subject saw a dot move horizontally and change direction by 45 deg upwards when the subject's eyes started to move. Electrodes, one fastened to the outer orbital ridge of one eye and the other to the ridge of the nose, signalled the beginning of the eye movement and caused the direction of the dot's motion to change. The sequence of horizontal and oblique motion was repeated 75 times. If learning causes the perceived direction of the pursuit phase to become like the direction of the image displacement, exposure to such conditions should cause the second phase of this motion sequence consisting of 45 deg motions to be gradually perceived as more horizontal. The effect of learning was measured by obtaining estimates of the apparent slope of the second motion phase under conditions where the direction change was only 25 deg or 10 deg, smaller than the one in the learning exposure. Such estimates were obtained before and after the 75 learning exposures. There was a mean change toward horizontal of 12 deg for the 25 deg test and a mean change of 9 deg for the 10 deg test. Since the slope angles were generally overrated, these changes amounted to only 38 and 57% of the given slope angles. A control experiment was also performed in which the image dispacement had the same slope of 45 deg as the pursuit phase. Here the tests registered no perceived slope change, a result significantly different from the result of the experimental condition at the 0.001 level.

This experiment demonstrated a connection between the motion perceived due to ocular pursuit and the preceding image displacement and, therefore, supported the notion that ocular pursuit becomes a condition of stimulation as a result of the frequent sequence of these stimulation conditions, either through learning or phylogenetically. But the experiment was not an analogue of a process that causes ocular pursuit to become a stimulation condition for perceived motion. The subject brought the capacity for using ocular pursuit as a stimulus for motion perception to the experiment. The experiment only demonstrated an assimilation of the direction of the motion resulting from ocular pursuit to the direction of the preceding image displacement.

1.4. The importance of smooth eye movement in motion perception

There is no evidence that ocular pursuit plays an important role in motion perception in ordinary, patterned visual environments. Unless an object moves in a homogeneous field, e.g., is luminous in total darkness, configurational change duplicates the information provided by ocular pursuit. The experiments by Wallach et al. (1982) and by Becklen and Wallach (1985), who confirmed their results, showed that configurational change is more potent than ocular pursuit. The high frequency with which induced motion is perceived when appropriate stimulation conditions are given, although they are in conflict with subject-relative stimulation conditions, confirms these findings. But that does not mean that ocular pursuit does not contribute when it provides the same information as configurational change, as happens in the great majority of instances of ordinary motion perception. The experiments by Wallach et al. (1985) show that the processes evoked by subject-relative displacement and configurational change readily combine even when they represent different motion paths, and there is no reason why the same should not happen when the two processes convey the same information and the combination changes nothing.

Summary Smooth ocular pursuit is only one of the three major stimuli which mediate motion perception, the most effective of which is configurational change. Most of the time, ocular pursuit and configurational change operate simultaneously, and the resulting redundant stimulation can have interesting consequences. The two stimuli may represent different kinematic components of the objective motions so that an object is seen to undergo simultaneously two motions. The two ensuing motion processes may or may not combine. That simultaneous motion processes resulting from different kinds of stimulation can combine to form a single experienced motion makes possible perceived motions which do not resemble either of the components causing the stimulation. Experienced motion paths may, for instance, be the psychological equivalent of Lissajous paths. That different stimuli often represent the same objective motion makes them candidates for the kind of perceptual adaptation that results from cue conflict.

2. Compensatory eye movements

Turning or nodding of the head causes an angular displacement of the environment relative to the eyes. Simultaneously an eye movement takes place in the direction opposite to the head movement, reducing the displacement of the projection of the environment on the retina by keeping the eyes relatively stationary at the same point in the environment while the head moves. "This compensatory movement is so much like the pursuit movement that one is tempted to regard them as identical."... But "there is one remarkable difference. The pursuit movement has a long latency, about 200 ms... But if you turn your head while fixating an object of interest... *the compensatory eye movement starts simultaneously with the active head movement.*" (Woodworth and Schlosberg, 1954, p. 518.) The compensatory eye movement is not visually caused but is a response to the head movement, and also takes place when one turns the head in the dark.

The compensatory eye movements can be modified by optical arrangements that alter the normal relationships between head motion and retinal image motion. Interesting results of long-term adaptation to left-right reversing prisms are reported in Volume 1 of this series (Berthoz and Melvill Jones, 1985). More rapid adaptation was obtained by Gauthier and Robinson (1975). Their subject wore 2.1 power magnifying lenses which approximately doubled the relative displacement of the environment caused by head movements. Therefore the extent of compensatory eye movements had to become twice as large if the projection of the environment on the retina was to remain stationary. After five days of adaptation to the lenses, compensatory eye movements were 50% larger than normal. Collewijn et al. (1983) obtained almost complete adaptation to modest (8–36%) visual magnification or minification after only 5 minutes of spectacle wearing. Earlier, Wallach and Bacon (1977) obtained changes in compensatory eye movements by having subjects track a fixation target that was made to move by 40% with each head movement, requiring eye movement 40% smaller than normal to keep the projection of a tracked point stationary on the retina. After 10 minutes of tracking the point during continuous head movements, compensatory eye movements measured in the dark were on average 1.93 deg, or 13%, shorter than before the exposure (10 subjects).

In the study by Wallach and Bacon (1977) compensatory eye movements were inferred by a psychophysical procedure in which subjects turned their heads in the dark as soon as a mark they were fixating disappeared. A stop limited the head movement to 15 deg. When the stop was reached, a flash gun behind a vertical slit lit the slit briefly and caused an afterimage. The slit was located directly beneath the mark the subject had initially fixated. A white screen with a fixation mark in its center was lit, and the experimenter marked the location of the afterimage the subject saw on the screen as he or she fixated the mark. If the compensatory eye movement was accurate, the location of the afterimage would be underneath the fixation mark because the compensatory eye movement would have caused the eye to remain directed toward the mark's original location. When the test was repeated after a 10-min exposure to the 'learning' condition, the afterimage had a different location, indicating a shortened compensatory eye movement. The shortening of the compensatory eye movement that continuous head movement yielded in 10 min amounted to 32% of the visual angle of 6 deg by which the relative environmental displacement was smaller during the exposure period, a very rapid change.

3. The role of eye movements in the constancy of visual direction

Wallach and Bacon (1977) did this experiment in the context of their investigation of the constancy of perceived visual direction, the compensating mechanism that prevents stimulation produced by the relative displacement between the environment and the eyes during head movements from resulting in motion perception. Whereas such stimulation would result in perceived motion of the environment if it were caused by an actual motion of the environment, the same stimulation does not result in perceived motion when it is caused by a head movement. Where sensory inputs are concerned, the two cases differ in that real environmental motion results only in visual stimulation, whereas the head movement is simultaneously represented by proprioceptive stimulation. Such information about head movements prevents the visual stimulation from having its normal effect. The result is analogous to position constancy, a compensation for the effect of the displacement of the images of stationary objects which results from eye movements.

Wallach and Kravitz (1965, 1968) developed a method of measuring the accuracy of the perceptual compensation for the relative motion of the environment caused by head movement. When the head is turned to the right by a certain angle, the environment moves to the left by the same angle, and that motion is not perceived. How much greater or smaller may that motion be and still not be perceived? Answering that question would be a measure of the accuracy of perceptual compensation. In order to increase or decrease the normal relative motion of the environment one would have to give it an objective motion that depended on the head movement, either against or with it. The smaller the range of such motion of the environment that is not detected the greater the accuracy of the compensation. The range will be called the immobility range and was measured with the following apparatus.

The subject wore a head gear with a vertical shaft located in the extension of the rotation axis of the head. This shaft was joined to the input shaft of a variable-ratio transmission mounted above the subject's head. The output of the transmission turned a small mirror mounted on a vertical shaft. The mirror intercepted the beam of a slide projector and reflected it onto a screen in front and at the eye level of the subject. The beam carried to the screen either a small light spot or a large pattern, either of which represented the environment (Fig. 5). The variable-ratio transmission made it possible to vary the ratio between the amplitude of the rotation of the en-

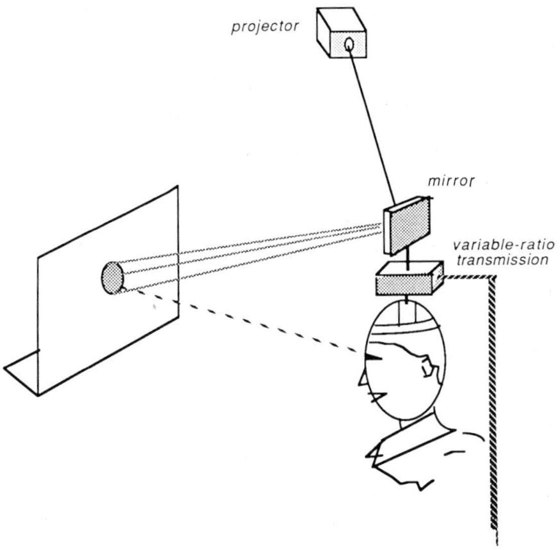

Fig. 5. Apparatus used to add or subtract from the relative displacement which the stationary environment undergoes during head turning. A vertical shaft attached to the head carries the head rotation to a variable-ratio transmission. The transmission imparted a proportion of the rotation to the subject's environment. It turned a mirror which reflected an image from a projector onto a screen in front of the subject, where it moved in some proportion to the head rotation, dependent on the setting of the transmission.

vironment and the amplitude of the rotation of the head. This ratio, called the displacement ratio, or DR, is equal to 0 in normal stationary environments and to 1 when the amplitude of the real objective displacement is equal to the amplitude of head rotation. DR was varied by changing the setting of the variable-ratio transmission. This setting determined how much a target spot, or a pattern on the screen in front of the subject, moved during every head turn, because the motion of the target spot depended on the rotation of a mirror controlled by the variable-ratio transmission, which, in turn, was activated by the subject's head turning. To measure the immobility range the setting of the variable-ratio transmission was such that head movements caused the pattern on the screen to move enough for the subject to perceive motion, say, *with* the head movement. Then the setting was changed in steps so that the pattern moved less and less until the motion was no longer noticeable. The amount of objective motion that was just not noticeable was one limit of the immobility range. The other limit was obtained in similar fashion by varying the objective motion in the direction *against* the head movement. The center of the immobility range usually coincided with objective immobility of the target pattern (Wallach and Canal, 1976).* The immobility range was found to have a width of 4–6% of the angle of the head rotation. The smallness of the immobility range made it possible to measure partial adaptation of the compensation process.

When such measurements are performed care must be taken that only the light spot, or the patterns that are made to move dependent on the head movement, arc visible. Compensation for environmental displacements caused by head movements takes place only in connection with subject-relatively given motion. When a stationary object is also present and configurational change takes place, every head movement will cause some perceived environmental motion. There is no compensation for motion that is mediated by configurational change.

One may be tempted to assume that the constancy of visual direction results from the compensatory eye movements that accompany turning head movements and keep the projection of the environment on the retina stationary (e.g., Hay, 1968). But stationary retinal images denote motion when they are associated with eye movements. It is the constancy of visual direction that prevents compensatory eye movements from resulting in perceived motion. Wallach and Bacon (1977) compared the

* This finding is of considerable interest when the target pattern is nearer than 2 m. Then, the relative displacement of the environment is effectively larger than the angle of the head rotation, because the eyes are about 10 cm in front of the head's rotation axis, and that gives them an added displacement relative to the stationary environment (Wallach and Kravitz, 1965). For short observation distances this added displacement is quite large. Nevertheless, the immobility range is centered on objective immobility, because a mechanism that takes observation distance into account and compensates for the added displacement participates in the constancy of visual direction (Wallach et al., 1972).

accuracy of normal compensatory eye movements measured with their afterimage technique and the width of the immobility range for 10 subjects and found no correlation (r=0.05).

3.1. Adaptation in the constancy of visual direction

That perception of the stationary environment during head movement adapts to artificially produced changes of the relative motions of the environment has been known since Stratton (1897) wore an inverting lens. An investigation of the consequences of such adaptation for perceived motion became possible only after the method of measuring the immobility range described in the previous section had been developed.

Wallach and Kravitz (1965) measured the effect of wearing lenses on the immobility range. They had subjects wear minifying lenses for 6 or for 2 hours. The lenses caused relative environmental motion to be diminished to a displacement ratio of 0.667, causing a displacement of the visual field by 33.3% of every head movement in the direction *with* the head movement. The subject's immobility range was measured before and after this adaptation period, with the lenses removed. After wearing the lenses for 6 hours, an environment that moved somewhat in the direction *with* the head movement was perceived as stationary by all 12 subjects. The center of the immobility range varied after adaptation between 0.102 and 0.345 DR. The mean shift of the center amounted to 0.175 DR, about half of complete adaptation, which would have resulted in a shift of 0.333 DR.

The adaptation period could be greatly shortened by having the subject turn his or her head without stopping. The apparatus used to measure the immobility range was also used to bring about adaptation. In the experiments to be described below, the pattern representing the environment was moved in the direction with the head movement at 0.4 DR, that is, at a rate of 40% of the head movement. After 10 min of continuous head turning under these conditions, motion of the environment in the direction of the head rotation in the amount of 13% of the head rotation was perceived as stationary (Wallach and Bacon, 1977). Since the immobility range was not wider after adaptation than it was before, an effect of this magnitude proved to be adequate to investigate the adaptation process.

A shift of the center of the immobility range is not the only manifestation of adaptation in the constancy of visual direction. As a result of adaptation the stationary environment is perceived to move during every turn of the head, and the extent of such an apparent motion also provides a measure of adaptation. Such a test has the advantage that, after adaptation, it needs to consist only of a single trial in which the subject gives an estimate of the extent of an apparent target motion. Before adaptation, Bacon, who developed this test, had every subject give estimates of the extents of a series of real target motions during a head turning of fixed extent. This series served as a baseline against which to evaluate the subject's post-adaptation estimate (Wallach and Bacon, 1977). The shift of the immobility range after adaptation can be understood to compensate for the apparent motion of the stationary environment.

It was in the context of such experiments that Wallach and Bacon (1977) changed compensatory eye movements by exposure to a mark that moved with each head turning and required smaller eye movements. However, the changed compensatory eye movements do not account for the perceptual adaptation that causes a tracked stationary point to appear to move, as has been explained above. Moreover, changed compensatory movements occurred only when subjects turned their heads in the dark.

3.2. Different adaptation conditions

It seems that if the cause of the apparent motion of the stationary environment resulting from adaptation were known, the nature of the perceptual adaptation, and along with it the compensation process, would be better understood. Does adaptation cause apparent motion of the environment because the normal eye movements needed to keep the eyes on a stationary point during a turning of the head are differently evaluated? In that case adaptation should occur if a fixation mark undergoes actual displacements during head turning, and it should not matter whether or not the visual environment also moves. Adaptation should develop only when a fixation mark undergoes the regular displacements during head movements that cause the adaptation, even when the rest of the environment remains stationary. On the other hand, adaptation may take place at a level of processing where, after eye movements have been take into account, the relationship of the environment to the head is represented. In that case, the abnormal shifts in visual direction of the whole environment that take place during head turning will cause adaptation. Then, it should not matter how the eyes move during adaptation; they may, for instance, track a stationary mark and undergo normal compensatory movements.*

Wallach and Canal (1976) obtained adaptation under both conditions. In one condition, called *eye movement adaptation*, the eyes tracked a mark whose movements were dependent on head movements while a large pattern surrounding the mark remained stationary. In another condition, called *field adaptation*, the environmental pattern moved in dependence on the head movement while the eyes fixated a stationary mark. Wallach and Bacon (1977) repeated these experiments with improved techniques and then investigated the nature of the adaptations that resulted. The visual environment filled the subject's field of view. Instead of a mirror turned by the output of the variable-ratio transmission (Fig. 5), a cylindrical arrangement of vertical rods could be connected to the output of the transmission. With a point source of light at their center, the rods cast a pattern of shadows on a circular screen surrounding the subject. During the 10-min adaptation period the shadow pattern moved at 0.4 DR in the direction of the subject's head turning. This arrangement produced ordinary adaptation, of the kind previously studied, when no stationary mark was present. With a stationary mark added, the same motion of the shadow pattern produced the conditions for field adaptation, when the subject was instructed to fixate the mark. Finally, when the shadow pattern was stationary and the mirror was connected to the output of the transmission and shifted a small mark in dependence on the subject's head movements, the arrangement yielded the condition for eye movement adaptation, provided the subject tracked the moving mark. Both adaptation tests were used in connection with the three adaptation conditions. Either the subject gave estimates of the extents of the apparent motion of the stationary mark while the head turned through a fixed angle, or the immobility range was measured before and after adaptation. The results of these tests can be found in the first two rows of Table 1. All adaptation effects listed in these rows were significant at the 0.001 level; all three adaptation conditions were thus highly effective.

It had been assumed that the eye movement adaptation consisted of a changed evaluation of the eye movements that compensate for the relative displacement of the stationary environment during head turning. What change in evaluation accounts for the reports of eye movement adaptation in Table 1? After exposure to the condition where the eyes tracked a mark that moved in the direction *with* the head turn, the mark was perceived as immobile when it moved with a mean of 0.072 DR in the direction *with* the head turning. When estimates for the apparent motion of a stationary mark were obtained, the mean extent of the perceived motion was 0.055 DR, and the apparent motion of a stationary mark was in the direction *against* the head turn. There is a fair match between the two results.

* One might wonder why the answer to these questions was not obtained by using the different arrangements in testing for adaptation rather than in producing adaptation. Such tests would have required that the tracked or fixated mark and the rest of the environment were presented in different motion states, and this would have resulted in configurational changes between the mark and the rest of the environment. The configurational changes would have caused perceived motions of the mark that were unrelated to adaptation and would have made the arrangements unsuitable for testing adaptation. As previously stated, the constancy of visual direction controls only the effects of subject-relative stimulation.

TABLE 1
Mean adaptation effects of 10-min exposure to three adaptation conditions, in DR units, and number of subjects (n).

Test	Adaptation conditions							
	Ordinary		Eye movement		Field		Field with saccades	
	DR	n	DR	n	DR	n	DR	n
Estimation	0.131	16	0.055	16	0.053	16		
Shift of immobility	0.098	12	0.072	28	0.056	28		
Pointing I	0.126	12	0.133	12	0.002	12		
Pointing II			0.106	18				
Forward direction	−0.004	12	−0.013	12	0.087	12	0.172	12

When in the estimation test the eyes track a stationary mark and undergo normal compensatory movements, the perceived motion of the mark during every head movement, which is the result of that test, is best explained as an overrating of these normal eye movements. Wallach and Bacon (1977) obtained independent evidence for such an overrating, by using a pointing response.

Pointing test I. In the dark, the subject turned his or her head to the left until a stop was reached at the end of an 18 deg turn. When this happened, a vertical line straight in front lit up, and the subject had to look at it and to point to it. Then the subject closed his or her eyes and the pointing direction was recorded. Three such tests were given before and three after each adaptation period. The difference between the average of the three tests before and the average after the adaptation period became the subject's pointing effect. The means of these pointing effects amounted to 2.27 deg for normal adaptation and 2.4 deg for eye movement adaptation. Changed into DR measures, they are listed in the third row of Table 1. As expected, there was no pointing effect after field adaptation, during which subjects presumably made normal compensatory eye movements.

That the pointing effect measured after ordinary adaptation is as great as the adaptation effect, and thus accounts for the effect of ordinary adaptation, suggests that ordinary adaptation consists in altered evaluation of eye movement. Both measurements of the adaptation effect after eye movement adaptation exposure showed a significantly smaller effect than after ordinary adaptation. The pointing effect after eye movement adaptation, however, was of the same magnitude as after ordinary adaptation. That the adaptation effect after eye movement adaptation exposures was, nevertheless, diminished, resulted most probably from the fact that, except for the tracked mark, the visual field was stationary during exposure. Its relative motion was normal and counteracted the changed evaluation of eye movements. The pointing effect, on the other hand, reflected only the abnormal motion of the tracked mark.

Another test of visual direction in which the subject causes a luminous point to be shifted to a position where it appears straight ahead turned out to show a change only after field adaptation. This forward direction test showed no effect, not only after eye movement adaptation but also after ordinary adaptation. This confirms that the ordinary adaptation obtained with a 10-min exposure to continuous head movements consisted in altered evaluation of eye movements.

3.3. *Saccadic eye movements during head turning*

The question arose whether a compensating process which corresponds to field adaptation participates in the constancy of visual direction and is modified when field adaptation takes place. The alternative, namely, that the field adaptation obtained by Wallach and Bacon (1977) is a product only of the procedure that yielded it, appeared unlikely. Because this procedure has no analogue in ordinary life, Wallach and Bacon asked under what conditions a compensation process might take place at the level where eye position has been taken into account and the visual environment is represented as it is related to the head. Compensatory eye movements are not the only eye movements that take place when the head is turned, particularly when the head movements are made to bring another part of the environment into view. Then, a compensatory eye movement is interspersed with a saccade in the direction of the head movement. A saccade that brings a point to the fovea may ordinarily be steered by the initial position of the point's retinal image. But when the saccade takes place during a compensatory eye movement, it is more likely that it is steered by the position of the point in the representation of the environment where the eye movement is taken into account than from its position on the retina. This consideration suggested to Wallach and Bacon that they should try an adaptation exposure where the subject turned his or her head back and forth and made a saccadic eye movement to the right during every head turn to the right. The subject faced an array of columns, each consisting of numerous rows of three letters. This array moved with a displacement ratio of 0.4 in the direction *with* every head turn. During each head turn to the right, the subject had to read the rows of letters in two neighboring columns, and this involved making a saccade from one column to the other. A forward direction test given before and immediately after such an adaptation period showed a strong effect: twelve subjects set the luminous point after the adaptation period to the right by a mean of 3.1 deg, which was equivalent to 0.172 DR and highly significant ($p<0.001$). Since the forward direction test had previously measured only field adaptation, Wallach and Bacon assumed that it did here also. If this assumption is correct, the procedure just described resulted in field adaptation. Wallach and Bacon (1977) obtained confirmation for this conclusion by showing that an effect of this procedure could be measured with another test which responded only to field adaptation, namely, a square test with fixation.

3.4. *Changed evaluation of saccadic eye movements*

After it had been found that rapid adaptation in the constancy of visual direction can consist in a changed evaluation of compensatory eye movements and that this changed evaluation can be measured by having subjects point to a target after they had turned their head (pointing test I), Wallach and Bacon (1977) asked whether eye movement adaptation also manifests itself in changed evaluation of eye movements which are not connected with head turning. Pointing test II resembled pointing test I except that the subject's head remained locked in normal position. Initially, 18 subjects fixated a mark straight in front. As the mark was extinguished another spot, 18 deg to the right of the mark, lit up. The subject was instructed to look at the spot as soon as it appeared and to point at it. (The pointing arm was, of course, not visible.) Here, too, the eye movement was overrated after the standard eye movement adaptation. The post-exposure pointings were farther to the right than those made before adaptation, with a mean difference of 1.9 deg, which was highly significant, $t(17) = 3.96$; $p = 0.001$. Transformed into a displacement ratio, the difference amounted to 0.106, a result not much different from that obtained with pointing test I. The two tests differed in that test I measured an overrating of a compensatory eye movement and test II an overrating of a saccade.

3.5. The nature of adaptation in the constancy of visual direction

In principle, three changes could account for adaptation in the constancy of visual direction: the compensation process might change, the evaluation of the proprioception that represents the head movement might be altered, or the evaluation of the visual stimulation that represents the displacement between the environment and the eyes might change. It was always found that the immobility range after partial adaptation is not wider than before adaptation. (See, e.g., Wallach and Kravitz, 1965; Wallach et al., 1969.) This fact is not compatible with the assumption that adaptation consists in a change in the compensation process. In this case, only after adaptation had become complete could one expect it to yield the narrowest immobility range.

If adaptation consisted in altered evaluation of proprioception, it should also make itself felt in auditory localization, but it did not. Wallach and Kravitz (1968) tested for a transfer of one-hour-long visual adaptation – they used 1.8 power lenses and had obtained visual adaptation of 0.132 DR with the same subjects – with negative results.

Wallach and Bacon found that ordinary perceptual adaptation was accompanied by a change in the evaluation of compensatory and saccadic eye movements and concluded that adaptation consisted in changed evaluation of eye movements. Since the magnitude of the effect measured with pointing test I equalled the magnitude of adaptation, changed evaluation of compensatory eye movements fully accounted for the rapid adaptation with which they experimented; there was no room for another form which adaptation might also take to operate.

No such direct evidence that it consists in a changed evaluation of visual stimulation is available for field adaptation, but it is nevertheless likely that it does. That rapid adaptation with saccades results in field adaptation suggests that adaptation to minifying or magnifying lenses, during which saccades frequently occur, resulted in part in field adaptation. In these experiments the immobility range had not been wider after partial adaptation than before and there was no transfer of adaptation to auditory localization, making it likely that field adaptation also consists in changed evaluation of visual stimulation.

4. The role of eye movements in shape perception

The question arose whether the changed evaluation of saccades that results from eye movement adaptation makes itself felt in shape perception. It has been suspected that the saccadic eye movements which take place when a visual object is inspected contribute to the perception of its shape (see Chapter 3). Altering temporarily the distances that saccades denote made it possible to obtain an indication of the contribution that saccades make to shape perception. Wallach and Bacon (1977) had subjects in the dark adjust the width of a luminous oblong so that its shape seemed to be square. Such adjustments were made before and after eye movement adaptation to target motion of 0.4 DR *with* the head turn. Adjustments were made under two viewing conditions; 12 subjects were allowed to inspect the adjustable oblong freely and another group of 12 subject had to fixate a stationary mark inside the oblong. The constant height of the oblong was 12.5 cm. Since the oblong was 28 cm from the subject's eyes, its height subtended a visual angle of 25 deg.

When, after adaptation, the extent of eye movements is overrated, eye movements may make the oblong look too wide to the degree to which they contribute to its perceived shape, and this would result in a diminished width setting after adaptation. Such a result was actually obtained. The subjects who were allowed eye movements set the width of the oblong 4.5 mm narrower after adaptation than before, a highly significant change, with $t(11) = 8.64$ and $p < 0.001$. On the other hand, adaptation had no effect on perceived shape when the subject had to fixate a stationary mark. Under that condition the mean width setting was an insignificant 0.4 mm wider after adaptation. The change of 4.5 mm measured when the subject was free to make eye movements corresponded to 0.036 DR, while, according to pointing test II, the adaptation had resulted in an overrating of saccades by the amount of 0.106 DR. This suggests that the apparent shape of the oblong depended by one-third on eye movements.

This contribution of eye movements to shape perception takes place only when shapes are large. When Wallach and Bacon repeated their experiment with a 110 cm distance of the adjustable oblong and its height subtended an angle of 6.5 deg, eye movements did not contribute to perceived shape; the square test measured no adaptation effect. Perceived shapes subtending moderate visual angles depend on image shape only. To find out at what larger image size eye movements start to contribute to perceived shape only requires varying the observation distance in the test. The adaptation procedure can also be easily combined with other ways of testing perceived shape, such as shape matching. For that purpose one of the shapes should be given with the subject's eyes fixating a stationary mark, while the other shape is inspected freely. Even a visual angle of 6.5 deg, though, corresponds to a large image size, and the information now available shows that eye movements play only a small role in ordinary shape perception.

References

Bacon, J. and Wallach, H. (1982) Adaptation in motion perception: alteration of motion evoked by ocular pursuit. Percept. Psychophys. 31, 251–255.

Becklen, R. and Wallach, H. (1985) How does speed change affect induced motion? Percept. Psychophys. 37, 231–236.

Berthoz, A. and Jones, G.M. (1985) Adaptive Mechanisms in Gaze Control. Elsevier, Amsterdam.

Collewijn, H., Martins, A.J. and Steinman, R.M. (1983) Compensatory eye movements during active and passive head movements: fast adaptation to changes in visual magnification. J. Physiol. 340, 259–286.

Duncker, K. (1929) Uber Induzierte Bewegung. Psychol. Forsch. 12, 180–259.

Gauthier, G.M. and Robinson, D.A. (1975) Adaptation of the human vestibuloocular reflex to magnifying lenses. Brain Res. 92, 331–335.

Hay, J.C. (1968) Visual adaptation to an altered correlation between eye movement and head movement. Science 160, 429–430.

Johansson, G. (1950) Configurations in Event Perception. Almqvist & Wiksells Boktryckeri AB, Uppsala.

O'Leary, A., McMahon, M.L. and Wallach, H. (1988) Perception of complex motion paths under three conditions of stimulation. Percept. Psychophys. 43, 339–345.

Stratton, G.M. (1897) Vision without inversion of the retinal image. Psychol. Rev. 4, 341–360, 463–481.

Wallach, H. (1935) Uber visuell wahrgenommene Bewegungsrichtung. Psychol. Forsch. 20, 325–380.

Wallach, H. (1976) On Perception. Quadrangle/The New York Times Book Co., New York.

Wallach, H. and Bacon, J. (1977) Two kinds of adaptation in the constancy of visual direction and their different effects on the perception of shape and visual direction. Percept. Psychophys. 21, 227–241.

Wallach, H. and Canal, T. (1976) Two kinds of adaptation in the constancy of visual direction. Percept. Psychophys. 19, 445–449.

Wallach, H. and Frey, K.J. (1972) Adaptation in distance perception based on oculomotor cues. Percept. Psychophys. 11, 77–83.

Wallach, H. and Kravitz, J. (1965) The measurement of the constancy of visual direction and of its adaptation. Psychonomic Sci. 2, 217–218.

Wallach, H. and Kravitz, J. (1968) Adaptation in the constancy of visual direction tested by measuring the constancy of auditory direction. Percept. Psychophys. 4, 299–303.

Wallach, H. and O'Leary, A. (1985) Vector analysis in rotary motion perception. Percept. Psychophys. 38, 47–54.

Woodworth, R.S. and Schlosberg, H. (1954) Experimental Psychology. Henry Holt & Company, New York.

Wallach, H., Frey, K.J. and Romney, G. (1969) Adaptation to field displacement during head movement unrelated to the constancy of visual direction. Percept. Psychophys. 5, 253–256.

Wallach, H., Yablick, G.S. and Smith, A. (1972) Target distance and adaptation in distance perception in the constancy of visual direction. Percept. Psychophys. 12, 139–145.

Wallach, H., Bacon, J. and Schulman, P. (1978) Adaptation in motion perception: alteration of induced motion. Percept. Psychophys. 24, 509–514.

Wallach, H., O'Leary, A. and McMahon, M.L. (1982) Three stimuli for visual motion perception compared. Percept. Psychophys. 32, 1–6.

Wallach, H., Becklen, R. and Nitzberg, D. (1985) Vector analysis and process combination in motion perception. J. Exp. Psychol. Hum. Percept. Performance 11, 93–102.

Eye movements and their role in visual and cognitive processes
E. Kowler, Editor

CHAPTER 7

Comparison of perception in the moving and stationary eye

George Sperling

Human Information Processing Laboratory, Department of Psychology and Center for Neural Sciences, New York University, New York, NY 10003, U.S.A.

1. Introduction

There are many different kinds of eye movement, each of which sweeps the image of the world across the retina in its distinctive way. Each kind of eye movement serves a unique function and in turn is served by a unique perceptual-motor process. Undoubtedly, the visual system has evolved special adaptations for this mode of operation. This chapter probes the question of to what extent these information-processing adaptations operate independently of the eye movements themselves.

Simulated eye movements: imposed motion. An important tool is the simulated eye movement: an image sequence which produces on a stationary retina precisely the same image motion that the moving eye would have produced. Comparing perception when image motion is produced by eye movements with perception under imposed motion offers substantial insights into both the mechanisms and the purposes of eye movements. To provide a frame of reference and to illustrate the general similarities between processing principles, all kinds of eye movements are considered briefly. The primary emphasis is on saccades because this is the domain the author has studied experimentally.

Restriction to eye-movement-induced image motion. Eye movements are usually measured in the laboratory with the body at rest and the head held stabilized by a 'biteboard' – an impression of the teeth of the observer which holds the observer's teeth, and thereby the head, in place. Of course, in normal viewing, the head and body move freely. The motion of images across the retina caused by uncompensated movements of the head and body is large compared to the image motion induced by some of the eye movements considered here. The nature and consequences of image motion produced by eye, head and body movements are considered in Ch. 3 of this volume (Steinman and Levinson). In the present chapter, only image motion caused by eye movements, principally saccadic eye movements, with the head and body held stationary is considered and compared with image motion produced by corresponding object movements. The descriptions of the eye movements themselves are very brief here because they are taken up in great detail in other chapters of this book.

2. Tremor

High-frequency tremor is a generic term applied to eye movements that are typically about 30–70 Hz, with amplitudes less than the width of a single cone, approx 0.5 min (Ratliff and Riggs, 1950; Yarbus, 1957). The blur circle under normal vision is about 2 min or more (Krauskopf, 1962; Westheimer and

Campbell, 1962), so the effects of tremor on the retinal image would be obscured by the much greater blur produced by the eye's optical imperfections. High-frequency tremor is probably irrelevant for normal vision. Occasional attempts to attribute some useful purpose to tremor, such as Yellott's (1987) proposal that tremor may act to smooth over irregularities in receptor spacing, have the aforementioned problem that the tremor is negligible compared to the much larger optical aberration.* Indeed, Krauskopf (1957, 1960) imposed tremor frequencies on retinally stabilized images and found that they did not improve the visibility of his test stimulus (a single line); in some instances imposed high-frequency motions were detrimental. Based on these measurements, I would predict that if normal tremor could suddenly be removed from vision, the change could probably not be noticed even in the fovea under psychophysical viewing conditions. Elsewhere in the visual field, or in the fovea under natural viewing with unrestrained head and body movements adding to retinal image motion, high-frequency tremor would seem to be far below the threshold of visibility.

3. Slow control movements

Slow control refers to the involuntary smooth motions of the eye that occur during steady fixation on a stationary target. A typical velocity for slow control movements, when the head is stabilized, is about 5–10 arc min per s (Ratliff and Riggs, 1950; Steinman et al., 1973), and a typical oscillatory frequency is about 2–3 Hz. Slow control movements may or may not be interrupted by small saccades, and the saccades may move the eye nearer or further from its intended fixation (see Ch. 1 of this volume for a more detailed review).

Are slow drift movements important for vision? When slow control movements and saccades are removed in stabilized vision, the image fades within several seconds. Visibility is restored to a stabilized image by imposing slow image oscillations. For optimal restoration of visibility, velocities higher than those typically observed in biteboard viewing are required (see Ch. 3 of this volume).

There are two issues here: (1) the role of drift image-motion in visibility, and (2) the appearance of movement in drifting images. I will consider first the appearance of movement in drifting images. Suppose that image drift were due to imperfect oculomotor control. Then, retinal drift would not be accompanied by signals of intentional motor movement; it would be residual image instability that was uncompensated by motor movement. Suppose also that proprioceptive information is unimportant when the eye is maintaining stable fixation. Then, if image drift were to be recorded from a subject and later produced as an imposed signal on a stabilized retina, the subject would have no way of discriminating the original drift due to image instability from the imposed motion. That is, image drift resulting from resolution failures of the oculomotor system logically cannot be discriminated from the same image drift imposed on a stabilized retina. Imposed drift will be discriminably different from natural drift when the amplitude of the imposed drift is artificially increased to be greater than natural drift. Just how much increase of artificial over natural drift is necessary for discrimination is not known. And we do not know to what extent typical drift movements, natural or imposed, produce apparent motion. This problem needs experimental study.

4. Slow drift with head free-moving

Not all head movements are intentional. Even when trying to hold the head as still as possible, as for example in walking, the head inevitably oscillates. The best possible compensation for retinal image slip with small head movements leaves a

* The suggestion that small eye movements might somehow overcome image perturbations induced by receptor irregularity, i.e., by higher visual centers assuming that the retinal receptors are embedded in a regular grid when they are not, encounters, additionally, a profound logical problem because receptors are typically as informative when they are spaced irregularly as regularly (Maloney, 1988, 1990; Yellott, 1987). The role of eye movements in correcting perception at a larger scale is considered later.

residual, uncompensated image slip of about 0.5 deg per s (Skavenski et al., 1979); with modest voluntary head rotation the image slip increases 10-fold to 5 deg per s (Steinman and Collewijn, 1980; Steinman and Levinson, Ch. 3 of this volume). In carefully controlled experimental situations, when motion of the head is induced by rotating the subject in a chair, the eye movements are invariably imperfect, and the proportion of compensation for head movement depends on the amplitude and frequency of the head movement (Skavenski et al., 1979). These authors found that the gain of compensatory movement decreased as the amplitude of oscillation decreased, and suggested an automatic adjustment of gain sufficient to maintain clear vision.

Despite the large image slip as the head moves around, the world does not appear to move, except in extreme situations. Remarkably, acuity for gratings hardly suffers: there is a slight decline in contrast sensitivy at high spatial frequencies and a slight improvement at spatial frequencies below 5 cycles/deg (Steinman et al., 1985).

When an image on the eye is stabilized, and image motions which mimic the large motions of normal unstabilized viewing are then imposed on this image, what does it look like? And how does the image movement affect acuity? Again, this experiment has not been carried out, although it seems obvious that the image would appear to move around. The effect of imposed motion on acuity has been studied only with very simple procedures. Kelly (1979) tested contrast sensitivity for sine gratings in stabilized vision with imposed constant image velocities, and found large acuity changes dependent on imposed velocity: a great decline in acuity at high frequency of imposed image movement, a small improvement at low frequencies. Steinman et al. (1985) tested acuity under comparable conditions of natural image motion in the same range of velocities and found smaller acuity losses. In Steinman et al.'s procedure, the image moved back and forth as the subjects moved their heads. In Kelly's procedure, the image moved at a constant velocity for several seconds before the subject responded. If Kelly's results with prolonged viewing of constant image velocities generalized to back-and-forth image motions, then we would have to conclude that imposed image motion is harmful to grating acuity over a range of image velocities that does not lead to acuity loss in natural viewing (see Ch. 3).

5. Smooth pursuit

Smooth pursuit refers to the smooth following of external image movement. Whether there is a significant distinction between the oculomotor subsystem responsible for following external image motion and the oculomotor subsystem that follows intrinsically caused image motion (produced, for example, by head or body movements) has been debated for many years. The velocity of smooth pursuit can be remarkably high, up to or exceeding 100 deg/s for large-amplitude motions (Collewijn et al., 1985; Meyer et al., 1985). The gain of smooth pursuit depends on many factors: notably the pattern of motion (waveform, frequency, amplitude, velocity of constant velocity motion, etc.) and on past history. The luminance contrast of the moving stimulus pattern seems not to be critical (Haegerstrom-Portnoy and Brown, 1979; Wintersonand Steinman, 1978).

5.1. Localization in smooth pursuit

Flashed targets. A flashed target seen during smooth pursuit is very accurately localized relative to the body (Hansen, 1979). Untracked objects seen during pursuit are also accurately localized. Taken together, Hansen's results establish that eye position is accurately known during smooth pursuit, and the knowledge of eye position is available to perceptual judgements relative to body position. However, the extent to which this extra-retinal knowledge is available to visual judgements of the relative positions of targets flashed during smooth pursuit is less clear (see Ch. 5 of this volume). The extent to which flash localization during real pursuit differs from localization during simulated pursuit is not known (cf. sections on spatial localization during saccades and simulated saccades.)

Reconstruction of the trajectories of moving objects. Suppose that a moving dot describes a perfect circle. When the eye is fixated, the circular trajectory is perceived veridically (correctly). During linear smooth pursuit of another target, the retinal projection of the circle becomes distorted. The perceptual system for computing localization of the eye relative to the body only partially solves this distortion problem. That is, the perceived path is a composite of the distorted retinal path and the true circular path in external space. (See the review by Mack, 1986, and Chs. 5 and 6 for further discussions of these illusions.) The issue of how spatiotemporal relations between stimuli that occur during eye movements might be reconstructed will be reconsidered in the section on saccades.

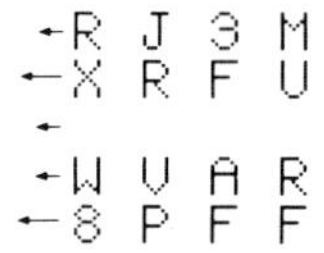

Fig. 1. Example of a display used by Khurana and Kowler (1987) Four rows of characters are visible at once. The arrows indicate the relative speeds of motion to the left. The subject is instructed to track an (invisible) point between the rows at the speed of one of the rows. The array contains two numerals among the letters: one in a fast row and one in a slow row. The subject's task is to report both numerals.

5.2. Simulated pursuit movements

Acuity. Brian Murphy (1978) produced, in stationary eyes, image velocities that were the same as the image slip velocities previously measured during pursuit movements. He measured contrast sensitivity for a 5 cycles/deg grating in both conditions and found no difference. Velocities above 2 deg/s produced equivalent acuity losses in both viewing conditions. Kelly's (1979) data cited above appear also to be related here, and to yield a conflicting conclusion.

5.3. Attention during smooth pursuit: search task

From many experiments (e.g. Dodge and Fox, 1928; Dubois and Collewijn, 1979; Kowler et al., 1984) we know that subjects can selectively choose which one of several retinal stimuli to track. Even when retinal position is controlled, the tracking instruction determines what is tracked. The question Khurana and Kowler (1987) sought to answer was: can a subject track one stimulus while attending to another?

The subjects in Khurana and Kowler's (1987) experiments tracked a moving 4×4 letter array with smooth-pursuit eye movements. During the movement interval, all the characters of the array were briefly changed, with two of the former letters being replaced by numerals; the subjects' task was to detect these target numerals. In various procedures, the odd rows (1 and 3) were moved at twice or at 1/2 the velocity of the even rows (Fig. 1). Two targets occurred: one target in the even rows, another in the odd rows. The subject was instructed to report both targets on every trial. On different trials, the subject was instructed to smoothly pusue either the even or the odd rows, always with fixation in the middle of the array.

The results of this procedure showed that the subject reported the letters in the tracked rows better than the untracked rows regardless of the actual retinal slip (because the retinal velocities were too low to degrade performance). That is, visual attention was naturally linked to the pursuit attempt.

In a control experiment, tracking and attention instructions were manipulated separately. Subjects were asked to smoothly pursue one set of rows while attending to the other. All the conditions taken together provide a cross-design in which the positively correlated factors of the main experimental condition (row-to-be-attended and row-to-be-tracked) are negatively correlated in the control condition. Thus, we can estimate the effect of the two separable independent variables (tracking instruction, attention instruction) upon the two dependent variables (tracking accuracy, search accuracy).

The results showed that tracking of pursued but unattended rows was slightly worse than tracking of these same rows when they were attended (attention instructions only slightly affect tracking). Search performance on the attended but untracked rows was slightly better than search in the unattended untracked rows, but never approached the performance on tracked, unattended rows, again, regardless of retinal slip (attention instructions only slightly affect search). In other words, the tracking instruction, not the attention instruction, controls the accuracy of visual search.

Attention is inextricably linked to tracking. The following picture emerges of the role of attention in tracking: tracking instructions have big effects, attention instructions have only small additional effects. For a given rate of retinal slip, the only way that tracking per se can influence search accuracy is indirectly through attention. That an attention-instruction has almost no effect independently of tracking-instruction implies that attention is inextricably linked to smooth pursuit.* Tracking a row depends on attentional selection and only an insignificant attentional residue remains to be assigned elsewhere.

In the imposed-motion control procedure for Khurana and Kowler's experiment, the eye remains stationary as the letter rows drift aross the field. The subject's attempt to fixate a stationary point while attending to one pair of moving rows leads either to a loss of fixation as the eye drifts in the movement direction or to a loss of search accuracy in the moving rows. Thus, the data obtained with eye movements and imposed movements are essentially equivalent. It follows that the attentional resources needed to maintain the eye fixated on a stationary point are not essentially different from those needed to maintain smooth pursuit at the image velocities Khurana and Kowler used. This result lends support to the view that fixation and smooth pursuit are governed by the same mechanisms (Nachmias, 1961).

* To have reached the conclusion that subjects *could not* disassociate attention from tracking (versus simply that they *habitually did not* disassociate attention from tracking) it was essential that Khurana and Kowler's subjects actually received training – feedback as to the correctness of the responses – and despite the training failed to learn to perform both tasks.

6. Saccades

Saccades are voluntary, quick, ballistic eye movements that take the eye from one fixation point to the next. Saccades range in extent from several minutes of arc to more than 70 degrees. A typical saccade of 4 degrees is well described as a ramp function of time in which the eye travels from its initial to its final position in about 15–20 ms, and then remains relatively still in the final position for 200 ms or longer. During active search of a display or scene, saccades may occur at a rate of 4 per second, but slower saccade rates are more typical. The effect of saccades is to convert the input to the visual system into a sequence of up to 3 or 4 relatively stationary images per second, with rapid transitions between the images.

There are many provocative issues concerning saccades. How is it that the world seems to remain stationary during a saccade even though the saccade-like image sequence would be perceived as a vigorous jump if it were imposed on a stationary retina. The visual image of the world is smeared across the retina during saccades yet, on the whole, we are unaware of seeing such a smear. Is this because visual sensitivity is reduced during saccades? Are there special perceptual mechanisms designed to utilize and link information acquired during successive saccades? For example, do saccades initiate visual processing episodes? And are relative spatial coordinates defined by saccadic eye movements or by head movements inherently more useful than coordinates defined equally accurately by image movements or by other more indirect means? Is attention inextricably linked to saccades (as it is to smooth movements) or can attention move oppositely to a saccade? In what sense are saccades an optimal solution to the ecological problem confronting a visual system?

Some of these issues have been with us almost since saccades were first described by Javal in 1878. For example, with respect to the issue of vision during saccades, an early demonstration is due to Woodworth (1906). He executed a saccade from one side of a rotating wheel to the other and observed that he was able to see clearly the spokes that happened to be traveling at the same rate as his eye. Thereby Woodworth demonstrated his capacity for sharp vision during a saccade. After a review of similar experiments in his textbook Experimental Psychology, he wrote *"given the same retinal stimulation, it makes no difference whether it is the eyes or the external field that moves"* (Woodworth, 1938, p. 593, italics in the original). Woodworth's conclusion was so intuitively unsatisfactory that the issue of visual suppression during saccades has been reexamined many times, and we examine it once again.

6.1. Is vision turned off during saccades?

The rumor that vision is dead during saccades is grossly exaggerated. Some time ago, eager to observe such an effect, I put together an apparatus for studies of vision during saccades. A gas discharge lamp illuminated a thin slit before, during, or just after saccades. The illumination flash was very brief, contained within 40 microseconds, so there would be no significant retinal smear of the slit during a saccade. Before conducting formal experiments, I wanted to check whether the apparatus actually triggered flashes during saccades. I quickly discovered that, in viewing the slit against a dark background, it was not possible to ascertain whether a flash had occurred during a saccade simply by noting the appearance of the flash. A flash that occurred during a saccade did not look any different from a flash that occurred before or after. Obviously, if there were a change in visual sensitivity during saccades, it was too small and too subtle to make an obvious difference in the appearance of a suprathreshold flash. Nevertheless, there have been many reports of raised thresholds for stimuli presented during saccades (for a review, see Volkmann, 1986). How can this be?

The question of whether visibility is altered during a saccadic movement must be resolved by the proper control experiments. In the control experiment, it is essential to produce on the stationary eye precisely the same sequence of stimuli that the saccading eye produces for itself when its threshold is tested during saccades. There are two reasons for this requirement. First, the movement of fixation points and other fixed stimuli across the retina during a saccade can affect the threshold for a dim test field, and the amount of this visual masking must be measured in the control experiment. Second, the apparent location of a stimulus flashed during, or slightly before or after a saccade, will not generally correspond precisely to its objective location. From the observer's point of view, there are locational *uncertainties*, indeed, even locational illusions, in which the test flash appears to have occurred at an unexpected location. Because, as is demonstrated below, there are many similarities in spatial localization during saccades and during the equivalant imposed image motion, control experiments may provide reasonable estimates for locational uncertainty and locational illusions as well as for incidental masking. We defer the issue of altered visibility during saccades until after considering localization.

6.2. Spatial localization during saccades

There are now many studies of the localization (in which observers indicate the apparent location) of test stimuli that are flashed briefly during saccades. I describe studies (Sperling and Speelman, 1964, 1965; Sperling, 1966) that have not been fully reported before in which data from appropriate non-saccade control stimuli are available. Subsequently, related experiments are considered in the light of these results.

6.2.1. Measuring and predicting localization errors

Objective and subjective foveal trajectories. In Sperling and Speelman's (1965) procedure, subjects view a display containing five marker spots (2×3 min), separated from each other by two degrees (Fig. 2a). These spots are called −2, −1, +1, +2. The observer is instructed to fixate spot −1, and then, upon an agreed-upon signal (a brief dimming of the spots), to fixate spot +1. About 200–250 ms after the signal, the observer's eye will execute a saccadic movement from position −1 to the neighborhood of position +1 (Fig. 2d). Observers' 4-degree saccades are quite individualistic; some observers have considerable overshoot; and all observers show corrective saccades after about 0.2 s (Fig. 2e). The objective trajectory of the fovea as a function of time $x_0(t)$ describes an observer's objective eye movement – the physical position of the fovea as a function of time referred to an external coordinate system.

Suppose that at some time during the saccade, a flash of light occurs and that it falls directly on the fovea. We ask the observer where this flash appears to fall relative to the external −2 to +2 coordinate system defined by the five spots of light. Obviously, when the flash occurs long before initiation of the movement, it is subjectively localized at location −1 (the initial fixation point); when it occurs long after the movement, it is localized at position +1 (the post-movement fixation). The subjective location assigned to a flash of light that strikes the fovea changes as a function of time; this function is called the subjective foveal trajectory $x_s(t)$, and it is measured in the same coordinates as the objective trajectory.

If it happened that the objective and subjective foveal trajectories were exactly equal $[x_0(t) = x_s(t)]$ then an observer would never mislocalize a foveal flash – the observer would always report its position correctly. In general, however, the observer makes localization errors for flashes that occur during, or shortly before and after saccades. This indicates that the objective and subjective foveal trajectories are not identical. For 4-deg eye movements, the subjective trajectory is usually not quite as quick as the objective trajectory.

Procedure. Some further details of the procedure are relevant. Subjects viewed the display with their heads fixed to a dental impression. Horizontal eye position was monitored by a limbus monitor (Fig. 2b,c). Initially, the monitor was dynamically calibrated with an artificial eye. During the experiment, it was calibrated between successive eye-movement trials. Dynamic eye position was resolvable to an accuracy of about 3 min (for 4-degree saccades) but was recorded for subsequent analysis only to an accuracy of 12 min because, in the limbus monitor, DC accuracy is not as good as dynamic accuracy. Upon a 10-ms interruption of the display (which appeared as a dark flash), subjects were instructed to shift their fixation as quickly as possible from spot −1 to spot +1 (Fig. 2d). A thin vertical test line was flashed during the display and subjects were instructed to report its position to an accuracy of 0.1 unit of the display distance. For example, if the test line appeared to strike midway between spots 0 and 1, subjects were to report '0.5'. Preliminary experiments to teach and test the use of this method of report (during fixation) had shown that subjects could report positions to within ± 0.1 unit. The apparatus could trigger a flash when the eyes crossed the midpoint of the display or at any later time. To obtain test flashes that occur before eye movements, the apparatus is set to trigger a flash at a predetermined delay from the warning stimulus. Trial-to-trial variations in this delay, together with subject variability in saccadic reaction time, yield a distribution of trials with times of occurrence before, during, and after the midpoint of the eye movement is obtained.

As a practical matter, in these experiments, all flashes occurred at precisely the same physical location, and hence at different retinal locations. The subjective foveal localization was computed from nonfoveal flashes on the assumption of a rigid translation of the central 4 deg of the perceptual coordinate system. (This assumption, and experiments by O'Regan (1984) testing it, are considered in detail later.) As a matter of convention, time is indicated relative to the moment at which the eye crosses the midpoint of the display. Four-degree eye movements typically take less than 20 ms; therefore the movement times are within ± 10 ms of zero (Fig. 2e).

Localization errors. Some data from an eye movement experiment in which the test flash was posi-

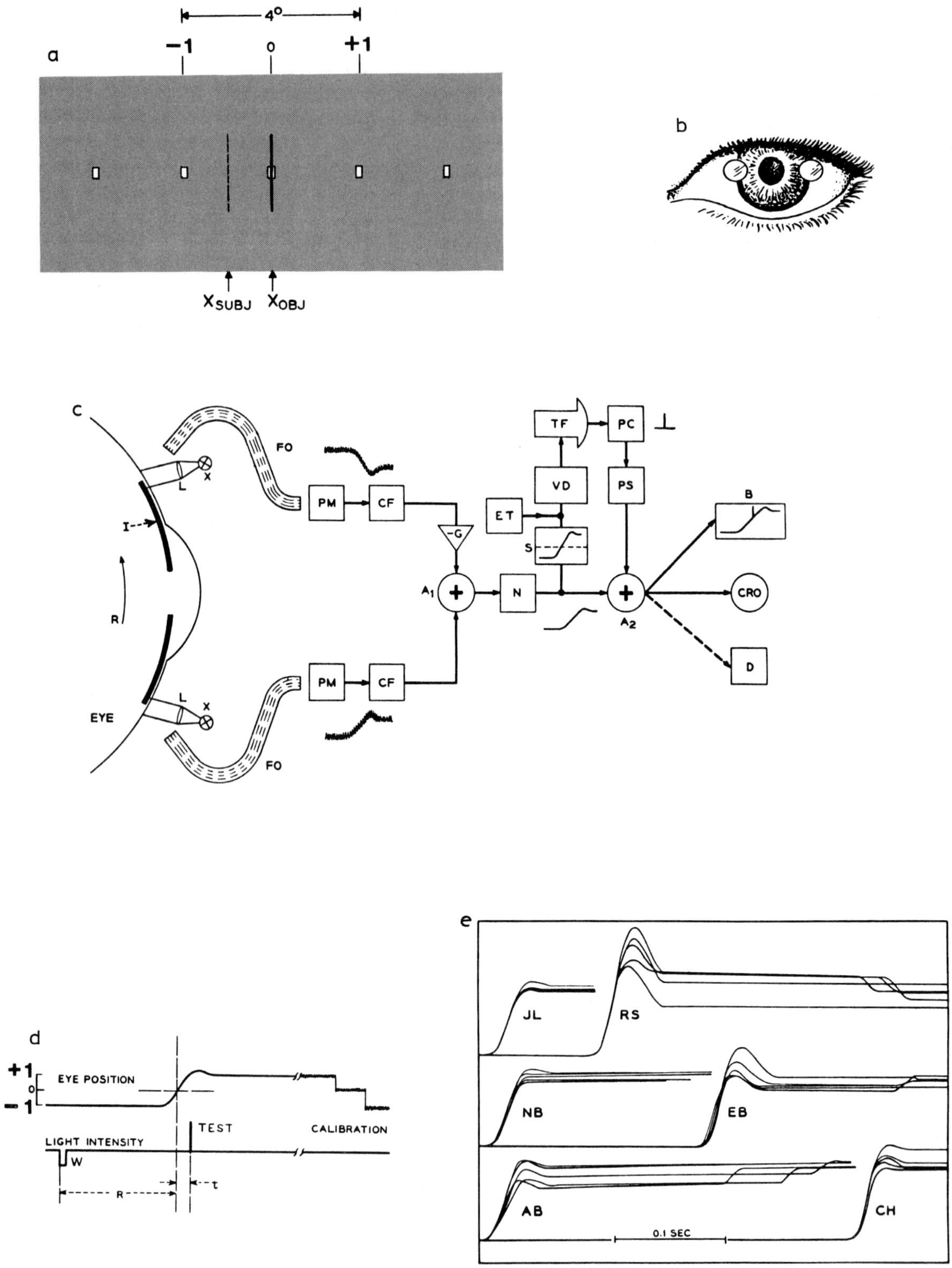
a
4°
−1
0
+1
X_SUBJ
X_OBJ
b
C
FO
L
X
I
R
EYE
PM
CF
-G
A1
N
ET
VD
TF
PC
PS
S
B
CRO
A2
D
d
+1
0
−1
EYE POSITION
TEST
CALIBRATION
LIGHT INTENSITY
W
R
t
e
JL
RS
NB
EB
AB
CH
0.1 SEC

tioned always to occur directly superimposed on the middle marker are shown in the leftmost column of Fig. 3. In this procedure, a correct report by the subject would always be '0.0' and would be indicated as 0 in the graph. This setup was chosen so that correct localization would be obvious – the test flash would appear directly superimposed on the center marker; its illusory appearance anywhere else clearly represented an error of localization. The abscissa of Fig. 3 indicates the time relative to the instant at which the eye crossed the middle marker. When the subject reports that the test flash appears displaced towards the final marker position, the error is indicated by an ordinate value greater than zero. For example, the greater-than-zero errors by subject 3 indicate that the perceptual spatial coordinates of the retina had already started to change to their new values, even before the eye had begun to move. Values below zero indicate that the retinal coordinates lag behind the physical movement.

Not all eye movements are precisely correct; some fall short of the intended mark and are corrected by a subsequent saccade. The data in the left column of Fig. 3 include all eye movements, those which reached their intended mark and those which did not. The advantage of mislocation errors as a dependent variable is that mislocation errors do not depend critically on the extent of the movement. It is reasonable to aggregate mislocation data from movements of somewhat different extents.

In terms of a computational theory to account for mislocation errors, the extent of the movement becomes a parameter, and for this purpose it is useful to restrict consideration to 4-deg eye movements which begin and end within 0.5 deg of the initial and final fixation markers. The data for each subject that describe the recorded eye positions as a function of time $x_0(t)$ can be reasonably well characterized by a 3-segment straight line: horizontal at position −1 until the start of the movement, linear slope (constant velocity) during the eye movement, and again horizontal with constant slope at the conclusion of the movement. Thereby, only two parameters are estimated, e.g., the starting time and the duration of a trajectory. These data are illustrated in the right column of Fig. 3.

The subjective foveal location (the location in space to which a test flash striking the fovea would be referred) is derived by adding the localization error $e(t)$ recorded in the experiment to the objective foveal location:

$$x_s(t) - x_0(t) + e(t)$$

Like objective foveal locations, subjective foveal locations $x_s(t)$ can be characterized by a 3-segment function. Fig. 3, right column, shows the observed objective and subjective eye position data for six subjects together with the 3-segment trajectories that maximize temporal prediction (minimize the

Fig. 2. (a) The display viewed by Sperling and Speelman's subjects in the saccadic movement experiments. Five bright spots of light were visible in a dark field. Initially, subjects fixed the spot labeled −1; upon a signal, they saccaded to the spot labeled +1. (Left/right was reversed from session to session.) Sometime before, during, or after the saccade, a thin bar centered on 'O' was illuminated by a stroboscopic flash. The subject's task was to report the apparent location of the bar relative to coordinates defined by the illuminated spots. (b) A limbus monitor illuminated rectangular spots at the iris/sclera border, and measured the amount of reflected light to indicate the eye's horizontal position. (c) The limbus monitor and the linked display system. R indicates the direction of saccadic rotation; I is the iris; X is a light source focussed on the iris/sclera border by a lens L; FO is a fiber-optic bundle that collects the reflected light and carries it to a photomultiplier detector PM; CF is an electronic (cathode follower) amplifier; G is a variable gain chosen to equate the amplitude of the left and right signals; A1 adds the right and the inverted left signals to yield an estimate of horizontal eye position; N is a low-pass linear filter which removes high-frequency noise; S is the threshold location in the saccade at which trigger is initiated; VD is a variable delay; TF is the stroboscopic flash gun that illuminates the target; PC and PS, respectively, are photodetectors which monitor the target and stimulus displays; A2 adds the display information to the position information to produce three records of the events of the trial; B, an ink-on-paper record; CRO, a CRT display; and D, a digital record on magnetic tape. (d) The sequence of events on a trial. A momentary darkening of the background spots is the signal to initiate the saccade; the test flash occurs at time t; and a calibration sequence of fixations on spots +1, 0 and −1 occurs between consecutive trials. The midpoint of the intended saccade is the point x=0, y=0, t=0. (e) Eye movement records obtained for six subjects. Five traces are superimposed in each record.

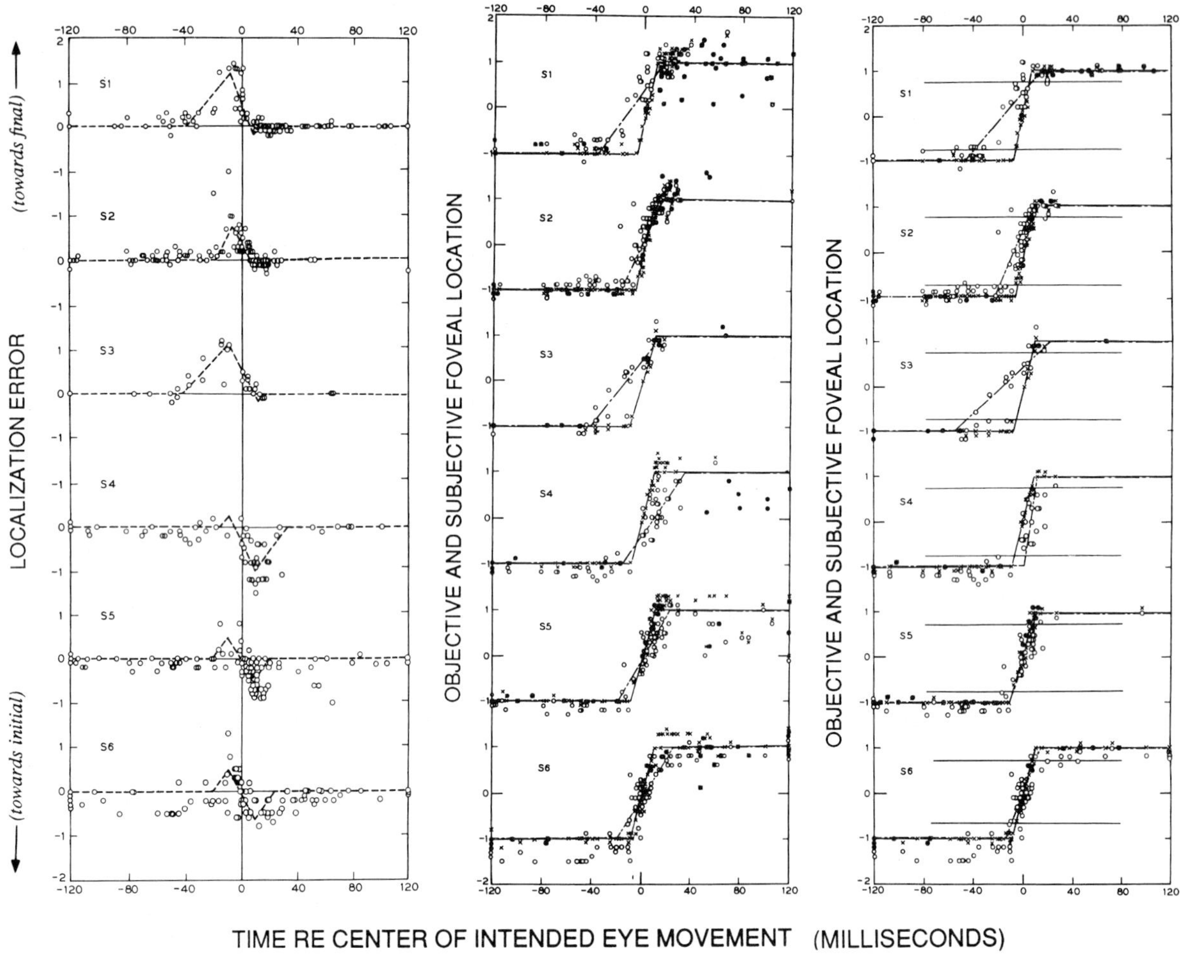

Fig. 3. Left. Errors in localization of a flash that occurs at location 0 as a function of its time of occurrence relative to the midpoint of the saccade. The ordinate is in display units: +1 represents a mislocalization of the target at the intended final location; −1 represents a mislocalization at the initial location. Each point represents one localization judgement. The dashed lines are the difference between the best-fitting objective and subjective eye trajectories shown in center. Right. Objective and subjective foveal location as a function of time relative to the midpoint of an intended 4-degree saccade. Data from all 'good' saccades that began and ended within 0.5 deg of the intended starting and final fixations are shown for six subjects. Each trial yields a paired objective foveal location (*) and subjective foveal location (open circle). The solid lines and dashed sloping lines minimize the squared horizontal distance from the objective and subjective location data, respectively, to the line within the middle three degrees of movement. Center. Same as right column except that all eye movements are included, and the three-segment functions minimize the vertical distance of the date to the function.

root mean square (rms) horizontal distances of the data to the trajectory) in the middle 3 degrees of the 4-degree movements. This treatment of the data is appropriate for the next section, 'A purely temporal analysis of saccadic localization'.

The center column of Fig. 3 illustrates objective and subjective foveal locations for all the attempted 4-degree saccades. These data include quite a few saccades that were substantially shorter and some that were longer than four degrees. The 3-segment functions which minimize the vertical rms distance of the data to the function are shown for both objective and subjective foveal locations. Strictly speaking, these objective (and subjective) foveal trajectories apply only to a homogeneous set of eye movements (e.g., movements between 3.9 and 4.1 degrees). However, the differences between objective and subjective trajectories, shown as dashed lines in the left column of Fig. 3, can be used to estimate mislocation errors even for a more heterogeneous collection of eye movements because saccadic extent cancels in the process of subtracting the objective from the subjective trajectory.

The estimated durations of the subjects' eye movements (objective foveal trajectories) vary from 16.4 to 20.8 ms. The durations of the optimized subjective foveal trajectories (those which best predict localization) vary from 29 to 56 ms (mean = 45 ms). There are considerable differences in the invidividual subjective trajectories; five subjects start the subjective movement before the objective movement, and one begins later.

The difference between the straight-line trajectory estimations of the observed objective and subjective foveal trajectories is the predicted localization error. These predictions are indicated by the dashed lines in the left column of Fig. 3. The objective-subjective trajectory difference gives a reasonable account of localization errors. Section 6.3 describes a saccade simulator: the data of Fig. 3 obtained with actual eye movements will be compared to data obtained with simulated eye movements. First, however, we consider an alternative analysis of the localization judgements.

6.2.2. A purely temporal analysis of saccadic localization

In the preceding section, errors in spatial localization were analysed in terms of the difference between the objective and subjective trajectories of the eye. Because localization errors are naturally measured as spatial localization errors, the spatial analysis was appropriate as an initial analysis. In this section, localization errors are considered not as spatial errors but as purely temporal errors. The reason is that spatial localization with stationary stimuli is extremely good, but, during rapid movements, small temporal errors would produce large spatial errors. Therefore, it seems most likely that the errors in spatial localization during saccades result indirectly from small temporal errors in when the saccade is estimated to have occurred relative to the test flash. Again, the temporal analysis is in terms of a mismatch between the objective and subjective trajectories of the eye but, in the purely temporal analysis, the trajectories are chosen to minimize the temporal prediction error (horizontal dimension in Fig. 3), not the spatial prediction error (vertical dimension in Fig. 3).

Temporally optimized trajectories. As was described above, ignoring overshoot, 4-deg saccadic eye movements are well described by a 3-segment function, a constant initial segment, a linear ramp, and a constant final segment. The duration of the movement, the ramp segment, is 18 ± 2 ms, and is constant for a particular subject.

The subjective foveal trajectories (derived from localization judgements) also are well fitted by three-segment functions. Earlier, in the left and center columns of Fig. 3, these functions were chosen to minimize the localization error – i.e., to minimize the vertical distance between the data points and the function on a graph of foveal trajectory versus time such as Fig. 3, center. Here, we are concerned with the hypothesis that all aspects of localization can be interpreted in terms of (a) temporal distortion of the movement trajectory and (b) irreducible temporal uncertainty (residual error). This requires estimating functions to maximize the goodness of temporal predictions, i.e., to minimize the horizontal distance between predictions and data.

Making horizontal (temporal) predictions is technically more difficult than vertical (spatial) predictions. Horizontal estimations can only be made in the middle sections of plots such as Fig. 3 (right). Basically, this requires selecting only good eye movements, those which finish within ± 12 min of the intended location, and making the estimates only at points between 0.25 and 0.75 of total traverse. This procedure considerably restricts the amount of data available; however, the statistics about objective and subjective location that we (Sperling and Speelman, 1965) computed for this subset of 'good movements' were, in fact, representative of the whole.

For three of six subjects (S4–6, Fig. 3, right), the duration of temporally optimized subjective trajectories was statistically within the range of objective saccade trajectory durations (11, 20, 27 ms). For the other three subjects (S1–3), the durations of subjective saccades (33, 60, 76 ms) were incontestably longer than objective saccades. Additionally, for these subjects, the midpoint of the subjective movement preceded the midpoint of the objective movement by 6–17 ms. Because of the overall similarity of localization judgements for real and simulated saccades for all subjects, the conclusion is that different subjects perceive rapid *visual* motion somewhat differently, and consequently make somewhat different localization judgements. (See, for comparison, the different time courses of visual persistence measured in different subjects by Weichselgartner and Sperling, 1985).

In addition to characterizing a subjective movement trajectory in terms of its duration, there is trial-to-trial variability in localization judgements. This variability can be conceptualized as resulting either from positional uncertainty or from temporal uncertainty. Positional resolution, as measured in control experiments, was extremely good in flash localization, with errors seldom exceeding $\pm$ 0.1 of the distance between markers. Therefore, we consider here to what extent localization errors can be modeled simply by temporal uncertainty in when the saccadic or simulated saccadic movement occurred.

Each objective eye position (Fig. 3, right) in the midrange between 0.25 and 0.75 of the total saccadic extent was interpreted in terms of the temporal (horizontal) deviation of the data point from the best-fitting trajectory. The root mean square deviation (rms, σ) of objective eye positions from the best-fitting objective eye trajectories varied only from 0.93 to 1.42 ms (for six subjects). Such small variations indicate that real eye movements follow a remarkably stereotypical time course. For the subjective foveal trajectories, the corresponding rms errors ranged from 4.0 to 8.2 ms, again a surprisingly small error and a small range of intersubject variation. There was no tendency for errors to vary with the duration of the subjective trajectory.

The purely temporal theory derived from the assumption that spatial localization errors in saccades are ultimately caused by temporal errors in the representation of the saccade relative to the test flash. This general principle led to the following specific conclusions concerning localization errors of a brief flash that occurred during a 4-deg saccadic eye movement with the visual reference stimuli continuously present:

(1) Flash-localization judgements in the presence of continuously present visual reference stimuli are determined primarily by visual factors.

(2) Half the subjects perceive the saccadic movement approximately correctly, and half perceive the movement to occur slightly too soon, and to be significantly longer than it actually is.

(3) Additionally, there is random temporal uncertainty with an rms value ranging from 4 to 8 ms (over subjects).

The irreducible *random* temporal errors in visual localization are somewhat greater than the temporal errors that can be estimated from Hansen and Skavenski's (1977 and 1985) motor localization tasks, which have the best experimentally observed temporal resolution. The main difference, however, is that the visual/perceptual representation of the movement is elongated relative to the objective eye movement for half the subjects in the present experiments, whereas Hansen and Skavenski (1977) found that the nonvisual (motoric) representation of the saccade in their motor task was uniformly accurate.

6.3. Simulated saccades

6.3.1. Saccadic motion smear

An eye movement simulator. To examine to what extent the visual stimulus, independent of the motor system, determined the observed localization judgements, we have to produce on the stationary eye precisely the same visual stimulus that the sac-

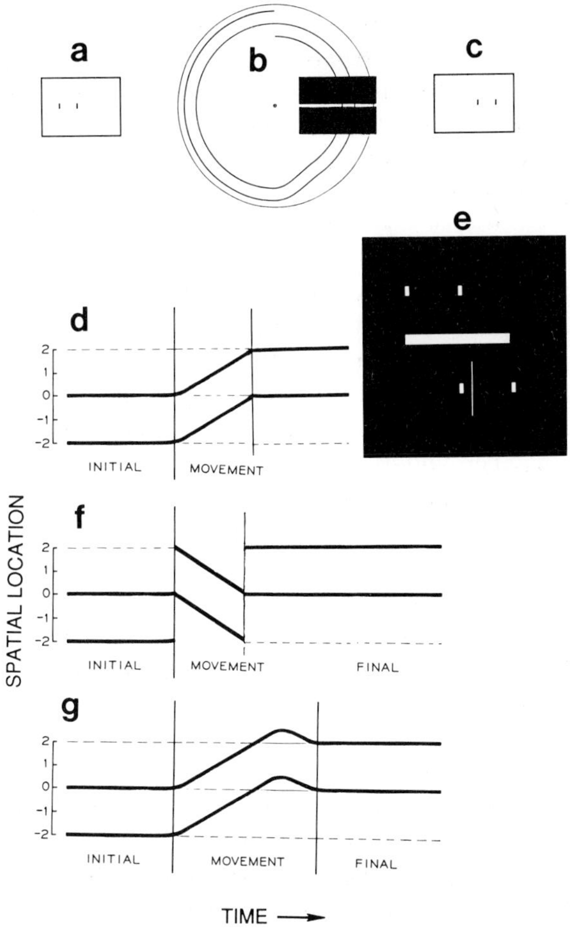

Fig. 4. Eye movement simulator: a mechanical device for generating saccadic images on a stationary eye. (a) The initial field. (b) The movement field. A large disk, rotating in the direction of the arrow, generates the moving component of the simulated saccade. The dark lines y1, y2 indicate translucent sections in the otherwise opaque disk, illuminated from behind. A masking partition M reveals only a narrow slit S to the observer. (c) The final field. (d) Representation of the position of spots y1 and y2 as a function of time for a linear saccade. The disk provides the moving field. A mirror tachistoscope, which illuminates only one field at a time, coordinates illumination of the movement field with the stationary initial and final fields. (e) The motion smear: a time-exposure photograph of the stimulus generated by the movement field. Also shown, markers in their initial and final positions, and the test flash. (f) A reversed eye movement. The direction of the motion segment is reversed relative to the initial and final fields. (g) A simulated saccadic trajectory with overshoot.

cadically moving eye produces. In the case of saccades, this is a formidable technical problem which was resolved as illustrated in Fig. 4. Again, the eye movement trajectory is composed of three parts: initial fixation, movement, and final fixation, produced in three fields of a tachistoscope. The initial stimulus is shown in Fig. 4a, the final fixation in Fig. 4c.

The moving stimulus was produced by a rotating a disk as shown in Fig. 4b. On an otherwise opaque disk, two transparent, approximately concentric, curves $c_1\ (\rho, \theta)$ and $c_2\ (\rho, \theta)$ are drawn. The disk spins continuously, is illuminated from behind, and is viewed through a narrow slit arranged along a horizontal radius. The observer sees two spots of light which move left or right as the radial distance ρ varies with θ. Almost any movement trajectory of the spots can be produced by appropriate choice of $c(\rho, \theta)$. When the disk spins at 6.3 rotations per second, the trajectory occupies 20 ms. Therefore, illumination of the moving field (Fig. 4b) has to be coordinated by elaborate temporal synchronization and optical superposition with illumination of the stationary initial and final fields (Fig. 4a and c).

A trial begins with the initial field displayed continuously. When the subject presses a key, at the first available rotation after 0.5 s, the initial field shuts off and the moving display turns on for 20 ms. After the movement section has passed, its illumination is shut off and the final field 3 is illuminated. In this setup, it was feasible to present only 2 of the 5 marker spots of the previous experiment, the −1 and +1 markers, corresponding to the initial and final fixations. A time-exposure photograph of the moving portion of the display is shown in Fig. 4e, as well as the initial and final fields. It illustrates the quite uniform motion smear produced by the simulated eye movement.

Finally, a Risley prism was inserted into the view path. By rotating the prism, the left/right orientation of the entire display could be reversed. By reversing the static initial and final positions and also reversing the entire display orientation (Fig. 4c), only the direction of movement remained reversed. Four conditions of movement trajectory were investigated: (a) normal motion trajectory (Fig. 4d), (b) reversed motion trajectory (Fig. 4f), (c) sampled motion trajectory – illumination of the moving field is turned off during the interval between initial and final fields – and (d) double reversed-direction sampled motion trajectory, i.e., this looks the same to the observer as the normal sampled motion trajectory. The temporal sequence of the normal initial and final fields is reversed, and the display is then reversed spatially with a Risley prism. This is a check for any undetected difference between initial and final fields that might affect the reversed motion trajectory. This apparatus was used to study continuous and sampled movements of various lengths and durations.

6.3.2. The appearance of motion smear

While the main purpose of the apparatus was to study spatial localization, I digress for a moment to consider the subjective appearance of the saccadically moving stimuli. The most surprising observation was that, even though the stimulus consisted of bright spots viewed against darkness, observers did not spontaneously discriminate the correct from the reversed movement trajectory when the imposed movements occupied 20 ms and the total distance traversed ranged from one to four degrees, according to the viewing distance. With the eye movement simulator, visual sensitivity to the various aspects of the retinal movement trajectory could be isolated. On alternate presentations, the illumination of the movement field was turned off, thereby eliminating the movement smear entirely and substituting 20 ms of darkness. Naive viewers did not spontaneously notice any difference between consecutive displays of continuous motion and sampled movement. Indeed, observers did not report a difference in the appearance of motion smear even when they were pressed, although many irrelevant aspects of the displays caught their attention.

When the difference between the normal-, reversed- and no-smear (sampled) displays is pointed out to viewers, they can notice a barely discriminable difference in the motion smear between continuous-movement and the sampled-movement trials but the direction-of-movement discrimination appears to be impossible. Of course, when the speed of the motion trajectory is slowed down by a factor of 10 or so, all the appropriate relations can easily be perceived.

Visual masking of motion smear. When the motion smear occurs alone (i.e., only Fig. 4b is shown and the initial and final fields (Fig. 4a and c) are turned off), the smear itself (Fig. 4e) is quite easy to detect. But the discrimination of motion direction in the smear remains difficult. MacKay (1970a), Campbell and Wurtz (1978) and Corfield et al. (1978) propose that the difficulty of detecting motion smear is due to visual masking by the visual stimulation that immediately precedes and follows the smear. In one experiment (Campbell and Wurtz, 1978), subjects initiated eye movements in the dark. During the eye movement, a light was turned on. When the light remained on only very briefly, subjects reported that the scene illuminated by the light was clearly visible and sharp (thereby reproducing once again the observation of clear vision during saccades). As the light remained on for 20 ms and longer during a long saccade, the scene appeared to become extremely blurred, much like the motion smear represented in Fig. 4e. On the other hand, if the light remained on for more than 40 ms *after* the saccade ended, the previous saccadic motion smear became invisible. Thus 40 ms of post-saccadic stimulation masked saccadic motion smear.

To study motion smear in the stationary eye, Corfield et al. (1978) represented saccadic motion smear by a stationary blank field, like that of Fig. 4e. They preceded and followed the blank field by different textured fields, principally sinusoid gratings and combinations of sinusoids. When the blank field was as brief as it would have been during normal saccadic eye movements, the blank field was not visible – it was completely masked by the preceding and following stimuli. While various parameters of masking were investigated, the process of visual masking itself was not elucidated in these experiments. However, whatever the masking process in the stationary eye may be, the experiments demonstrate that it is also sufficient to account for the invisibility of motion smear in the saccadically moving eye.

6.3.3. The effect of motion smear on spatial localization

Spatial localization during imposed saccade-like movements. The difficulty of observing motion smear during real and simulated saccades even under optimal conditions for its appearance (i.e., a scene consisting of bright spots on a dark background) suggests that motion smear would not contribute to other kinds of psychophysical judgements. Nevertheless, I (Sperling, 1966) used the saccadic motion simulator shown in Fig. 4 to investigate spatial localization. The motion trajectory on the retina and the psychophysical procedure were analogous to those of the saccadic spatial localization task described above in section 6.2.

The saccadic movement simulator was arranged to provide the linear saccadic movement stimulus illustrated in Fig. 4d. During the movement trajectory, a thin test line was flashed briefly, and the subject was asked to localize the flash relative to the position of moving spots at the instant of the flash. The localization judgement was similar to that illustrated in Fig. 2a, with the subject initially fixated on the spot labeled −1, except that the only other spot visibe was +1. The subject maintained fixation rather than moving his eyes, and the display moved quickly so that, after the movement, the spot +1 was at the fixation point.

The movement trajectory was a linear translation between initial and final positions which traversed the distance in 20 ms (Fig. 2d). In this experiment, the viewing distance was increased so that the total length of the movement trajectory was 95 min of visual angle. The movement was somewhat slower than a natural saccade and somewhat shorter than the saccades studied in the previous section. These experimental parameters were chosen to maximize the number of localization judgements between – rather than at – the end points in order to give the imposed trajectories the maximum opportunity to exert differential effects. Normal continuous movements, reversed movements (Fig. 4f) and sampled (no smear) movements were tested. The test line, rather than flashing at different retinal locations, as in the saccadic movement experiment, always occurred displaced slightly from the fixation point (the fovea) in the direction of the simulated movement (0.2 of the movement distance as shown in Fig. 4e).

The results can be described succinctly. No subject showed any significant difference between the normal and reversed movement conditions with respect to spatial localization of the test flash. In other words, the direction of the saccade-like image smear did not influence spatial localization judgements – they were determined by the pre- and post-movement fields.

There were minor localization differences between continuous-movement (normal or reversed) and sampled movement for some subjects and not for others. When there was a difference, it was a greater tendency in the sampled movement displays for the test flash to be localized at the initial or final positions, not in between. Data representing each type of performance are shown in Fig. 5. For example, S4 hardly ever localizes a flash at locations between −1 and 0 in the sampled control (top and bottom panels, Fig. 5), but does so frequently in both smear conditions (middle panels, Fig. 5).

Spatial localization during much slower-than-saccadic simulated movements. The saccadic simulator can be used to impose retinal motion at velocities that are higher or lower than saccadic velocities. Subjects viewed the moving stimuli while maintaining fixation on a stationary fixation point. In order that subjects did not correctly anticipate the image motion and move their eyes, the direction of motion was random from trial to trial. As in the case of movements at saccadic speeds, subjects were asked to judge the location of a brief flash relative to the moving coordinate system defined by the dots.

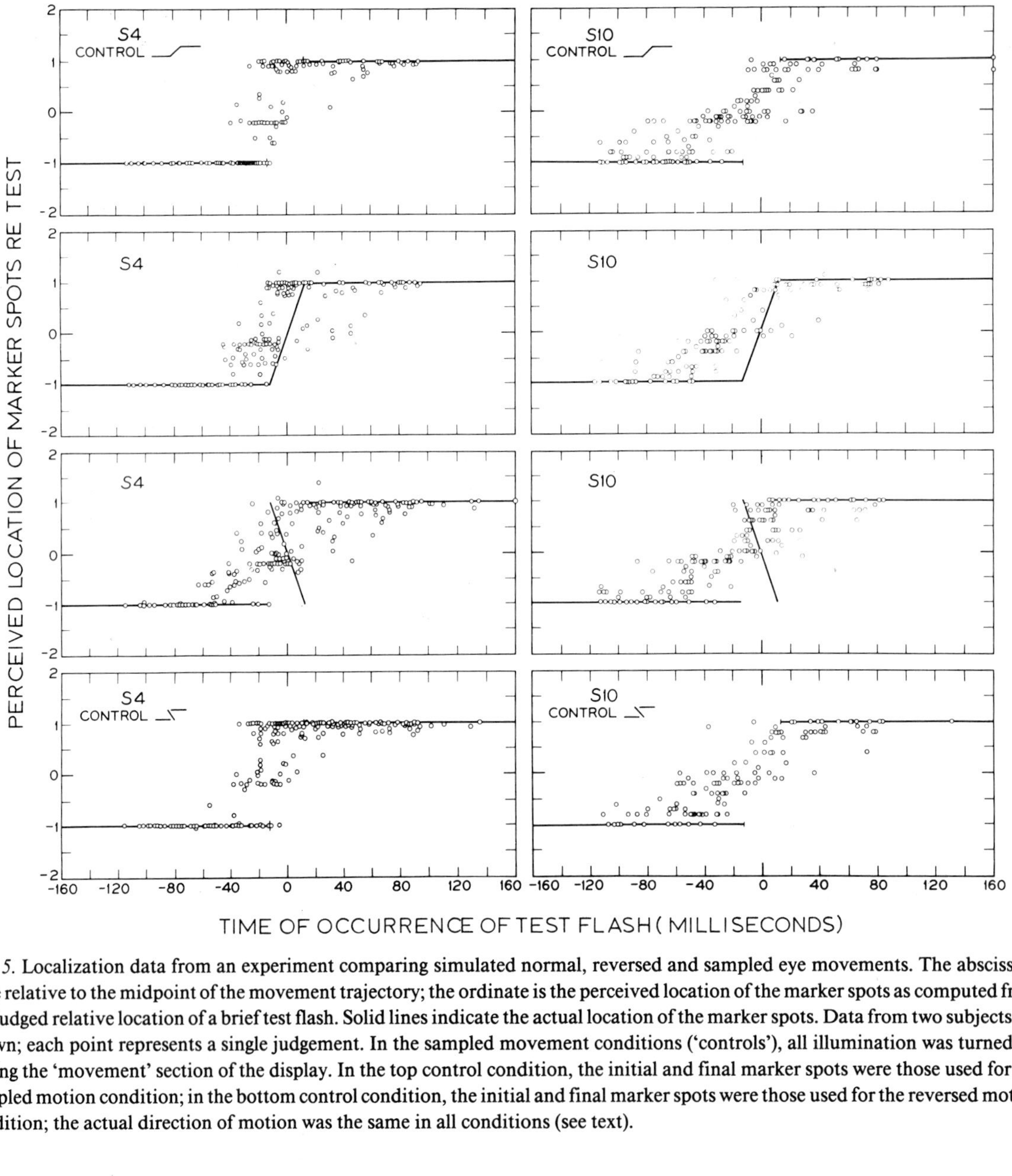

Fig. 5. Localization data from an experiment comparing simulated normal, reversed and sampled eye movements. The abscissa is time relative to the midpoint of the movement trajectory; the ordinate is the perceived location of the marker spots as computed from the judged relative location of a brief test flash. Solid lines indicate the actual location of the marker spots. Data from two subjects are shown; each point represents a single judgement. In the sampled movement conditions ('controls'), all illumination was turned off during the 'movement' section of the display. In the top control condition, the initial and final marker spots were those used for the sampled motion condition; in the bottom control condition, the initial and final marker spots were those used for the reversed motion condition; the actual direction of motion was the same in all conditions (see text).

The left half of Fig. 6 shows the localization of the test flash relative to the moving coordinate frame during 4-deg continuous movements, with durations of 50, 125, 250 and 500 ms. The right half of Fig. 6 shows localization during no-smear (sampled) movements. As in the previous experiment, the test line occurred slightly displaced from fixation in the direction of movement (Fig. 4e).

As the duration of the movement component of a trajectory is stretched out in time so that it is much slower than saccadic eye movements, there eventually come to be quite obvious differences in appearance between a display with a normal movement trajectory and one with the movement trajec-

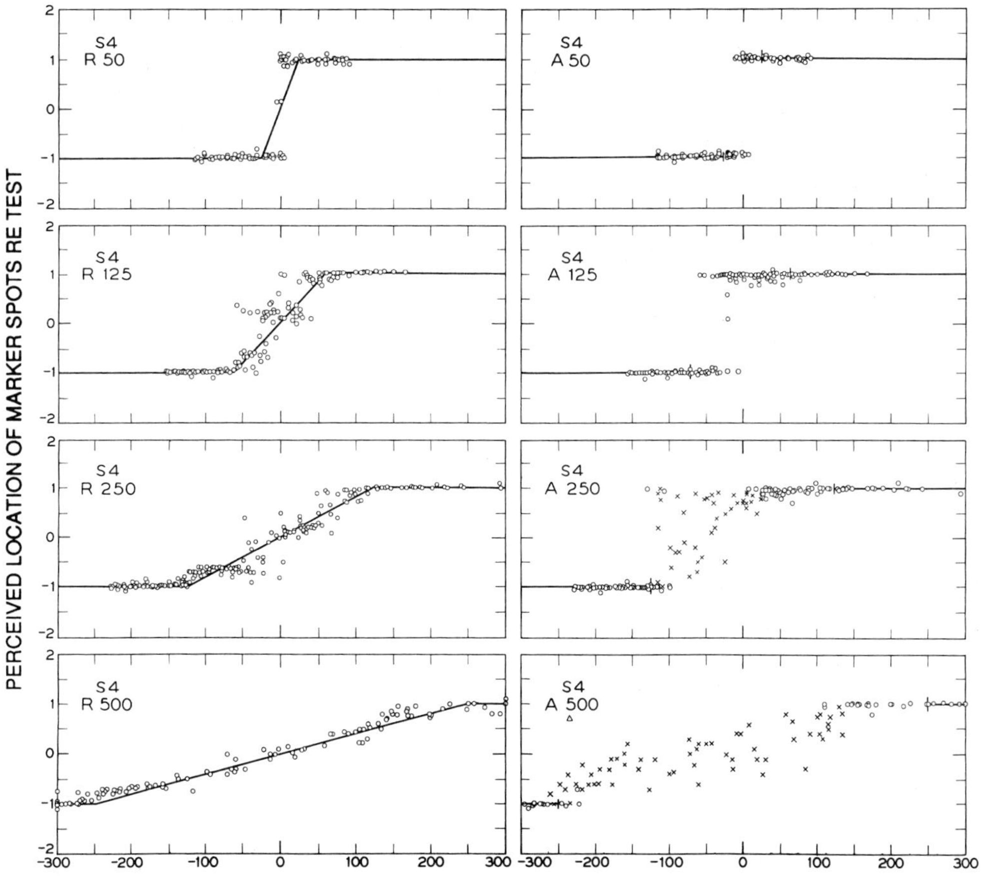

Fig. 6. Spatial localization compared in continuous and sampled motion stimuli of various speeds. The solid lines indicate the actual motion trajectory; the coordinates are as in Fig. 5. Left panels show continuous motion stimuli, right panels show sampled (sometimes called *apparent*) motion stimuli. Open circles indicate the perceived location of the moving marker spots as computed from the judged location of a brief test flash; x's indicate that the marker spots were temporarily eclipsed at the instant of the test flash and the location judgement was made relative to an *inferred* trajectory.

tory turned off. The trajectory between the initial and final position is correctly perceived as a slow translation; when it is absent, a blank period is perceived (e.g., blank times of 250 and 500 ms are quite obvious). With long blank times, the localization task for sampled-motion (interrupted) stimuli is ambiguous. When the localization task is redefined as 'judge the flash relative to where you believe the markers would be if they were visible,' the results of localization experiments with continuous-movement and with sampled-movement stimuli are quite similar. (Localization judgements made when the coordinate frame appeared to be invisible at the instant the test flash occurred are indicated by x in Fig. 6.) Because the linear interpolation of visual motion is so natural, even when there is an obvious blank period between initial and final positions, the localization task is not appropriate for revealing the differences in appearance.

Localization judgements during movements of various speeds yield some obvious and predictable results and some surprising ones. (1) For practical purposes, flash localization judgements do not distinguish between continuous and sampled motion at saccadic and near-saccadic velocities, i.e., 1.6 deg, 20 ms imposed movement (Fig. 5) and the 4.0 deg, 50 ms imposed movement (Fig. 6). (2) When markers spaced by 4 degrees traverse the inter-marker space in 50 ms, flashes are nearly always localized only at their initial and final locations. This strictly bimodal distribution of localization judgements obtains for greater spaces or quicker traverses. (3) For motions of 125 ms (less than 1/6 of saccadic velocity), the localization judgements for continuous and sampled movements are profoundly different. For continuous movements, test flashes are localized quite accurately along the continuous motion trajectory. For sampled movements, test flashes are localized only at the endpoints of the trajectory. Bimodal localization judgements accurately reflect the fact that the motion trajectory is bimodal. However, bimodal localization judgements fail to reflect the phenomenology: the 125-ms sampled motion stimulus appears to jump across the space and to take a non-zero interval of time doing so. (3) With long blank times, localization judgements made during the interval in which the moving reference stimulus was turned off indicate remarkably accurate predictions of position. While these 'cognitive' localization judgements based on an invisible stimulus are somewhat more variable than 'perceptual' judgements based on an actual moving stimulus, they are nevertheless remarkably similar.

Spatial localization with overshoot trajectories. Saccadic trajectories typically have brief overshoots at the end of the movement in which the line of sight briefly extends beyond the intended endpoint and then returns back to the steady inter-saccadic position. One of our subjects typically showed overshoots as large as 50 percent of the movement. To determine whether such a trajectory might influence perception, we (Sperling and Speelman, 1965) simulated a trajectory with 33% overshoot on the movement apparatus (Fig. 4g). In order to give the unusual trajectory the maximal opportunity to affect localization, it was run much slower than real time: the linear component from start to first arrival at the final location was 80 ms, and the overshoot duration was an additional 40 ms (see Fig. 4g). Stimulus conditions were similar to the previous simulated-motion experiments. As before, the subjects' task was to judge the location, relative to the moving coordinate frame, of a test flash that occurred during the movement.

Two motion extents (from initial to final) were investigated: (1) 95 arc min, and (2) 9.4 arc min. This small extent of movement was produced by means of an inverting telescope which reduced the 95 arc min by a factor of 10. Data for one typical subject are shown in Fig. 7. Two aspects of the data are noteworthy. Test flashes are never localized outside the initial-to-final interval in spite of the large, simulated saccadic overshoot. Indeed, even with these slow simulated movements (which are at least 3 times slower than real time) there is no evidence that the overshoot has any effect on perception.

The stimulus to study overshoots also revealed another important characteristic of localization. With the small displays (and correspondingly slow, small movements), there was no difference between localization in continuous-movement displays and in sampled movement displays with the motion segment turned off. However, with the 1.6-deg movement, the difference between continuous and sampled motion is overwhelming: test flashes during continuous movements nearly always appear at locations between the initial and final markers; with sampled movements, the test flashes are localized only at the endpoints. These data extend the top panels of Fig. 6, showing that the continuous–sampled motion difference can be made to vanish with sufficiently small displays, just as Fig. 4 showed that the continuous–sampled motion difference vanished with sufficiently brief (20 ms) motion periods (Fig. 6). All these differences between continuous and sampled motion follow immediately from a Fourier frequency analysis of the stimuli (Watson et al., 1986). Obviously, the parameters of visual motion exert a controlling influence on how test flashes are localized relative to a saccadic-like moving reference stimulus. This will be important in interpreting test flash localization during real saccades.

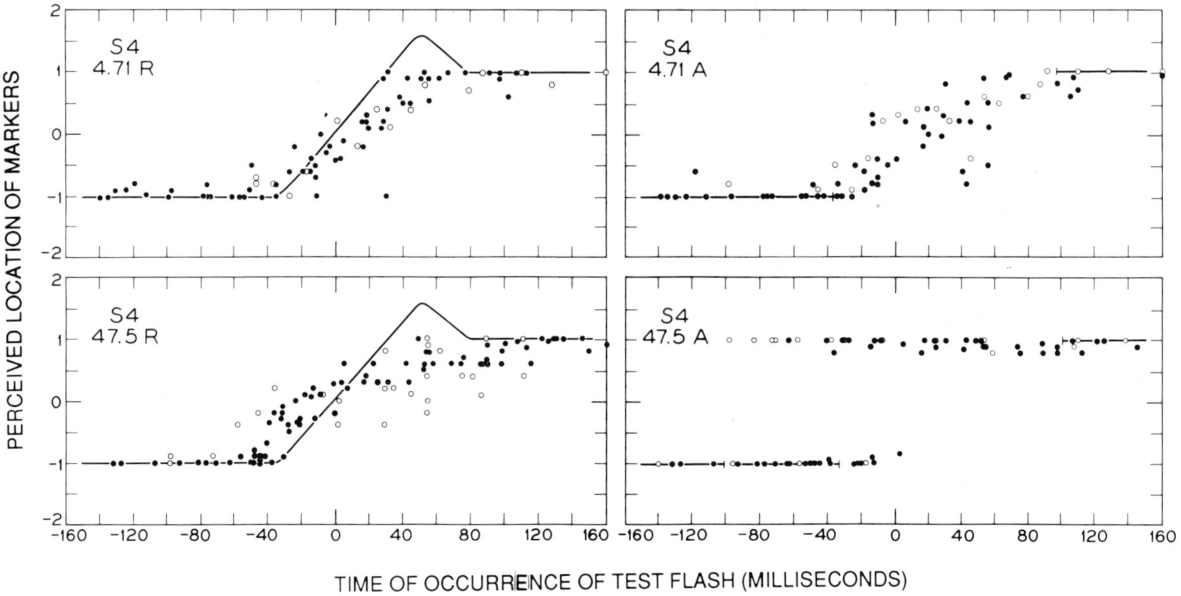

Fig. 7. Location judgements with continuous and sampled motions of two sizes. In the lower panels, the moving markers traversed from 47.5 min on one side of fixation to 47.5 min on the other side. In the upper panels, the display size was reduced by a factor of 10. The movement was a much-slower-than-real-time simulated saccade-with-overshoot (see text). Overshoot appears not to matter at these motion speeds. Turning off the movement field (saccadic *smear*) matters only for the larger movement.

All these observations indicate that the invisibility of high-velocity motion smear, which is present naturally during saccades, and errors of test flash localization relative to continuously moving images are not unique to saccades, but reflect visual responses to moving retinal images. With respect to motion smear, the visual system may have developed insensitivity to rapid-motion smear as a way of dealing with saccadically induced stimulation. However it may have evolved and developed, the visual system that we now have seems to respond in the same way to the same retinal stimulation – whether the stimulation is saccade-produced or object-produced. The following sections investigate the extent to which the mechanisms of spatial localization, which include nonvisual mechanisms, operate similarly in real and simulated saccades.

6.3.4. *What determines the subjective foveal trajectory $x_s(t)$ during eye movements?*

Comparisons of spatial localization in real and simulated saccades. The saccadic simulator was designed to imitate the retinal stimulation produced by objective movements. While it is possible to reproduce the trajectory of any particular eye movement, it is not practical nor necessary to reproduce the normal variation of saccadic trajectories in this experiment. Since we now know that saccadic motion smear does not importantly affect visual localization judgements, it is sufficient to use one typical trajectory in the imposed-motion control experiment – a 20 ms, 4 deg, linear motion trajectory. How does spatial localization with this simulated eye-movement trajectory on the stationary retina compare to localization during real saccades?

To compare real and simulated saccades, a subset of all the saccades was selected for which the simulated trajectory was a good approximation, i.e., saccades that began and ended within 12 min of their intended locations. For each saccade in this subset of 'good' saccades, the retinal location of the test flash relative to the saccade was noted. In the simulated saccade condition, the test flash was produced at precisely the same retinal location relative to the moving reference points, and the observer made the corresponding location judgement of the test flash relative to the marker spots.

In the simulated saccade experiment, the subject sees two stationary spots (−1, +1, Fig. 2a) with a 2-degree separation between adjacent spots. When the subject is ready, the subject initiates a trial by pressing a button. After a variable delay, the lines quickly move to replicate the saccade-induced sweep of the grid across the retina. During this sequence of events, the brief test flash occurs, and the subject's task is to report the location of the flash relative to the moving coordinate system.

Twin procedure. Each trial in the simulated saccade experiment is the twin of an earlier saccadic trial. The stroboscopic flash in the simulated movement trial always occurs at the same coordinate point relative to the moving reference stimulus (0.0) and the same time relative to the movement as did the original flash in the saccadic trial. The order of the simulated trials duplicates the order of the original 'good' saccadic trials. The perceived location of the brief flash relative to the saccadically simulated moving coordinate system on the stationary eye is precisely analogous to the flash location relative to the real saccade-induced moving coordinate system. That is, if localization with eye movement and simulated movement trajectories were entirely equivalent, observers would make precisely the same localization judgements in the two conditions.

Five of the six subjects whose saccadic localization data were shown in Fig. 3 served in the simulated saccade experiment. On the whole, the localization data from the simulated eye movement condition were similar to the data from real saccades. The main significant differences were a few instances in which observers judged a test flash in the simulated display at an endpoint when they had previously, in the real saccade, judged the flash at an intermediate position. Were these differences due to residual physical differences between the real- and simulated-movement images? For example, the display for the real saccadic movements (Fig. 2) showed five marker spots, whereas the simulated saccadic movement image showed only the −1 and +1 marker spots (Fig. 5).

Whether the slight differences in localization judgements between these real and simulated movements were due to residual differences between the displays in saccadic and simulated conditions or to differences in the process of localization between real saccades and simulated saccades was not determined for 4-degree saccades. However, if there are differences in localization between real and simulated 4-deg saccades, they are certainly not much larger than the trial-to-trial and subject-to-subject variability for the displays studied here.

To help resolve the issue of saccadic versus simulated saccadic localization differences, data were obtained with one subject using 8 (rather than 4) degree real and simulated saccades. With the larger motion extent, the localization differences between real and simulated saccades increased strikingly: there was much more localization of the test *between* endpoints for the 8-deg real saccade, and more localization *at* the endpoint for the simulated saccade. The change in simulated saccadic localization with scale followed basically the pattern illustrated in the sampled motion conditions of Fig. 7. Another indicator of a change in the localization process with saccadic size was that the duration of the 8-deg subjective trajectory $x_{s,8}(t)$ was briefer than the duration of the 4-deg subjective trajectory $x_{s,4}(t)$, although the objective 8-deg saccade took about twice as long as the 4-deg saccade. While such data were obtained with only one subject, they suggest that, even when visual information is prominent in the visual field, in larger saccades the motor movement itself importantly influences localization judgements in larger saccades. This issue is considered in the next section.

Visual versus nonvisual factors. As noted above, dynamic visual stimulation during saccades – certainly during brief saccades – is unimportant because it is effectively masked by stimulation arising from the static pre- and post-saccadic fields. Therefore, the static pre- and post-saccadic stimuli are the primary contributors to dynamic visual localization judgements, a matter illustrated in Fig. 5 (insensitivity to trajectory) and whose consequences will be taken up in more detail later. By contrast, nonvisual (motor system) factors might become more prominent in localization for large eye movements (e.g., 8 deg for the kinds of displays considered above; see also Pola, 1972). In addition to size of a saccade, the most obvious factor that determines the role of nonvisual factors is the visibility of the visual scene itself. As the scene becomes dimmer and thereby less visible, and ultimately invisible, spatial localization of a test flash will be determined more and more, and finally exclusively, by nonvisual knowledge of eye position.

A number of experimenters, among them Bischof and Kramer (1968), Mateeff (1978) and MacKay (1970b, 1973), have studied spatial localization during saccades in the presence of background stimuli. O'Regan (1984) points out, in effect, that the failure to use an adequate simulated saccadic control may invalidate conclusions about possible localization mechanisms from these earlier studies. In his own experiments, O'Regan (1984) did use a simulated saccadic control. While he found similarities between real and simulated saccades, his data were not collected in a twin procedure and they do not allow one to detect small differences that might exist. Even so, O'Regan's data, like the data reported in the previous section, show a tendency to localize test flashes at intermediate points more often for real than for simulated saccades.

The conclusion, based on the data described here and from published data in which judgements were made of the spatial location of a visual test flash against a structured visual background, is that, in normal viewing, visual factors predominantly determine test flash localization, whether the eye or only the image is moving. However, when visibility is reduced (darkness is an extreme case) or when nonvisual components are enhanced (as in large eye movements), or when the test flash is judged relative to the body rather than relative to another visual stimulus (Hansen and Skavenski, 1977, 1985) then nonvisual factors become more and more important.

6.3.5. Visual localization in the dark

Spatial localization after a visual frame of reference is extinguished. What is the perceived location of a test line flashed while the eye is executing a saccadic movement in the dark? For example, the observer views a fixation point *A*. It goes off and subsequently a point *B* appears which is the target of an intended saccade. The observer is instructed to saccade from *A* to *B*, but the *B* is turned off 100 ms after it appears, before the eye begins its movement. A stroboscopic flash is programmed to strike the fovea sometime before, during, or after the movement. The observer perceives this flash as originating from some point in the environment. Where? And how does the observer indicate where?

The test flash is judged relative to the memory of the extinguished markers, *A, B*. Obviously, just as in the light, a flash striking the fovea would be localized first at the initial location and then, sometime after the end of the saccade, at the final location. During, and shortly before and after the saccade, flashes are localized at intermediate points. For this experiment, there is no equivalent control experiment in the stationary eye. Spatial localization in the absence of visual stimuli must be controlled by nonvisual factors. The computation of the location of the fovea could rely on efferent outflow signals or upon proprioceptive feedback, but, in the absence of visual stimuli, it cannot rely on vision. This procedure allows one to measure the quality of visual localization information that is available via the motor system.

Experiments show that the perceived location of a foveal flash during a saccadic movement in the dark changes very slowly relative to the speed of perceived location of a foveal flash viewed against a visually structured environment. It takes hundreds of milliseconds for the perceived location of flashes in the dark to move from *A* to *B* compared to the few tens of milliseconds needed to execute the saccade (see Matin, 1986, for a review).

Hypothesis: feedback determines the frame of reference. In a closely related experiment in which the task of the observer is not to judge the test flash relative to a previously remembered location but to strike the flash directly with a hammer, Hansen and Skavenski (1977, 1985) find extraordinarily accurate localization. In their experiments, subjects have almost perfect, almost instantaneous, nonvisual knowledge of position relative to the body of the saccadically moving eye. Why does this knowledge not manifest itself when the subject is asked locate a visual flash relative to a remembered visual location? Skavenski (Ch. 5) proposes that the subject adopts a different frame of reference in the two tasks.

Adopting a task-dependent frame of reference means that the weight the subject assigns to different sources of information in arriving at a response depends on the task. This matter will be considered in the next section. Here we note that for the subject to achieve an optimal weighting of information sources in any of these complex tasks requires practice with feedback. All humans practice all their lives coordinating saccadic eye movements with body movements. Therefore, it is not surprising to discover that a subject is aware of the position of the eye relative to the body. However, people never practice making a purely visual judgement, which does not involve any body movement, in circumstances in which illumination is suddenly extinguished. The hypothesis put forward here is that, because all information necessary to perform this task is available to the subject, with practice a subject should be able to learn the purely visual task. The critical aspect for all the visual localization experiments considered here is that they measure what the subject habitually does, not the subject's capacity. To make an inference about capacity – an intrinsic *inability* to visually localize stimuli when a visual frame of reference is extinguished – requires that a subject *fails to learn* in an experiment with feedback (Sperling et al., 1990).

6.4. Models for spatial localization during eye movements

This section considers theories for the data that have been presented concerning the localization of flashes which occur during or proximal to eye movements. (The issue of how information from successive saccades is combined is considered in a later section.) Basically two kinds of information are involved; purely visual and visuo-motor. Visual information ('retinal factors' in the literature) refers exclusively to information carried by light, and it is the same in real and in simulated eye movements. Visuo-motor information includes efferent or afferent motor-system information ('extra-retinal factors') linked to vision. Here *visuo-motor* information is abbreviated to *nonvisual* although it makes no sense to consider nonvisual information alone – without vision – in a visual localization task.

Obviously, only nonvisual factors distinguish between real and simulated eye movements. (This requires that the simulated events are truly equivalent to the retinal images during eye movements, a technical requirement that has often been violated because it it difficult to achieve.) To evaluate the role of purely visual and visuo-motor factors in spatial localization, it is useful to have in mind at least one specific model for how each kind of information might be processed. We consider here a model for each process.

6.4.1. Model for purely visual localization during saccadic-like image sequences

Attention gating model: events, glimpses, episodes. The mechanism of the attention gating model of Reeves and Sperling (1986) and Sperling and Weichselgartner (1989) is the core building block of all the proposed models. The gating model deals with the mental representation of external stimulus events that occur in close temporal and spatial proximity to each other. According to the model, such closely contiguous events are not stored or accessed individually in memory; they are packed into an attentional *glimpse*. The glimpse is the smallest attentional unit. Its contents result from a single opening and closing of an attentional gate. The events that comprise a glimpse define its space-time window, much as the location where a camera is pointed and the time its shutter is open determine the space-time window of a photograph. A glimpse may incorporate events that span from about 1/4 s up to about 1 s. One or more glimpses may be bundled into an episode. The episode is the unit that is accessed when information is retrieved from long-term memory.

The gating model (Reeves and Sperling, 1986) describes the computational mechanism that creates attentional glimpses. In the environment in which it was developed and tested (highly controlled stimulus sequences which give the experimenter full control over the sequence of events) the gating model has great predictive power. The time course of attentional glimpses was found to be highly constrained and constant for an individual. The basic premise of the attention gate is that the *amount* of information recorded internally about an external stimulus event is proportional to the amount of attention received by the stimulus event at its time of occurrence, which, in turn, is determined by where within the glimpse the event occurs. The amount of information recorded about an event is characterized by a positive real number, its *strength*. The computational concept of *strength* represents the structural concept of the *strength of a link* which connects an event to the node designating the episode to which the event is attached.

To arrive at an observable response, information recorded in a glimpse must be interpreted. Here, the following assumptions are made. In the decision algorithm, information is weighted according to its strength. In arriving at a decision, it is not critical whether information is acquired from one or from several glimpses.

According to Weichselgartner and Sperling (1987), there are two kinds of glimpse, automatic and voluntary. In automatic glimpses the opening of the attentional gate is determined by the contents of the glimpse itself. For example, in the glimpse that records the test flash in a localization experiment, the attentional gate admits information about the test flash itself, about the visual field in proximity to the test flash, and about other events that may have occurred in close temporal proximity to the test flash.

In a voluntary attentional glimpse, information is admitted according to an attentional gate which is triggered by events external to the glimpse itself. For example, if the occurrence of a test flash were a cue to the observer to begin remembering the configuration of a complex background, the test flash would be remembered in the first glimpse and background information would be recorded in a subsequent glimpse.

Attentional gating functions are derived empirically from experiments in which a subject is asked to remember a single test event embedded in a visual field populated with other events (Reeves and Sperling, 1986; Weichselgartner and Sperling, 1987). The spatial and temporal location of events that the subject extracts along with the test can be used to derive the spatio-temporal gating function. Fig. 8 illustrates the time courses of an automatic and voluntary glimpse derived from such an experiment. The trigger event was the brief flash of an outline square, much like the test flash in the spatial localization experiments. The other events that the observer attempted to remember along with the outline square were flashes of letters, superimposed in a rapid stream inside the square. The voluntary attentional glimpse was quite slow compared to an automatic attentional glimpse – just as slow as if it had required a spatial shift of attention. Such voluntary attentional glimpses have been studied in a great variety of contexts (Reeves, 1977; Sperling and Reeves, 1980; Reeves and Sperling, 1986) and been found to be remarkably constant for a particular individual over a variety of conditions. The properties of the automatic attentional glimpses have not yet been quite as well defined.

Sources of information for localizing test flashes during saccade-like image movements. In a localization experiment, there are four stimulus events: (i)

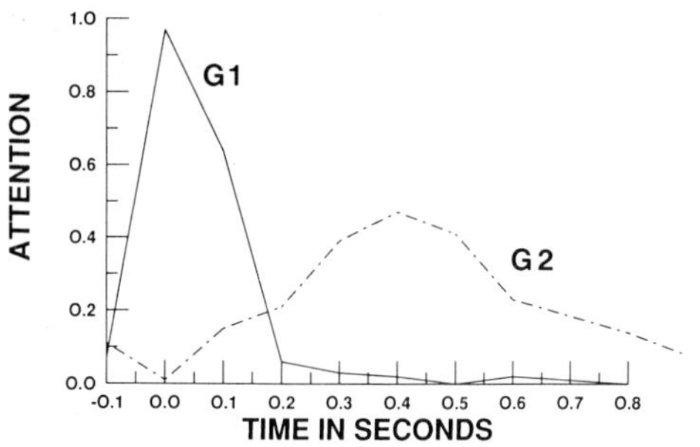

Fig. 8. Time course of attention triggered by the occurrence of a brief flash of an outline square. Two glimpses are distinguishable: G1, an automatic glimpse which records the flash and closely neighboring events, and G2, a controlled glimpse which mainly records events 200–600 ms later. The abscissa is time relative to the trigger event which occurred at time 0.0; the ordinate is the instantaneous amount of attention. (After Weichselgartner, 1984, Fig. 4.19a.)

the premovement field (a visual image of the retinal stimulus as it existed before the movement); (ii) the movement flowfield (a representation of the movement and, possibly, a visual respresentation of motion smear caused by the retinal sweep of the background), (iii) the post-movement field (an image of the retinal stimulus after the movement), and (iv) the test flash to be localized. When the test flash occurs during or in close temporal proximity to the movement, these events are represented in three glimpses: (1) a controlled glimpse which contains the premovement field plus weak representations of subsequent events, (2) an automatic glimpse triggered by the test flash which contains the test flash and possibly all the other events, pre-field, movement, and post-field, and (3) a controlled glimpse which contains primarily the post-field. It is assumed that, at the level of processing where a localization judgement is made, the automatic episode in which the test flash is recorded will be given the primary weight in determining the localization judgment.

Content analysis of the visual component events. There are two separate kinds of motion information: motion smear (a static retinal image) and the *motion flowfield.* In the case of saccadic movements, because of masking by pre- and post-saccadic fixation fields, motion smear is usually invisible and therefore unavailable for any subsequent processing (see section 6.3.2.). Therefore, motion smear is retained explicitly as 'null' in Glimpse ii. In the case of test flash localization in much-slower-than-saccadic movement, the motion smear takes on non-zero values.

The motion perception system calculates the motion flowfield, an assignment of motion velocity (a vector) to each point in two-dimensional space (Clocksin, 1980; Hoffman, 1982; Koenderink and van Doorn, 1986; Longuet-Higgins and Prazdny, 1980; Sperling et al., and Perkins, 1989). The neural computations of image motion are assumed to be the same whether the flowfield is produced by saccades or by image movements and whether the motion is continuous or sampled (e.g., Adelson and Bergen, 1985; Heeger, 1987; van Santen and Sperling, 1984, 1985; Watson and Ahumada, 1983; Watson et al., 1986). In the automatic glimpse containing the test flash, the temporal and spatial proximity of the saccadic image-velocity vectors to the test flash determine the weight of image motion in the localization judgment. This weight, expressed by the area (w_2 in Fig. 9a) under the test flash's attention glimpse function, represents the belief: 'The test flash occurred during the movement'. The computation of the weights of the various events that comprise the test-flash glimpse is illustrated in Fig. 9.

Visual persistence and test flash localization. While pre- and post-saccadic fields mask saccadic motion smear, the test flash in localization experiments is typically not masked. Therefore, because of its visual persistence (e.g., Efron 1970a,b; Sperling, 1960, 1967), the test flash becomes a de facto component of subsequent stimuli. Unless the test occurs long before the movement, it will persist into the post-saccadic background stimulus. In computing spatial relationships within an image, the persisting visual image of the test flash is treated in the same way as a physically present test image would be. Therefore, the persistence of a test flash

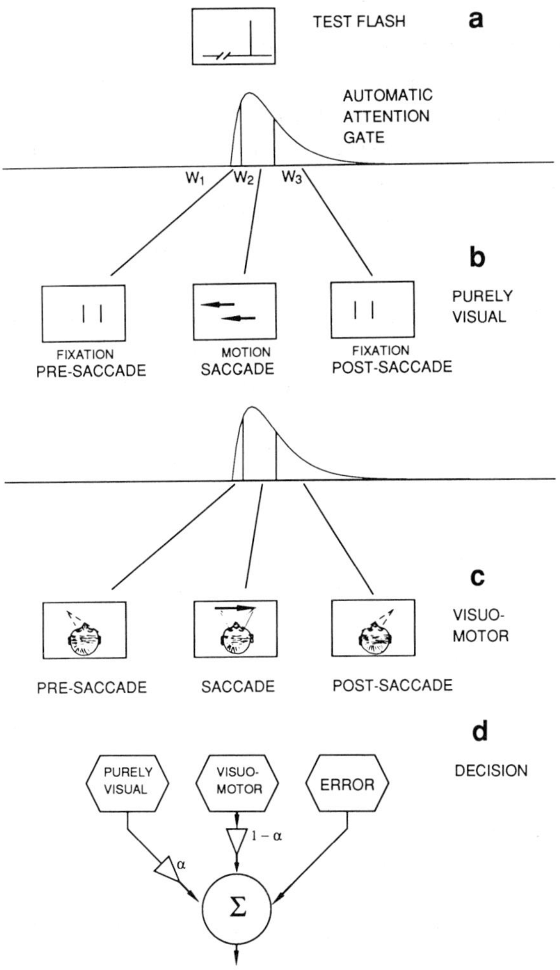

Fig. 9. Models for purely visual localization, visuo-motor localization, and for the combination of different sensory cues. (a) The intensity of a nearly instantaneous test flash as a function of time, and the attentional window of the episode in which the flash is recorded. (b) Representation of the retinal images of a stationary background before, during, and after a saccade. In purely visual localization, the images, weighted by their proximity to the test flash (w_1, w_2, w_3), are the only information available for the judgement/decision process. The particular weights shown here are appropriate for a test flash that occurs early in a saccade. (c) In visuo-motor localization, the representations of the pre-saccadic eye position, the moving eye positions and the post-saccadic eye position are weighted to derive the eye position to be linked with the test flash. (d) A simple model for the combination of cues from different sensory sources that has been found to accurately predict the data from multi-cue experiments. Data from various sources, weighted according to the task requirements ($0 \leq \alpha \leq 1$) are summed together with irreducible sensory noise (*ERROR*) to generate a response on each trial.

at particular location of the post-saccadic field is interpreted as very strong evidence (large weight) for occurrence of the test at that location. Visual persistence is probably the most important factor in the tendency of most observers to locate test flashes that occur shortly before saccades relative to the post- (rather than pre-)saccadic visual environment (O'Regan, 1984).

The entire rise and decay of visual persistence was mapped for individual subjects by Weichselgartner and Sperling (1985). Large individual variations in visual persistence functions were found. It would be of great interest to determine whether the duration of an individual's persistence function is correlated with the tendency toward localization errors in the post-saccadic direction.

When multiple tests are flashed during a saccade, their location is judged as though they all occurred at the same time (Mateeff, 1978; O'Regan, 1984).* That is, they are judged at their actual retinal positions without taking into account that the eye and the background retinal image were moving. This is explained by the persistence of all the flashes in the post-saccadic image. The simultaneous persistence of many flashes allows their retinal spatial relationships to be computed in the same way as if they had actually occurred at the same time. Such internal evidence of consistent spatial relationships is compelling, and overwhelms evidence of a differential time of occurrence during movement.

Nondistortion of images flashed during saccades. It was mentioned above that complex images briefly flashed during eye movements do not appear distorted. This observation has a long history (e.g., Woodworth, 1906, 1938; Campbell and Wurtz, 1978). One might expect images to appear distorted because the latency of visual responses varies with retinal location, as well as with stimulus contrast and with spatial frequency. In the stationary eye, this variation in the precise arrival time of sensory information at some more central process-

* Mateef has a different interpretation of his data.

ing center might be irrelevant. In the saccadically moving eye, small time differences represent large location differences. Again, it is not that time differences in sensory processing are somehow compensated for during saccades. When stimuli are flashed in isolation, retinal location and intensity influence perceived location (O'Regan, 1984). However, in the face of visual persistence that is long relative to the difference in onsets, there is a long period when all the stimulus information is simultaneously available. As with test flashes produced in rapid succession during saccades, the computation of spatial relationships between simultaneously available stimulus components provides evidence which is given overwhelming weight relative to evidence of difference in arrival times. Small differences in arrival times are used with extraordinary sensitivity in motion computations. During saccades, however, object motion is *masked* by saccadically produced image motion and perhaps also *suppressed* (see below, section 6.5). Small arrival time differences *un*associated with stimulus motion are not generally treated as significant data. It requires unusual stimulus conditions to demonstrate that uncompensated sensory processing times can enter into perceptual computations.

Saccadic versus simulated saccades. In the preceding discussion, it has been taken for granted that statements made about moving images in saccades would hold for simulated saccades in the stationary eye. For example, flashing a complex scene during a saccade from one marker spot to another is simulated by flashing a complex scene during the movement of two marker spots on a stationary retina. It seems so obvious that moving two marker spots would not alter the appearance of the flashed scene that it has not been explicitly tested. Similarly, it seems likely that two quickly consecutive flashes striking the fovea during the sweep of a moving background would both be localized at the same place. But this, too, still needs to be tested.

Computing visual evidence. Ultimately all sources of localization information are combined and a decision is reached. Of the various glimpses in which the test flash is represented, the automatic glimpse triggered by the test flash itself will be the main determiner of localization, and this is illustrated in Fig. 9. Fig. 9a and b illustrates the weights of the pre-saccadic, motion, and post-saccadic events in the automatic glimpse. The test flash also may occur in the pre- and post-saccadic glimpses. Their weights in the overall computation, which are disregarded in this illustration, would be determined by the attentional strength of the test flash within these events.

A full computational model requires specification of the following major component processes (as well as many subsidiary ones). (a) It must specify the gating function that computes the precise weighting of events in the temporal neighborhood of the test flash. It has been assumed here that the gating function is similar to the automatic attentional glimpse of Weichselgartner and Sperling (1987). In these experiments, a visual test flash of an outline square was linked primarily to visual events within ± 50 ms of its occurrence (Fig. 8). (b) A formal specification is needed of the decision rule – how the weighted mixture of events linked to the test flash is interpreted to generate a response. For example, if a test-flash glimpse assigned 20% of the weight to the prefixation field, 45% to the motion field, and 35% to the post-fixation field, what localization response would be generated?

The simplest decision rule occurs when the link of the test flash to the motion segment is very weak, i.e., when the motion segment in Fig. 9b is very brief and its weight w_2 is negligible. This usually occurs in displays in which the test flash is far away in space or time from the nearest test marker spot. A reasonable initial hypothesis for this decision rule is that such a location judgement is binary – appropriate either to the pre- or to the post-fixation background, depending on which has greater strength. With a significant motion weight, intermediate location responses become more plausible. An intermediate location response would be generated, reflecting the relative strengths of the pre- and post-fixation backgrounds. However, at saccadic velocities, the motion is so fast that even when motion enters into the localization computation, it enters only as a weight to determine whether an intermediate response is appropriate and not as a cue to localization.

Close proximity of the test flash to a background marker yields more convincing, and hence more persistent, spatial evidence of test location than when the test flash is far away from the nearest marker. (The definition of near/far depends on distance from the fovea.) While this can be formally modeled as a distortion of spatial localization in the neighborhood of spatial markers, it represents an inherent complexity of vision. The perceived spatial location of a test flash during image motion depends critically on the nature of the moving image itself.

6.4.2. Model for visuo-motor localization during saccadic eye movements

The model for visuo-motor (extra-retinal, nonvisual) localization during real, rather than simulated, saccades is basically analogous to the model for purely visual localization. Instead of linking the test flash to three visual events, it is linked to three corresponding nonvisual events: (1) a representation of eye position relative to the head position before the saccadic movement; (2) a representation of the saccadic movement command itself (outflow) or the saccadic movement itself (inflow); and (3) a representation of eye position relative to head position after the movement. As in the purely visual model, the glimpse in which the visual test flash is contained assigns weights to each of these nonvisual representations; the relative strength of the link is determined by the degree of temporal overlap of the test flash with the nonvisual event. Indeed, in the nonvisual as in the purely visual computation, a simple weighting function which uses overlap with the motion segment only to determine whether or not intermediate location judgements might be justified, and then uses the ratio of strengths of post- to pre-fixation links to determine the location, might suffice to account for the data. The advantage of this kind of computation is that it offers good resolution of position of test flashes which occur during saccades without requiring any correspondingly fast visual processing. We will return to the issue later.

6.4.3. A model for resolving conflicting cues

A natural question to ask is: when both purely visual and nonvisual information are available, how are these sources of information utilized in the performance of various tasks? A linear model based on Thurstone's Case V (Thurstone, 1927) for the combination of perceptual cues has been found to work remarkably well in a variety of tasks involving visual judgements (Dosher et al., 1986; Bruno and Cutting, 1988). Predictions work equally well when cues agree (add) and when they conflict (subtract).

Weighing the evidence. In the case of two perceptual alternatives (such as two different perceptual interpretations of a rotating Necker cube), each perceptual alternative is represented by a pan on balance scale. Each cue represents evidence, and a weight proportional to the weight of its evidence in favor of an alternative is placed on the balance pan of that alternative. The relative importance of a particular cue depends not only on the abstract quality of information provided by the cue itself but also on how each subject weights that quality in the particular task. The final perceptual decision is determined by the algebraic addition of the strengths of all the cues plus a random error that reflects the variability of judgement (Fig. 9d).

For localization judgements during real saccades, the present evidence suggests that visual information is given greatest, perhaps exclusive, weight in making visual judgements (Hansen, 1979). For example, in localizing one visual event (a flash) relative to other visual events (the saccadically moved background), visual information appears to dominate. With increasing saccade size the situation may be different because two factors come into play. First, if the background markers against which a test flash is localized are not size scaled, they become less effective stimuli as they become more peripheral. For this reason, saccade size would be best varied by varying the viewing distance and keeping the display constant. Otherwise, placing markers and test flashes more peripherally alters the early computations of visual spatial relations. Usually the alteration is in the direction of weakening the contribution of the spatial visual information. On the other hand, it seems obvious that nonvisual information would be stronger for larger saccades than for smaller saccades. Thus, even in purely visual localization judgements, nonvisual information may come to play a role in larger saccades. This relative increase in nonvisual influences on localization in large saccades does not involve a change in strategy (decision weights) but rather a change in the strengths of sensory inputs.

Motor localization reponses. In localizing targets by means of motor responses (versus making perceptual judgements) visuo-motor information is given greatest weight (versus purely visual information). For example, as was noted above, when an observer is asked to strike the location of a flash seen during a saccade with a hammer, the response is extremely accurate (Hansen and Skavenski, 1977, 1985). In this experiment, visual cues to flash localization were removed so that the observers were forced to rely on nonvisual information. Indeed, in localizing the flash relative to their body position, the observers did not succumb to the mislocalizations that they would have made if they were judging the flash's location relative to its visual environment. For further evidence that different sources of information are used in purely visual and visuo-motor saccadic localization tasks, see Ch. 5 of this volume.

6.5. Motion perception during saccadic eye movements

Suppose that, during a saccadic movement, the experimenter tricks the subject and shifts the visual field. To what extent can the subject detect such trickery? This question devolves into several component questions.

(1) When the retinal image sequence that would have been produced by a saccadic motion is artificially perturbed by extraneous motion, how detectable is the perturbation? (Motion masking.)
(2) How well can the observer detect that his eye has not landed where it intended? (Saccadic calibration.)
(3) Given that motion is a perceptual primitive, why is image motion not experienced during saccades? (Motion suppression.)

Motion detection and discrimination during saccades. Earlier, this chapter considered the detection of a simple flash during a saccade. Early investigators had claimed there was great loss of sensitivity during a saccade. Once the proper control experiments were conducted with simulated saccades, it became clear that the actual sequence of images on the retina produced visual masking and positional uncertainty of the test stimulus that was sufficient to account for threshold changes observed during saccades. There was no residual threshold change that could be attributed to the saccade per se. The problem of detecting and discriminating visual motion during saccades seems to be similar. There are several reports of an impaired ability to detect or discriminate motion during saccades (e.g. Bridgeman et al., 1975; Mack, 1970; Stark et al., 1976; Whipple and Wallach, 1978). However, when Brooks and her collaborators (Brooks and Fuchs, 1975; Brooks et al., 1980a,b; Brooks and Impelman, 1981) produced equivalent motion perturbations in real and in simulated saccades, they found them to be equally detectable.* Their answer to the motion masking question raised above is that any inability to detect motion perturbations during eye movements is explained entirely by the sequence of images on the retina. To this it must be added that in both real and simulated saccades, Brooks et al.'s subjects discriminated nor-

* While Brooks et al. (1980a) mostly found identical thresholds in real and simulated saccades, in a few of their conditions there were slight differences that could have been caused by residual, uncontrolled differences in procedure.

mal from perturbed motion on the basis of the shape of the perceived motion blur – not on the basis of perceived motion of the perturbation (Brooks, personal comunication).

In Brooks et al. (1980b) and in every other instance up to this point, when a psychophysical discrimination was based on retinal images, it has not mattered whether these images were viewed in a stationary or saccadically moving eye provided that the retinal images were equivalent. However, the problem of *motion* detection and discrimination during saccades is more complex than the problem of simple object detection because the *sensation of image motion obviously is suppressed during saccades.*

The sensation of motion: saccadic motion suppression. Consider Question 3: saccadic trajectories are excellent stimuli for the motion perception system. That is, moving an image in the trajectory of a simulated saccade on a stationary retina produces a strong sensation of apparent motion.* Why do we not experience visual apparent motion during the same retinal image movement when it is saccadically induced? Notice that the sensation question is a fundamentally different question from the discrimination question raised above. Sensation refers to how an observer describes his experience, and does not involve a right or wrong answer as does a discrimination task.

It is helpful to place the suppression of motion sensations during saccades into the broader context of other voluntary movements. For example, the otolith signals acceleration with respect to gravity: why don't we experience a sensation of falling whenever we voluntarily sit down? When we voluntarily turn our head, the vestibular and visual systems should signal vertigo, but we do not experience it. The other side of the coin is the shock we experience when we expect one sensory input, for example, strawberry mousse, and encounter another, sour cream with salmon roe. However, merely observing that the interpretation of sensory input quite generally depends on voluntary movements and on the corresponding sensory expectations does not answer any specific questions about the processes that are invoked. We first consider Question 2 (Saccadic calibration) and then the issues concerning the types and levels of sensory processing.

Saccadic calibration: piano analogy. The answer to Question 2 concerning sensitivity to environmental displacement during saccades depends on the size of the displacement as a fraction of intended eye movement, and on the suspicions of the observer. Sperling and Speelman (1965) observed that a stimulus displacement of 2 deg during a 4-deg saccade was reliably detected (cf. Bridgeman et al., 1975; Stark et al., 1976; Whipple and Wallach, 1978).

The issue of sensitivity to visual displacements can be easily understood by an analogy. Imagine a pianist performing a difficult piece on a piano. While his hands are in the air, we move the piano. Indeed, on grand pianos, the soft pedal accomplishes just such a movement, moving the keyboard by about a quarter the width of a key so that the hammers strike only two of three strings. Such small keyboard movements usually go unnoticed. Suppose, instead, that while the pianist's hands are in the air, we move the piano the width of a key. The unfortunate pianist would strike wrong notes and probably infer that he was out of practice. But, suppose we moved the piano a foot, so that the pianist's hands struck completely unbelievable notes. Not only would such trickery be shocking and instantly recognized, but the pianist would attribute every subsequent wrong note to external interference. In a psychophysical procedure, the pianist's ability to discriminate real mistakes from induced mistakes would follow roughly a Weber fraction of the lateral hand movement. The situa-

* The motion perception of objects moving at saccadic speeds has been studied almost exclusively with part-field stimuli. Saccades move the entire retinal field and, except in the laboratory, the entire retinal field is usually filled with stimuli. The author is not aware of any study that examines whether full-field stimuli moving at saccadic velocities produce as strong a perception of motion as part-field stimuli.

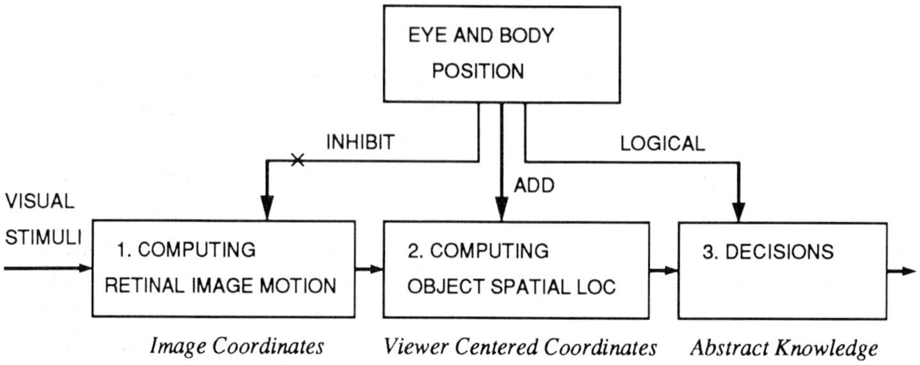

Fig. 10. Processing of visual and nonvisual information. Three stages at which nonvisual information interacts with visual information: the label on the arrows indicates the mode of interaction.

tion with saccadic eye movements is not essentially different. Whether we move the hand or the eye, we know what to expect when we arrive. The cognitive processes by which we build up representations of the external world and derive predictions from the representations are quite complex; they are considered briefly later in this chapter.

The experiments on the spatial localization of flashes during eye movements are analogous to the localization of tactual stimulation during ballistic hand movements. As with the eye, when the hand is stimulated as it is moved rapidly over a surface, the source of stimulation is projected onto a location on the surface. The subject's hand trajectory can be compared quantitatively to the objective trajectory, just as with eye trajectories, and it is undoubtedly subject to similar illusions. Indeed, comparisons of motor programming in vision with motor programming in other modalities promise to yield insights into both domains of study.

Determining the level of visual–nonvisual interaction in the perception of image motion. To analyse the processing of visual motion during saccades, we consider the visual and nonvisual inputs and the three levels at which they can interact. Specifically, the inputs are (1) the retinal images generated by the saccades and (2) the nonvisual eye movement and body position signals. The computational levels are (1) computing retinotopic image motion, (2) computing object spatial position, and (3) a decision level (Fig. 10). At each level, we consider computations that could inhibit the sensation of motion during saccades.

At the level of computing retinotopic motion, the effect of nonvisual input from a saccade would have to be inhibitory and nonspecific. That is, because all parts of the visual field may be stimulated by saccadic motion, motion signals would have to be suppressed throughout the visual field. The question of whether motion signals that represent directions of motion counter to or perpendicular to the saccade are also suppressed (Stark et al., 1976; Whipple and Wallach, 1978) is left open because, it will be argued, the retinotopic inhibitory mechanism is itself implausible.

A higher level of saccadic visual–nonvisual interaction is at the level of computing the position of a visual object relative to the head. (For specificity, we take head direction to be the direction the nose is pointing.) Computing object position requires adding two angles: (1) the retinal angle between the object and the fixation point – the line of regard – and (2) the angle between the line of regard and the nose. Saccadic motion suppression at this level implies that spatial position rather than the retinotopic motion is used to infer perceived motion.

At the decision level, a decision is made about whether or not object motion may have occurred during a saccade. Consider the piano analogy. The pianist's hands land on the piano but on a wrong note. Ordinarily, the pianist does not entertain the hypothesis that the piano has moved, and so the sensory signal is logically re-interpreted to indicate that the hands must have erred in executing their intended movement. The case of visual objects whose position is perturbed during a saccade is similar. All the systems up to the point of decision may be sending appropriate signals, but they are discarded at the point of decision. However, when the new game is pointed out to subject or pianist, the decision rule can be quickly revised.

Modifiability, the critical role of feedback. It is assumed here that the modifiability of processing is related to level: the higher the level, the more easily processing is modified.

Full-field inhibition of retinotopic motion computations during saccades would generally be assumed to be an unmodifiable genetically determined process. At the level of computing coordinates, the ability to calibrate eye movements is genetic, but saccadic extent (and many other motor components of eye movements) can be recalibrated in a few minutes to a few hours of observation time (Keller and Zee, 1986). The situation is not essentially different from the case of a pianist switching from a standard piano to a harpsichord which has narrower keys or, in the second case, having different dynamic properties so that key-press movements have to be recalibrated.

The issue of modifiability is critically related to experimental method. Feedback means that a subject is told and/or experiences the consequences of correct versus incorrect responses. When they are correctly carried out, experiments without feedback are essentially ecological investigations; they determine how sensory inputs are habitually computed. Experiments with full feedback can determine the computational limits. For example, to establish that there is retinotopic motion inhibition requires an experiment with feedback. From experiments without feedback one can learn only that subjects habitually ignore motion signals during saccades. To determine that the failure to perceive motion during saccades is not merely a habit but an unmodifiable deficiency would require the experiment with feedback to fail to train subjects to use retinotopic motion signals.

To understand the limits of motion perception during saccades requires at least two conditions: (1) comparing real saccades with simulated saccadic controls and (2) experiments with feedback. The numerous reports of saccadic motion suppression cited above fail one or both of these criteria. We consider saccadic motion perception below in the section on correlating successive saccadic images.

The issues suggested by the flow diagram in Fig. 10 are, in principle, resolvable. For example, a possible generalized loss of sensitivity to image motion during saccades can be investigated experimentally by presenting visual motion stimuli (motion probes) before, during, and after saccades. There are the masking and suppression questions: the ability to experience the perception of motion of the probe and the ability to discriminate different probe motions. Generality of suppression is studied by determining to what extent perception and discrimination of motion are inhibited by temporal proximity of the motion probe to a saccade, and determining whether the direction of motion matters. The problems in pursuing this research are great technical requirements in eye movement recording and even greater technical difficulties in producing the proper simulated-saccade controls.

One argument against motion suppression occurring early in visual processing is the autokinetic effect. Stationary points of light in the dark, even when fixated, appear to make small movements from time to time (see Mack, 1986, for references). Autokinesis seems like an obvious failure of motion suppression for small eye movements, although it is not unexpected, given that nonvisual information appears to be quite weak for small saccades. On the other hand, with normal full field stimulation in the light, the world as a whole does not appear to jump around, suggesting that more stringent perceptual criteria are applied to large-field than to small-field motions. In summary, the question of "At what processing level, and by what mechanisms are the sensations of motion re-interpreted during saccades?" remains unresolved.

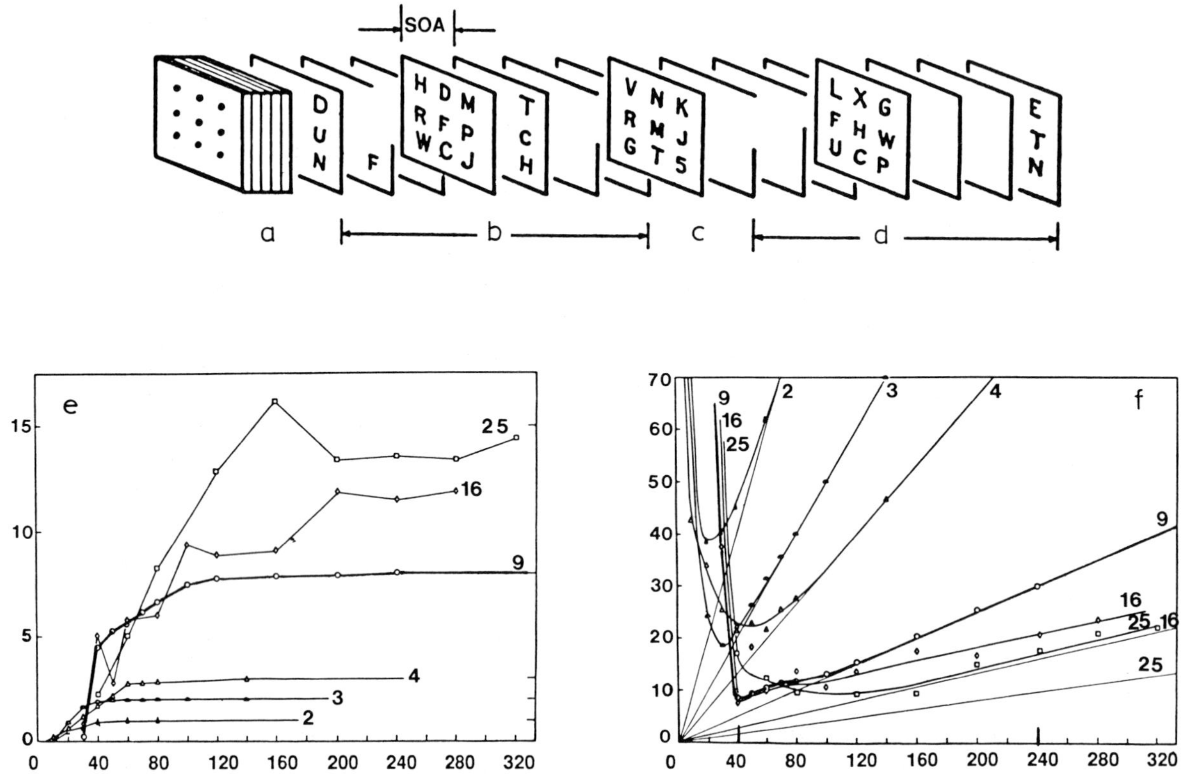

Fig. 11. Simulated saccadic search. A fixation field (a) is followed by a variable number (b) of arrays which contain letter distractors. The critical array (c) is embedded near the middle of the sequence. It contains a numeral target, and is followed by (d) letter arrays. The time between successive arrays is SOA (stimulus onset asynchrony). (e) The estimated number of characters in each array successfully searched by the subject as a function of the SOA. Data for the 9-character array illustrated above are emphasized by a heavy connecting line. The lack of improvement with SOAs longer than about 120 ms for arrays of 16 and 25 ms indicates that the second half of the exposure interval is wasted when the interval is as long as the intersaccadic interval. (f) The same data replotted to show the estimated scan time per character. 40 ms indicates the quickest scan times for 9- and 16-letter arrays; 240 ms indicates the minimum intersaccadic interval. (Redrawn from Sperling et al., 1971. Data from subject J.S.)

7. Sequences of saccades

7.1. Visual search

7.1.1. Simulated search: saccades are not always the optimum information-gathering strategy

By the definition of 'survival of the fittest', the visual system that we now have, which includes a high-resolution fovea, a low-resolution periphery and saccadic eye movements, is the optimum visual system under the set of constraints under which humans evolved. In this light, it is informative to consider a simple search task in which the saccadic mechanism is nonoptimal because it is too slow.

Consider a simple search task such as scanning a large array of letters (distractors) for an embedded numeral (the target). Normally, this search would be carried out by means of saccades, each saccade positioning the eye in a different region of the array. To simulate this search task in the stationary eye, the new information is presented to the stationary eye at regular intervals, as illustrated in Fig. 11. The subject views a long sequence of stimulus frames; all except the critical frame contain arrays of letters. In the critical frame, a number is embedded at an unknown position of the array. The subject's task is to detect the number. As a purely technical matter, the subject is also required to press a reaction-time key as quickly as possible upon detection, to give the position in the array at which the number occurred, and to state a confidence for the identification task. These additional bits of information are useful in discriminating true from accidentally correct detections.

The results of such an experiment are the percentages of correct detections as a function of the parameters of the experiment (Fig. 11e). The percentage of correct detections is most usefully transformed into a search rate – the number of distractors that must be searched each second in order to support the observed percent correct (Fig. 11f). The parameters include the time interval from one array to the next (stimulus onset asynchrony, SOA), the size of the arrays to be searched, the sets of items used as targets and distractors, the size and discriminability of the items, the advance knowledge that the subject may have about possible targets, and so on (Sperling and Dosher, 1986).

The parameter of interest with respect to simulated eye-movement search is the interval between arrays. Saccades do not occur faster than about 4/s; this corresponds to a presentation time of 250 ms per array in the simulated search procedure. Indeed, when arrays of characters are presented every 240 ms, the observed search rate is about 50 characters per second, which is equivalent to 20 ms per character (Sperling et al., 1971). About the same search rate is observed in natural search (Neisser, 1963, 1964; Neisser et al., 1963). However, when the interval between arrays is reduced, the search rate can be substantially higher. The highest rate of search, more than 100 characters per second (less than 10 ms per character), occurs when new arrays occur every 40–50 ms, a presentation rate five times faster than the rate of eye movements. The simple empirical conclusion is that eye movements, which limit the time between bursts of new information to one per 250 ms, limit the rate of search to half of what it can be when the presentation rate is increased.

Why is this particular search task (a numeral among letters) slower with natural eye movements than in the simulated search procedure? According to analyses by Fisher (1982) and Sperling and Dosher (1986) there are two interlocked reasons. First, the visual system seems to be able to execute the search in parallel in at least three of four locations of the visual field. Second, foveal search is faster than peripheral search. To some extent, foveal/peripheral search differences can be overcome by appropriate size scaling of stimuli to be searched. However, mixing character sizes in arrays to be searched slows search down rather than speeding it up (Sperling and Melchner, 1978). Therefore, the fastest search occurs when arrays of four or more characters are presented to the fovea at a rate consistent with its information-processing capacity. For highly legible characters, central vision can process 25 batches of four characters per second. This mode is two times more efficient (in terms of the number of characters searched) than saccadically driven search, which processes only 3 or 4 batches per second.

7.1.2. When is saccade rate a limiting factor in performance?

There is enormous flexibility in visual processing. The only task in which saccades have been a limiting factor was the simulated search for a relatively large, highly familiar target (a numeral) among letter distractors (Fig. 11). This is contrary to intuition, which suggests that saccades would limit performance when searching for tiny targets which could be discriminated only in the fovea. The problem is that, when a target is made so difficult to detect that it requires foveal acuity, the processing time to detect that target, even in the fovea, is likely to become so long that processing time itself, rather than intersaccade time, becomes the limiting factor. All this merely indicates that the capacities of the motor and processing components of the visual system are matched to each other, which is as it should be.

7.2. Do saccades initiate processing episodes? The optimal duration of inter-saccadic fixations

When the retinal image is artificially kept motionless, independent of eye movements, it fades, and information-processing from that image ceases (Ditchburn and Ginsborg, 1952; Riggs et al., 1953; Yarbus, 1957). Saccades can maintain or restore an image to visibility; however, they are not necessary – smooth eye movements are perhaps even more effective (e.g., Gerrits and Vendrik, 1974; see Kowler and Steinman, 1980, for a review). These observations have induced vision scientists to speculate that smooth eye movements are especially associated with continuous information-processing whereas saccades are associated with discontinuous, episodic information-processing. Saccades are assumed to initiate processing episodes. The visual system is assumed to be especially adapted to process the kinds of image sequences that saccades provide: tens of milliseconds of smear followed by hundreds of milliseconds of steady image, repeated over and over. Undoubtedly the visual system is adapted to this saccadic mode of operation. This chapter continues, with more complex stimuli and tasks than before, to deal with the question raised at the onset: to what extent do the information-processing adaptations to saccadic vision operate independently of the saccades themselves? In particular, to what extent are adaptations to saccadic vision exhibited equally when the simulated saccadic sequence of images is presented to a stationary eye?

7.2.1. In natural saccadic viewing, are long-duration fixations 'better' than brief ones?

Loftus (1972) investigated this question experimentally using natural saccadic movements in a recognition memory experiment. In the learning phases of the experiments, subjects viewed a sequence of photographs of natural scenes; each scene was exposed for a fixed time interval. Later, subjects were tested for their ability to discriminate previously viewed scenes from new (distractor) scenes. Loftus found that the best predictor of later recall was the number of saccades that a subject made in the initial viewing. Exposure duration itself had an effect upon recall only in controlling the number of saccades: given the same number of saccades, the inter-saccadic durations themselves had no influence on recall.

Loftus's finding that increasing inter-saccadic duration has no effect on recognition accuracy invites the inference that each saccade initiates a processing episode which is completed in less time than the shortest inter-saccadic duration. The possible difficulties with this conclusion illustrate the problem of studying saccades naturally without also using an appropriate simulated-saccade control. The problem is that saccadic viewing strategies are determined by the subject, not the experimenter. Therefore the viewing strategy may be perfectly confounded with the intrinsic memorability of a picture. Easy-to-remember pictures induce short inter-saccadic durations. Without further embellishments, Loftus's procedure would admit no conclusions about the effectiveness of saccades as a function of the inter-saccadic durations. This kind of difficulty in studying natural saccadic viewing is very difficult to overcome because inter-saccadic duration is a dependent variable rather than an independent variable. Loftus himself ultimately found it necessary to study approximately-simulated saccades (Loftus, 1981). Sometimes, it is desirable, additionally, to use artificially constructed stimulus materials to give still better experimental control, as in the attempt to answer the following question.

7.2.2. In a search task, are two short saccades better than a long one?

The question of whether saccades initiate processing episodes that are quickly over – even before the onset of the next saccade – suggests several experiments with simulated saccades. For example, in a simulated search task, are two saccades better than one long saccade? And, if two short saccades are indeed better than one long one, must the information presented in the two successive exposures fall on different retinal coordinates?

Letter arrays. Kowler and Sperling (1980) studied simulated search for a numeral embedded in a 5×5 letter array viewed with either single or double exposures of various durations. Each stimulus sequence was terminated with exposure of a visual noise field. The stimulus array was either flashed once (a), or twice (b), or twice with a lateral translation between exposures (c), or the array was presented continuously (d), or continuously with a lateral translation in mid-exposure (e). Search accuracy depended little on the viewing condition when the total duration of visual availability (onset of the stimulus to onset of the noise field) was less than about 100 ms. For longer exposures,the order of conditions, from best to worst, was d > e > b > c > a. That is, displacements were not helpful, two flashes were better than one, but a single continuous exposure was always best. Even for the longest simulated fixations (800 ms), dividing the long fixation into two short ones was harmful under the parameters of this search task.

Natural scenes. To complement his study of natural scenes viewed by natural eye movements, Loftus (1981) studied natural scenes viewed by successive bursts of illumination, each burst followed by a visual noise field. His procedure was not a saccadic simulation because the time interval between successive exposures was long enough to permit real saccades to reposition the eyes. Like Kowler and Sperling (1980), Loftus (1981) found that breaking a long flash into several shorter ones did not improve recognition memory. However, when fixation changed voluntarily between flashes, performance did improve with the number of fixations. Loftus concluded that the critical component in later recognition is the number of picture-features that a subject remembers from a scene. For example, generally, performance improves with number of flashes. But, "when the number of places looked is held constant, the effect of number of flashes vanishes, thereby indicating that additional flashes are only useful insofar as they permit acquisition of information from additional portions of the picture" (Loftus, 1981, p. 373). Memorable features in Loftus's natural scenes were less dense and more widely spread out than were characters to be searched in Kowler and Sperling's 5×5 arrays, so subjects benefited from successive images that fell on different retinal locations in the scene experiment and not in the character search experiment.

7.2.3. Are sudden onsets (such as might be provided by saccadic eye movements) necessary or beneficial for information-processing?

To directly test the utility of abrupt stimulus onsets for information-processing, Kowler and Sperling (1983) used a simulated saccadic sequence of images in a search task for a numeral embedded in a sequence letter arrays, as shown in the top panel of Fig. 12. Additionally, in various conditions of their experiment, the temporal waveform of the successive images was varied. They measured search accuracy with both abrupt (step) and gradual (sawtooth) onsets and offsets of images in the sequence, at two presentation rates (Fig. 12).

Search accuracy was the same, independent of the waveforms shown in Fig. 12; search accuracy depended only on the time between successive arrays. That is, only the time available to process the stimulus items influenced performance, not how that time was apportioned into dark and light phases of the cycle. These results are quite different from those obtained with stimuli at the threshold of detection or discrimination. When visual process-

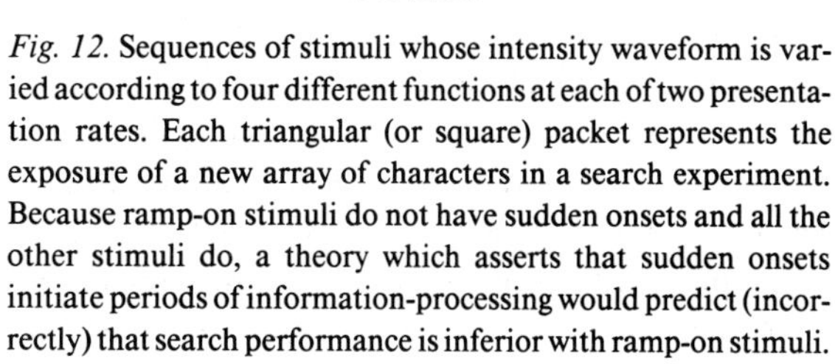

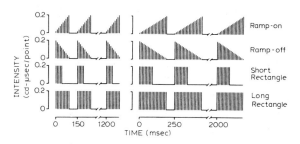

Fig. 12. Sequences of stimuli whose intensity waveform is varied according to four different functions at each of two presentation rates. Each triangular (or square) packet represents the exposure of a new array of characters in a search experiment. Because ramp-on stimuli do not have sudden onsets and all the other stimuli do, a theory which asserts that sudden onsets initiate periods of information-processing would predict (incorrectly) that search performance is inferior with ramp-on stimuli. (From Kowler and Sperling, 1983.)

ing is limited by the energy in the stimulus, the temporal waveform of the stimulus matters critically for performance (Watson and Nachmias, 1979). However, when stimuli contain sufficient energy to be easily discriminated processing is time-limited, not energy-limited, and the temporal waveform becomes relatively unimportant (Kowler and Sperling, 1983; Sperling, 1979).

The conclusions are that, under good visibility conditions, the physical parameters of image onsets imposed by saccades are relatively unimportant, presumably because of the great efficiency of visual preprocessing. For a particular stimulus and a particular task, high-level processes of feature encoding (in recognition memory experiments) and of feature matching (in search experiments) determine where the eye should be placed and when it should be moved for optimal performance.

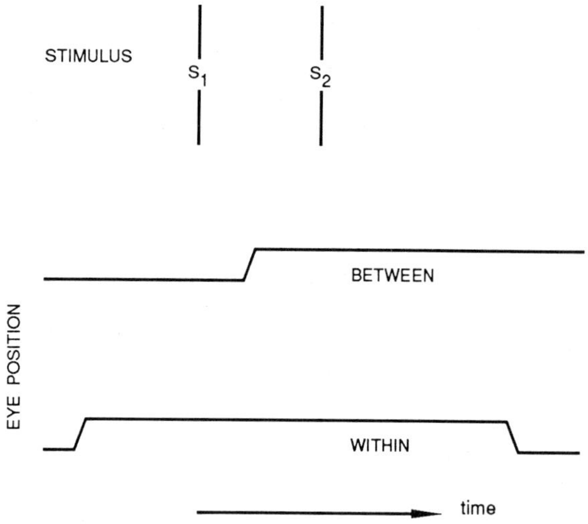

Fig. 13. The two-flash procedure. S_1 and S_2 represent stimuli illuminated by the first and second flashes, respectively, and the horizontal coordinate represents time. In the Between-fixation condition, a saccade occurs during the interval between the flashes; in the Within-fixation condition, both flashes occur within the same fixation.

7.3. Two-flash displays: masking, localization, movement, memory

The two-flash paradigm. Experiments with a two-flash stimulus have been particularly productive in the analysis of information-processing within and between fixations. The observer views two consecutive, brief flashes separated by a time interval δt. Either both flashes are confined to within a single fixation (the Within condition, Fig. 13) or a saccadic eye movement occurs between the flashes (the Between condition). Comparison of performance in Within and Between fixation conditions yields insight into saccadic information-processing. The ability of the observer to correlate the contents of the two images is tested by memory tests or by psychophysical tests that involve, for example, the ability to perceive motion between the images. The previous section considered search experiments in the within-fixation but not the between-fixation variant of the paradigm. The two-flash paradigm has also been used to study spatial localization and visual masking.

The great technical advantage of the two-flash procedure is that the simulated eye movement control experiment does not require producing a complex eye movement streak on the retina, merely two flashes. As with other eye movement paradigms, there are two disadvantages of the two-flash paradigm. The exact time of occurrence of a saccadic eye movement cannot yet be perfectly predicted. Many trials must be conducted in order to obtain a few critical trials with the eye movement centered between the flashes. To control for possible effects of the context of imperfect trials on performance in the critical trials, an equivalent imperfect context has to be provided for the within-fixation control experiment. The second problem is that the eye position must be known exactly at the time of the two flashes in order to ensure that the control presentation in the within-fixation presentation is truly equivalent to the between-fixation presentation – for both the 'same-retinal-coordinates' and 'same-spatial-coordinates' variations. While the problem of positional accuracy is endemic to all eye movement recordings, the apparent simplicity of the two-flash paradigm has seduced experimenters into attempting it with less-than-adequate eye movement recording.

7.3.1. Visual masking

Visual masking in a two-flash paradigm with an interleaved saccade was studied by Davidson et al. (1973) and Irwin et al. (1988), with roughly similar procedures and results. In Irwin et al.'s experiment, subjects were presented first with a 10 ms exposure of a row of five letters. This was followed by a 40–70 ms blank interval during which, on some trials, a saccade occurred. After the saccade, a masking pattern was superimposed on one of the letters. The masking pattern was found to exert its masking effect primarily when it occurred at the same retinal location, not the same spatial location, as the letters.

Does interposing a saccade between the first and second flash alter the masking effect of the masking pattern? With a δt between onsets of the first and second flashes of 40–70 ms, retinotopic masking results suggest that an eye movement would make no difference for this kind of masking. However, neither Davidson et al. (1973) nor Irwin et al. (1988) report a no-movement control condition, so we can only conjecture that masking is the same in real and simulated saccades.

7.3.2. Spatial localization

To compare masking and spatial localization during saccades, Irwin et al. (1988) used a two-flash background presentation like that described above. Again, the first flash was a 5-letter array; the second flash was a bar marker rather than a masking field. The bar marker was a short vertical line segment which instructed the subject to report the name of the letter below it (Averbach and Sperling, 1961). These experiments are essentially spatial localization experiments completely analogous in many details of procedure, theory and results to those described in the section on spatial localization during saccades (section 6.2). Irwin et al.'s results show that the bar marker changes its apparent location relative to the stable letter array with approximately the same time course during the saccade as did Sperling and Speelman's (1965) short-line segment relative to their dot array in the localization experiments described earlier. The comparison between experiments is only approximate because Irwin et al. did not make precise measurements of the time course.

Irwin et al. observed that, even though a masking flash that masks an earlier letter was at the same retinotopic location, the apparent spatial location of the masking pattern corresponds to its new spatiotopic retinal coordinates. That is, the apparent spatial location of a masking pattern is computed in the same way as the apparent location of other spatial patterns, such as bar markers.

7.3.3. Motion detection and perception

The two-flash paradigm naturally lends itself to the study of motion perception between the two flashes. Perceiving motion requires some form of correlation to be computed between the first and second stimulus, so motion perception implies at least an elementary form of pattern memory. The issues that arise in the two-flash paradigms are precisely the same as those which emerged in section 6.5. However, in experiments that measured the ability of subjects to detect object displacements during saccades, no attempt was made to ascertain whether detection was based on perceived motion or on perceived change in location.

Shioiri and Cavanagh (1989) attempted to determine whether motion could be perceived during a saccade by using random-dot patterns which offered good motion cues but only weak locational cues when they were displaced. When pattern displacements occurred between two fixations in an explicit two-flash paradigm, their subjects failed to discriminate displacement from no-displacement trials. The subjects were also unable to use apparent motion to correctly identify the direction of displacements that occurred around the time of saccades.

Unfortunately, Shioiri and Cavanagh's procedures illustrate the hazards of violating the three methodological precepts proposed above. They did not measure eye movements accurately enough to know the actual retinal placement of their stimuli. Perhaps for this reason, they did not use feedback to teach the observers to use all the available movement information. Therefore, the most we can know is that their observers habitually do not use retinal movement information to determine whether stimuli have moved during saccades – not that motion information is unavailable or suppressed. And the investigators did not run the simulated-movement control experiment within a fixation to permit comparisons of movement perception in retinally matched sequences of displays within and between saccade-separated fixations. Thus, while it is clear that people tend not to report perceiving motion between two saccade-separated flashes, the question "To what extent *can* motion be perceived between two saccade-separated fixations?" remains unanswered.

7.3.4. Recognition memory for images related by translations

While motion perception is an elementary computation that compares two (or more) views of the world, there may well be analogous higher-level computations. Consider that saccadic eye movements convert the visual input into essentially a series of still frames at a typical rate of about two or three frames per second. When the environment is stationary, all these successive images are related by simple translation. Might there be a specialized memory for recognizing and storing images which differ only by translation? How are the relationships between images coded to enable the observer to build up a coherent internal model of the world.

Recognition memory for translated images in the stationary eye. Let two successive images, such as might be produced by successive saccades, be produced on the stationary eye. Does the observer have any special ability to recognize relationships between such successive images? In one procedure, Roseanne Speelman and I presented subjects with two successive images, each consisting of ten shapes. One shape was changed; the remaining ones were the same in both presentations. The subject's memory was tested by asking which shape was different. Shapes were chosen that were not as easily named as alphanumeric characters, and brief exposure durations were used in order to selectively probe visual memory (and to reduce the role of verbal memory). The ten shapes were arranged in a horizontal row, and translated upward or downward. The direction of translation (up or down) and the distance between frames was varied randomly.

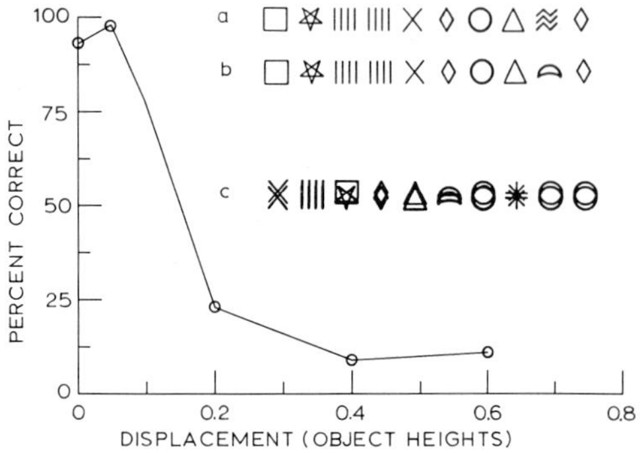

Fig. 14. Stimuli and results from a two-flash, simulated saccade memory experiment. The first stimulus is *a*; the second stimulus is *b*; the subject's task is to locate the changed position. Stimuli *a* and *b* occur in quick succession separated vertically, as shown. (*c*) Two stimuli that overlap by about 0.2 object heights. This small shift reduced performance from near perfect to less than 25% correct. The graph shows recognition accuracy (identification of changed locations) from an experiment in which displacement between memory and test stimuli was varied. The data points are the average of three subjects; the accuracies have been corrected for chance guessing. (Sperling and Speelman, unpublished data, AT&T Bell Labs, 1968.)

Fig. 14 shows typical results of the study in which the second flash immediately followed the first and the duration of each was 167 ms. When the shapes moved, strong motion cues were produced by the movement. In addition, the changed target item produced dramatically more local flicker and random apparent motions. The combined flicker/motion cue allowed the subjects easily to identify the location of the changed shape. However, the subjects had no special ability to identify the first of the two shapes in a location. Virtually identical results were obtained when shapes were moved horizontally or diagonally, when they were viewed from different distances, and when the subject knew in advance the probable direction of movement. There is a potential technical problem in studying large displacements which place the two rows one above the other, because visual persistence of the first array facilitates comparison with the second. However, under conditions that minimize visual persistence or when post-stimulus masks are used (Sperling, 1963), performance continues to decline monotonically with the magnitude of displacement regardless of its direction.

When the shapes moved for 1/5 of their extent or more, or there was a sufficiently long interstimulus interval so that motion cues did not selectively point to the altered shape, subjects did quite poorly. Subject's asymptotic performance can be characterized as indicating a memory of slightly more than one of the ten shapes. If the altered stimulus was the stimulus they had memorized, they detected the change; if not, they guessed randomly. There was no indication whatever of a special memory for translated images.

7.3.5. Trans-saccadic perceptual fusion

The perceptual fusion paradigm. Perceptual fusion refers to the phenomenon in which two consecutive displays are perceptually combined and perceived as a unitary display. For example, in the two-flash display of Eriksen and Collins (1967), some subareas of a stimulus letter are displayed in the first flash and the remaining ones in the second flash. When the first and second flashes occur in extremely close succession, the resulting stimulus is not discriminably different from a single exposure of the whole stimulus, and the letter is clearly identifiable. As the time between flashes is increased, perceptual fusion becomes increasingly difficult and, at around 100 ms of separation, depending somewhat on stimulus conditions, accuracy of letter identification drops to chance. In the two-flash stimulus developed by Hogben and DiLollo (1974), the first flash contains 12 dots randomly chosen from a 5×5 square array; the second flash contains 12 of the remaining 13 dots; and the subject's task is to locate the missing dot. Again, when the two flashes are presented in extremely close succession, the subject perceives 24 dots simultaneously, and the location of the missing dot is found effortlessly. As the interval between flashes is increased, performance eventually drops to chance levels. How does interposing a saccade between the two flashes affect perceptual fusion?

Fusion requires retinal, not spatial, superposition. An early study (Jonides et al., 1982) of perceptual fusion in the missing-dot paradigm erroneously reported that when flash 1 was presented in the periphery before a saccade, and flash 2 in the fovea after the saccade, there was good perceptual fusion. That is, the two flashes in the same physical location, but different retinal locations, could be combined to solve the missing-dot problem. Subsequently, this result was discovered to be an artifact of luminous persistence in the CRT display (Jonides et al., 1983).*

With correctly constructed displays, there is not more perceptual fusion in the between-fixation (interposed saccade) condition than in the within-fixation control. This was demonstrated in a letter-fusion paradigm by O'Regan and Levy-Schoen (1983) and in missing-dot paradigms by Bridgeman and Mayer (1983), Irwin et al. (1983) and Rayner and Pollatsek (1983). With an interposed saccade, two flashes that originate at the same physical location strike different retinal locations, but perceptually they seem to have originated from the same physical location. In the control condition in the stationary eye, flashes that fall on the same two retinal locations appear to have occurred at quite different physical locations. Each of these perceptions is correct. However, correctly perceiving retinally separated flashes to have occurred in the same spatial location does not imply useful trans-saccadic perceptual fusion.

Can perceptual fusion occur when two flashes strike the same retinal location but a saccade has intervened so that they appear to have occurred at different spatial locations? This question is quite similar to the two-flash motion question posed in

* Jonides et al. (1982) are not the only investigators to have erroneously reported trans-retinal perceptual fusion. See Irwin et al. (1983) for a critique.

an earlier section. In both cases (achieving perceptual fusion, detecting small retinal displacements) to succeed in the trans-saccadic task, the subject must succeed in ignoring or cancelling the nonvisual signals arising from the saccade. And because in both cases there are formidable technical and procedural difficulties in conducting the experiments, we do not yet have adequate answers.

7.3.6. Other tests of trans-saccadic memory: conclusion

Among the contexts in which the notion of a special trans-saccadic memory has been proposed is reading (McConkie and Rayner, 1976). Here, too, experimental attempts to demonstrate such a specific memory have failed (McConkie and Zola, 1979; Rayner et al., 1980; McConkie et al., 1982). Psychophysical discriminations which require memory for line length and for the shape of rectangles demonstrate that there is trans-saccadic memory (Palmer and Ames, 1989). However, that subjects remember length or shape from one fixation to the next is hardly a novel discovery. The particular issue that concerns us here is whether a saccade, as compared to a simulated saccadic display in the fixated eye, facilitates or inhibits performance in the memory task. The reading and psychophysical experiments have not been designed to answer this question.

The two-flash experiments have not yielded any data to suggest that interposing a saccade facilitates performance relative to the simulated saccade in the stationary eye. Indeed, there remains the as yet unproved possibility that when a task requires the subject to ignore nonvisual signals generated by a saccade, performance may suffer relative to the simulated saccade.

7.4. Organizing information from sequences of saccades

7.4.1. Spatially coordinating successive retinal images

A failure to coordinate successive images. Subjects with extreme tunnel vision are unable to coordinate the information from successive eye movements. A similar failure to coordinate images in the stationary eye was found by Hochberg (1968). Subjects viewed a sequence of frames that represented successive views of a complex shape. The subjects were unable to deduce the overall shape from these views. Apparently, the information about relative locations of points in successive views is not easily derived from a sequence of images.

7.4.2. Both image content and spatial location are represented symbolically

Spatial location as a tag. In the retina and visual cortex, spatial location is coded retinotopically and anatomically. It is taken as axiomatic that at higher levels of processing, spatial location is ultimately coded as a tag, not as an anatomical brain location. That is, successive views are stored not in a topological arrangement corresponding to their two-dimensional relationships in the environment, but in more complex symbolic form in which information about relative positions in space is carried as a tag or feature in the representation. A visual object is described by a set of visual features and the relationships between them.* The representation of spatial location of the object relative to other objects, to the body, and to the environment is not logically different from the representation of other relationships. In this respect, the representation of visual space is not essentially different from the representation of tactual space defined, for example, by the hands moving over a surface and attempting to learn about it.

Must spatial tags be derived from eye and body movements? One interesting question is whether the information about spatial position that is derived from the position of the body, head and eyes can be replaced with position information derived from other modalities. For example, can a repre-

* See Ballard (1987) and Feldman (1985) for discussion of the frames of reference within which observer-object relationships are best represented.

sentation of the environment be built up when the information about location is provided by the position of the hand rather than the eye. To investigate this question, the eye is fixated on a display screen. The subject places a finger at various spots on a surface and an image is produced corresponding to the neighborhood of each spot pointed at. To the extent that the subject can learn to substitute finger movements for eye movements, the visual processing of successive saccadically produced visual images is not uniquely linked to the oculomotor system but can utilize other channels which provide reliable spatial information.

8. Summary and conclusions

Smooth and saccadic eye movements are uniquely adapted to acquire information via an eye that is organized into a specialized fovea and a wide periphery. The most useful working hypothesis is that, while both visual sensory processes and motor control have evolved to a high degree of specialization to deal with the eye movements, modality-specific processes yield to content-specific processes as early as practicable in the processing hierarchy. Thus, in processing information acquired by pursuit and saccadic eye movements, the earliest link between the retinal and extra-retinal components of the eye movement appears to occur at high levels of processing. As a consequence, when differences on psychophysical tests of perception in responses to self-produced image motion and to imposed image motion were observed they were attributed, for the most part, to failures to provide truly equivalent retinal stimuli in the moving and the stationary eyes. For example, acuity seems to be determined by retinal slip, and it makes no difference whether the object or the eye is moving. Similarly, the visual system is designed so that the kind of motion smear produced during saccades is not perceived even when it is produced on a stationary retina by a simulated saccade. The many reports of changes of visual sensitivity during saccades are adequately explained by the masking effect of the actual sequence of stimuli on the retina and by the uncertainty in where a test stimulus that is flashed during a saccade will appear to be located.

Spatial localization of flash seen during a 4-degree saccadic eye movement did not differ from localization of a flash during the equivalent imposed image movement. Errors of localization could be explained by assuming that there was a temporal uncertainty of about 6 ms in when a visual test flash occurs relative to saccadically produced image movement. Additionally, for some subjects, the subjective duration of their saccadic image movement was somewhat longer than its objective duration, and the subjective movement began too soon (relative to a test flash). This slightly inaccurate internal representation of the imposed image movement produced characteristic localization errors. For larger saccades, there were significant differences between localization judgements in eye movements and imposed movements because extra-retinal information contributed significantly to saccadic localization.

Extra-retinal information about the time of saccadic occurrence is used to suppress sensations of visual apparent motion, which would otherwise occur with saccadic image motion on the retina. This saccadic motion suppression is similar to re-interpretation of sensory inputs following voluntary movement in other modalities. The extent to which subjects can learn to ignore extra-retinal information in making visual judgements during saccades is not yet known.

Other than the ability to compute apparent motion between related images (based on correlations between elementary local features), subjects have no special memory for images that are related by simple translation. To coordinate images produced by successive fixations, the visual/cognitive system needs spatial information about the direction of gaze. This directional information cannot easily be extracted from the image sequence but is normally provided by the oculomotor system in conjunction with the head and body. Possibly even this oculomotor directional information could be replaced by equivalent directional information acquired from other modalities.

While saccades are usually remarkably efficient, it was possible to create a search task in which performance was substantially improved by eliminating saccades and presenting stimuli at a rate five times faster than saccades (25 new search arrays per second). Sudden onsets of stimulation such as might be caused by saccades were shown not to be necessary to initiate information-processing episodes; gradual ramp onsets served equally well.

Most of these results should not have been surprising – hindsight is easier than insight – from the point of view of processing efficiency. Both the visual sensory system and the oculomotor system have evolved extremely specialized and extraordinarily sensitive processing capacities near their respective receptors and effectors. In the brain, however, motor signals concerned with eye movements and visual signals, the result of post-retinal image processing, apparently interact only at high levels where the visual signal, at least, is far removed from its sensory origin. Because visuo-motor interactions occur at a high level, it suggests that they may be modifiable and substitutable. For example, when the extent of saccadic eye movements is optically modified, visuo-motor recalibration quickly occurs.

The hypothesis that emerged was that direct sensory control of vision by the oculomotor system is unnecessary. For example, in order to avoid confounding motion signals produced by eye movements with real object motion, it is not necessary to desensitize the retina during saccades. It is sufficient to process all such motion signals equally, and then to disregard saccadic motion outputs at what might be regarded as an 'interpretive' level. On the other hand, to avoid noticing saccadic motion smear, the visual system has evolved to ignore smear-followed-by-clear signals independently of how they are generated. Again, there is no visuomotor interaction here, merely an effective adaptation of the visual system to a mode of seeing.

Acknowledgements

The preparation of this chapter was supported by The Air Force Office of Scientific Research, Life Sciences Directorate, Visual Information Processing Program Grant 88-0364 and by the Office of Naval Research, Cognitive and Neural Sciences Division, Grant N00014-88-K-0569. The author wishes to express his appreciation for the assistance provided by the late Roseanne G. Speelman in the experiments reported herein.

References

Adelson, E.H. and Bergen, J. (1985) Spatiotemporal energy models for the perception of motion. J. Opt. Soc. Am. A, 2, 284–299.

Averbach, E. and Sperling, G. (1961) Short term storage of information in vision. In: C. Cherry (Ed.), Information Theory. Butterworths, Washington DC, pp. 196–211.

Ballard, D.H. (1987) Eye movements and spatial cognition. Technical Report 218, University of Rochester Computer Science, 50 pp.

Bischof, N. and Kramer, E. (1968) Untersuchungen und Ueberlegungen zur Richtungswahrnehmung bei Willkuerichen sakadischen Augenbewegung. Physiol. Forsch. 32, 185–218.

Bridgeman, B. and Mayer, M. (1983) Failure to integrate visual information from successive fixations. Bull. Psychonomic. Soc. 21, 285–286.

Bridgeman, B., Hendry, D. and Stark, L. (1975) Failure to detect displacement of the visual world during saccadic eye movements. Vision Res. 15, 719–722.

Brooks, B.A. and Fuchs, A.F. (1975) Influence of stimulus parameters on visual sensitivity during saccadic eye movement. Vision Res. 15, 1389–1398.

Brooks, B.A. and Impelman, D.M. (1981) Suppressive effects of a peripheral grating displacement during saccadic eye movement and during fixation. Exp. Brain Res. 42, 489–492.

Brooks, B.A., Impelman, D.M. and Lum, J.T. (1980a) Influence of background luminance on visual sensitivity during saccadic eye movements. Exptl. Brain Res. 40, 322–329.

Brooks, B.A., Yates, J.T. and Coleman, R.D. (1980b) Perception of images moving at saccadic velocities during saccades and during fixation. Exp. Brain Res. 40, 71–78.

Bruno, N. and Cutting, J.E. (1988) Minimodularity and the perception of layout. J. Exp. Psychol. Hum. Percept. Performance, 117, 161–170.

Burr, D. (1980) Motion smear. Nature 284, 164–165.

Campbell, F.W. and Wurtz, R.H. (1978) Saccadic omission: why we do not see a grey-out during a saccadic eye movement. Vision Res. 18, 1297–1303.

Clocksin, W.F. (1980) Perception of surface slant and edge labels from optical flow: a computational approach. Perception 9, 253–269.

Collewijn, H., Steinman, R.M. and van der Steen, H. (1985) The performance of the smooth pursuit eye movement system during passive and self-generated stimulus motion. J. Physiol. 366, 19P.

Corfield, R., Frosdick, J.P. and Campbell, F.W. (1978) Grey-out elimination: the roles of spatial waveform, frequency and phase. Vision Res. 18, 1305–1311.

Davidson, M.L., Fox, M.J. and Dick, A.O. (1973) Effect of eye movements on backward masking and perceived location. Percept. Psychophys. 14, 110–116.

Ditchburn, R.N. and Ginsborg, B.L. (1952) Vision with a stabilized retinal image. Nature 170, 36–37.

Dodge, R. and Fox, J.C. (1928) Optic nystagmus. I. Technical introduction with observations in a case with central scotoma in the right eye and external rectus palsy in the left eye. Arch. Neurol. Psychiatry 20, 812–823.

Dosher, B.A., Sperling, G. and Wurst, S.A. (1986) Tradeoffs between stereopsis and proximity luminance covariance. Vision Res. 26, 973–990.

Dubois, M.F.W. and Collewijn, H. (1979) Optokinetic reactions in man elicited by localized retinal motion stimuli. Vision Res. 19, 1105–1115.

Efron, R. (1970a) The relationship between the duration of a stimulus and the duration of a perception. Neurophysiologica 8, 37–55.

Efron, R. (1970b) The minimum duration of perception. Neurophysiologica 8, 56–63.

Eriksen, C.W. and Collins, J.F. (1967) Some temporal characteristics of visual pattern perception. J. Exp. Psychol. 74, 476–484.

Feldman, J.A. (1985) Four frames suffice: a provisional model of vision and space. Behav. Brain Sci. 8, 265–289.

Fisher, D.L. (1982) Limited-channel models of automatic detection: capacity and scanning in visual search. Psychol. Rev. 89, 662–692.

Gerrits, H.J.M. and Vendrik, A.J.H. (1974) The influence of stimulus movements on perception in parafoveal stabilized vision. Vision Res. 14, 175–180.

Haegerstrom-Portnoy, G. and Brown, B. (1979) Contrast effects on smooth-pursuit eye movement velocity. Vision Res. 19, 169–174.

Hansen, P.M. (1979) Spatial localization during pursuit eye movements. Vision Res. 19, 1213–1221.

Hansen, R.M. and Skavenski, A.A. (1977) Accuracy of eye position information for motor control. Vision Res. 17, 919–926.

Hansen, R.M. and Skavenski, A.A. (1985) Accuracy of spatial localizations near the time of saccadic eye movements. Vision Res. 25, 1077–1082.

Heeger, D.J. (1987) A model for the extraction of image flow. J. Opt. Soc. Am. A, 4, 1455–1471.

Hochberg, J. (1968). In the mind's eye. In: R.N. Haber (Ed.), Contemporary Theory and Research in Visual Perception. Appleton-Century-Crofts, New York.

Hoffman, D.D. (1982) Inferring local surface orientation from motion fields. J. Opt. Soc. Am. 72, 888–892.

Hogben, J.H. and Di Lollo, V. (1974) Perceptual integration of brief visual stimuli. Vision Res. 14, 1059–1069.

Irwin, D.E., Yantis, S. and Jonides, J. (1983) Evidence against visual integration across saccadic eye movements. Percept. Psychophys. 34, 49–57.

Irwin, D.E., Brown, J.S. and Jun-Shi Sun. (1988) Visual masking and visual integration across saccadic eye movements. J. Exp. Psychol. Gen. 117, 276–287.

Javel, L.E. (1878) Essai sur la physiologie de la lecture. Ann. d'Oculistique 82, 242–253.

Jonides, J., Irwin, D.E. and Yantis, S. (1982) Integrating visual information for successive fixations. Science 215, 192–194.

Jonides, J., Irwin, D.E. and Yantis, S. (1983) Failure to integrate visual information for successive fixations. Science 222, 188.

Keller, E.L. and Zee, D.S. (Eds.) (1986) Adaptive Process in Visual and Oculomotor Systems. Pergamon Press, Oxford.

Kelly, D.H. (1979) Motion and vision. II. Stabilized spatio-temporal threshold surface. J. Opt. Soc. Am. 69, 1340–1349.

Khurana, B. and Kowler, E. (1987) Shared attentional control of smooth eye movement and perception. Vision Res. 27, 1603–1618.

Koenderink, J.J. and van Doorn, A.J. (1986) Depth and shape from differential perspective in the presence of bending deformations. J. Opt. Soc. Am. A, 3, 242–249.

Kowler, E. and Sperling, G. (1980) Transient stimulation does not aid visual search: implications for the role of saccades. Percept. Psychophys. 27, 1–10.

Kowler, E. and Sperling, G. (1983) Abrupt onsets do not aid visual search. Percept. Psychophys. 34, 307–313.

Kowler, E. and Steinman, R.M. (1980) Small saccades serve no useful purpose: reply to a letter by R.W. Ditchburn. Vision Res. 20, 273–276.

Kowler, E., van der Steen, J., Tamminga, E.P. and Collewijn,H. (1984) Voluntary selection of the target for smooth eye movement in the presence of superimposed, full-field stationary and moving stimuli. Vision Res. 24, 1789–1798.

Krauskopf, J. (1957) Effet of retinal image motion on contrast threshold for maintained vision. J. Opt. Soc. Am. 47, 740–744.

Krauskopf, J. (1960) Effect of target oscillation on contrast resolution. J. Opt. Soc. Am. 50, 1306.

Krauskopf, J. (1962) Light distribution in human retinal images. J. Opt. Soc. Am. 52, 1046–1050.

Lennie, P. and Sidwell, A. (1978) Saccadic eye movements and visual stability. Nature 275, 766–768.

Loftus, G.R. (1972) Eye fixations and recognition memory. Cognitive Psychol. 3, 525–551.

Loftus, G.R. (1981) Tachistoscopic simulations of eye fixations on pictures. J. Exp. Psychol. Hum. Learn. Mem. 7, 369–376.

Longuet-Higgins, H.C. and Prazdny, K. (1980) The interpretation of a moving retinal image. Proc. R. Soc. Lond. Ser. B, 208, 385–397.

Mack, A. (1970) An investigation of the relationship between eye and retinal image movement in the perception of motion. Percept. Psychophys. 8, 291–298.

Mack, A. (1986) Perceptual aspects of motion in the frontal plane. In: K. Boff, L. Kaufman and J. Thomas (Eds.), Handbook of Perception and Performance, Vol. 1, Wiley, New York, Ch. 17, pp. 1–38.

MacKay, D.M. (1970a) Elevation of visual threshold by displacement of retinal image. Nature 225, 90–92.

MacKay, D.M. (1970b) Mislocation of test flashes during saccadic image displacements. Nature 227, 731–733.

MacKay, D.M. (1973) Visual stability and voluntary eye movements. In: R. Jung (Ed.), Handbook of Sensory Physiology, Vol. 7. Springer Verlag, Berlin, pp. 307–331.

Maloney, L.T. (1988) Spatially irregular sampling in combination with rigid movements of the sampling array. Invest. Ophthalmol. Vis. Sci. 1988, 29, 58.

Maloney, L.T. (1990) The consequences of discrete retinal sampling for vision. In: M.S. Landy and A.J. Movshon (Eds.), Computational Models of Visual Processing. Cambridge, MIT Press, Cambridge, MA.

Mateeff, S. (1978) Saccadic eye movements and localization of visual stimuli. Percept. Psychophys. 24, 215–224.

Matin, L. (1986) Visual localization and eye movements. In: K. Boff, L. Kaufman and J. Thomas (Eds.), Handbook of Perception and Performance, Vol. 1, Wiley, New York, Ch. 20, pp. 1–45.

McConkie, G.W. and Rayner, K. (1976) Identifying the span of the effective stimulus in reading: literature review and theories of reading. In: H. Singer and R.B. Ruddell (Eds.), Theoretical Models and Processes of Reading. International Reading Association, Newark, DE.

McConkie, G.W. and Zola, D. (1979) Is visual information integrated across successive fixations in reading? Percept. Psychophys. 25, 221–224.

McConkie, G.W., Zola, D., Blanchard, H.E. and Wolverton, G.S. (1982) Perceiving words during reading: lack of facilitation from prior peripheral exposure. Percept. Psychophys. 32, 271–281.

Meyer, C.H., Lasker, A.G. and Robinson, D.A. (1985) The upper limit of human smooth pursuit velocity. Vision Res. 25, 561–563.

Murphy, B. (1978) Pattern threshold for moving and stationary gratings during smooth eye movements. Vision Res. 18, 521–530.

Nachmias, J. (1961) Determiners of the drift of the eye during monocular fixation. J. Opt. Soc. Am. 51, 761–766.

Neisser, U. (1963) Decision time without reaction time: experiments in visual scanning. Am. J. Psychol. 76, 376–385.

Neisser, U. (1964) Visual search. Sci. Am. 210.

Neisser, U., Novick, R. and Lazar, R. (1963) Searching for ten targets simultaneously. Percept. Motor Skills 17, 955–961.

O'Regan, J.K. (1984) Retinal versus extraretinal influences in flash localization during saccadic eye movements in the presence of a visible backround. Percept. Psychophys. 36, 1–14.

O'Regan, J.K. and Levy-Schoen, A. (1983) Integrating information from successive fixations: does trans-saccadic fusion exist? Vision Res. 23, 765–768.

Palmer, J. and Ames, C.T. (1989) Measuring the effect of multiple eye fixations on size and shape discrimination. Invest. Ophthalmol. Vis. Sc. ARVO Suppl. 30, 159.

Pola, J. (1972) The relation of visual direction to eye position during and following a voluntary saccade. Unpublished doctoral dissertation. Columbia University.

Ratliff, F. and Riggs, L.A. (1950) Involuntary motions of the eye during monocular fixation. J. Exp. Psychol. 40, 687–701.

Rayner, K. and Pollatsek, K. (1983). Is visual information integrated across saccades? Percept. Psychophys. 34, 39–48.

Rayner, K., McConkie, G.W. and Zola, D. (1980) Integrating information across eye movements. Cognitive Psychol. 12, 206–226.

Reeves, A. (1977) The identification and recall of rapidly displayed letters and digits. Unpublished doctoral dissertation, City University of New York.

Reeves, A. and Sperling, G. (1986) Attention gating in short-term visual memory. Psychol. Rev. 93, 180–206.

Riggs, L.A., Ratliff, F., Cornsweet, J.C. and Cornsweet, T.N. (1953) The disappearance of steadily fixated visual test objects. J. Opt. Soc. Am. 43, 495–501.

Shiori, S. and Cavanagh, P. (1989) Saccadic suppression of low-level motion. Vision Res. 29, 915–928.

Skavenski, A.A., Hansen, R., Steinman, R.M. and Winterson, B.J. (1979) Quality of human retinal stabilization during small natural and artificial body rotations in man. Vision Res. 19, 675–683.

Sperling, G. (1960) The information available in brief visual presentations. Psychol. Monogr. 74, No. 11 (Whole No. 498).

Sperling, G. (1963) A model for visual memory tasks. Hum. Factors 5, 19–31.

Sperling, G. (1966) Comparisons of real and apparent motion. J. Opt. Soc. Am. 56, 1442.

Sperling, G. (1967) Successive approximations to a model for short-term memory. Acta Psychol. 27, 285–292.

Sperling, G. (1979) Critical duration, supersummation, and the narrow domain of strength-duration experiments. Behav. Brain Sc. 2, 279–282.

Sperling, G. and Dosher, B.A. (1986) Strategy and optimization in human information processing. In: K. Boff, L. Kaufman and J. Thomas (Eds.), Handbook of Perception and Performance, Vol. 1, Wiley, New York, Ch. 2, pp. 1–65.

Sperling, G. and Melchner, M.J. (1978) The attention operating characteristic: some examples from visual search. Science 202, 315–318.

Sperling, G. and Reeves, A. (1980) Measuring the reaction time of a shift of visual attention. In: R. Nickerson (Ed.), Attention and Performance, Vol. VIII. Erlbaum, Hillsdale, NJ, pp. 347–360.

Sperling, G. and Speelman, R.G. (1964) Spatial localization

during eye movements. Am. Psychol. 19, 526–527.

Sperling, G. and Speelman, R.G. (1965) Visual spatial localization during object motion, apparent object motion, and image motion produced by eye movements. J. Opt. Soc. Am. 55, 1576.

Sperling, G. and Weichselgartner, E. (1989) Movement dynamics of spatial attention. Mathematical Studies in Perception and Cognition, 89–14. Department of Psychology, New York University.

Sperling, G., Budiansky, J., Spivak, J.G. and Johnson, M.C. (1971) Extremely rapid visual search: the maximum rate of scanning letters for the presence of a numeral. Science 174, 307–311.

Sperling, G., Landy, M.S., Dosher, B.A. and Perkins, M. (1989) Kinetic depth effect and identification of shape. J. Exp. Psychol. Hum. Percept. Performance 15, 826–840.

Sperling, G., Dosher, B.A. and Landy, M.S. (1990) How to study the kinetic depth effect experimentally. J. Exp. Psychol. Hum. Percept. Performance 16, 445–450.

Stark, L., Kong, R., Schwartz, S., Hndry, D. and Bridgeman, B. (1976) Saccadic suppression of image displacement. Vision Res. 16, 1185–1187.

Steinman, R.M. and Collewijn, H. (1973) Binocular retinal image motion during active head rotation. Vision Res. 20, 415–429.

Steinman, R.M., Haddad, G.M., Skavenski, A.A. and Wyman, D. (1973) Miniature eye movement. Science 181, 810–819.

Steinman, R.M., Levinson, J.Z., Collewijn, H. and Steen, J. van der (1985) Vision in the presence of known natural retinal image motion. J. Opt. Soc. Am. A, 2, 226–233.

Thurstone, L.L. (1927) A law of comparative judgment. Psychol. Rev. 34, 273–386.

van Santen, J.P.H. and Sperling, G. (1984) A temporal covariance model of motion perception. J. Opt. Soc. Am. A, 1, 451–473.

van Santen, J.P.H. and Sperling, G. (1985) Elaborated Reichardt detectors. J. Opt. Soc. Am. A, 2, 300–321.

Volkmann, F.C. (1986) Human visual suppression. Vision Res. 26, 1401–1416.

Watson, A.B., Ahumada, A.J. and Farrell, J.E. (1986) The window of visibility: a psychophysical theory of fidelity in time-sampled motion displays. J. Opt. Soc. Am. A, 3, 300–307.

Watson, A.B. and Ahumada, A.J. (1983) A look at motion in the frequency domain. NASA Tech. Memo. 84352.

Watson, A.B. and Nachmias, J. (1977) Patterns of temporal interaction in the detection of gratings. Vision Res. 17, 1143–1149.

Weichselgartner, E. (1984) Two processes in visual attention. Unpublished doctoral thesis. Department of Psychology, New York University, pp. 141.

Weichselgartner, E. and Sperling, G. (1985) Continuous measurement of visible persistence. J.Exp. Psychol. Hum. Percept. Performance 11, 711–725.

Weichselgartner, E. and Sperling, G. (1987) Dynamics of automatic and controlled visual attention. Science 238, 778–780.

Westheimer, G., and Campbell, F.W. (1962) Light distribution in the image formed by the living human eye. J. Opt. Soc. Am. 52, 1040–1045.

Whipple, W.R. and Wallach, H. (1978) Direction-specific motion thresholds for abnormal image shifts during saccadic eye movement. Percept. Psychophys. 24, 349–355.

Winterson, B.J. and Steinman, R.M. (1978) The effect of luminance on human smooth pursuit of parafoveal and foveal targets. Vision Res. 18, 1165–1172.

Woodworth, R.S. (1906) Vision and localization during eye movements. Psychol. Bull. 3, 68–70.

Woodworth, R.S. (1938) Experimental Psychology. Henry Holt and Co., New York.

Yarbus, A.L. (1957) The perception of an image fixed with respect to the retina. Biofiz. (USSR) 2, 703–712. (Translated by J.E.S. Bradley.)

Yellott, J.I. Jr. (1987) Consequences of spatially irregular sampling for reconstruction of photon noisy images. Invest. Ophthalmol. Vis. Sci. ARVO Suppl. 28, 137.

Eye movements and their role in visual and cognitive processes
E. Kowler, Editor

CHAPTER 8

Eye movements in visual search: cognitive, perceptual and motor control aspects

Paolo Viviani

Faculty of Psychology and Educational Sciences, University of Geneva, 24 rue du Général Dufour, CH-1211 Geneva, Switzerland

1. Introduction

The main problem considered in this chapter is: what can we learn from eye movement data about the cognitive and perceptual processes involved in the exploration of the visual world? In the first section of the chapter I will examine critically the assumptions that one would have to make in order to lend scientific credibility to the stated problem. I will argue that there are several serious (perhaps fatal) difficulties with many received beliefs in this field, and in particular with the assumption that mental processes can be inferred inductively on the sole basis of experimental findings about eye movements. However, I will also argue that, under certain conditions, eye movement data may be useful in evaluating specific theories of visual and cognitive processes. Specifically, the kind of eye movement data that I believe to be more conducive in this respect are those which address the following two issues:

(1) What are the empirical, indisputable properties of the sequences of scanning eye movements? Each of these properties, or some combination of them, may eventually translate into the specific constraints that must be satisfied by any perceptual and cognitive theory which postulates a principled organization of eye movements.

(2) What are the computational problems that the oculomotor system must be able to solve in order (a) to behave as it does, and (b) to meet the very general requirements that are likely to be imposed by any sensible set of controlling psychological processes?

The rest of the chapter (with the exception of section 8) will review a few representative studies selected to illustrate specific aspects of these two questions. Thus, what follows does not provide a comprehensive coverage of current research on exploratory eye movements. In particular, reference to the detailed properties of the oculomotor system and to the psychophysical aspects of its functioning will only be made insofar as it is relevant to the analysis of visual search. Some of these topics are discussed in this volume, and the recent review by Hallet (1986) provides excellent coverage of this field. Moreover, I will only touch marginally upon the large and in many respects special field of reading eye movements, which is fully covered in Ch. 9.

I will begin (section 3) by describing those spatial and temporal properties of the eye fixations in the scanning of a static scene which are independent of the frame of reference in which movements are organized. These properties, it has been argued, place some constraints on the visual, cognitive and motor processes involved in visual search. The next section (4) addresses the question of what is an appropriate frame of reference for planning eye movements, and, in particular, how to set up such a frame under static conditions. Then (section 5) I will consider the peculiar computational problems that arise when visually searching a scene which is in relative motion with respect to the observer. Two following sections are devoted to motor planning during search. First (section 6), the two-saccade sequence is considered, with special reference to (a) the planning of such movements and (b) the integration of perceptual information across successive fixations. Second (section 7), I will take up the general case of longer saccade sequences. Are they planned as a unit, as the study of other forms of motor behavior suggests, or are they basically stimulus-driven on a step-by-step basis? The last section (8) returns to the main conceptual problem tackled in this chapter. It presents an overview of those very few instances in which the properties of exploratory eye movements across complex and naturalistic scenes have been demonstrably related to psychological and cognitive processes. In discussing these instances I will try to substantiate the general epistemological position expounded in the first section.

The point of view that will emerge from this critique is pessimistic. I believe that the hope of progressing inductively from experimental data on exploratory eye movements to a theoretical description of the underlying cognitive processes is ill-founded. Eye movements will only become useful in the context of a deductive approach: not until we conjure up a reasonably articulated theory of these processes will data on overt behavior truly contribute to our understanding by verifying or disproving the predictions of the theory.

2. An examination of the hypothesis that eye movements can help us to understand higher psychological processes

In his inquiry into the history of scientific ideas Kuhn (1970) defines 'paradigms' as "those accepted instances of actual scientific practice which include law, theory, application, and instrumentation together, that provide models from which spring particular coherent traditions of scientific research" (p. 10). According to Kuhn, the notion of a paradigm is closely related to that of 'normal research' which refers to those canons and beliefs implicitly or explicitly adopted by the practitioners of a specific discipline in defining the rules of the game for that discipline (pp. 23–42). By virtue of their status, the canons and beliefs, once established, are no longer questioned and become preconceptions in the strict sense of the word.

The rather specialized field of eye movement research may afford a particularly nice instance of scientific paradigm. Admittedly, the domain in question is not on the same grand scale as those considered by Kuhn, yet all the ingredients seem to be there. The instrumentation and the experimental procedures have become fairly standardized (which reputable journal would accept a report based only on an introspective assessment of what the eyes do, à la Wundt?). Also, the information-processing parlance and its recent cognitive flavoring supply the intellectual scaffolding to support the data. Last but not the least, a central dogma is at hand which provides the initial motivation for much of the work in the domain. The dogma takes several forms and disguises, most of which can, however, be summarized by the following quote from a leading scientist in the field: "[Exploratory saccadic] eye movements can at the very least be considered as tags or experimentally accessible quantities that scientists can observe to understand underlying processes of cognition". Once such a view has been adopted, the motivation for studying visual search by humans follows syllogistically from the (uncontroversial) belief that the study of human cognition is a worthy endeavor, both for its own sake, and for the possible practical outgrowths.

A noticeable cleavage emerges from the literature when one considers the intellectual posture of those active in the oculomotor field vis à vis the belief expressed by the above quote. On the one side, many behavioral researchers seem to believe that it is truly a self-evident dogma and, as such, above all reasonable doubt. On the other side, I suspect that many scientists concerned mainly with the 'hardware' of the oculomotor system do worse than challenge the dogma: they just couldn't care less. Both postures appear overly simplistic and potentially dangerous. Exploratory eye movements are not sensorimotor reflexes. Therefore, they must reflect to some extent the inner working of higher mental events. Conversely, it should also be clear that the relationship between the observable eye and the mind's eye is less an empirical fact established on the basis of solid experimental evidence than a petition of principle (Nissen, 1979). In fact, several lines of experimental evidence point to a significant degree of independence between eye movements and cognitive activities (e.g., Teichner et al., 1978; Rothkopf, 1978; Fisher et al., 1983; Sigman and Coles, 1980). Clearly, a critical assessment of the central dogma would be of some value. However, such an evaluation cannot rest on the mere observation of cases in which eye movements do and do not correlate with cognitive activities. It would be of greater value instead to delve into this crucial issue at a more analytical level, by trying to dissect the several interrelated components of the dogma.

2.1. Evaluation of the central dogma: the assumption of seriality

To begin with, it is obvious that eye movements, qua measurable motor sequences, represent a strictly serial behavior. Thus, to posit a close connection between this overt behavior and some identifiable cognitive process amounts to postulating that at least the most significant aspects of these processes unfold sequentially in time. Indeed, suppose that the mental events associated with a given perceptual experience were instead, in some real, functional sense, the emerging result of the concomitant activation of several parallel processess (cf. Kolers, 1976; Fodor, 1983). For instance, recent influential theorizing on both the early stages of visual processing (Marr, 1982) and on the conceptual categorization of percepts (e.g., Ackley et al., 1985; von der Malsburg and Bienenstock, 1986; Rumelhart et al., 1985; Rumelhart and McClelland, 1986) suggests that apperception of the external world is mediated by an array of concomitant processes hierarchically coordinated. Then, the sequential pick-up of information by visual scanning either (1) would be related to just one of the component processes rather than to the total event, or (2) would be subserving, on a time-sharing basis, several distinct processes at the same time. In the first case, any insight into the component process will remain worthless until we have an idea of the role that this component has in the total event. In the second case, observed motor sequences would afford a cross-sectional representation of the dynamic status and requirements of the individual components, and no isomorphism could be established between the properties of the motor sequences and the structure of the global mental process. In neither case would one be justified in claiming that 'the experimentally accessible quantities' can be used to 'understand the underlying processes of cognition'.

Chess-playing affords an interesting example of this essential difficulty in relating eye movements to complex mental procedures. It is known that expert players perceive the very many alternatives that are normally open in the middle game almost as though they were actually displayed on the board. In-depth analysis is then carried out only for very few among these alternatives. Clearly, in such a complex mental task we find aspects that suggest parallel processing and others that suggest serial processing, the two modes being intimately intertwined. Even if we assume that each eye movement between two cases on the board corresponds to a hypothetical move, it would still be impossible to know which mode is actually active. Moreover, several different developments may include the same move. Not surprisingly, only the analysis of on-line verbal reports has, in a few cases, justified a posteriori the corresponding pattern of eye movements (De Groot, 1978).

The foregoing argument can be summarized as follows:

(1) The central dogma would be valid if we knew a priori that a given cognitive process unfolds sequentially, but we did not know the specific sequences of mental events that take place in a given task. Eye movements could then afford a clue to discovering the unknown sequence.

(2) The central dogma is false whenever several concurrent processes can be suspected, unless we have a theory about how eye movement commands emerge from the various processes. Of course, no

such theory is in sight. Moreover, we are not going to be able to produce one solely on the basis of empirical evidence.

It appears then that the heuristic validity of the central dogma hinges upon the crucial issue: what can we say about the structure of the cognitive processes? The debate on this issue is quite open (cf. Fodor, 1975, 1983; Johnson-Laird, 1983; Gardner, 1985), and I will not even attempt to present the competing points of view. At any rate, it does not seem unfair to say that the central dogma possesses precious little of that quality of self-evidence that one would like a dogma to have.

2.2. Evaluation of the dogma: does attention coincide with the line of sight?

The second component of the dogma is somewhat more technical. By recording eye movements we measure the direction of line of sight either in space, or with respect to the head. In trying to infer from these measures the information sampled from the visual scene, we implicitly assume that the fovea is the most important field of functional significance. Indeed, while there is general agreement that the peripheral retina has important roles (to be considered later), the analysis of the distribution of fixations is almost always based on the assumption that the information being sampled is contained in a narrow (< 2 degrees) field symmetrically centered on the fovea. This assumption makes good sense in many important cases such as reading and close inspection of a figural detail. Nonetheless, there are now strong indications that the area of the visual field where focal attention is concentrated may occasionally be dissociated from the foveal field. The most spectacular demonstration of such dissociation has been provided by Zinchenko and Vergiles (1972). With the aid of a suction cup device mounted on the eye, they projected on the retina a stabilized image of a square array of digits. In the control situation where exploratory eye movements were prevented, they obtained the expected result that only the digits at the center of the matrix could be seen. When the subject was allowed to move the eyes, a normal scanning sequence was recorded. These movements, of course, did not change the retinal projection of the stimuli, and yet the subject was then able to read off correctly digits which were well into the peripheral field and should have not been visible. This amazing result can only be explained by postulating a 'functional' fovea which is driven around as a search-light under the indirect guidance of the efferent motor commands.

The fact that eye movements, albeit ineffectual from the point of view of the retinal projection, are instrumental in producing attentional shifts may be related to the illusory visual displacements that occur shortly before and during the execution of a saccade (Mateeff, 1978; Matin et al., 1970). In fact, one possible interpretation of these illusions is that, in order to compensate for the retinal displacement produced by the saccade and preserve phenomenal stability, impending motor commands shift the retinal system of reference in a direction opposite to the eye rotation. In both cases we would then have evidence of a perceptual effect due to efferent commands.

Further evidence that fixations do not always coincide with the points on the scene that are being attended to by the higher mental processes comes from the work on allocation of attentional resources (Engel, 1971, 1974; Edwards and Goolkasian, 1974; Posner, 1980; Posner and Cohen, 1980; Sperling and Reeves, 1980; Reeves and Sperling, 1986; Remington, 1980; Shaw, 1983). It appears in fact that, under appropriate conditions of pre-cueing, visual attention can be directed almost everywhere in the visual field, irrespective of the actual direction of the line of sight.

As a final remark on this point, I would like to call attention to the fact that, for technical reasons, almost all recordings of scanning eye movements have only considered the exploration of static scenes (one exception will be discussed at length in a later section). We have no way of ascertaining what bias, if any, this limitation has induced in our appreciation of the role of eye movements for the perception of the visual world. Be that as it may, the fact remains that in real life a good deal of visual exploration occurs in a dynamic environment, and that many concepts developed from the analysis of laboratory situations may not be terribly relevant to even such mundane circumstances as watching a soccer game.

2.3. Requirements of a theory relating eye movements to cognitive processes

So far I have been concerned with two major assumptions implicit in the central dogma of visual search studies. The first one was that visual scanning can be construed as the overt manifestation of a strictly serial algorithm (such as one that might drive a sophisticated TV camera endowed with all the known functional properties of the retina; cf. Just and Carpenter, 1976). The second assumption was that the direction of the line of sight coincides with the direction of attention. To continue the TV camera analogy, this assumption states that the camera points faithfully to whatever area of the visual scene happens to be important for the ongoing operation of the algorithm, and that no special qualifications are necessary to handle the case of a moving scene. Neither assumption can be completely rejected, but some evidence against both of them has been cited.

I now turn to a different and more general issue. To press my point as simply and as forcefully as possible, I will assume that all the criticisms leveled so far against the central dogma can demonstrably be dismissed, and that the two assumptions summarized above hold true. Then, one can ask: under what conditions is it proper to assume that the sequence of fixations conveys information? I will argue that this is a very difficult question mainly because the notion of information, despite its widespread usage in all arguments concerning visual perception, remains largely ambiguous. On the one side we have the rigorous measure-theoretic definition due to Shannon (cf. Reza, 1961) which has gained currency almost exclusively in the field of electrical communication (the analysis of response times is a notable exception; cf. Laming, 1968; Luce, 1986). On the other side, 'intuitive' definitions are rife in the human sciences, but in many cases amount to little more than equating information with the distal stimulus (the so-called 'stimulus fallacy'). Clearly, what is needed before attempting an answer to our question is a restatement of the formal machinery of information theory that can be embodied in a plausible set of cognitive processes. What follows is only a very sketchy outline of such a restatement.

Whenever an observer explores the visual world in order to solve a specific problem, there are at least three cognitive operations whose involvement seems inescapable:

(1) Activating a set of a priori beliefs concerning the possible states of the world. Virtually every problem that can be solved with the help of sensory information is in fact phrased as a selection among competing hypotheses. The set must be complemented with a full probability scheme: in general not all hypotheses are equally likely. Note that only subjective probabilities are relevant in this context, and that they may differ considerably from their objective counterparts.

(2) Breaking up the complex, holistic hypothesis that normally regulates our commerce with the world into an appropriate hierarchy of simpler alternatives. The alternatives need not be figural in nature. It is only required that a univocal correspondence exists between each alternative and an appropriate visual configuration in the field.

(3) Translating the alternatives into an actual sequence of locations in visual space whose content is most likely to disambiguate each alternative. These locations become targets for eye fixations. The selection of these visual targets may not be entirely preordained, and an essential part of the task is to update the selection principle on the basis of the current alternatives under consideration and their corresponding likelihoods.

The usual accounts of the visual search task to be found in many textbooks mostly expand on the last of these three points and tend to overlook the key role of a priori beliefs in the process of information acquisition. I maintain that this can lead to serious misconceptions concerning the very notion of information and that the true difficulties in the cognitive restatement of classical information theory can only be exposed by a careful consideration of all three points (for a more general and extensive treatment of these issues, see Viviani, 1987).

Much of the faith in the possibility of investigating higher cognitive processes via the analysis of eye scanpaths rests on the (false) identification of the information acquired by the observer with the visual stimulation that impinges on the retina (see above). Since, by assumption, cognitive processes are 'powered' by information, the sequences of fixations are supposed to provide us with both the input stimuli and the overt ongoing response of the cognitive processes to these stimuli. The trouble is that information *is not* out there in the visual field. It only comes into being when a visual configuration is able to eliminate the a priori uncertainty that exists at the very moment that we explore the world. Moreover, the amount of information thus acquired depends only on the subjective probabilities assigned to the alternatives that we happen to entertain. From the fact that a given point of the scene has been fixated we can only infer that some information *might* have been gleaned. To assess quantitatively how much information was actually taken in, however, it would be necessary to have an idea of the set of beliefs the onlooker has, and this is the real crux of the matter. In man-made communication systems this set of beliefs is usually predetermined and fixed. By contrast, a distinctive feature of most cognitive processes is that the beliefs (internal states) which set the frame for interpreting sensory stimulations are themselves updated on the basis of the incoming information. In particular, the likelihoods attached to the a priori beliefs are modified continuously. Since information and internal states influence each other, we seem to be trapped in a circular argument.

To be sure, similar chicken-and-egg predicaments also occur in other domains. In the general theory of systems, for instance, the difficulty can be resolved within the framework of the so-called State Approach (cf. Zadeh and Desoer, 1963). In essence, the idea is to separate the description of the system behavior into two components. One component describes the observable reaction of the system to an incoming stimulus, assuming a certain internal state. The other describes the evolution of the internal state, which, in general, is not observable. If we were able to assess the evolution of the set of a priori beliefs of the observer under the continuous flow of incoming information a similar approach could also be adopted in the case of visual exploration.

We have seen that neglecting the role of a priori beliefs entails the stimulus fallacy, which consists in equating discriminatory information with the distal stimulus. As a natural consequence of the fallacy, it has often been assumed that 'informativeness' is an objective quality which is distributed more or less evenly across the scene. Several attempts have been made to single out the aspects of the distal stimulus which are responsible for this distribution, and eye movement data have been cited as supporting evidence for the resulting criteria. The import of these attempts will now be discussed briefly.

Ever since Attneave's early work (Attneave, 1951, 1954; Attneave and Arnoult, 1956), it has been maintained frequently that information of two-dimensional shapes is concentrated along contours, and more specifically at points where changes in the direction of the contours are sharpest (e.g. Locher and Nodine, 1973). Moreover, points of intersection of line segments, sharp changes in texture gradients, the number of closed subpatterns within the external contour, and several other geometrical features have also been cited as particularly informative (cf. Zusne, 1970; Marr, 1982), and their effect on visual scanning has been investigated (e.g., Mackworth and Morandi, 1967). It has been suggested (cf. also section 8) that scanning eye movements tend to cluster around those places with high 'informativeness values' (Antes, 1974), and that this can be taken to support the claim implicit in the central dogma. Once again, however, I am afraid that the claim is logically flawed. No doubt the presence of details or any form of structure in the visual scene has, in general, the potential to carry more information than a uniform field. There are, however, exceptions. If I'm sure that I have stained my shirt with tomato sauce, my anxious eye's scanpath across the miraculously immaculate fabric will falsify a hypothesis endowed with high likelihood. Therefore, it will convey a lot of information. At any rate, while it is true that anything that helps to discriminate visual forms and consequently discriminate between alternative hypotheses can, *under certain circumstances*, carry information, it is equally true that one cannot infer from the intrinsic properties of the visual stimulus or from movements of the eye what these circumstances are, and how much information really gets taken in.

The notion that 'informativeness' is an intrinsic quality of the visual stimulus, distributed across the scene and scooped out by eye movements, is also inconsistent with the well-known phenomenon of instantaneous recognition. When we look at simple visual scenes or at familiar faces, recognition may actually occur at the first glance (Eriksen and Eriksen, 1971; Biederman et al., 1973, 1974; Intraub, 1981), suggesting some kind of holistic matching of the visual configuration with a stored set of templates (Ellis, 1981). Considering that information about facial expression can be identified from a 20-ms view as reliably as from much longer exposures (Simpson and Crandall, 1972), eye movements recorded for any extended period of time (Yarbus, 1967; Walker-Smith et al., 1977; Groner et al., 1984) may have little to do with the pick-up of information and the associated mental events. (Characteristically, Groner et al. (1984) in their experiment on visual scanning of photographic portraits were forced to eliminate one subject who could consistently recognize faces with just one fixation.) The clustering of eye fixations around specific features of the image after recognition has occurred may be taken to suggest the existence of stereotyped scanpaths. Thus, for instance, the fact that in looking at faces the gaze mostly concentrates on the eyes and the mouth even after recognition has occurred (Yarbus, 1967) could be due to the innate consciousness that *in general* these two features of the face are most important for discriminating the feelings of the observed person. The mere occurrence of such a scanpath *in a specific instance* will not tell us much that we do not know already from the well-known psychophysical studies on face recognition (Shepherd et al., 1981).

So far, I have been concerned exclusively with the dominant, exteroceptive function of vision whereby we perceive the properties of the external world. However, it should be stressed that vision may also have a proprioceptive function. The dynamic invariances of the optic flow do in fact afford an accurate measure of the relative state of motion of the body with respect to the environment (Gibson, 1950, 1966, 1979), as well as some vitally important information for organizing behavior, such as the time-to-contact with an external obstacle (Lee, 1980; Lee and Reddish, 1981). Very little is known about the interaction of the exteroceptive and proprioceptive functions of vision in the exploration of the real world, but the importance of this interaction cannot be questioned. In a later section, for instance, I will argue that visual scanning of a dynamic environment requires the discrimination of self-motion and object motion, which is itself contingent on the contribution of proprioceptive visual information. With respect to the foregoing critique of the use of information theory in the analysis of perceptual mechanisms, the proprioceptive mode differs sharply from its exteroceptive counterpart. In fact, a peculiar aspect of this mode is its apparent independence of cognitive beliefs and processes (Lishman and Lee, 1973). For instance, in the well-documented phenomenon of vection (Brandt et al., 1973; Berthoz et al., 1975; Lestienne et al., 1977; Tardy-Gervet et al., 1984) the illusory sensation of self-motion overrides the conscious knowledge of being objectively still. In as much as proprioceptive visual inputs are truly context-insensitive, the analysis of their role in the overall planning of visual exploration may escape some of the logical difficulties that I have discussed in this section. Such analysis, however, remains largely to be done.

I have examined the possibility of peering into the cognitive underpinnings of exploratory eye movements. Three reasons were cited for entertaining a sobering pessimism about this possibility: (1) the fact that a logical prerequisite for interpreting eye movement data is the knowledge of the architecture of the very same underlying cognitive processes that we wish to elucidate; (2) the fact that measuring what meets the fovea is only a part of what meets the (mind's) eye; (3) the fact that the acquired visual information cannot be measured reliably. Is there any value then in measuring eye movements during visual search? Yes. As long as a specific hypothesis is set forth which can, in principle, be falsified by a set of empirical data, the analysis of eye movements will have a heuristic value. The next section will be devoted to the simplest type of measurements that can provide such an empirical data-base.

3. Fixations

Fixations are the pauses between saccades. For a few hundreds of milliseconds the gaze is virtually stilled with respect to the head (position drifts and microsaccades may occur during longer fixations, but their amplitude does not exceed 10 minutes of arc (Nachmias, 1959; Bennet-Clark, 1964; Steinman, 1965) and their functional significance is open to question (Ditchburn, 1980; Kowler and Steinman, 1980)). Of course, fixations are also the more important aspect of visual scanning, the 'basic unit of encoding' as Loftus (1972) puts it. Much of what we can hope to understand about such movements comes from the analysis of (a) how long these pauses last and (b) where they occur. These two questions are not independent (see later). However, for the sake of clarity they will be considered separately. Point (a) is dealt with in this section. Discussion of point (b) is deferred until section 8.

At least three processes may be assumed to take place within the 300 milliseconds or so of a typical visual search fixation (cf. Ditchburn, 1973; Viviani et al., 1982): the analysis of the visual stimulus in the foveal field, the sampling of the peripheral field, and the corresponding planning of the next saccade. The minimum duration of the stimulus-processing has been estimated at about 100–150 ms (e.g., Eriksen and Eriksen, 1971; Spencer, 1969), but further processing may take place after correct identification. Thus, the estimate of the minimum time necessary to guide further movement (Salthouse et al., 1981) or to memorize the stimuli (Potter, 1975) might be revised upward. It is most likely that the three processes mentioned above are carried out concurrently, with several nervous structures acting in parrallel (Eriksen and Schultz, 1979; see also sections 2.3.3 and 3.7.1.6 in Hallet, 1976, and section III in Potter, 1983), but the amount of overlap among them is largely unknown. Actually, the encoding of the visual stimulus may exceed the duration of a fixation (Intraub, 1980). We do know, however, that the time spent for each process, which can be construed as a reaction time, is affected by several contextual factors. In order to discuss these factors it is appropriate to begin by distinguishing the statistical properties of fixation durations in normal exploratory scanning from those which can be measured in the laboratory.

3.1. Perceptual sampling and motor planning

With the help of carefully contrived experimental paradigms, investigators have attempted to manipulate the analysis, sampling and planning processes mentioned above. In particular, the visual detection and motor programming processes involved in the capture of a peripheral target have been studied extensively with classical reaction-time (target 'step-tracking') paradigms in which the visual processing of the foveal field is minimized by having the subject fixate a featureless point (e.g., Saslow, 1967b; Wheeless et al., 1966). Some of the findings are not specific to the oculomotor system. These include: compatibility effects (reaction times are shorter when stimulus and response are spatially homologous than when they are not, e.g., Hallet, 1978; Hallet and Adams, 1980), single vs. choice reaction times (single reaction times are generally shorter; e.g., Viviani and Swensson, 1982), and preparatory effects (a signal which pre-cues the required movement reduces its latency; cf. the 'pulse-

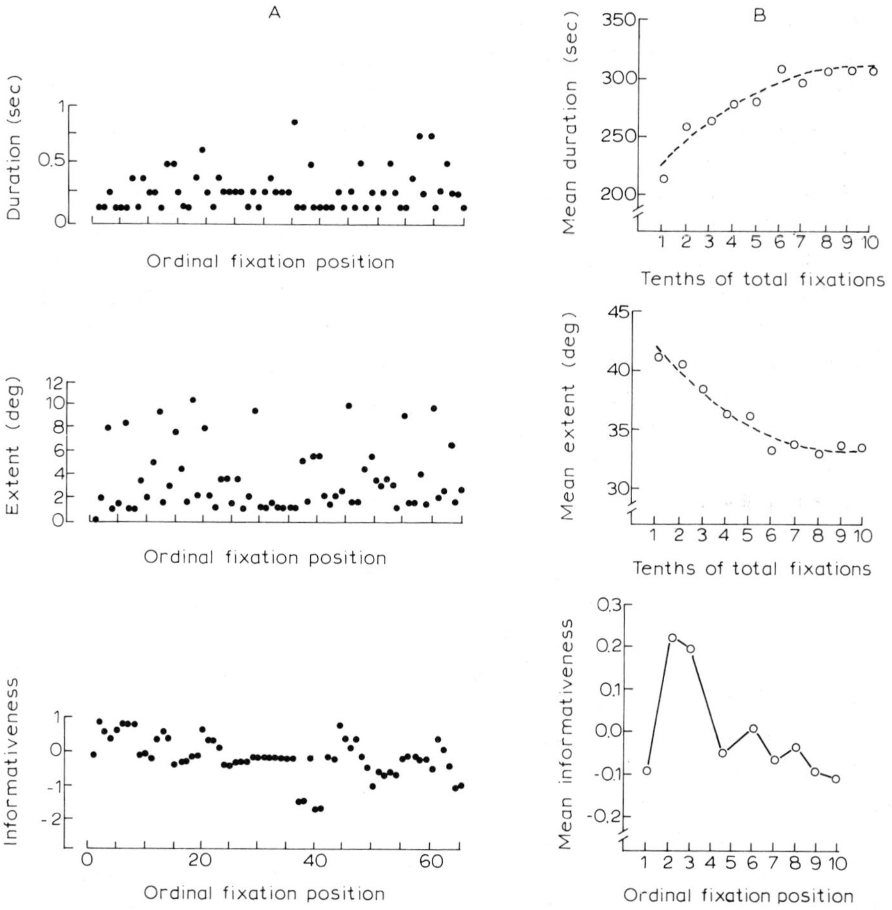

Fig. 1. Time-varying properties of exploratory eye movements. Ten pictures were freely explored for 20 seconds. Saccade amplitudes (extent) and fixation durations were measured. Each picture was then divided into regions where the fixation density was approximately constant. The mean subjective 'informativeness' of each region was measured with a rating technique. A: analysis of one trial (one subject scanning one picture). Each panel describes the actual sequence of values of the indicated parameters in the course of the trial. B: averages across all subjects and all pictures. Each panel describes the evolution of the indicated quantities as a function of tenths of the total number of fixations. Dashed lines through the data points are least-square approximations. How far the exploration has proceeded affects independently mean duration, mean extent and informativeness. Notice, however, that, within a trial, the duration of a fixation and the size of the following saccade are only weakly correlated. (Adapted from Antes, 1974)

forward' condition in Komoda et al., 1973); a non-specific visual warning before target onset reduces saccadic latencies (Saslow, 1967a; Becker, 1972; Ross and Ross, 1981). For obvious reasons I cannot deal here with all these general issues in motor control. I will concentrate instead on the processes related to the presence of a visual input and, more specifically, on those which precede the actual onset of the saccade. Two particular aspects of the oculomotor latencies appear to be most relevant to the description of visual scanning.

(1) The average latency of small saccades is almost constant. Instead, for larger movements there is a positive correlation between the eccentricity of the target and saccadic latency (Cohen and Ross, 1977; Miles, 1936; Saslow, 1967a,b; White et al., 1962, Viviani and Swensson, 1982). This is a robust effect, but it is not clear yet what fraction of it should be ascribed to the perceptual processes and what to the motor planning, nor, indeed, whether a

clear temporal separation of the two is warranted (Sanders, 1980; Townsend, 1976). At any rate, in actual sequences of scanning movements the correlation between the duration of a fixation and the size of the following saccade is much weaker (see Fig. 1A (from Antes, 1974)). There might be at least three reasons for that. (1) The effect of eccentricity only appears for saccade amplitudes greater than those usually found in free scanning. Perhaps the increasing difficulty of calibrating large saccades, which is responsible for the long latencies, discourages the use of such movements. (2) The duration of the fixations while scanning a meaningful scene includes the processing of the visual stimulus, which is absent in the reaction-time paradigm. The correlation may be weakened by the presence of this independent, additive component. (3) More generally, the requirements of a typical step-tracking task differ considerably from those of a visual scanning task in as much as the latter normally involves a more complex processing of visual information. Thus, inferences drawn from step-tracking need not apply also to the case of unconstrained visual search.

(2) The latency increases with the a priori uncertainty about the location of the target (Boyce, 1965). For instance, the latency of the saccade is significantly shortened if the eccentricity of the target is specified, and only the angular direction has to be determined from visual inputs (Viviani and Swensson, 1982). Thus, analysis of the latencies during free scanning, conditional on a specific size of the following saccade, might reveal something about the subjective expectancies of the viewer.

3.2. *Analysis of the visual stimulus*

The single most important event taking place during a fixation is the analysis of the visual array within the foveal field. Also, the duration of this process, as that of perceptual sampling and motor planning (see above), is somewhat variable and flexible. It has been argued (Gould, 1973; Just and Carpenter, 1980; Massaro and Schmuller, 1975; Rayner, 1978; Blanchard, 1985) that these variations reflect the varying computational load for processing the information acquired foveally. The notion of 'Process Monitoring' has been proposed in this context (Rayner, 1978) to describe a general class of models for fixation control. In Vaughan's words "the term implies that the central control mechanisms that control the duration of fixations ordinarily monitor the acquisition and interpretation of the visual information acquired in each fixation, and initiate the saccade that will end this fixation only after this information has been processed" (Vaughan, 1982, p. 710). Support for this view has come from at least two independent observations:

(1) Normally, the gaze is not aimed at a very specific location, for anything falling within the foveal and parafoveal field can be perceived satisfactorily. However, if the task requires an accurate fixation of point-like targets, the duration of the pauses can increase by as much as 100 ms with respect, for instance, to typical reading fixations (Bouma, 1978, p. 137). Perhaps this increase is the consequence of the additional perceptual load for centering the gaze accurately. Moreover, if the discriminability of the target in a visual search task is reduced (see Fig. 2 (from Jacobs, 1986), the observed increase is even larger.

(2) The second observation concerns the distribution of the processing of visual input over two fixations. It is known that some preprocessing of a target area occurs while the gaze is still fixating elsewhere and the target is therefore in the peripheral field (Dodge, 1907; Rayner, 1975; Levy-Schoen, 1981). The amount of preprocessing is inversely proportional to the discriminability of the target (Fig. 3 (from Levy-Schoen, 1981)). Thus, the Process-Monitoring hypothesis would predict a positive correlation between the duration of the fixation when the target is reached and the size of the saccade that leads to it. This prediction has been verified experimentally by Kapoula (1983), who asked subjects to count the number of target symbols contained in a line of distractors. The patterns of reading movements used to perform the task exhibited a significant increase of fixation duration

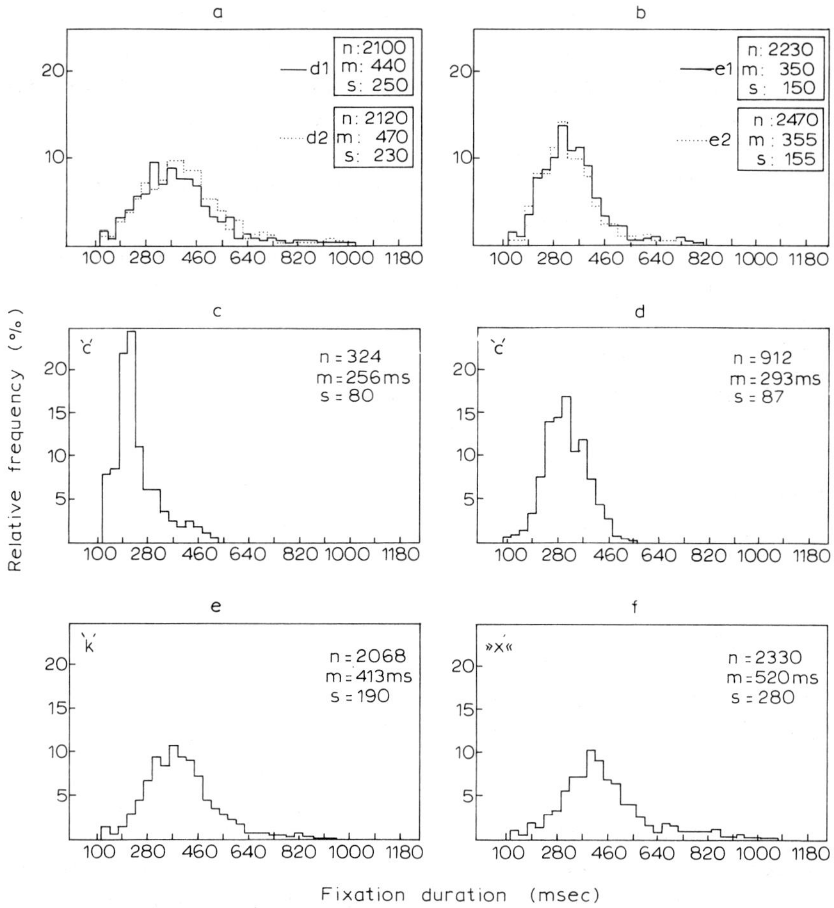

Fig. 2. Fixation durations during visual search. An experiment investigated the properties of eye movements when subjects scanned lines of distractors searching for a target character. Each panel shows the relative frequency for fixation duration under various experimental conditions. *n*, sample size; *m*, mean; *s*, variance. In all cases the results are relative to searching movements over lines that did not contain targets. (a) Comparison between small (d1) and large (d2) viewing distance. (b) Comparison between small (e1) and large (e2) character spacing. (c–f) Results for the four target characters shown inset. As the characters become more difficult to discriminate from the distractors, both mean and variance increase. Since the subjects scanned in fact physically identical lines (i.e. lines which contained no targets), the results suggest that cognitive expectations about target presence enter into the specification of saccadic latencies. (Reproduced from Jacobs, 1986)

as a function of the size of the preceding saccade. By contrast, a recent analysis of the eye movements during free scanning of a complex dynamic display (Ellis and Smith, 1985) has demonstrated just the opposite: a large (200 ms) reduction in mean fixation duration as the size of the preceding saccade varies between 1 and 8 degrees. It is difficult to reconcile these opposing findings other then by noting that the experimental conditions in the study by Ellis and Smith are much less constrained and may be more relevant for understanding real-life operations.

In any case, some other lines of evidence are also damaging for the Process-Monitoring idea. For instance, near-normal reading remains possible when the duration of the exposure to a portion of text is controlled by the experimenter (Bouma and de Voogd, 1974; Potter et al., 1980). This observation

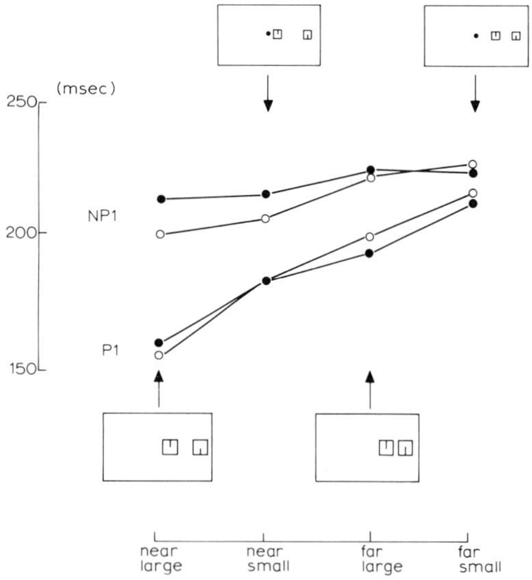

Fig. 3. Influence of peripheral preprocessing on fixation duration. A comparison task required the successive fixation of two stimuli (square outlines) differing only by the orientation of the small segment within the squares. Data points describe the relationship between the time spent fixating the first stimulus (ordinate) and the discriminability of the stimuli (abscissa, ordinal scale). When the discriminatory feature appeared only after the saccade to the first stimulus (condition NPI), the latency was weakly affected by stimulus discriminability. A large increase in the latency appeared instead when the discriminatory feature was already present at stimulus onset (condition PI). Conditions were either kept invariant (filled symbols) or randomized (empty symbols) across trials, but the differences in latencies were not very large. The results support the hypothesis that preprocessing of peripheral stimuli can curtail fixation times, and that the amount of preprocessing is inversely proportional to target discriminability. (Adapted from Levy-Schoen, 1981)

weakens the claim made by the Process-Monitoring model of a strict relationship between exposure duration and acquired information. Moreover, direct testing of the hypothesis has yielded somewhat inconclusive results. If a delay is introduced between the beginning of a fixation and the presentation of the stimulus in a visual discrimination task, the total fixation time remains almost constant up to delays of 120 ms. (Rayner and Pollatsek, 1981; Vaughan and Graefe, 1977; Salthause et al., 1981; Vaughan, 1978, 1982). Thus, visual processing time may be compressed by as much as one-third of the total fixation duration. However, for delays longer than 120 ms the fixation is increasingly lengthened as though no further compression were possible. These results are incompatible both with the Process-Monitoring hypothesis and with the competing hypothesis that the fixation duration is already predetermined at the end of the saccade (in this case, one assumes that the selected duration is always long enough to accomodate whatever visual processing may be necessary).

To conclude this brief discussion of the duration of the fixations in highly controlled laboratory conditions, it should be stressed that great prudence must be exercised in trying to infer the nature of the planning of sequences of eye movements from the study of simple fixation-saccade pairs. As discussed in a later section, some of these sequences represent higher units of oculomotor planning which are coordinated and executed as a whole. Thus, the properties of their components may reflect more the overall organization of the sequence than anything else.

3.3. Fixation durations during free scanning

Several studies have indicated that the statistical properties of fixation durations during free scanning of a complex scene are not stationary. Antes (1974) has shown, for instance, that the average duration over successive tenths of a 20-s period of free scanning increases from about 220 ms at the beginning of the exploration to about 300 ms at the end (Fig. 1B (from Antes, 1974)). Apparently, the first moments of observation are spent concentrating on the salient features of the scene with relatively short fixations. Later on, other (perhaps less important?) features are examined for longer times. Also, Nodine (1982) recorded eye movements while subjects compared original and altered versions of famous paintings and observed a similar concentration of early fixations on the most salient features of the image. Friedman and Liebelt (1981) confirmed the trend of increasing fixation durations with viewing time. However, they showed that this lengthening is not the result of shifting the attention

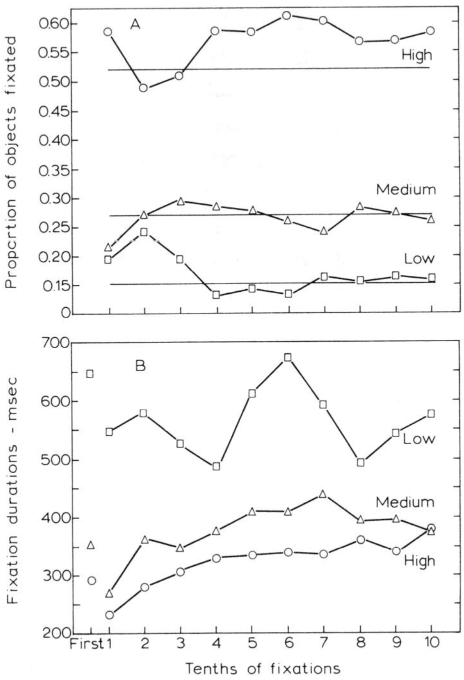

Fig. 4. Fixations during free scanning. Average results from a population of subjects who freely scanned a series of naturalistic pictures. The objects in the pictures had various degrees of contextual 'likelihood'. A: the spatial distribution of fixations is constant across successive tenths of their total number. The proportion of fixations on high, medium and low probability objects reflects the percentage of these three types of object in the pictures. Thus, unlikely objects draw the same attention as highly expected ones. B: fixation durations depend on both the degree of contextual likelihood and their serial order. (Adapted from Friedman and Liebelt, 1981)

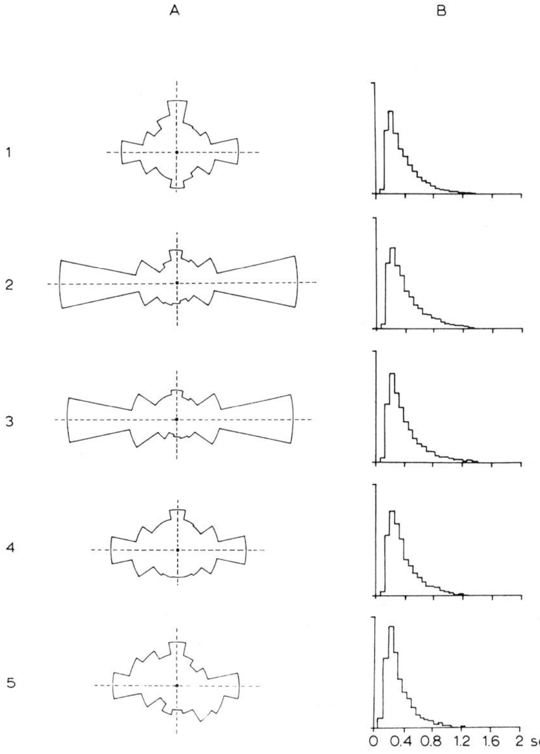

Fig. 5. Global characteristics of exploratory eye movements. A set of 25 naturalistic scenes were scanned freely for 40 seconds by 25 observers. Individual differences in scanning strategies proved to be less marked than the differences across scenes. The set of scenes was then partitioned into 5 (unequal) groups on the basis of some global parameters of the exploratory movements. The polar distributions for 16 orientations of one of these parameters, namely the number of saccades, are shown in column A for each group of scenes. Data are pooled over all subjects. Because of the large sample size, all pairwise comparisons between distributions, with the exception of 4–5 and 2–3, show significant differences. Equally large differences existed in the distributions of saccade amplitudes (not shown here). In column B are shown the histograms of the fixation durations for the same groups of scenes. The distribution of fixation durations is almost identical in all groups. (Adapted from Viviani et al., 1982)

from more salient to less salient features. In their experiment subjects were asked to inspect pictures containing objects whose presence in the context of the picture varied from highly likely to very unlikely. The results showed (Fig. 4A) that fixations were distributed evenly over all objects, and, in contrast with Antes' results (see above), their distribution remained invariant across viewing time. Although fixation durations were found to depend strongly on the contextual likelihood of the object being fixated (Fig. 4B), a trend of increasing durations was present for each level of likelihood.

Despite such non-stationary behavior, and the very many factors discussed above that may enter into the specification of the fixation duration, the probability distributions of these durations are surprisingly simple. In an experiment designed to determine the general characteristics of exploratory eye movements 25 subjects scanned 25 naturalistic color scenes freely for 30 seconds (Viviani et al.,

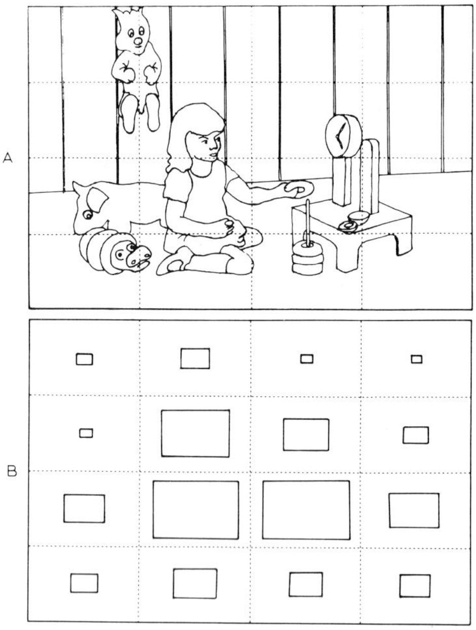

C

387	378	391	287
333	557	424	346
420	388	377	382
453	296	298	339

Fig. 6. Global characteristics of exploratory eye movements. A: simplified outline of one of the 25 scenes used in the experiment. For the purpose of the analysis, the scene is partitioned into 16 quadrants (dashed lines). B: the total number of fixations in each quadrant is indicated by the perimeter of the corresponding rectangle. Data for all subjects. C: average duration of the fixation (in ms) for each quadrant. Notice that, in contrast with the observation by Antes (1974), fixations on the more evocative parts of the scene (in this case, the face of the girl) are much longer than all the others. Generally, the maximum density of fixations does not occur in that quadrant. (Adapted from Viviani et al., 1982)

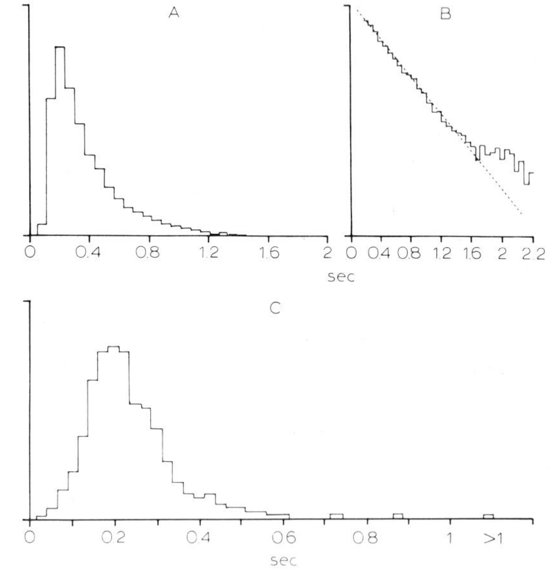

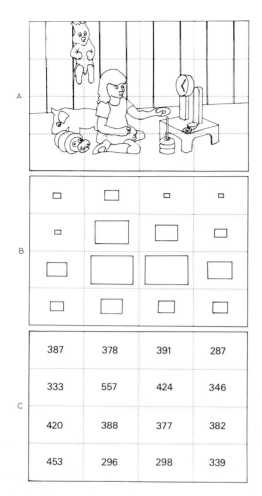

Fig. 7. Histograms of fixation duration. A: results for all subjects and all scenes. Pooling over scene groups is justified by the great similarity of the results for each group (see Fig. 5). B: tail of the distribution of fixation durations shown in A in logarithmic scale (ordinates). A straight-line approximation of the data points is quite satisfactory over most of the range of interest. (Adapted from Viviani et al., 1982.) C: data from reading eye movements (adapted from O'Regan and Levy-Schoen, 1978). Reading fixations are, on average, faster than exploratory fixations, and their distribution is less positively skewed. Individual differences do, however, exist. Notice that in this, as well as in many other instances in the literature, some of the differences between histograms of fixation duration are due to the computer algorithms used to measure the fixation (cf. Karsh and Breitenbach, 1983).

1982). The scenes were selected with the empirical criterion that the distribution and type of figural features should be such as to induce systematic differences in some of the scanning parameters which would emerge over and above the idiosyncratic habits of the viewers. A typological analysis of the results (Desaraty, 1976) showed that in fact the 25 images could reliably be partitioned into five groups on the basis of three criteria: the number and the amplitude of saccades in the various spatial directions, and the spatial distribution of fixations. Spatial distributions will be discussed later. Suffice here to demonstrate (a) that considerable quantitative differences exist in the scanning saccades for the five groups of scenes (see amplitude histograms in Fig. 5A) and (b) that equally large differences exist within any one scene for the average fixation durations in different parts of the field. This is illustrated by the typical example of Fig. 6. The point I want to make then is illustrated by the histograms of fixation durations for each group shown in Fig. 5B. Apart from insignificant differences, these global distributions of probability are indistinguishable. Actually, one can describe the statistical properties of the durations with just one histogram for all subjects and all scenes (Fig. 7A).

What can be inferred from the shape of these distributions? To begin with, the distributions include data which, at least in principle, should be rather heterogeneous. Even if one admits that many of the effects found in particular experimental conditions become marginal in free scanning, the substantial differences in mean latency in the course of the exploration (cf. above) and across different parts of the scene should show up as a tendency toward normality in the probability distributions. Instead, as shown in Fig. 7B, the long asymmetric tail of the distribution is very nearly a negative exponential and there is a sharply defined minimum latency. Recent measurements of the distribution of fixation durations from infants and free-viewing adults (Harris et al., 1988) have confirmed the presence of an exponential tail and set the minumum latency at about 50 ms for infants and 100 ms for adults. Thus, if indeed the histograms of Fig. 5B are a mixture of distributions with different means, all these distributions must have the same exponential form with identical minimum latency. Differences in means reflect the analogous differences in the slope of the upper tail.

A number of hypothetical mechanisms may be compatible with this general form of the distribution of fixation durations (Snodgrass and Townsend, 1980; Harris et al., 1988). Following the suggestion originally put forward by Sternberg (1967), it may be interesting to conceptualize the encoding of the visual stimulus during a fixation as a two-stage operation. The first stage affords an abstracted representation of its physical properties, and its duration may be assumed to be stimulus-independent and fixed. The second affords conceptual identification by comparing the stimulus representation with a memory representation, in the same way as someone searching through the stacks of a library for a specific title. If books are shelved at random, the duration of the search will be a random

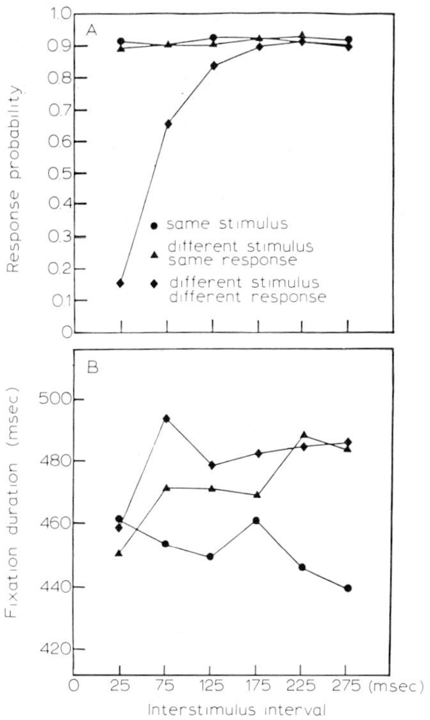

Fig. 8. Evidence for the existence of two levels of visual processing. Subjects were asked to make a saccade to an asterisk in the center of the field. As soon as the eye movement was detected, the asterisk changed into a randomly chosen digit (0 to 9). After a variable delay, the digit changed. If subjects perceived an odd (even) digit, they had to make a second saccade to an asterisk in the left (right) field. Since all ten digits were equally likely, in 10% of the trials the first and second digits were the same (data points 0), in 40% of the trials the digits were different but they were both odd or both even so that they required the same saccades (both leftward or both rightward) (data points ▲), and in 50% of the trials the digits were different and required opposite saccades (data points ■). A: probability of a correct response as a function of asynchronies between digit onsets. Notice that, when the response remained unchanged, performance was almost perfect for all asynchronies. In the case of conflicting stimuli, good performance was only attained after the masking effect had subsided. B: fixation duration for the three trial types. Latencies are greatly increased when the two digits are different. Further processing is needed to elaborate the correct response even for asynchronies that ensure almost perfect discrimination. (Adapted from Salthouse et al., 1981)

variable with a negative exponential distribution (cf. Papoulis, 1965). Salthouse et al. (1981), using a delayed interference paradigm, have provided some experimental support for this idea of distinguishing at least two stages of visual processing (Fig. 8). Although their interpretation of the stages is not the same as the one proposed above (the authors distinguished stimulus 'registration' at a low level of processing, and stimulus 'comprehension' at a higher cognitive level), the difference is not essential at this point. Moreover, this hierarchical representation need not be limited to foveal processing, and may also be relevant for describing the time course of visual sampling for the peripheral field.

By contrast with the above analysis of the fixation components, much less can be said about the statistical properties of the time course of the motor planning stage and the amount of overlap with the purely visual processes. A simple hypothesis is that all these processes are strung up in series, that each process has the same probability of being terminated in a time interval δt, and that the total fixation duration is just the time necessary to complete them all. In this case the resulting distribution should be of the Erlang type (Hastings and Peacock, 1974). The fitting, however, is not quite satisfactory, probably because only the visual sampling (both foveal and peripherical) but not the motor program stages can be construed as self-terminating processes (cf. Reed, 1973). In other words, it is possible that, irrespective of the moment when the specification of the motor plan is attained, the stage responsible for the planning must run though a number of mandatory duty cycles. A better approximation can be obtained by relaxing the condition of equality of the time constants. One then obtains a distribution which is the weighted algebraic sum of exponentials (McGill, 1963) and is itself not too different from an exponential. Despite the large difference in the time scales involved, it may be interesting to note that search-time distributions for small three-digits numbers embedded in a field of distractors have been modeled in this way (McGill, 1960).

The shape of the distributions of fixation durations in free scanning is considerably different from the distributions of fixation durations during reading (Fig. 7C). Since it seems reasonable to believe that the motor planning component of the latencies and the purely visual processes are the same in the two cases, the difference should then reflect some specific characteristics of the analysis component. This component corresponds to the second stage in Sternberg's model (see above), which supposedly encodes visual information at some higher cognitive level.

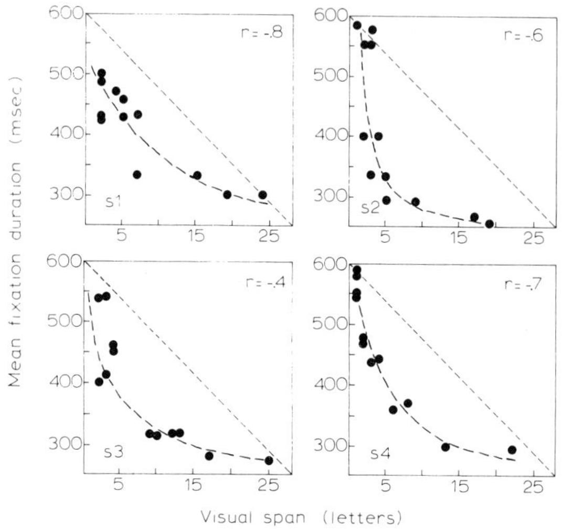

Fig. 9. Latencies and visual span. Results from the visual search experiment of Jacobs (1986) already referred to in Fig. 2. Plots show individual data for four subjects. A clear relation exists between visual span (eccentricity in number of characters on either the left or the right side of the fixation point at which the target letter can be identified with 50% correct responses) and the mean fixation duration. Each data point corresponds to a different combination of target size, target confusibility, and interletter spacing. Dashed interpolating lines (added by me) suggest a continuous, nonlinear decrease of the latency with increasing discriminability. This result can be taken to suggest that in a letter-detection task fixation durations depend mainly on the ease of perceptual processing. (Adapted from Jacobs, 1986)

The difference between free scanning and reading calls to mind the distinction proposed by Groner (1978) between *scanning fixations*, which are associated with stimulus search and are relatively short (100–200 ms), and *processing fixations*

(300 ms and more), which are supposed to take place when a visual stimulus must be analysed to answer specific perceptual queries. It may be supposed that, in examining an image, scanning fixations tend to occur early in the viewing period to provide a general descriptive frame, while processing fixations intervene at a later stage. Thus, Groner's distinction is in keeping with the progressive increase of the fixation duration observed by Antes (1974) in the course of prolonged free scanning (see Fig. 1). To the extent that this distinction applies to reading fixations, it may imply that the high level of redundancy of written language favors the use of the fast scanning mode during reading. This hypothesis can be further qualified on the basis of the results of a recent experiment on visual search by Jacobs (1986) (Fig. 9). Jacobs observed that mean fixation duration while searching for the target symbol decreased as a function of target discriminability (as measured by the visual span within which target letters can be identified with 50% success rate). From these data Jacobs inferred that fixation durations can be separated into two different classes: (1) short and constant duration if span is greater than 5 characters and, (2) longer and variable durations for shorter spans. In fact, the hypothesis of a continuous trade-off between discriminability and duration is probably more in keeping with the results. In any case, the important point is that, given the experimental conditions of the study, this trade-off appears to depend on a priori expectations and on the level of uncertainty about the target presence, and not on sensorimotor processes (cf. Fig. 2). Since most searching saccades exceeded 1 degree of visual angle, it seems unlikely that the effect observed by Jacobs reflects the longer times required for the planning of small ($\leq 30'$) saccades (Wyman and Steinman, 1973; Kowler and Anton, 1987).

In summary, analyses of distribution of fixation duration and the change in the parameters with type of task suggest three sub-processes: the sampling of visual information, the analysis of this information, and the motor planning of the subsequent saccade. In all three cases the identification of the component was based on the effects that the contextual conditions had on the total duration. Thus, the identification is somewhat contingent on the hypothesis that the underlying processes are arranged serially in time. However, since there is reason to suspect an unspecified amount of overlap among them, most of the quantitative results presented in this section are subject to caution. In the coming section I will touch upon some of the problems that must be solved by the oculomotor system in order to move from one fixation to another.

4. Setting up an invariant frame of reference

When we transport our whole body by walking or by car, the places to be reached and the path that is followed are defined with respect to the stable frame of reference provided by the external world. It took a while before investigators in the field of motor control came to appreciate fully the fact that, whenever an action requires the accurate positioning of many body segments with respect to each other, the availability of such a stable frame of reference cannot be taken for granted. Actually, there is now a large consensus that in these cases the selection of an appropriate reference is one of the main aspects of motor planning. This, of course, is also true for exploratory eye movements, as discussed here. I have already remarked in section 2 that the vast majority of investigations on scanning eye movements are concerned with the exploration of a visual scene which is fixed with respect to the viewer. Thus, it is appropriate to begin the discussion of the frame of reference problem in this rather special case and defer to the next section the consideration of the general dynamic situation.

The specific problem that arises in the case of the eye is due to the peculiar fact that the localizing device (the retina) moves with the aiming device (the fovea). Thus, each aiming movement alters the very system of coordinates that is supposed to code its target. Leaving aside for the moment the perceptual correlates of eye movements (see later), this fact per se would seem to be inconsequential as far as the capture of isolated visual targets is concerned. Indeed, if a point-like stimulus appears in the dark, it is quite easy to bring the stimulus into the foveal field with an accurate saccade, despite the absence of all external frames of reference. Actually, even if the stimulus is switched off at the onset of the saccade, the localization error does not exceed 0.5 degree (Miller, 1980). Thus, a precise transformation must occur between the coding of the target position on the retina (the so-called retinal error) and the set of oculomotor commands necessary to make the axis of the gaze coincide with the spatial direction of the stimulus (Robinson, 1973; Schiller and Koerner, 1971; Schiller and Stryker, 1972). If one makes an abstraction of the problem of how to code a specific force vector in the non-orthogonal frame of reference which results from the complex insertion of extraocular muscles (Ostriker et al., 1985), the nulling of the retinal error could in principle be realized simply by a one-to-one sensori-motor homeomorphism. Not surprisingly then, the idea of a simple transformation from retinal error into gaze position has provided one of the earliest principles for describing the control of all types of goal-directed eye movement.

However, the visual exploration of a scene obviously entails much more than capturing a light spot in the dark. To begin with it is easy to show (1) that, even when the eyes do not move, we do in fact establish a spatio-centric frame of reference for locating visual objects,and (2) that this cannot be done by using retinal information alone. For instance, in the absence of contextual clues, a visual target located 15 degrees to the right of the sagittal plane when the gaze is in the sagittal plane gives rise to the same retinal excitation as a target in the saggittal plane when the gaze is off by 15 degrees to the left. Nevertheless, we can reliably tell the difference between the two situations. Thus, the nervous system has access to some extraretinal eye position information (EEPI) about the absolute direction of the gaze in space. Here I will not discuss in detail the origin and nature of EEPI (for a complete review, see Matin 1986). For the moment, it will be sufficient to note that the absolute location of visual targets in space can be obtained simply by combining vectorially the position of the retinal image with respect to the fovea and the direction of the gaze.

A spatio-centric reference is also vital when we do move the eyes. In fact EEPI, which is responsible for establishing such a reference, is also instrumental in maintaining perceptual stability, that is, in maintaining us blissfully unaware of the fact that any eye movement produces a concomitant shift of the retinal image. Without perceptual stability the visual world would appear to us to be moving around continuously. Even more important in the present context is the fact that, if we did not have a frame of reference for the scene which remains invariant when the eye moves in the orbit, we could not plan temporal sequences of exploratory saccades. The argument runs like this: if each exploratory saccade were independent of all the preceding saccades, it could in principle be planned on the basis of the retinal error between the current position of the gaze and the location of an interesting spot in the field *as seen in the temporary reference associated with that location.* By contrast, no sequence of more than one saccade could be planned because each successive movement alters the viewpoint and makes the retinal errors computed previously totally inadequate. Thus, the evidence to be presented later that pre-planned sequences do indeed occur in free scanning provides further confirmation that the retinal error signal must be complemented by some other information in order to obtain a reference that is invariant with respect to the displacements of the eye. Actually, the requirement of invariance is often even more stringent, since it involves possible movements of the head with respect to the body and of the whole body in space (see section 5). For this reason it is sometimes necessary to distinguish further between orbital-centric and spatio-centric references, which coincide only when the head is held fixed. Moreover, the notion of EEPI must really be construed as the sum total of many different afferent and efferent data on the relative positions of eye, head and trunk. In any case, it seems unlikely that a sensori-motor mapping based exclusively on retinal coordinates can explain per-

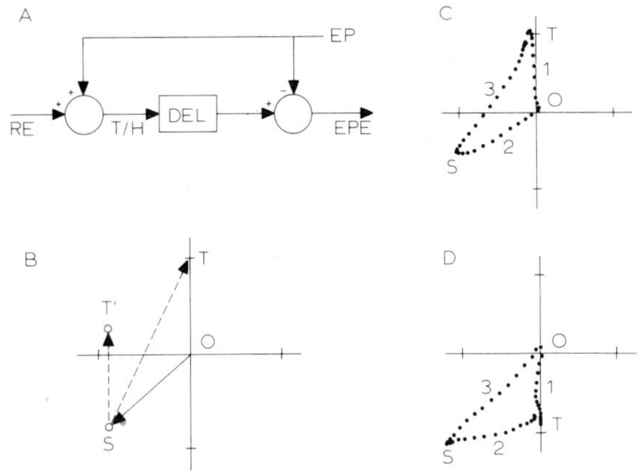

Fig. 10. Retinocentric vs. spatiocentric systems of coordinates. A: a simple scheme to compute saccade vectors in non-retinocentric coordinates (redrawn from Zee et al., 1976). The position of a target in the peripheral field is coded as a retinal error (RE) vector. Adding to this vector the eye position signal (EP) produces a coding of the target position with respect to the head (T/H). The saccade necessary to fovealize the target (Eye Position Error, EPE) is obtained by subtracting from T/H the eye position EP. Thus, if EP does not change during the latent period (DEL) from target onset to the saccade, the latter coincides with RE. Spatiocentric coding, however, ensures a correct fovealization of the target T even if EP changes (panel B). If the gaze is displaced from the original fixation O to a secondary fixation S, a purely retinocentric system of coordinates would result instead in an erroneous movement to T′. C,D: experimental evidence in support of the spatiocentric hypothesis (redrawn from Mays and Sparks, 1981). Each *X–Y* plot represents two trials. Saccades labelled 1 are direct movements to a 100-ms target (T) 10 deg above (C) or below (D) the fixation point. Saccades labelled 2 to a secondary fixation S were induced by stimulating the superior colliculus of the monkey. Traces labelled 3 are the final, correct saccades to the target.

ceptual invariance any better than, say, binaural phase differences per se can account for the accurate localization of an acoustic target in space.

Hansen and Skavenski (1976) demonstrated that accurate information about the position of the eye in the head is available and can be used to direct saccades towards stable external targets. More recently, an elegant demonstration that saccades are indeed planned in an orbital-centric system of reference has been provided with neurophysiological techniques (Mays and Sparks, 1980; Sparks and Mays, 1983) (When the head is fixed as in these experiments, orbital and spatio-centric systems of reference coincide. A distinction between the two must be made only when the head is unconstrained.) Monkeys were trained to fixate in the dark a location were a brief light flash had been presented. In experimental trials, during the latent period before the saccade, the initial direction of the gaze is displaced by an involuntary saccade elicited by electrical stimulation of the superior colliculus. Nevertheless, the final destination is reached in the absence of all visible stimuli as accurtely as during training (Fig. 10C,D). This cannot be explained in terms of retinal error alone (Fig. 10B). Apparently, the animal keeps track of the target position relative to its head (i.e., locates the target in a stable external frame of reference) by compounding the retinal error information with an accurate, real-time estimate of the eye position in the orbit (Fig. 4A). The putative role of proprioceptive ‘inflow’ from extraocular muscles vs. efferent copy ‘outflow’ in supporting perceptual invariance has been debated ever since Helmoltz’s (1866) original suggestion (see Merton, 1964; Festinger and Cannon, 1965; MacKay, 1973) and will be reviewed in another chapter in this volume. Suffice it here to say that, in the context of the experiments described above, proprioception does not appear to represent the decisive factor in the Mays and Sparks experiment because section of the ophthalmic branch of the trigeminal nerve did not impair the animal’s ability to locate the target (Guthrie et al., 1983). This leaves us with just one plausible explanation, namely, the outflow (or efference copy) hypothesis according to which each motor command to the eyes elicits centrally a faithful representation of the expected result of the command on the position of the gaze (Skavenski, 1972; Skavenski and Steinman, 1970; Skavenski et al., 1972; Shebilske, 1984).

Recent results in humans (Viviani and Velay, 1986) have confirmed this hypothesis and clarified further the respective role of retinal error and efferent commands in the programming of saccades. Fig. 11 illustrates the paradigm used for this study and the basic findings. Panel A in this figure describes the first experiment. A short (50 ms) flash

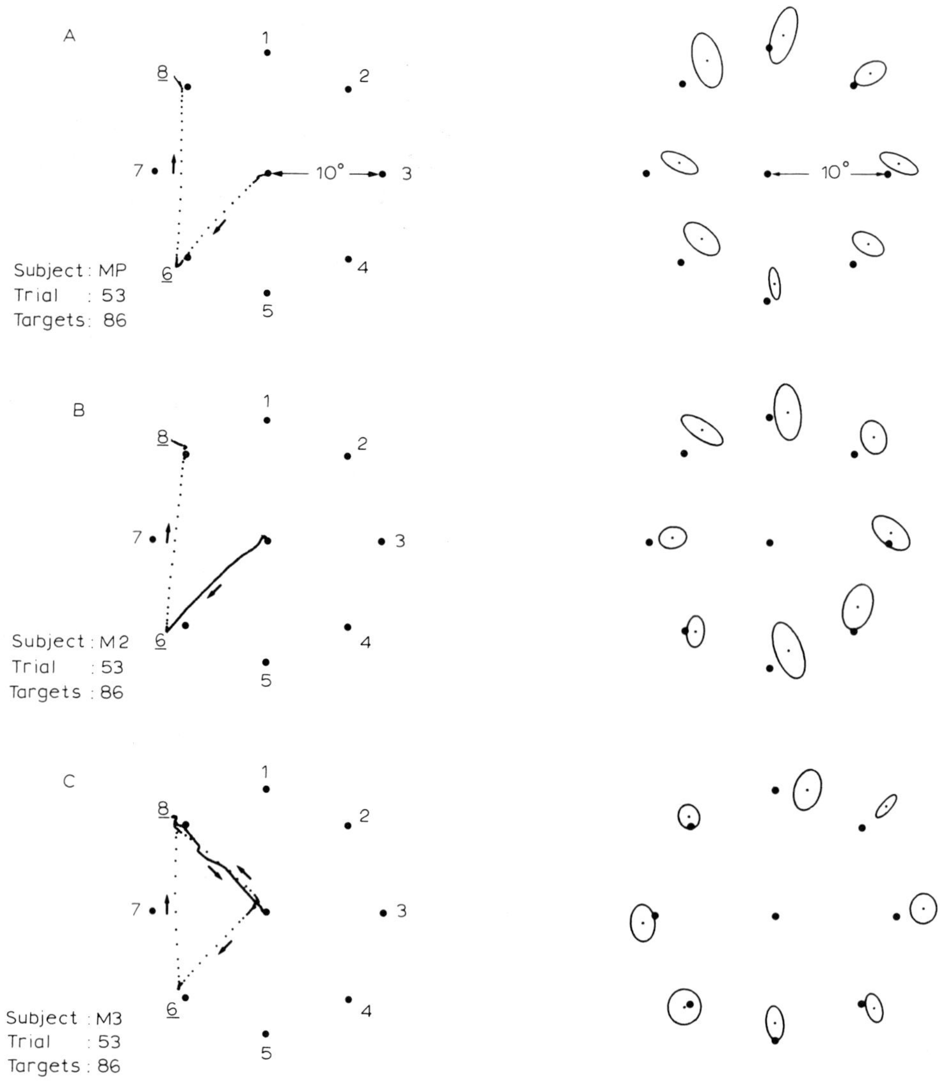

Fig. 11. Spatial coding of voluntary saccades in man. In the left panels typical trials are used to define the three paradigms used in the study. The right panels illustrate the basic findings through the average data of one subject. A: a brief (50 ms) spot is flashed in one of the eight possible positions (number 8 in these examples). Then the subject must fixate an 800-ms spot which appears in another random position (number 6 in these examples). When this spot goes off, leaving a totally dark field, the subject must try and reach the position in space where the first spot had been flashed. B: same as in A, the only difference being that the intermediate random position (6) is reached with a smooth pursuit (7.14 deg/s) of the initial fixation point. Fixation on the final pursuit position is maintained for 400 ms. C: first the final position to be reached (8) is indicated by driving the gaze there with a smooth pursuit of the fixation point. Thereafter, the trial continues as in A. The average final position of the eye and the corresponding ellipses of confidence (right panels) demonstrate that spatial localization is quite accurate in all conditions. (Adapted from Viviani and Velay, 1986).

selects randomly a spatial location among eight possible ones arranged symmetrically around the fixation point. The observer must only take notice of the location selected without leaving the central fixation. A second, longer (800 ms) stimulus appears in a different location and must be fixated with a saccade. When this stimulus also disappears, leaving a completely dark field, the subject must try and reach – again with a saccade – the location where the first flash had appeared. In other words, the role of the electric stimulation in the animal experiment is taken here by a voluntary saccadic fixation. The results show that the accuracy of localization is equivalent to that observed when one must fixate directly in the dark a remembered location (Skavenski, 1971; Miller, 1980). Thus, in keeping with the orbital coding hypothesis, the second and final saccade is our experiments is calculated by summing vectorially the retinal error with the displacement induced by the first saccade.

The second (B) and third (C) panel in Fig. 11 illustrate the more novel contribution of the study. The notion of efferent copy in the field of oculomotor research has been evoked mainly in the context of saccadic movements. As for smooth pursuit, contrasting reports exist concerning the effectiveness of extraocular information for providing an orbital frame of reference during these movements. Some authors (Festinger et al., 1976) maintain that "the perceptual system takes into account very little about smooth pursuit eye movements" (p. 1384). Others (Hansen and Skavenski, 1977; Hansen, 1979) disagree with this conclusion. In particular, Hansen proposes that a distinction should be drawn between spatial localization *with a motor act*, which would have access to accurate extraretinal information, and *conscious* spatial localization, which would rely exclusively on information about retinal image motion and would therefore be inaccurate. Miller (1980) tested this hypothesis but did not find any evidence that the oculomotor system has access to eye movement information that is unavailable to the central perceptual system.

In order to find out whether the efferent copy idea can also be extended to smooth-pursuit movements, the same experiment described above was replicated by replacing the first saccade with a smooth pursuit of the fixation point. No significant difference could be detected with respect to the first condition. This can be taken to suggest that all eye movements, irrespective of their nature, are continuously monitored by an internal reafference. However, one cannot exclude the possibility that proprioception does play a role in the monitoring of slow movements (as far as I am aware, the deafferentation paradigm used by Guthrie et al. (1983) in the case of saccades has not been replicated for smooth pursuit). At any rate, the accuracy of orbital coding during pursuit must be at least as good as that afforded by retinal signals alone under static conditions. This can be inferred from the results of a third experiment illustrated in Fig. 11C. In this experiment a location in space is first selected by bringing the gaze to it with a smooth pursuit. After homing back to the central fixation, the sequence of events is the same as in the first experiment, and again the final localization is just as good. In this paradigm, a retinal error is never present. Both the first and the second target have been localized on the sole basis of motor commands and, possibly, of sensory feedback. Thus, not only is retinal error information not in general sufficient to account for the observed behavior, but in some cases it is not actually necessary. As discussed in the next section, this capacity of the oculomotor system to rely only on outflow information for locating the gaze in space is instrumental in an effective visual scanning of a moving scene.

5. Scanning under dynamic conditions

We have just seen that, in principle, the frame of reference problem for the stationary case can be solved by keeping the control system informed of the effect of the saccadic and smooth-pursuit commands. However, while no data seem to be available on the subject, it would be surprising if the percentage of time spent in scanning stationary scenes turned out to be a significant fraction of our total viewing time. Indeed, in most real-life situations, with the exception of reading and other activities which require close scrutiny, the presence of a relative motion between the scene and the observer is quite common. Therefore, we move now to consider in some detail the specific requirements that must be met by the oculomotor system to en-

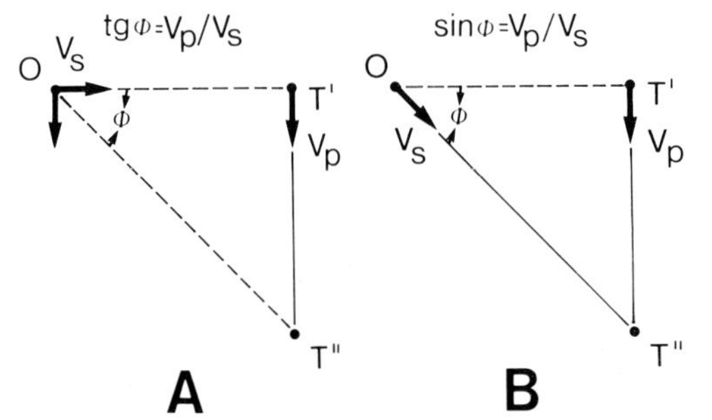

Fig. 12. Two possible strategies for the dynamic capture of a peripheral target. The gaze is pursuing the movement of the point O and must proceed to fixate a peripheral target T′ moving with the same speed (V_p) and direction as O. A: if a saccade velocity vector V_s directed to T′ is superimposed on the smooth-pursuit velocity vector, accurate interception of the target at T″ is automatically ensured by the principle of vector summation. In this case the ratio of the pursuit to the saccade velocity is equal to the tangent of the saccade direction Φ. According to this hypothesis the vertical component of the eye movement should not contain saccadic (high-velocity) components. B: if the smooth pursuit is temporarily discontinued, position T″ can be reached with an oblique saccade whose amplitude and direction must be computed from V_p, target distance and main sequence characteristics. In this case the ratio of V_p and V_s must be equal to the sinus of the saccade direction (see Fig. 7B). (Reproduced from Viviani, 1982).

sure accurate scanning in this more general condition.

Suppose one wants to explore a portion of the visual scene that is moving across a stable background. In order to be able resolve details within this moving scene, it is necessary to keep them in the foveal field by compensating for the external movement (humans do indeed have the capacity to accurately and smoothly pursue targets moving across stationary backgrounds; cf. Ch. 1 of this volume). While the visual system is processing the information in the portion of the scene that is being fixated, the oculomotor system must plan the saccade to the next target. If the pursuit velocity matched the velocity of the scene, the localization of the target in retinocentric coordinates could proceed as in the static case because the scene is stationary on the retina.

Nevertheless, the situation is not entirely the same as that of the static scene. In fact the capturing saccade cannot be planned simply by inverting the retinal error vector because (1) the displacement of the scene is not in general collinear with this retinocentric vector, and (2) the retinal displacement of the scene during the latency interval of the saccade and during the saccade itself must be taken into account. Both the amplitude and the direction of the saccade must instead be planned to reach the point in space where the target will be *after* the saccade. The error that would result if the displacement of the scene during the saccade were not taken into account can be substantial. For instance, according to recent measurements of amplitude/duration characteristics (Patla et al., 1985), a 15 deg horizontal saccade across a scene moving at 40 deg/s would miss the target by as much as 5 deg.

Fig. 12A,B illustrates schematically the two simplest hypotheses for explaining how an appropriate planning of the saccade can be achieved. The first hypothesis (A) is based on the suggestion (Jürgens and Becker, 1975; Jürgens et al., 1981) that when a goal-directed saccade occurs during a smooth pursuit, and in the same direction, the two velocities summate algebraically. The hypothesis is as follows. Suppose that saccadic commands to the eye muscles can be issued without discontinuing the pursuit commands, and that the resulting velocities summate vectorially. Suppose further that the velocity of the pursuit matches the velocity of the scene (i.e. pursuit gain is 1). Then, the position T″ of the target after the saccade will be reached accurately irrespective of the duration of the movement. The second hypothesis (B) is that the pursuit is temporarily suppressed or strongly attenuated, and an oblique saccade is aimed directly to the point where the target is expected to be at the end of the movement. Assuming again that the relative velocity of the image (V_i) can be confounded with that of the pursuit (V_p), the direction Φ of the movement is given by the relation: $\sin \Phi = V_p / V_s$, where V_s is the velocity of the saccade.

To discriminate experimentally between these two hypotheses subjects were asked to read a text which was moved sinusoidally in the vertial direction ($V_i = 38 \cdot \sin(2\pi \cdot 0.6 \cdot t)$ deg/s) (Viviani, 1982).

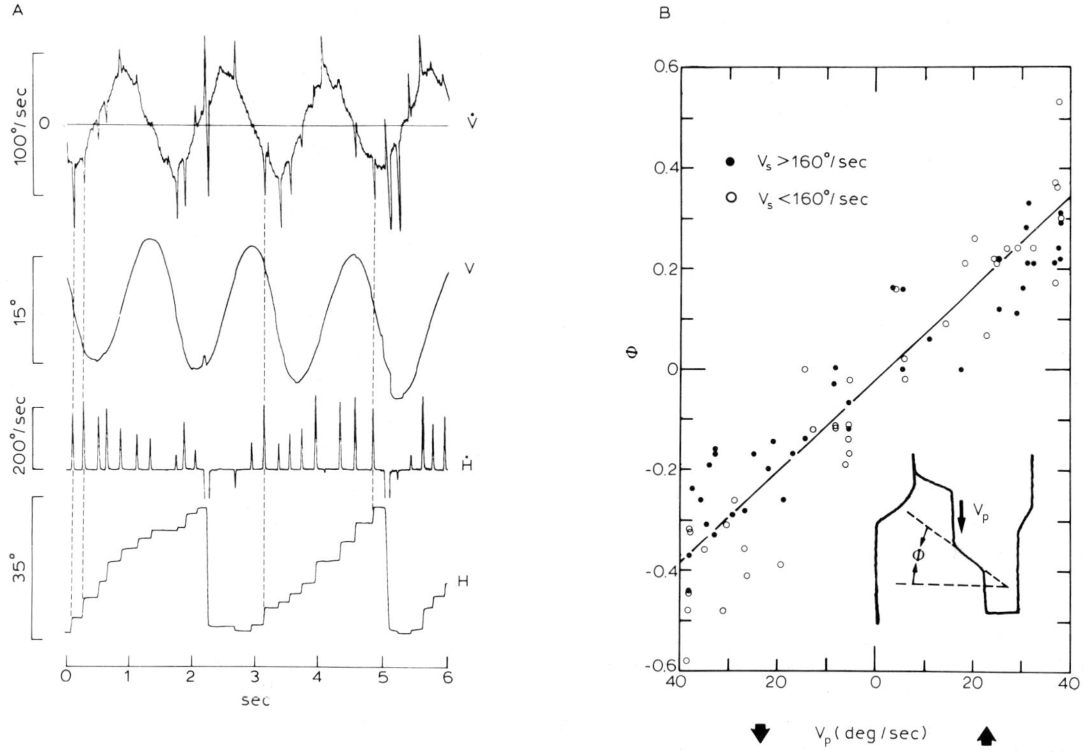

Fig. 13. Interaction of smooth pursuit and saccadic capture. A: eye movements during reading a text that moves sinusoidally in the vertical direction (amplitude, ± 10 deg; peak velocity, 38 deg/s). Horizontal (*H*) and vertical (*V*) components of the displacement illustrate the remarkable fact that the two main oculomotor modes (smooth pursuit and saccadic capture) can be used independently for the two principal directions of the movement. Both velocity components (*H* and *V*) contain saccadic (high-velocity) components. This proves that the task is accomplished using the strategy schematically described in panel B of Fig. 12. B: quantitative confirmation that visual capture of a moving target involves the programming of one oblique saccade. Data points describe the relation between the instantaneous velocity of the pursuit (abscissa) and the sine of the direction of the oblique saccade (ordinate). The continuous line describes the theoretical relation $\sin \Phi = V_p/V_s$ (Fig. 12B) for $V_s = 160$ deg/s. Because of the small spread of saccadic velocity in the experimental conditions only two classes of velocity have been distinguished (solid symbols: $V_s > 160$ deg/s; open symbols: $V_s < 160$ deg/s). (Adapted from Viviani, 1982).

Fig. 13A shows a typical record of the horizontal and vertical components of displacement and velocity of the eye. Saccadic components are conspicuously present in the vertical displacement and clearly demonstrate that the oblique movements necessary to reach each succesive target are bona fide saccades as stated by the second hypothesis, and not the vectorial composition of a smooth pursuit and a saccade. Moreover, as shown in Fig. 13B, the relation between the angle Φ and the velocities V_p and V_s closely approximates the theoretical expression derived from the second hypothesis.

Superimposing saccadic and smooth-pursuit commands would seem much simpler than the alternative – demonstrated by the results of Fig. 13 – of shutting down or attenuating pursuit during saccades. The reason why this simple solution is not adopted is not clear. Maybe it is impossible to activate saccades and pursuit simultaneously, but such explanation could best be verified with neurophysiological techniques. Whatever the reason, it may be interesting to investigate the complexity of the control space implied by the hypothesis outlined in Fig. 12B and verified experimentally in Fig.

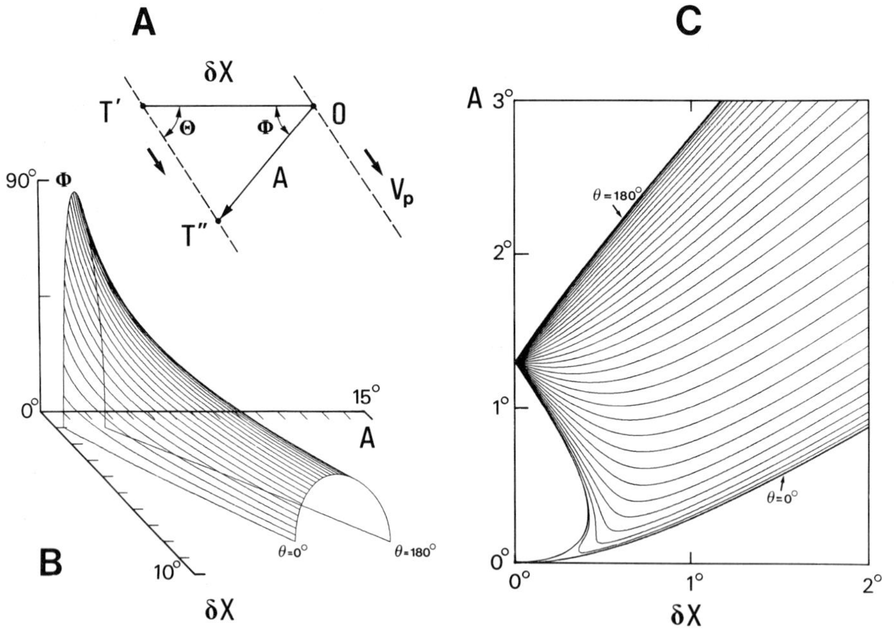

Fig. 14. Control space for dynamic capture of peripheral targets. A: schematic description of the quantities involved in the analysis of the general case. While pursuing the movement of O with velocity V_p in the direction θ, the gaze must reach the target T′ whose eccentricity is δx. The amplitude A and the direction Φ of the saccade necessary to reach the target in the position T″ can be computed by taking into consideration the empirical relation between saccade size and saccade duration (main sequence). B: theoretical values of saccade amplitude and direction for various values of eccentricity δx and pursuit direction θ. C: detailed description of the A–δx relation in the small movement range. For this simulation we have assumed $V_p = 40$ deg/s. The ordinate of the point where all curves converge is $(\alpha V_p)^{1/1-\beta}$. If one makes a saccade of this size while pursuing a target, it will find the target again at the end of the movement. For small values of θ and δx the interception problem has three solutions. One corresponds to $\Phi = 0$ (moving toward the target). The other two solutions correspond to $\Phi = 180°$, that is, to saccades in the same direction as the target movement. Rather paradoxically, it is the target that catches up with the gaze.

13. To avoid unnecessary complications it is convenient to make three assumptions: (1) the relative velocity of the image is approximately constant over one saccade duration, (2) the pursuit gain is 1 ($V_p = V_i$) and (3) the relationship between saccade amplitude (A) and duration (T) can be described as a power law: $T = \alpha \cdot A^{\beta}$ (Robinson, 1964; Yarbus, 1967; Stark, 1968). With reference to the schematic diagram of Fig. 8A, let us suppose that the eccentricity δx of the target T′ with respect to the fixation 0, the relative velocity of the scene V_i, and the direction θ of the movement with respect to the reference 0T′ can be estimated by the visual system. Then, the amplitude A and the direction Φ of the saccade can be derived by solving a system of non-linear equations (Viviani, 1982). Fig. 14B shows the relationship between A, Φ and δx that obtains over the range of target eccentricities 1 to 8 deg for a relatively fast pursuit movement ($V_p = 40$ deg/s). In this simulation, the parameters α and β ($\alpha = 0.0195$, $\beta = 0.41$) have been estimated by fitting a power law model to Yarbus's data for oblique saccades (see Fig. 75, p. 134, in Yarbus, 1967). These values of the parameters also fit well more recent main-sequence data (Eizenman et al., 1984; Smit et al., 1987).

The influence of the direction of the movement θ on the relationship between target eccentricity and saccade size is better appreciated in Fig. 14C, which offers a close-up view of the control space in the range of small saccade amplitudes. Notice that, because of the non-linearity of the equations involved, some of the features of the control space are quite peculiar. For instance, in some cases the graph predicts three possible solutions to the capture problem (see figure legend). To be sure, the oculomotor behavior for such small movement sizes is not likely to be relevant to the organization of visual scanning. However, the fact remains that, in spite of the simplifying assumptions made to derive the control space in dynamic conditions, the picture that emerges, even in the usual range of saccadic sizes, is still quite complex relative to that of the static scene. The latter case could be handled by assuming that saccadic commands keep the system informed of their effects. To handle the case where there is relative motion between the viewer and the scene one must in addition estimate the velocity vector field associated with this motion. As long as the pursuit mode is operating with a unit gain, such an estimate can be provided by also feeding forward to the control system the smooth-pursuit commands. Thus, one and the same scheme based on the use of efferent signals for establishing an orbital frame of reference could work in both the static and the dynamic case. However, when the pursuit gain is less then one, either because the scene velocity is too high, or because positional cues are insufficient (if the oculomotor system must rely only on velocity inputs, 10–20% eye–target mismatches are not unusual, even at very low velocities (Puckett and Steinman, 1969; Williams and Fender, 1979), it is also necessary to take into account the retinal slip signal. Because of such complexity, it is possible, and should be verified experimentally, that exploratory eye movements across a moving scene are subject to more constraints than those recorded under static conditions.

6. Integrating information across saccades

In section 2 I suggested that one of the key conceptual difficulties in the understanding of visual exploration is the relationship between the sequential nature of exploratory eye movements and the unknown nature of the underlying mental processes. A conceptual device – the 'buffer' – has been invoked repeatedly to partially overcome this difficulty.

In its more generally accepted form the term buffer stands for any memory device which is capable of maintaining information at a particular stage of processing. Obviously, the larger the number of buffers that we are led to postulate on the road from the eye to the mind, and from there to the muscles, the larger the capacity of these buffers, the easier it will be to ensure compatibility between the strictly serial nature of eye fixation sequences and the unknown architecture of the mental processes. It is equally obvious, though, that the beneficial effects of interposing many capacious buffers between the eye and the mind will be paid for in terms of our ability to infer mental events from eye movement data. Indeed, the very significance of the buffers is to introduce some degree of uncoupling between stimuli and their central effects. Potter (1983) has provided a very detailed review of the various types of buffer (input, central, output) that can be assumed to exist, and of the arguments that can be brought to bear to qualify their properties. Here I will only consider a special and yet important aspect of this issue, namely the possibility of integrating in a perceptual (central) buffer visual information across the smallest possible sequence of eye movements, that composed of just two fixations. It should be stressed again that in commenting on the available experimental results I will always make the implicit assumption of seriality discussed in section 2.

Suppose I am fixating a location A and something in location B at, say, 5 degrees to the right attracts my attention. Then, a saccade brings the fovea on B and leaves A in the left peripheral field. If indeed a stable, orbital-centered system of reference is available to the oculomotor system (see sections 4 and 5), and if we disregard possible head movements, I should know that what is now in sharp focus on the fovea is in the same spatial location occupied by the stimulus that had occasioned the saccade. Conversely, what was imaged on the fovea in A has become a somewhat blurred image in the left field, but has not changed its spatial position. As long as one believes that the basic cycle of operation of the perceptual mechanism that integrates information in the course of scanning is one fixation long, there is no difficulty in accepting the view that "all that is really required of the human perceptual system is the capability to ignore retinal image shifts. . ." and that "there may be no need to postulate an integrative visual buffer to explain visual stability" (Irwin et al., 1983, p. 57). To be sure, such a short cycle of operation is not something that can be accepted lightly. To begin with, a number of simple visual tasks such as comparing the length of two adjacent line segments imply, by definition, the integration of at least two fixations (cf. for instance the pattern of eye movements in the Mueller-Lyer illusion; Yarbus, 1967; Boyce and West, 1967). Moreover, several studies involving linguistic (McConkie and Rayner, 1975; Rayner, 1975; Rayner and McConkie, 1976; Rayner et al., 1978), figural (Pollatsek et al., 1984; Levy-Schoen, 1981; Levy-Schoen and Rigaud-Renaud, 1980; Kapoula, 1983) and psychophysical (Wolf et al., 1978, 1980; Ritter, 1976; Breitmeyer, 1983; Breitmeyer et al., 1982; Jonides et al., 1982) stimuli all suggest that preprocessing of a stimulus while it is still located in the peripheral field can be compounded with the more detailed processing that takes place during the fixation.

While it is not a logical necessity, it certainly makes sense to infer from such cooperation of pre- and post-fixation processing the necessity of a common representational level and the possibility of integrating information across at least two fixations. It should be clear in any case that constraining the sequence of fixations by a zero-degree Markov condition (see later) would all but deprive the analysis of scanpath movements of much of its heuristic value. Not surprisingly then, some authors (cf. Potter, 1983), following the original suggestion by Hochberg (1968), have entertained the notion of an integrative visual buffer, that is, of a visual registry (not to be confounded with short-term or iconic memory) where information from successive fixations is pasted together to provide a coherent alignment of the individual snapshots. Unfortunately, finding supporting evidence for this hypothesis proved difficult. Carefully planned, independent experiments (O'Regan and Levy-Schoen, 1983; Rayner and Pallatsek, 1983; Irwin et al., 1983) reported chance-level performances in conditions in which the extraction of discriminatory information is critically dependent on the possibility of superimposing two snapshots from successive fixations. This seems to rule out a strong interpretation of the buffer hypothesis, which implied both the actual summation of low-level visual features from *independent* images, and perceptual availability of the result.

Successive samples of a visual scene are seldom uncorrelated, as in the three experiments mentioned above. In fact, if the movement is not too large, two overlaps can occur in the hypothetical buffer when moving from location A to B: one between the blurred image of B and its sharp version after the saccade, the other between the sharp image of A before the saccade and its subsequent blurred version. Despite the low-pass filtering due to the loss of resolution in the periphery, the sharp and blurred versions of A and B will still be highly correlated. Detecting such correlation might be the specific role of the buffer and indeed could provide a powerful way of calibrating the oculomotor system (cf. Marr, 1982). In fact, only when the motor output produces precisely the intended movement is there a mutual consistency between the motor command on the one side, and the retinocentric displacement vector that maximizes the two-dimensional cross-correlation between the pre- and post-saccadic visual field, on the other side. A similar argument involving attentional shifts has also been used to explain phenomenal stability in purely visual terms, without calling into play motor reafferences (Wolff, 1984).

Clearly, neither this line of reasoning nor any information-processing at the purely visual level can explain the priming effects observed in experiments involving figural and linguistic stimuli. The fact that a letter string presented in the peripheral field can facilitate the naming of a visually similar word which later appears in foveal vision (Rayner et al., 1978), while the actual features of the text font can be manipulated in real time without disrupting reading (McConkie and Zola, 1979), suggests that these effects originate at a more abstract level, after the visual stimulation has been translated in some symbolic system. Notice that the hypothesis of a level of representation more general than the analog visual code available on the retina has also been evoked by O'Regan and Levy-Schoen (1983) to explain the phenomenal stability and continuity of the visual world. These authors suggest that our mental representation of a visual scene is essentially semantic rather then 'photograph-like'. This kind of representation based on 'tags' (the image of a chair is coded as 'chair') and spatial relational terms ('near', 'far', 'in front of', and so on) has the obvious advantage of not requiring complex shifting or aligning of successive 'snapshots'. Moreover, it may contain enough relative-position clues to guide eye movements whenever more specific spatial information must be extracted from the visual field.

Having entertained (but not proved) the hypothesis of a *perceptual* buffer for integrating sequential information before further processing, it becomes tempting to speculate on the implications that this might have for the *motor* specification of saccade sequences. The properties of the hypothetical buffer delimit the class of perceptual problems that can be addressed by visual search. Thus, for instance, a problem whose solution requires integrating the information from k successive fixations can only be solved if the buffer capacity is at least equal to k. By the same token, the decay rate of the buffer content necessarily prescribes a maximum time interval within which the data collection from successive fixations must be comprised. In analogy with the general argument already put forward in other domains (e.g. perception and production of speech), we may then surmise that fixation sequences are specified, both spatially and temporally, by the implicit constraint that they produce inputs which the integrative buffer can deal with meaningfully. However, I would like to stress that the hypothetical utilization of successive snapshots for calibrating eye movements is fully compatible with the 'null' hypothesis that hopping from one fixation to the next is a zero-memory Markov process (see above). This null hypothesis can only by falsified by direct measurements of the many-steps transition probabilities, or by demonstrating the existence of preplanned sequences. To this subject I now turn.

7. Sequences of fixations

Many human movements are so complex that, when we state formally the associated control problem in terms of independent simple commands, real-time simulation exceeds the capability of even today's most powerful computers. On the other side, to code our huge repertoire of learned motor skill as strings of unrelated commands would probably require an extravagant amount of motor memory. Ever since Bernstein's (1967) and Lashley's (1951) pioneering work, much effort to escape this conceptual impasse has revolved around the pivotal concepts of *motor sequence* and *unit of motor action*. Under the assumption that motor skills are memorized and executed as a whole, that 'the brain does not control muscles, but movements', as a famous quote claims, the focus of attention has shifted from the elementary components of these movements toward their abstract, relational properties.

With respect to this general issue, searching eye movements are special on at least two counts. First, fixation sequences are not intrinsically as complex as, for instance, finger movements in piano playing. In the latter case, reference to a superordinate plan is forcefully suggested by the very existence of a melodic line. In the former, the existence of such an underlying plan is entirely speculative. Second, searching movements are unique in as much as each component of the sequence may bring in information that completely alters the a priori expectations. In this section I will review some experimental evidence suggesting the existence of internal organization within saccade sequences.

We have seen that a popular view some fifteen years ago was that size and direction of goal-directed saccades are determined exclusively by the retinocentric coordinates of the target (Young,

1981; Vossius, 1960; Robinson, 1973). An alternative, namely that saccades are planned in orbital coordinates, has also been discussed previously. Here I simply call attention to the fact that, if correct, the retinocentric view implies that only one saccade can be planned at a time. This is because the retinal location of a target is not known until the preceding saccade is over. As argued in section 2, this would place serious limitations on the kind of cognitive processes that could be related to the concurrent exploratory eye movements. Thus, anyone interested in establishing such relationships should eagerly look for experimental evidence that, at least in some circumstances, sequences of fixations are planned as a whole and therefore constitute a self-contained unit of motor action.

Clear-cut evidence of this kind is not easy to obtain in a free-scanning situation. The only general strategy for ascertaining the unitary nature of a sequence of motor acts consists in defining some abstract relational properties among the sequence parameters and demonstrating that these properties remain invariant across changes in the value of the parameters (Viviani, 1986). Indeed, this type of strategy has proved effective in the case of other voluntary motor behaviors related to cognitive processes, such as typing (Terzuolo and Viviani, 1980) and handwriting (Viviani and Terzuolo, 1983). It presupposes, however, the possibility of controlling the input stimuli and subject's intentions to an extent that is seldom, if ever, attainable in the case of free visual exploration. One must, therefore, settle for evidence derived from situations with more constraints on the sequence of movements than are actually present in real-life scanning.

The simplest possible sequence, that composed of just two fixations and two saccades, has been extensively investigated with the so called 'double-step' technique. In this technique a target is flashed at an eccentric position and is then displaced to a second position while the subject is still preparing or executing the first saccade (Westheimer, 1954; Bartlett et al., 1961; Wheeless et al., 1966; Levy-Schoen and Blanc-Garin, 1974; Carlow et al., 1974; Lisberger et al., 1975; Becker and Jurgens, 1979; Aslin and Shea, 1987). Under certain circumstances, one then gets two closely spaced saccades. As the interval between the two targets is reduced, the time between the saccades eventually becomes smaller than the typical minimum oculomotor latency (about 150 ms) (below a certain interval, only one saccade is made directly to the second target, but this need not concern us here). These short intersaccadic intervals have been taken to suggest that the two saccades are executed by a 'Grouped Program' (Levy-Schoen and Blanc-Garin, 1974). Alternatively, it has been maintained that "the saccadic system consists grosso modo of a chain of processing elements each having a time delay, and that operations associated with different saccades are carried out simultaneously" (Becker and Jurgens, 1979, p. 967). In either case, however, since very few fixations in free scanning are shorter that 100 ms (see Fig. 7A; cf. also Bahill et al., 1975) it is not clear whether these instances of organized sequences prove anything other than the capacity of the oculomotor system to compensate on-line for occasional poor aiming (Viviani and Swensson, 1982).

A more direct approach toward demonstrating the unitary nature of some saccade sequences has been proposed recently by Zingale and Kowler (1987). Taking inspiration from the influential report of Sternberg et al., (1978) on the timing of speech and typing sequences, these authors investigated sequences of eye fixations on simultaneously displayed sets of point targets. The important result of the study, which is relevant to the issue discussed here, is the demonstration that both the fixation durations and the saccade sizes during the scanning of the targets depend idiosyncratically on the length of the sequence and on the ordinal position of the movement within the sequence. In other words, each subject produces a stable motor pattern which, to some extent, is preplanned before the inception of the movement. In analogy with the interpretation proposed for other forms of patterned motor activity (cf. Viviani and Terzuolo, 1983), it can then be argued that these sequences of fixations and saccades also constitute units of motor action in the

A

Target position

	1	2	3	*	*	*	10	11	*	13	*	19	*	22	*	*	25
1	*	*	*	*	*	*	*	*	*	*	*	*	*	*	*	*	*
2	0	0	0				.9	0		0		0		0			.1
3																	
*																	
*																	
*																	
10	.1	0	0				0	0		0		.9		0			0
11	0	.9	0				0	.1		0		0		0			0
*																	
13	0	0	.2				0	.8		0		0		0			0
*																	
19	0	0	0				0	0		0		.2		.8			0
*																	
22	1	0	0				0	0		.9		0		0			0
*																	
*																	
25	*	*	*	*	*	*	*	*	*	*	*	*	*	*	*	*	*

B

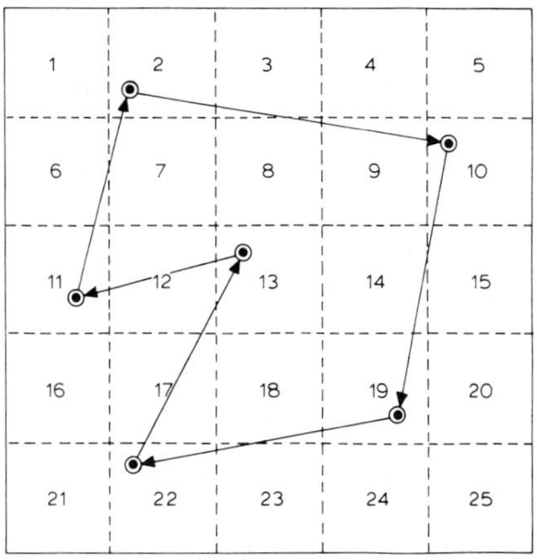

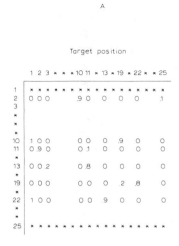

Fig. 15. Markovian analysis of scanpaths. A hypothetical example in which the visual scene has been subdivided into 25 regular regions $R_1, R_2, \ldots, R_{25}$. A: a portion of the (25×25) square probability matrix that describes the sequential regularities of an experimental scanpath (asterisks indicate unspecified values). Each entry P_{ij} of this matrix represents the conditional probability that a fixation in the region R_i of the scene (starting position) is followed by a fixation in the region R_j (target position). These probabilities must be estimated as the ratio between the number of transitions $i \rightarrow j$ and the total number of saccades during the period of exploration. Once the gaze has left a position it must necessarily land somewhere. Thus, the probabilities in a row sum to one. The basic feature of the Markovian model is that the probability with which the gaze will move from the current location to other regions is independent of the previous path followed to reach that location. A transition probability matrix can always be calculated from actual data. However, simple inspection of the matrix will not reveal whether or not the scanpath is Markovian. This can only be ascertained through the analysis of the *n*-steps transitions (see text). In this example it is assumed that from each indicated starting position the gaze could only reach two targets, one of the two being, however, highly preferred. B: the scanpath that would result if, starting from one of the regions, the gaze always selected the preferred target. Notice that, despite the high transition probabilites associated with the arrows, the predicted probability of observing the complete cycle is only 0.41 and drops to 0.16 for two successive cycles. Thus, in order for repeated cycles to actually be present in the scanpath, each transition in the cycle must be extremely probable.

sense proposed by Lashley (1951). These results are both relevant for the study of oculomotor control and encouraging for the cognitive perspective in as much as they demonstrate the necessity of establishing a link between overt behavior and (unobservable) higher mental activities, namely the presence of temporal structure in the fixation sequences. Of course they provide no guarantee about the sufficiency condition, which, as discussed in Section 2, hinges on the serial vs. parallel dilemma. In other words, the mere existence of a specific sequence of fixations does not demonstrate that a meaningful mapping can be established between that sequence and a chain of mental events. An array of point-like targets in an otherwise empty field is hardly the kind of visual stimulus that is likely to elicit an intense cognitive activity.

When the selection of the targets is imposed by the experimenters, as in the study by Zingale and Kowler, only the timing, size and duration of the saccades need be taken into account. In the presence of more complex, naturalistic scenes an internal organization could also emerge in the actual sequence in which targets are selected. Noton and Stark reported that subjects viewing a naturalistic picture tend in fact to look at a particular idiosyncratic sequence of features called a 'scanpath' (Noton, 1970; Noton and Stark, 1971a,b). However, scanpaths are difficult to identify because exploratory movements are intrinsically variable: no specific sequence can be expected to occur, repeatedly or interspersed with other sequences, with exactly the same parameters. Thus, since no quantitative criterion was proposed to discriminate scanpaths from other saccadic sequences, the original formulation of 'Scanpath Theory' has proved of limited value. More recently, Stark and Ellis (1981) have described a probabilistic approach for defining such a criterion (see also Ellis and Smith, 1985, for some preliminary data). The approach is based on a mathematical tool, the transition probability matrix, which is routinely used for the description of discrete Markov processes (Bharucha-Reid, 1960). Specifically, let us suppose that, by a preliminary analysis of the scanning movements, we have been able to identify some regions of the scene where fixations tend to cluster (in the next section we will see that this is a sensible supposition). Let $R_1, R_2, \ldots, R_n$ be these regions (states, in the Markov parlance). Then, a sequential analysis of the visual scan permits us to estimate a $(n \times n)$ square matrix, P_{ik}, whose entries represent the probability that a fixation on R_i is followed by a fixation on R_k (Fig. 15A). The peculiar merit of this formalism is to expose directly and operationally the transition between the static description of the scanpath and the description of its dynamic properties. In particular, if only a few entries in each row dominate all the others (the sum of the entries in a row is always 1), scanning movements should contain cyclic sequences (Fig. 15B). Every time the movement enters one of these cycles, it has a high probability of going through the entire sequence. Subcycles of a main sequence can also be defined by particular combinations of entries in the transition matrix, and their probability of occurrence can be calculated.

The existence of cycles in the scanpath is neither necessary nor sufficient for demonstrating the existence of coherent units of motor action (see later). However, if higher units of motor action do indeed exist within exploratory eye movements, and are represented by cyclic or subcyclic sequences of fixations, the Markov formalism affords a most congenial tool for identifying these units. By definition, the transition between any two states in a true Markov process is independent of all previous transitions. Then the probability of reaching R_k from R_i after n intermediate steps is uniquely determined by the (i, k) entry of the n-th power of the one-step transition probability matrix (Bharucha-Reid, 1960). Thus, the extent to which actual exploratory movements are dependent on past history (as one would suspect if these movements were to reflect the unfolding of complex cognitive activities) can be gauged by comparing the actual n-steps transition probabilities calculated from the scanpath with the predictions of a pure Markovian process. If the large number of data necessary to work out the predictions of the Markov model are not available, simpler methodological approaches to the analysis of fixation sequences are also possible. In particular, Groner et al. (1984) have recently demonstrated the possibility of discriminating individual styles in face scanning by considering only the relative frequency of fixation triplets.

The relationship between Scanpath Theory and the underlying cognitive processes will be discussed again in the next section. To conclude the present discussion, I would simply comment on the previous remark that the hypothetical presence of probabilistic sequential effects is neither sufficient nor necessary for claiming that a sequence of fixations and saccades constitutes a unit of motor action. As for sufficiency, it is possible that repetitive scanpaths across a complex scene arise because of stimulus-driven processes. By this term I am referring to the hypothesis that the size of saccades in a searching task depends on the size of the perceptual (visual) span around the fixation (Bouma, 1978; Levy-Schoen et al., 1984). In particular, the extreme 'visual span control hypothesis' (e.g., Jacobs, 1986) posits that each saccade brings the eye to the zone where new information can be gathered, i.e. somewhere to the edge of the area covered by the visual span. (Actually, Jacobs provided support for the weaker notion that the coupling between saccade size and visual span is inversely proportional to the visual span itself.) Even so, it is clear that the spatial distribution of salient features in the scene can then induce probabilistic regularities in the scanpaths which are strongly stimulus-driven and not related to high-order oculomotor planning. Conversely, it is also clear that true instances of global sequence programming need not occur frequently enough to be captured by a probabilistic Markovian description. Moreover, such a description ignores altogether the temporal aspects of the sequences, which, as mentioned before, may turn out to be very important for identifying the underlying units of oculomotor programming.

8. The quest for a link

In section 2 I discussed in general terms the central dogma that motivates, directly or indirectly, many investigations on exploratory eye movements. Recall that, according to the central dogma, eye movements provide observable indicators of underlying cognitive processes. From the argument and evidence presented so far, I derived a considerable skepticism about the validity of this belief, at least in its strong version. However, it should be obvious that weaker versions of the dogma stand a better chance of resisting criticism than the strong one. Thus, in this final section I will consider some of these weak restatements of the dogma that have motivated actual experimental work. The possibility of establishing a link between experimental observations and higher mental functions will be discussed with the help of a few selected examples of such work.

Possibly the weakest version of all is implicit in the work of Yarbus (1967). His general belief that "eye movements reflect the human thought processes" (page 190) was in fact immediately qualified. Through the analysis of the celebrated sequence of scanpaths of Rapin's 'The Unexpected Visitor' we are convincingly shown that the gross regularities of the eye movements depend, to a very large extent, on what the observer was told to discover in the picture. However, the thought processes Yarbus alluded to in the quote clearly do not refer to the actual computations that, in real time, evaluate the incoming visual input and organize the scan. Indeed, the scanpaths that result from different verbal instructions to the viewer are radically different, and yet one and the same basic set of mental processes (inferences, memory search and retrieval, causation, comparison, etc.) is likely to be involved in every case. To use a metaphor, it is one thing to observe that different motivations result in different verbal productions, and quite a different thing to infer from this observation (1) the invariant rules (grammar) of the language, and (2) why a specific content is expressed in a specific format. So, what Yarbus meant is that something about an observer's interest might be inferred from the scanpath. But the scanpath, by itself, does not show how visual details are apprehended or used to plan subsequent movements.

Another weak version of the cognitive dogma posits a relationship between the distribution of fixations and the distribution of 'informativeness' within the scene (Antes, 1974; Baker and Loeb, 1973; Mackworth and Morandi, 1967). The term 'informative', however, has not been used in a consistent manner. On one hand, as mentioned in section 2, informativeness has been related to some purely physical aspects of the scene. For example, it is well documented (e.g., Mackworth and Morandi, 1967) that fixations tend to cluster around places with high gradients of change in the luminance distribution. Undoubtedly, these structural details may happen to coincide with the targets the viewer needs to capture to test his a priori beliefs. However, one should not ignore the fact that the known anatomo-functional properties of the oculomotor system do provide the basis for accounting, at least in part, for the tendency to fixate visually salient features of the field. In fact, while the superficial layers of the superior colliculus receive retinotopically arranged visual stimuli (e.g., Cynader and Berman, 1972; McIlwain, 1977), the underlying layers have a corresponding saccadic motor map (e.g., Wurtz and Goldberg, 1972; Sparks, 1978). The alignment of these maps could then mediate the observed correspondence between the location of salient features and the concentration of fixations (notice that this 'classical' view of the visuo-motor organization is not uncontroversial (e.g., Mohler and Wurtz, 1976); for a review of the possible models, see Schiller (1984)).

On the other hand, the term informativeness has

also been associated with those parts of the visual field which help the viewer to interpret the *meaning* of the scene (Yarbus, 1967; Antes, 1974). In particular, in the case of human faces, as already discussed in section 2 (Walker-Smith et al., 1977; Luria and Strauss, 1978; Groner et al., 1984), the eyes and the lips get most of the attention, and the notion of meaning refers mostly to the attitude and feelings expressed by the person depicted. Attending to these clues is a behavior that is deeply rooted in our anthropological heritage, and whose importance for survival and social intercourse need not be emphasized. Once again, the analysis of eye movements in these cases can hardly do more than reaffirm the existence of specific forms of stimulus-driven behavior. Finally, informativeness of a detail has (correctly) been defined as being related to the subjective likelihood of finding just that detail within the context of the scene (Loftus and Mackworth, 1978; Frideman and Liebelt, 1981; Yarbus, 1967; Berlyne, 1958; Russo, 1978). Loftus and Mackworth maintain that objects with low contextual 'belongingness' are fixated earlier, more often, and with longer durations. Friedman and Liebelt failed to replicate the first two findings, but confirmed that fixations on subjectively unlikely objects are almost twice as long as the average fixation (Fig. 4B). Antes and Penland (1981) found that first fixations on expected objects were shorter when they occurred in an appropriate context.

Over and above these discrepancies, it seems safe to conclude that unexpected, bizarre, improbable details elicit almost immediately a fixation reaction. This may not be an extremely exciting result, but it is a robust one. When it comes instead to stronger claims about the relationship between eye movements and cognitive processes, clear-cut results are hard to come by. A case in point is provided by visual search situations where the viewer must identify a target feature in a distracting context (cf. Bouma, 1978). Robust results are only available for very global measures of performance, such as the effect of stimulus characteristics on the average scanning rate (Neisser, 1967), or for the effects of psychophysical factors, as in the phenomenon of lateral inhibition, on visual search (Bouma, 1970).

Important questions remain instead unanswered. Consider, for instance, the case of embedded, hidden or ambiguous figures (Nodine and Kundel, 1982; Nodine et al., 1979; Gale and Findlay, 1983; Holcomb et al., 1979; Ellis and Stark, 1978). Both identification and reversals in these figures are known to occur 'catastrophically': hidden figures pop out from apparently meaningless patterns; perceptual solutions are suddenly found for organizing the figural elements in ways that could not be suspected at a first glance; perspective views flip back and forth for no apparent reason. These phenomena are not understood. In order to understand them it would be essential to know whether they are induced in a 'bottom-up' fashion from the incoming sensory datum, or in a 'top-down' fashion in which the perceptual reorganization is triggered by and contingent upon the availability of the corresponding visual concept at a higher cognitive level (Nodine and Kundel, 1982; Magnussen, 1970). Unfortunately, attempts to answer this question have remained so far inconclusive. The only unexpected and interesting finding in this domain is the increase in fixation duration in conjunction with perspective reversals in ambiguous figures (Ellis and Stark, 1978). However, this result, by itself, does not permit one to decide whether the reversal is provoked by the eye position (a 'bottom-up' process) or whether the change in eye position reflects the fact that a reversal has already taken place.

I have repeatedly stressed that exploratory eye movements are largely dependent on the options, points of view, intentions and goals that the observer happens to entertain when he looks around, as well as on his specific competencies. This cognitive background of the viewer dictates which visual feature needs to be attended to. Then, the only possible rationale for trying to relate eye movements to the purely structural features of the visual field is to find out why, in a specific context, a specific set of features happens to be pertinent for the search. There are only a few cases when the feature selection process can be related to clearly discriminable mental states. The basic results can be summarized in a few statements:

(a) When the two (or three) perceptual solutions of a polysemous figure have well-known attractors (such as the eyes and lips in Boring's 'Young Woman/Old Woman' and in Fisher's (1971) 'Two Women/Old Women' images), fixations cluster around these attractors, wherever they happen to be within a particular solution.

(b) A similar shift of attention occurs in the case of hidden figures. As soon as the target pattern pops out, the eye quickly fixates the salient features of the new gestalt. Of course, the term 'feature' is this case does not refer to any physical property of the visual field. Because a new configuration has emerged, some hitherto meaningless blobs acquire representational meaning, 'stand for' something, and are fixated only because of their new role.

(c) Some technical images (chest X-rays, sonograms, radar displays, etc.) contain details which are only meaningful and important in the context of an expert, conceptual description of what is represented. Skilled professionals immediately concentrate fixations on these details (Carmody et al., 1980; Kundel and Nodine, 1983), whereas laymen tend to scan the whole image in a random, uniform way. A similar phenomenon occurs in the analysis of chess positions (cf. De Groot, 1978).

Clearly, even these findings – interesting as they are – do not directly address the important top-down vs. bottom-up question. Both possibilities, as well as any combination of them, are compatible with these eye movement data.

The evidence presented up to this point is only compatible with the uncontroversial belief that exploratory eye movements and cognitive processes have a mutual influence. To conclude, I will now discuss in some detail the experimental support that can be brought to bear for stronger versions of the central oculomotor dogma, which, as we recall, postulates a direct connection between sequences of eye movements and concurrent cognitive processes. The best-known example of a detailed theory for such a connection is the Scanpath Theory by Noton and Stark (Noton, 1970; Noton and Stark, 1971a,b; Stark and Ellis, 1981), which I have already mentioned in the preceding section. The initial impetus for the theory came from the well-documented fact that, during extended exploration of a scene, the observer's eye repeatedly returns to the same elements in the picture (Yarbus, 1967; Zusne and Michels, 1964; Jeannerod et al., 1968; Buswell, 1935). In section 6 I have mentioned the hypothesis that during the exploration of a complex scene the sequence of foveal glimpses is integrated into a coherent percept with the help of the corresponding eye movement information (Hochberg, 1968). In line with this hypothesis, the existence of these recurrent cycles of fixations has been taken to indicate that, in perceiving a novel scene, we create and store in memory cycles of visuo-motor traces ('feature rings' and 'feature networks'; see the discussion on Markov models in section 7). With respect to this general idea, the Scanpath Theory introduces two further qualifications:

(a) Feature rings and feature networks are pattern-specific and idiosyncratic. However, once established, they remain unchanged.

(b) For recognition of a figure to occur, it is necessary and sufficient to run through the corresponding feature cycles established on first viewing.

This second, crucial hypothesis is obviously akin to the radical motor theory of visual perception defended by Festinger (e.g., Festinger and Eaton, 1974), who held that form perception is determined by the set of saccadic programs placed in readiness by the visual input.

Scanpath Theory has been criticized on logical grounds that need not be detailed here (cf. Fisher et al., 1983; Groner et al., 1984; Groner and Menz, 1985). However, the most devastating objection to this (and to many other) motor theory of perception is the fact that accurate recognition of complex figures remains possible even when eye movements are prevented by reducing the viewing time to a few hundred milliseconds. Essentially the same objection has been used to deny that eye movements are responsible for some visual illusions such as the misjudging of the double arrow length in the classical Mueller-Lyer illusion (Yarbus, 1967; Boyce and West, 1967; Festinger et al., 1968). To escape the criticism in the case of visual illusions, it has been conjectured that, when eye movements do not occur, the synthesis of the conscious percept results from the mere intention to make those movements, which is supposed to be irrepressible (Burnham, 1968; Festinger et al., 1967). However, this countermove appears to me as close to unrestrained handwaving as anything can be, and I would not recommend it to rescue Scanpath Theory (for additional criticism of the motor theory of perception see Murphy et al. (1974), who demonstrate no correlation between the stabilized position of the line of sight and the structure or appearance of simple forms).

If scanpaths are not always necessary to recognize pictures, how often do they occur when eye movements are permitted? In their original reports, Noton and Stark claimed that in 65% of the cases the same sequence occurred in both memorization and recognition of a pattern. However, they gave no quantitative criterion for recognizing a scanpath. Locher and Nodine (1974) used instead a more precise criterion. A subject was said to exhibit scanpath behavior if 50% of the fixations from the recognition phase matched the correspondingly numbered fixations in the learning phase. Only about 50% of the subjects satisfied this rather lenient criterion. It is of note that finding that 50% of the subjects do not exhibit a behavior which is supposed to be fundamental for perceiving is more disturbing than, say, finding that everybody exhibits the behavior 50% of the times. Finally, Walker-Smith et al., (1977), studying face recognition, observed short sequences (two, three saccades) which were common to both the examination and recognition phases. However, the sequences did not remain invariant across the different contexts in which the faces were examined.

Even if the experimental validations of the theory were more encouraging, the presence of regular sequences of eye movements would still not be the decisive argument in support of the theory: the sequences could arise simply as a matter of motor strategy rather than a component of recognition memory. For Scanpath Theory to hold, it remains to be proved that if the exploratory sequence is *not* followed during recognition, the performance is affected. Lochner and Nodine (1974) tested this crucial prediction and found no correlation between the occurrence of a scanpath and the proportion of correct recognition.

The above discussion of the Scanpath Theory and of the other weaker versions of the central dogma was undertaken to support the contention that empirical evidence from eye movement research, by itself, has been insufficient to specify models for the perceptual and cognitive processes involved in the visual exploration of the world. Furthermore, the nature of the arguments raised in section 2 makes me believe that the underdetermination is not a consequence of technical limitations. It is rather a serious case of essential inadequacy. The possibility of moving the eyes is an integral part of the human visual system, but there is a lot more to the system that is independent of this possibility. It is somewhat ironical that a fitting concluding remark in the same vein can be borrowed from a source that is usually much more optimistic than I am:

"Because of the superior importance given to concepts in the mind's dialogue with visual data, it is not surprising that eye fixations that reflect data gathering do not by themselves help us to understand how subjects come to perceive the pictures [. . .]. The psychological event that leads to the perception of a picture is largely conceptual, not perceptual" (Kundel and Nodine, 1983, p. 367).

References

Ackley, D.H., Hinton, G.E. and Sejnowski, T.J. (1985) A learning algorithm for Boltzmann Machines. Cognitive Sci. 9, 147–169.

Antes, J.R. (1974) The time course of picture viewing. J. Exp. Psychol. 103, 62–70.

Antes, J.R. and Penland, J.G. (1981) Picture context effects on eye movements patterns. In: D.F. Fisher, R.A. Monty and J.W. Senders (Eds.), Eye Movements: Cognition and Visual Perception. Lawrence Erlbaum Associates, Hillsdale, NJ.

Aslin, R.N. and Shea, S.L. (1987) The amplitude and angle of saccades to double-step target displacements. Vision Res. 27, 1925–1942.

Attneave, F. (1951) The relative importance of parts of a contour. US Human Resources Research Center, Research Note P&MS No. 51–8.

Attneave, F. (1954) Some informative aspects of visual perception. Psychol. Rev. 61, 183–193.

Attneave, F. and Arnoult, M.D. (1956) The quantitative study of shape and pattern perception. Psychol. Bull. 53, 452–471.

Baker, M.A. and Loeb, M. (1973) Implication of measurement of eye fixations for a psychophysics of form perception. Percept. Psychophys. 13, 185–192.

Bahill, A.T., Adler, D. and Stark, L. (1975) Most naturally occurring saccades have magnitudes of 15 degrees or less. Invest. Ophthalmol. 14, 468–469.

Bartlett, N., Eason, R.G. and White, C.T. (1961) Latency of ocular fixation upon the second of two successive stimuli. Percept. Motor Skills 13, 259–268.

Becker, W. (1972) The control of eye movements in the saccadic system. Bibl. Ophthalmol. 82, 233–243.

Becker, W. and Jurgens, R. (1979) An analysis of the saccadic system by means of double step stimuli. Vision Res. 19, 967–983.

Bennet-Clark, H.C. (1964) The oculomotor response to small target replacements. Opt. Acta 11, 301–314.

Berlyne, D.E. (1958) The influence of complexity and novelty in visual figures on orienting responses. J. Exp. Psychol. 55, 289–256.

Bernstein, N.A. (1967) The Co-ordination and Regulation of Movements. Pergamon Press, Oxford.

Berthoz, A., Pavard, B. and Young, L.R. (1975) Perception of linear self-motion induced by peripheral vision (linear vection). Basic characteristics and visual-vestibular interactions. Exp. Brain Res. 23, 471–489.

Bharucha-Reid, A.T. (1960) Markov Processes and their Applications. McGraw-Hill, New York.

Biederman, I., Glass, A.L. and Stacy, E.W. (1973) Searching for objects in real world scenes. J. Exp. Psychol. 1973, 97, 22–27.

Biederman, I., Rabinowitz, J.C., Glass, A.L. and Stacy, E.W. (1974) On the information extracted from a glance at a scene. J. Exp. Psychol. 103, 597–600.

Blanchard, H. (1985) A comparison of some processing time measures based on eye movements. Acta Psychologica 58, 1–15.

Bouma, H. (1970) Interaction effects in parafoveal letter recognition. Nature 226, 177–178.

Bouma, H. (1978) Visual search and reading: eye movements and functional visual field: a tutorial review. In: J. Requin (Ed.), Attention and Performance VIII. Lawrence Erlbaum Associates, Hillsdale, NJ, pp. 115–146.

Bouma, H. and de Voogd, A.H. (1974) On the control of eye saccades in reading. Vision Res. 14, 273–284.

Boyce, P.R. (1965) The visual perception of movement in the absence of an external frame of reference. Opt. Acta 12, 47–54.

Boyce, P.R. and West, D.C. (1967) A perceptual effect on the control of fixation. Opt. Acta 14, 213–217.

Brandt, T., Dichgangs, J. and Koenig, E. (1973) Differential effects of central versus peripheral vision on egocentric and exocentric motion perception. Exp. Brain Res. 16, 476–491.

Breitmeyer, B.G. (1983) Sensory masking, persistence, and enhancement in visual exploration and reading. In: K. Rayner (Ed.), Eye Movements in Reading: Perceptual and Language Processes. Academic Press, New York, pp. 3–30.

Breitmeyer, B.G., Kropfl, W. and Julesz, B. (1982) The existence and role of retinotopic and spatiotopic forms of visual persistence. Acta Psychol. 52, 175–196.

Burnham, C.A. (1968) Decrement of the Mueller-Lyer illusion with saccadic and tracking eye movements. Percept. Psychophys. 3, 424–426.

Buswell, G.T. (1935) How People Look at Pictures: A Study of the Psychology of Perception in Art. University of Chicago Press, Chicago.

Carlow, T., Dell'Osso, L.F., Troost, B.T., Daroff, R.B. and Birkett, J.E. (1975) Saccadic eye movement latencies to multimodal stimuli. Intersubject variability and temporal efficiency. Vision Res. 15, 1257–1262.

Carmody, D.P., Nodine, C.F. and Kundel, H.L. (1980) Global and segmented search for lung nodules of different edge gradients. Invest. Radiol. 15, 224–233.

Cohen, M.E. and Ross, L.E. (1977) Saccade latency in children and adults: effects of warning interval and target eccentricity. J. Exp. Child Psychol. 23, 539–549.

Cynader, M. and Berman, N. (1972) Receptive field organization of monkey superior colliculus. J. Neurophysiol. 35, 187–201.

Desaraty, B.V. (1976) SMART: Similarity measure anchored ranking technique for the analysis of multidimensional data arrays. IEEE Trans. Syst. Man Cybernet. 6.

De Groot, A.D. (1978) Thought and Choice in Chess. Mouton, The Hague.

Ditchburn, R.W. (1973) Eye-movements and Visual Perception. Clarendon Press, Oxford.

Ditchburn, R.W. (1980) The function of small saccades. Vision Res. 20, 271–272.

Dodge, R. (1907) An experimental study of visual fixation. Psychol. Rev. Monogr. Suppl. 35, 1–95.

Edwards, D.C. and Goolkasian, P.A. (1974) Peripheral vision location and kinds of complex processing. J. Exp. Psychol. 102, 244–249.

Eizenman, M., Frecker, R.C. and Hallet, P.E. (1984) Precise noncontactive measurements using the corneal reflex. Vision Res. 24, 167–174.

Ellis, H.D. (1981) Theoretical aspects of face recognition. In: G. Davies, H.D. Ellis and J. Shepherd (Eds.), Perceiving and Remembering Faces. Academic Press, London, pp. 171–196.

Ellis, S.R. and Stark, L. (1978) Eye movements during the viewing of Necker cubes. Perception 7, 575–581.

Ellis, S.R. and Smith, J.D. (1985) Patterns of statistical dependency in visual scanning. In: R. Groner, G.W. McConkie and C. Menz (Eds.), Eye Movements and Human Information Processing. North-Holland, Amsterdam, pp. 221–238.

Engel, F.L. (1971) Visual conspicuity, directed attention and retinal locus. Vision Res. 11, 563–576.

Engel, F.L. (1974) Visual conspicuity, and selective background interference in eccentric vision. Vision Res. 14, 459–471.

Eriksen, C.W. and Eriksen, B.A. (1971) Visual perceptual processing rates and backward and forward masking. J. Exp. Psychol. 89, 306–313.

Eriksen, C.W. and Schultz, D.W. (1979) Information processing in visual search: a continuous flow conception and experimental results. Percept. Psychophys. 25, 249–263.

Festinger, L. and Cannon, L.K. (1965) Information about spatial location based on knowledge about efference. Psychol. Rev. 72, 373–384.

Festinger, L. and Easton, A.M. (1974) Inferences about the efferent system based on a perceptual illusion produced by eye movements. Psychol. Rev. 81, 44–58.

Festinger, L., Burnham, C.A., Ono, H. and Bamber, D. (1967) Efference and the conscious experience of perception. J. Exp. Psychol. Monogr. (Whole No. 637).

Festinger, L., White, C.W. and Allyn, M.R. (1968) Eye movements and decrements in the Mueller-Lyer illusion. Percept. Psychophys. 3, 376–382.

Festinger, L. Sedgwick, H.A. and Holtzman, J.D. (1976) Visual perception during smooth pursuit eye movements. Vision Res. 16, 1377–1386.

Fisher, D.F., Karsh, R., Breitenbach, F. and Barnette, B.D. (1983) Eye movements and picture recognition: contribution or embellishment. In: R. Groner, C. Menz, D.F. Fisher and R.A. Monty (Eds.), Eye Movements and Psychological Functions: International Views. Lawrence Erlbaum Associates, Hillsdale, NJ, pp. 193–210.

Fisher, G.H. (1971) Perception and art: why do we see the world as we do? Aspects Educ. 13, 63–90.

Fodor, J. (1975) The Language of Thought. Thomas Y. Crowell, New York.

Fodor, J. (1983) The Modularity of Mind. MIT/Bradford Press, Cambridge, MA.

Friedman, A. and Liebelt, L.S. (1981) On the time course of viewing pictures with a view toward remembering. In: D.F. Fisher, R.A. Monty and J.W. Senders (Eds.), Eye Movements: Cognition and Visual Perception. Lawrence Erlbaum Associates, Hillsdale, NJ, pp. 137–155.

Gale, A.G. and Findlay, J.M. (1983) Eye movement patterns in viewing ambiguous figures. In: R. Groner, C. Menz, D.F. Fisher and R.A. Monty (Eds.), Eye Movements and Psychological Functions: International Views. Lawrence Erlbaum Associates, Hillsdale, NJ, pp. 145–168.

Gardner, H. (1985) The Mind's New Science: A History of the Cognitive Revolution. Basic Books, New York.

Gibson, J.J. (1950) The Perception of the Visual World. Houghton Mifflin, Boston.

Gibson, J.J. (1966) The Senses Considered as Perceptual Systems. Houghton Mifflin, Boston.

Gibson, J.J. (1979) The Ecological Approach to Visual Perception. Houghton Mifflin, Boston.

Gould, J.D. (1973) Eye movements during visual search and memory search. J. Exp. Psychol. 98, 184–195.

Groner, R. (1978) Hypothesen im Denkprozess. Grundlagen einer verallgemeinerten Theorie auf der Basis elementarer Informationsverarbeitung. Huber, Bern, Stuttgart, Wien.

Groner, R. and Menz, C. (1985) The effect of stimulus characteristics, task requirements and individual differences on scanning patterns. In: R. Groner, G. McConkie and C. Menz. (Eds.), Eye Movements and Human Information Processing. North-Holland, Amsterdam, pp. 239–250.

Groner, R., Walder, F. and Groner, M. (1984) Looking at faces: local and global aspects of scanpaths. In: A.G. Gale and F. Johnson (Eds.), Theoretical and Applied Aspects of Eye Movement Research. Elsevier, Amsterdam, pp. 523–533.

Guthrie, B.L., Porter, J.D. and Sparks, D.L. (1983) Corollary discharge provides accurate position information to the the oculomotor system. Science 221, 1193–1195.

Hallet, P.E. (1978) Primary and secondary saccades to goals defined by instructions. Vision Res. 18, 1279–1296.

Hallet, P.E. (1986) Eye movements. In: K.R. Boff, L. Kaufmann and J.P. Thomas (Eds.), Handbook of Perception and Human Performance. Vol. 1, Sensory Processes and Perception. John Wiley & Sons, New York, pp. 10.1–10.112.

Hallet, P.E. and Adams, B.D. (1980) The predictability of saccadic latency in a novel voluntary oculomotor task. Vision Res. 20, 329–339.

Hansen, R.M. (1979) Spatial localization during pursuit eye movements. Vision Res. 19, 1213–1221.

Hansen, R.M. and Skavenski, A.A. (1977) Accuracy of eye position information for motor control. Vision Res. 17, 919–926.

Hastings, N.A.J. and Peacock, J.B. (1974) Statistical Distributions. Butterworths, London.

Helmoltz, H. von (1866) Handbuch der Physiologischen Optik Leipzig: Voss. (English translation in: J.P.C. Southall, Ed. and Transl.) A Treatise on Physiological Optics, Dover, New York.

Hochberg, J. (1968) In the mind's eye. In: R.N. Haber (Ed.), Contemporary Theory and Research in Visual Perception. Holt, Rinehart & Winston, New York, pp. 309–331.

Holcomb, J.M., Holcomb, H.H. and De la Pena, A. (1977) Selective attention and eye movements while viewing reversible figures. Percept. Motor Skills 44, 639–644.

Harris, C.M., Hainline, M., Abramov, I., Lemerise, E. and Camenzuli, C. (1988) The distribution of fixation durations in infants and naive adults. Vision Res. 28, 419–432.

Intraub, H. (1980) Presentation rate and the representation of briefly glimpsed pictures in memory. J. Exp. Psychol. Hum. Learn. Mem. 6, 1–12.

Intraub, H. (1981) Identification and processing of briefly glimpsed visual scenes. In: D.F. Fisher, R.A. Monty and J.W. Senders (Eds.), Eye movements: Cognition and Visual Perception. Lawrence Erlbaum Associates, Hillsdale, NJ, pp. 181–190.

Irwin, D.E., Yantis, S. and Jonides, J. (1983) Evidence against visual integration across eye movements. Percept. Psychophys. 34, 49–57.

Jacobs, A.M. (1986) Eye-movement control in visual search: how direct is visual span control? Percept. Psychophys. 39, 47–58.

Jeannerod, M., Gerin, P. and Pernier, J. (1968) Deplacements et fixations du regard dans l'exploration libre d'une scène visuelle. Vision Res. 8, 81–97.

Johnson-Laird, P.N. (1983) Mental Models: Towards a Cognitive Science of Language, Inference and Consciousness. Harvard University Press, Cambridge, MA.

Jonides, J., Irwin, D.E. and Yantis, S. (1982) Integrating visual information from successive fixations. Science 215, 192–194.

Jürgens, R. and Becker, W. (1975) Is there a linear addition of saccades and pursuit movements? In: G. Lennerstrand and P. Bach-y-Rita (Eds.), Basic Mechanisms of Ocular Motility. Pergamon Press, Oxford, pp. 525–529.

Jürgens, R., Becker, W. and Rieger, P. (1981) Different effects in the interaction of saccades and the vestibulo-ocular reflex. Ann. N. Y. Acad. Sci. 374, 744–754.

Just, M.A. and Carpenter, P. (1976) Eye fixations and cognitive processes. Cognitive Psychol. 8, 441–480.

Just, M.A. and Carpenter, P. (1980) A theory of reading: From eye fixation to comprehension. Psychol. Rev. 87, 329–354.

Kapoula, Z. (1983) The influence of peripheral preprocessing on oculomotor programming in a scanning task. In: R. Groner, C. Menz, D.F. Fisher and R.A. Monty (Eds.), Eye Movements and Psychological Functions: International Views. Lawrence Erlbaum Associates, Hillsdale, NJ, pp. 101–114.

Karsh, R. and Breitenbach, F.W. (1983) Looking at looking: the amorphous fixation measure. In: R. Groner, G. McConkie and C. Menz (Eds.), Eye Movements and Human Information Processing. North-Holland, Amsterdam, pp. 53–64.

Kolers, P.A. (1976) Buswell discoveries. In: R.A. Monty and J.W. Sanders (Eds.), Eye Movements and Psychological Processes. Lawrence Erlbaum Associates, Hillsdale, NJ, pp. 373–395.

Komoda, M.K., Festinger, L., Phillips, L.J., Duckman, R.H. and Young, R.A. (1973) Some observations concerning saccadic eye movements. Vision Res. 13, 1009–1020.

Kowler, E. and Anton, S. (1987) Reading twisted text: implications for the role of saccades. Vision Res. 27, 45–60.

Kowler, E. and Steinman, R.M. (1980) Small saccades serve no useful purpose: Reply to a letter by R.W. Ditchburn. Vision Res. 20, 273–276.

Kowler, E., van der Steen, J., Tamminga, E.P. and Collewijn, H. (1984) Voluntary selection of the target for smooth eye movements in the presence of superimposed, full-field stationary and moving stimuli. Vision Res. 24, 1789–1798.

Kuhn, L.S. (1970) The Structure of Scientific Revolutions. The University of Chicago Press, Chicago.

Kundel, H.L. and Nodine, C.F. (1983) A visual concept shapes image perception. Radiology 146, 363–368.

Laming, D.R.J. (1968) Information Theory of Choice-Reaction Times. Academic Press, London.

Lashley, K.S. (1951) The problem of serial order in behavior. In: W.A. Jeffress (Ed.), Cerebral Mechanisms in Behavior: The Hixon Symposium. Wiley, New York, pp. 112–136.

Lee, D.N. (1980) The optic flow: the foundation of vision. Phil. Trans. R. Soc. Lond. B, 290, 169–179.

Lee, D.N. and Reddish, E. (1981) Plummeting gannets: a paradigm of ecological optics. Nature 293, 293–294.

Lestienne, F., Soechting, J. and Berthoz, A. (1977) Postural readjustments induced by linear motion of visual scenes. Exp. Brain Res. 28, 363–384.

Lévy-Schoen, A. (1981) Flexible and/or rigid control of oculomotor scanning behavior. In: D.F. Fisher, R.A. Monty and J.W. Senders (Eds.), Eye Movements: Cognition and Visual Perception. Lawrence Erlbaum Associates, Hillsdale, NJ, pp. 299–314.

Lévy-Schoen, A. and Blanc-Garin, J. (1974) On oculomotor programming and perception. Brain Res. 71, 443–450.

Lévy-Schoen, A. and Rigaud-Renard, C. (1980) Préperception ou activation motrice au cours du TR oculomoteur? In: J. Requin (Ed.), Fonctions Anticipatrices du système nerveux et Processus Psychologiques. Editions CNRS, Paris, pp. 205–217.

Lévy-Schoen, A., O'Regan, J.K., Jacobs, A.M. and Coeffe, C. (1984) The relation between visibility span and eye movements in various scanning task. In: A.G. Gale and F. Johnson (Eds.), Theoretical and Applied Aspects of Eye Movement Research. North-Holland, Amsterdam, pp. 133–142.

Lisberger, S.G., Fuchs, A.F., King, W.M. and Evinger, L.C. (1975) Effect of mean reaction time on saccadic responses to two-step stimuli with horizontal and vertical components. Vision Res. 15, 1021–1025.

Lishman, J.R. and Lee, D.N. (1973) The autonomy of visual kinaesthesis. Perception 2, 287–294.

Locher, P.J. and Nodine, C.F. (1973) Influence of stimulus symmetry on visual scanning patterns. Percept. Psychophys. 13, 408–412.

Locher, P.J. and Nodine, C.F. (1974) The role of scanpaths in the recognition of random shapes. Percept. Psychophys. 15, 308–314.

Loftus, G.R. (1972) Eye fixations and recognition memory for pictures. Cognitive Psychol. 3, 525–551.

Loftus, G.R. and Mackworth, N.H. (1978) Cognitive determinants of fixation location during picture viewing. J. Exp. Psychol. Hum. Percept. Performance 4, 565–572.

Luce, R.D. (1986) Response Times: Their Role in Inferring Elementary Mental Organization. Oxford University Press,

Oxford.
Luria, S.M. and Strauss, M.S. (1978) Comparison of eye movements over faces in photographic positives and negatives. Perception 7, 349–358.
MacKay D.M. (1973) Visual stability and voluntary eye movements. In: R. Jung (Ed.), Handbook of Sensory Physiology, Vol. 7, Part 3A. Spinger Verlag, Berlin, pp. 307–331.
Mackworth, N.H. and Morandi, A.J. (1967) The gaze selects informative details within pictures. Percept. Psychophys. 2, 547–552.
Magnussen, S. (1970) Reversibility of perspective in normal and stabilized viewing. Scand. J. Psychol. 11, 153–156.
Malsburg, van der C. and Bienenstock, E. (1986) Statistical coding and short-term synaptic plasticity: a scheme for knowledge representation in the brain. In: E. Bienenstock, F. Fogelman and G. Weisbuch (Eds.), Disordered Systems and Biological Organization. Springer Verlag, Berlin, pp. 247–272.
Marr, D. (1982) Vision: A Computational Investigation into the Human Representation and Processing of Visual Information. Freeman, San Francisco.
Massaro, D.W. and Schmuller, J. (1975) Visual features, perceptual storage, and processing time in reading. In: D.W. Massaro (Ed.), Understanding Language. An Information-Processing Analysis of Speech Perception, Reading, and Psycholinguistics. Academic Press, New York.
Mateeff, S. (1978) Saccadic eye movements and localization visual stimuli. Percept. Psychophys. 24, 215–224.
Matin, L. (1986) Visual localization and eye movements. In: K.R. Boff, L. Kaufmann and J.P. Thomas (Eds.), Handbook of Perception and Human Performance. Vol. 1, Sensory Processes and Perception. John Wiley & Sons, New York, pp. 20.1–20.45.
Matin, L., Matin, E. and Pearce, D.G. (1969) Visual perception of direction when voluntary saccades occur: I. Relation of visual direction of a fixation target extinguished before a saccade to a flash presented during the saccade. Percept. Psychophys. 5, 65–80.
Matin, L., Matin, E. and Pola, J. (1970) Visual perception of direction when voluntary saccades occur: II. Relation of visual direction of a fixation target extinguished before a saccade to a subsequent test flash presented before the saccade. Percept. Psychophys. 8, 9–14.
Mays, L.E. and Sparks, D.L. (1980) Saccades are spatially, not retinocentrically, coded. Science 208, 1163–1165.
Mays, L. and Sparks, D. (1981) The localization of saccade targets using a combination of retinal and eye position information. In: A.F. Fuchs and W. Becker (Eds.), Progress in Oculomotor Research. Elsevier North-Holland, Amsterdam, pp. 41–47.
McConkie, G.W. and Rayner, K. (1975) The span of the effective stimulus during a fixation in reading. Percept. Psychophys. 17, 578–586.
McConkie, G.W. and Zola, D. (1979) Is visual information integrated across successive fixations in reading? Percept. Psychophys. 25, 221–224.
McGill W.J. (1960) Search distribution in magnified time. In: Visual Search Techniques. National Academy of Science – National Research Council, Washington, DC, Publication No. 712, pp. 50–58.
McGill, W.J. (1963) Stochastic latency mechanisms. In: R.D. Luce, R.R. Bush and E. Galanter (Eds.) Handbook of Mathematical Psychology. John Wiley and Sons, New York, pp. 309–360.
McIlwain, J.T. (1977) Topographic organization and convergence in corticotectal projections from areas 17, 18 and 19 in the cat. J. Neurophysiol. 40, 189–198.
Merton, P.A. (1964) Human position sense and sense of effort. Symp. Soc. Exp. Biol. 18, 387–400.
Miles, W.R. (1936) The reaction time of the eye. Psychol. Monogr. 47 (2, Whole No. 212).
Miller, J.M. (1980) Information used by the perceptual and oculomotor systems regarding the amplitude of saccadic and pursuit eye movements. Vision Res. 20, 59–68.
Mohler, C.W. and Wurtz, R.H. (1976) Organization of monkey superior colliculus; intermediate layer cells discharging before eye movements. J. Neurophysiol. 39, 722–744.
Murphy, B.J., Haddad, G.H. and Steinman, R.M. (1974) Simple forms and fluctuations of the line of sight: implications for motor theories of form processing. Percept. Psychophys. 16, 557–563.
Nachmias, J. (1959) Two dimensional motion of the retinal image during monocular fixation. J. Opt. Soc. Am. 49, 901–908.
Neisser, U. (1967) Cognitive Psychology. Appleton, New York.
Nissen, M.J. (1979) The mind's eye. Contemp. Psychol. 24, 630–631.
Nodine, C.F. (1982) Compositional design as a perceptual determinant of aesthetic judgment. Rev. Res. Vis. Arts Educ. 15, 43–54.
Nodine, C.F. and Kundel, H. (1982) Hidden figures, eye movements, and the perception of art. In: R. Groner and P. Fraisse (Eds.), Cognition and Eye Movements. VEB, Berlin, pp. 34–47.
Nodine, C.F., Carmody, D.P. and Herman, E. (1979) Eye movements during visual search for artistically embedded targets. Bull. Psychonomic Soc. 13, 371–374.
Noton, D. (1970) A theory of visual pattern perception. IEEE Trans. Syst. Sci. Cybernet. 6, 349–357.
Noton, D. and Stark, L. (1971a) Scanpaths in eye movements during pattern perception. Science 171, 308–311.
Noton, D. and Stark, L. (1971b) Scanpaths in saccadic eye movements while viewing and recognizing patterns. Vision Res. 11, 929–942.
O'Regan, J.K. and Levy-Schoen, A. (1978) Les mouvements des yeux dans la lecture. Ann. Psychol. 78, 459–492.
O'Regan, J.K. and Levy-Schoen, A. (1983) Integrating visual information from successive fixations: does trans-saccadic

fusion exist? Vision Res. 23, 765–768.

Ostriker, G., Pellionisz, A. and Llinas, R. (1985) Tensorial computer model of gaze. I. Oculomotor activity is expressed in non-orthogonal natural coordinates. Neuroscience 14, 483–500.

Papoulis, A. (1965) Probability, Random Variables and Stochastic Processes. McGraw-Hill, New York.

Patla, A.E., Frank, J.A., Allard, F. and Thomas, E. (1985) Speed-accuracy characteristics of saccadic eye movements. J. Motor Behav. 17, 411–419.

Pollatsek, A., Rayner, K., Collins, W.E. (1984) Integrating pictorial information across eye movements. J. Exp. Psychol. Gen. 113, 426–442.

Posner, N.I. (1980) Orienting of attention. Q. J. Exp. Psychol. 32, 3–25.

Posner, M.I. and Cohen, Y. (1980) Attention and the control of movement. In: G.E. Stelmach and J. Requin (Eds.) Tutorials in Motor Behavior. North-Holland, Amsterdam, pp. 243–258.

Potter, M.C. (1975) Meaning in visual search. Science 187, 965–966.

Potter, M.C. (1983) Representational Buffers: The Eye-Mind hypothesis in picture perception, reading, and visual search. In: K. Rayner (Ed.), Eye Movements in Reading: Perceptual and Language Processes. Academic Press, New York, pp. 413–437.

Potter, M.C., Kroll, J.F. and Harris, C. (1980) Comprehension and memory in rapid sequential reading. In: R.S. Nickerson (Ed.), Attention and Performance VIII. Lawrence Erlbaum Associates, Hillsdale, NJ, pp. 395–418.

Puckett, J. de W. and Steinman, R.M. (1969) Tracking eye movements with and without saccadic correction. Vision Res. 9, 695–703.

Rayner, K. (1975) Parafoveal identification during a fixation in reading. Acta Psychol. 39, 271–282.

Rayner, K. (1978) Eye movements in reading and information processing. Psychol. Bull. 85, 618–660.

Rayner, K. and McConkie, G.W. (1976) What guides a reader's eye movements? Vision Res. 16, 829–837.

Rayner, K., McConkie, G.W. and Ehrlich, S. (1978) Eye movements and integrating information across fixations. J. Exp. Psychol. Hum. Percept. Performance 4, 529–544.

Rayner, K. and Pollatsek, A. (1981) Eye movement control during reading: evidence for direct control. Q. J. Exp. Psychol. 33, 351–373.

Rayner, K. and Pollatsek, A. (1983) Is visual information integrated across saccades? Percept. Psychophys. 34, 39–48.

Reed, K.R. (1973) Psychological Processes in Pattern Recognition. Academic Press, New York.

Remington, R.W. (1980) Attention and saccadic eye movements. J. Exp. Psychol. Hum. Percept. Performance 6, 726–744.

Reza, F.M. (1961) An Introduction to Information Theory. McGraw-Hill, New York.

Ritter, M. (1976) Evidence for visual persistence during saccadic eye movements. Psychol. Res. 39, 67–85.

Robinson, D.A. (1964) The mechanics of human saccadic eye movements. J. Physiol. (Lond.) 174, 245–264.

Robinson, D.A. (1973) Models of the saccadic eye movement control system. Kybernetik 14, 71–83.

Ross, S.M. and Ross, L.E. (1981) Saccade latency and warning signals: effects of auditory and visual stimulus onset and offset. Percept. Psychophys. 29, 429–437.

Rothkopf, E.Z. (1978) Analyzing eye movements to infer processing styles during learning from text. In: J.W. Senders, D.F. Fisher and R.A. Monty (Eds.), Eye Movements and the Higher Psychological Functions. Lawrence Erlbaum Associates, Hillsdale, NJ, pp. 209–223.

Rumelhart, D.E., Hinton, G.E. and Williams, R.J. (1985) Learning internal representations by error propagation. Institute for Cognitive Science Report 8506, University of California, San Diego.

Rumelhart, D.E. and McClelland, J.L. (Eds.) (1986) Parallel Distributed Processing: Explorations in the Microstructure of Cognition. MIT Press, Cambridge, MA.

Russo, J.E. (1978) Adaptation of cognitive processes to the eye movement system. In: J.W. Senders, D.W. Fisher and R.A. Monty (Eds.), Eye Movements and the Higher Psychological Functions. Lawrence Erlbaum Associates, Hillsdale, NJ, pp. 89–112.

Salthouse, T.A., Ellis, C.L., Diener, D.C. and Somberg, B.L. (1981) Stimulus processing during eye fixations. J. Exp. Psychol. Hum. Percept. Performance 7, 611–623.

Sanders, A.F. (1980) Stage analysis in reaction processes. In: G.E. Stelmach and J. Requin (Eds.), Tutorials in Motor Behavior. North-Holland, New York, pp. 331–354.

Saslow, M.G. (1967a) Effects of components of displacement-step stimuli upon latency for saccadic eye movements. J. Opt. Soc. Am. 57, 1024–1029.

Saslow, M.G. (1967b) Latency for saccadic eye movements. J. Opt. Soc. Am. 1967, 57, 1030–1033.

Schiller, P.H. (1984) The superior colliculus and visual function. In: J.M. Brookhart and V.B. Mountcastle (Eds.), Handbook of Physiology, The Nervous System, Volume III. American Physiological Society, Bethesda, MD, pp. 457–505.

Schiller, P.H. and Koerner, F. (1971) Discharge characteristics of single units in superior colliculus of the alert rhesus monkey. J. Neurophysiol. 34, 920–936.

Schiller, P.H. and Stryker, M.P. (1972) Single unit recording and stimulation in the superior colliculus of the alert rhesus monkey. J. Neurophysiol. 35, 915–924.

Shaw, M. (1984) Division of attention among spatial locations: a fundamental difference between detection of letters and detection of luminance increments. In: M. Posner (Ed.), Attention and Performance X. Lawrence Erlbaum Associates, Hillsdale, NJ, pp. 109–121.

Shebilske, W.L. (1984) Context effects and efferent factors in perception and cognition. In: W. Prinz and A.F. Sanders

(Eds.), Cognition and Motor Processes. Springer Verlag, Berlin, pp. 99–119.

Shephard, J., Davies, G. and Ellis, H. (1981) Studies in cue saliency. In: G. Davies, H. Ellis and J. Shepherd (Eds.), Perceiving and Remembering Faces. Academic Press, London, pp. 105–130.

Sigman, M. and Coles, P. (1980) Visual scanning during pattern recognition in children and adults. J. Exp. Child Psychol. 30, 267–276.

Simpson, W.E. and Crandall, S.J. (1972) The perception of smiles. Psychonomic Sci. 29, 197–200.

Skavenski, A.A. (1971) Extraretinal correction and memory for target position. Vision Res. 11, 743–746.

Skavenski, A.A. (1972) Inflow as a source of extraretinal eye-position information. Vision Res. 12, 221–229.

Skavenski, A.A. and Steinman, R.M. (1970) Control of eye position in the dark. Vision Res. 10, 193–203.

Skavenski, A.A., Haddad, G.M. and Steinman, R.M. (1972) The extraretinal signal for the visual perception of direction. Percept. Psychophys. 11, 287–290.

Smit, A.C., van Gisbergen, J.A.M. and Cools, A.R. (1987) A parametric analysis of human saccades in different experimental paradigms. Vision Res. 27, 1745–1762.

Snodgrass, J.G. and Townsend, J.T. (1980) Comparing parallel and serial models: Theory and implementation. Journal of Exp. Psychol. Hum. Percept. Performance 2, 330–354.

Spencer, T.J. (1969) Some effects of different masking stimuli on iconic storage. J. Exp. Psychol. 81, 132–140.

Sperling, G. and Reeves, A. (1980) Measuring the reaction time of a shift of visual attention. In: R.S. Nickerson (Ed.), Attention and Performance VIII. Lawrence Erlbaum Associates, Hillsdale, NJ, pp. 347–380.

Sparks, D.L. (1978) Functional properties of neurons in the monkey superior colliculus: coupling of neuronal activity and saccade onset. Brain Res. 156, 1–16.

Sparks, D.L. and Mays, L.E. (1983) Spatial localization of saccade targets. I. Compensation for stimulation-induced perturbations in eye position. J. of Neurophysiol. 49, 45–63.

Stark, L. (1968) Neurological Control Systems. Plenum, New York.

Stark, L. and Ellis, S.R. (1981) Scanpath revisited: cognitive models direct active looking. In: D.F. Fisher, R.A. Monty and J.W. Senders (Eds.), Eye Movements: Cognition and Visual Perception. Lawrence Erlbaum Associates, Hillsdale, NJ, pp. 193–226.

Steinman, R.M. (1965) Effect of target size, luminance and color on monocular fixation. J. Opt. Soc. Am. 55, 1158–1165.

Sternberg, S. (1967) Two operations in character recognition: some evidence from reaction time measurements. Percept. Psychophys. 2, 45–53.

Sternberg, S., Monsell, S., Knoll, R. and Wright, C. (1978) The latency of rapid movement sequences: comparison of speech and typewriting. In: G.E. Stelmach (Ed.), Information Processing in Motor Control and Learning. Academic Press, New York, pp. 117–152.

Tardy-Gervet, M.F., Gilhodes, J.C. and Roll, J.P. (1984) Perceptual and motor effects elicited by a moving visual stimulus below the forearm: an example of segmentary vection. Behav. Brain Res. 11, 171–184.

Teichner, W.H., LeMaster, W.D. and Kinney, P.A. (1978) Scanning patterns during inspection and recall. In: J.W. Senders, D.F. Fisher and R.A. Monty (Eds.), Eye Movements and the Higher Psychological Functions. Lawrence Erlbaum Associates, Hillsdale, NJ, pp. 259–278.

Terzuolo, C.A. and Viviani, P. (1980) Determinants and characteristics of motor patterns used for typing. Neuroscience 5, 1085–1103.

Townsend, J.T. (1976) Serial and within-stage independent parallel model equivalence on the minimum completion time. J. Math. Psychol. 14, 219–238.

Vaughan, J. (1978) Control of visual fixation duration in search. In: J.W. Senders, D.W. Fisher and R.A. Monty (Eds.), Eye Movements and the Higher Psychological Functions. Lawrence Erlbaum Associates, Hillsdale, NJ, pp. 135–142.

Vaughan, J. (1982) Control of fixation duration in visual search and memory search: another look. J. Exp. Psychol. Hum. Percept. Performance 8, 709–723.

Vaughan, J. and Graefe, T. (1977) Delay of stimulus presentation after the saccade in visual search. Percept. Psychophys. 22, 201–205.

Viviani, P. (1982) The coordination of pursuit and saccadic eye movements in the scanning of a visual scene. In: Roucoux, A. and Crommelinck, M. (Eds.), Physiological and Pathological Aspects of Eye Movements. Junk Publishers, The Hague, pp. 51–76.

Viviani, P. (1986) Do units of motor action really exist? In: H. Heuer and C. Fromm (Eds.), Generation and Modulation of Action Patterns. Springer Verlag, Berlin, pp. 201–216.

Viviani, P. (1987) Fonctions de prise d'information et d'exploration. In: J. Piaget, P. Mounoud and J.P. Bronckart (Eds.), Encyclopédie de la Plèiade: La Psychologie. Gallimard, Paris, pp. 1663–1711.

Viviani, P. and Swensson, R.G. (1982) Saccadic eye movements to peripherally discriminated visual targets. J. Exp. Psychol. Hum. Percept. Performance 8, 113–126.

Viviani, P. and Terzuolo, C.A. (1983) The organization of movement in handwriting and typing. In: B. Butterworth (Ed.), Language Production, Vol. 2. Academic Press, London, pp. 103–146.

Viviani, P., Monot, A., Sallio, P. and Kretz, F. (1982) Caractéristiques générales des mouvements exploratoires oculaires d'images fixes. Rév. Radiodiffusion-Télévision 71, 30–39.

Viviani, P. and Velay, J.L. (1986) Spatial coding of voluntary saccades in man. In: K. O'Regan and A. Levy-Schoen (Eds.), Eye Movements: From Physiology to Cognition. Elsevier North-Holland, Amsterdam, pp. 69–78.

Vossius, G. (1960) Das System der Augenbewegung. Z. Biol. 112, 27–57.

Walker-Smith, G.J., Gale, A.G. and Findlay, J.M. (1977) Eye movement strategies involved in face perception. Perception 6, 313–326.

Westheimer, G. (1954) Eye movement responses to a horizontally moving visual stimulus. Arch. Ophthalmol. 52, 932–941.

Wheeless, L. Jr., Boynton, R.E. and Cohen, G.H. (1966) Eye movement responses to step and pulse-step stimuli. J. Opt. Soc. Am. 56, 956–960.

White, C.T., Eason, R.G. and Bartlett, N.R. (1962) Latency and duration of eye movements in the horizontal plane. J. Opt. Soc. Am. 52, 210–213.

Williams, R.A. and Fender, D.H. (1979) Velocity precision in smooth pursuit eye movements. Vision Res. 19, 343–348.

Wolf, W., Hauske, G. and Lupp, U. (1978) How presaccadic gratings modify postsaccadic modulation transfer function. Vision Res. 18, 1173–1179.

Wolf, W., Hauske, G. and Lupp, U. (1980) Interaction of pre- and postsaccadic patterns having the same coordinates in space. Vision Res. 20, 117–125.

Wolff, P. (1984) Saccadic eye movements and visual stability: Preliminary considerations toward a cognitive approach. In: W. Prinz and A.F. Sanders (Eds.), Cognitive and Motor Processes. Springer Verlag, Berlin, pp. 121–137.

Wurtz, R.H. and Goldberg, M.E. (1972) Activity in the superior colliculus in behaving monkey. III. Cells discharging before eye movements. J. Neurophysiol. 35, 575–586.

Wyman, D. and Steinman, R.M. (1973) Latency characteristics of small saccades. Vision Res. 13, 2173–2175.

Yarbus, A.L. (1967) Eye Movements and Vision. Plenum, New York.

Young, L.R. (1981) The sampled data model and foveal dead zone for saccades. In: B.L. Zuber (Ed.), Models of Oculomotor and Control, CRC Press, Boca Raton, FL, pp. 43–74.

Zadeh, L.A. and Desoer, C.A. (1963) Linear System Theory: The State Space Approach, McGraw-Hill, New York.

Zee, D.S., Optican, L.M., Cook, J.D., Robinson, D.A. and Engel, W. (1976) Slow saccades in spinocerebellar degeneration. Arch. Neurol. 33, 243–251.

Zinchenko, V.P. and Vergiles, N.Y. (1972) Formation of visual images: Studies of stabilized images. Consultant Bureau. Plenum Press, New York.

Zingale, C.M. and Kowler, E. (1987) Planning sequences of saccades. Vision Res. 27, 1327–1341.

Zusne, L. (1970) Visual Perception of Forms. Academic Press, New York.

Zusne, L. and Michels, K.M. (1964) Nonrepresentational shapes and eye movements. Percept. Motor Skills 18, 11–20.

Eye movements and their role in visual and cognitive processes
E. Kowler, Editor

CHAPTER 9

Eye movements and reading

J. Kevin O'Regan

Groupe Regard, CNRS, Université René Descartes, EPHE,
EHESS, 28 rue Serpente, 75006 Paris, France

1. Introduction

1.1. Why study eye movements in reading? Reading as a domain in its own right and as a microcosm of visual perception

The main characteristics of eye movements in reading have been known since Lamare (1893) and Javal (1878) placed what was essentially a stethoscope on the closed eyelid, and heard the clicks made by saccades. Ever since, researchers have studied the sequence of fixations and saccades that characterize eye movements in reading, either with a view to understanding the underlying perceptual processes (the earliest work, in particular by Dodge and Huey) or in order to find the most favorable conditions for reading (work in the 1950s: Tinker, Buswell) or in the last decade, because of interest in linguistics and psycholinguistics, to use eye movements as an indicator of the reader's cognitive processes. This latest trend has been particularly active, because eye movements appear to be an ideal, unobstrusive probe of the mind: unlike the more classic tools of the psychologist, e.g., manual button presses or oral responses, they are the very means by which information is extracted and require no conscious action by the reader; they are also continuously present, and so are a moment-to-moment index of processing.

In addition to being interesting in itself, the study of eye movements in reading is also a convenient place to start studying visual perception in general. Whereas reading has its own specificities, perhaps involving scanning routines and types of (linguistic) processing not found in scene understanding, it is nevertheless a microcosm whose objects (letters, words, sentences,. . .) are more easily described than the tables, faces, scenes, of everyday life. We have a set of units (letters) which can be used to describe the visual world of reading; we have the rules (of lexical structure and grammar) that govern how the units can combine to form larger units (words, sentences). Finally, psycholinguists provide us with knowledge about the processes that underlie language comprehension. We have no such units or grammar for visual scenes; we have no such well-developed theory of scene understanding.

1.2. Organization of the chapter

Comprehensive reviews have appeared in the past years on recent work on eye movements in reading (Rayner, 1978; Rayner and Inhoff, 1981; Lévy-Schoen and O'Regan, 1979; O'Regan and Lévy-Schoen, 1979; McConkie, 1983; Rayner and Pollatsek, 1987; Jacobs and Lévy-Schoen, 1987). These reviews show that our knowledge has reached a 'Mendeleevian' state: data have been organized and statistical regularities discovered. But what is lacking is the equivalent of a theory of atomic structure to explain the observed facts. We would like a more mechanistic explanation of why each individual saccade goes where it goes and why each fixation lasts the length of time it lasts. The present chapter will attempt a step in this direction by proposing a 'strategy-tactics' theory of eye movement control in reading. The theory derives its main inspiration form a recent discovery showing that in each word there is a position, called the 'optimal viewing position', which the eye must fixate first in order to recognize the word most rapidly. An efficient eye movement strategy in reading must take account of the existence of this optimal viewing position, and the fact that it may be different in different words. In addition, the strategy must take into account a number of purely motor or visuo-motor constraints that place limitations on saccade accuracy and fixation durations. These low-level constraints have not been adequately considered in the past.

The present chapter will trace again the steps which led me to the optimal viewing position phenomenon and the strategy-tactics theory. Before starting, however, there are two preliminary subsections: one that recalls the basic characteristics of reading eye movements and some problems of definition, and a second sub-section which gives a brief historical overview. Section 2 will then start the main line of argument by discussing the notion of 'perceptual span'. This notion has been central to eye movement work since the introduction of computer-controlled eye-movement registration systems. Its importance derives from the supposition that eye movements in reading might be intimately linked to perceptual span: the eye might at each new saccade be moving so that successive spans just touch. However, I will show that, as generally used, the notion of perceptual span is not sufficiently precise. Section 2.6 remedies this by distinguishing 'visual' span from 'perceptual' span, and then gives conclusive evidence that eye movements in reading are actually not directly linked to perceptual span: other factors must be active in determining eye movements. Sections 3 and 4 consider some low-level spatial and temporal visuo-motor factors that might be active, of which some will prove to be useful for the strategy-tactics theory. Section 5 then presents the optimal viewing position phenomenon and section 6 the strategy-tactics theory. Section 7 confronts the theory with evidence in the literature, thereby providing an opportunity to review some recent work on the relationship between linguistic processing and eye movements.

One consequence of the decision to organize this review chapter around the strategy-tactics theory is that the chapter will not do full justice to the impressive work that has been done by other research groups, in particular those of K. Rayner and G. McConkie. Also, two important issues are not discussed directly, but only appear incidentally as needed in the text. These are: types of eye guidance model, and the use of parafoveal information. For better treatment of these issues, and for a less theoretically oriented account, the review articles cited above should be consulted.

1.3. Eye movement characteristics in reading

Fig. 1A shows a typical record of the horizontal eye movements during reading, obtained using a photoelectric eye movement recording device. The most striking and well-known aspect of such records is the staircase-like sequence of intersaccadic pauses, called 'fixations', separated by saccades (which are generally rightwards or 'progressive', but sometimes also leftwards or 'regressive'), terminated at the end of each line by a large leftwards 'return sweep' that takes the eye to the beginning of the next line of print. The return sweep is often rapidly followed by a correction saccade intervening after a shorter latency than the average fixation duration. This is similar to the undershoot found for large ($>$ 10 deg) saccades in other visual tasks (c.f. Frost and Pöppel, 1976). Several microscopic aspects of the eye movements are also visible in Fig. 1A, such as dynamic overshoot and post-saccadic drift, but these are usually disregarded in reading research, since they presumably do not contribute to, or appreciably modify, the information-extraction process.

The eye movement parameters which are generally used to quantify reading behavior are derived from the basic fixation-saccade sequence: the number of fixations, the number of regression movements, the size of saccades (regressive and progressive), the duration of fixations, and their precise positions in the line. However, controversy has

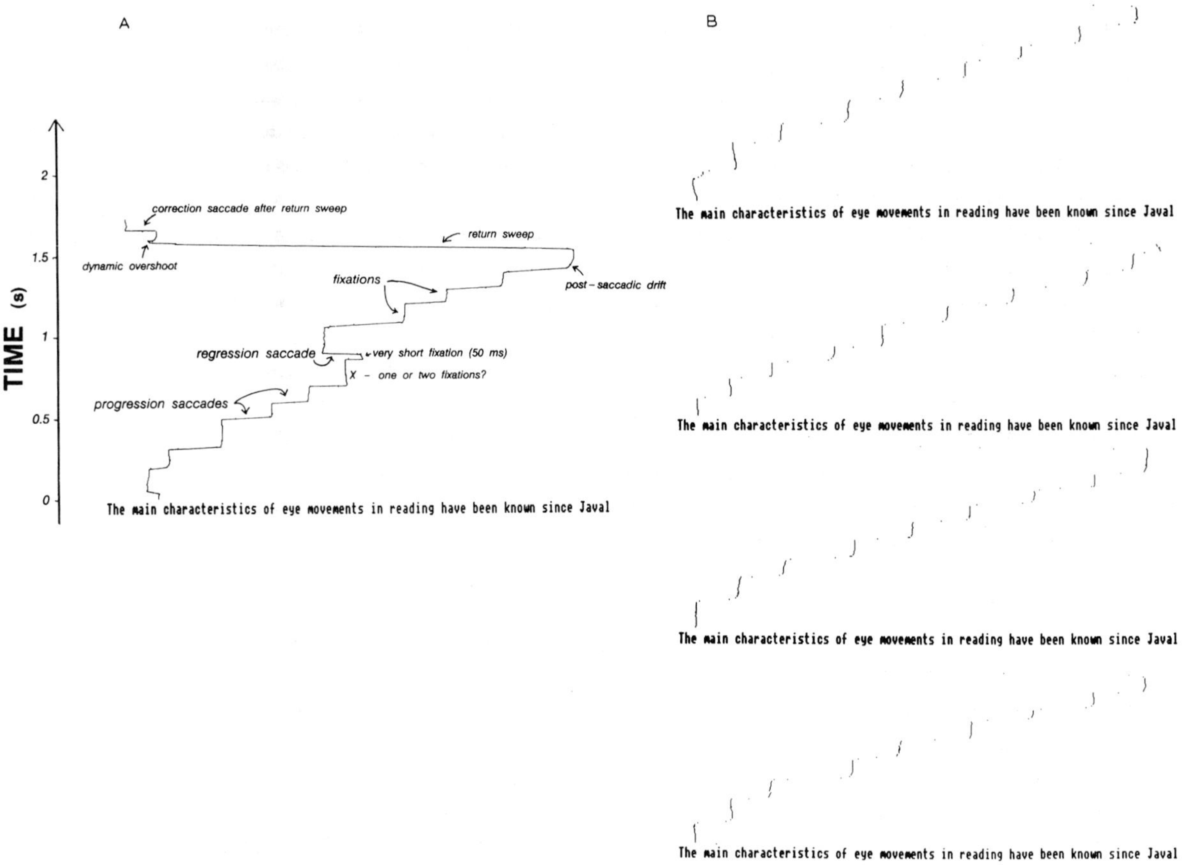

Fig. 1. Records, obtained by an infra-red photo-electric scleral reflection technique, of eye movements while reading the sentence shown on the abscissa. Sampling was done every 10 ms. Time (in seconds) increases vertically along the ordinate, so to recreate the eye's movement the traces should be read from bottom to top. A. A record showing various typical aspects of eye movements in reading. For visibility individual eye position samples have been connected with lines. B. Records of the author reading the same sentence four times in succession. The positions of the samples with respect to the sentence are shown by small dots (visible particularly in saccades). Note that while average saccade sizes and fixation durations are comparable in all the records, the exact places where the eye stopped are not the same across the four records.

arisen around the question of which measures are the 'correct' ones to use. 'Correctness' can only be relative to some purpose, in this case that of using eye movements as an indicator of cognitive processes in reading.

An initial, fundamental, debate concerns fixations. What is a fixation? Looking very closely at the record in Fig. 1A, it might be possible to argue that the long fixation marked X is in fact two shorter fixations separated by a very small saccade, only a fraction of a letter in size, visible as a discontinuity in the record near the X. Such very small saccades certainly exist: in fact Cunitz and Steinman (1969), Haddad and Steinman (1973) and Steinman et al. (1967) claim that the processes controlling small saccades are not different from those controlling the large saccades that occur during reading. Further, during long fixation of stationary targets, Boyce (1967) observed that the smallest (< 1.5 min arc) saccades are the most numerous (for further discussion of fixational eye movements, see Ch. 1 of this volume). If there is no lower limit to saccade size, then the notion of fixation becomes vacuous, since we can never be sure that what we call a fixation is not in fact a number of shorter fixations separated by invisibly small saccades. The solution to this problem is to realize that one's definition of 'fixation' must depend on one's theoretical motivations. Thus, if one believes, as seems reasonable, that saccades smaller than a fraction of a letter are irrelevant to information-extraction processes in reading, then these can be ignored. This is the view taken by most authors, and we will also henceforth (and somewhat arbitrarily) use the term 'fixation' to mean the time during which the eye makes no saccades, and 'saccade' to mean a movement of more than half a letter taking place in less than 20–30 ms. Note, however, that this is not the only possibility: there is another theoretical approach, taken first by Just and Carpenter (1980), which dispenses entirely with the notion of fixation. Under this approach it is supposed that the unit of processing in reading is not the letter, but the word or small group of words. Saccades within these units are considered irrelevant, and what counts is only the total time or 'gaze duration' spent by the eye in such regions.

A second debate concerns the units in which saccade sizes should be measured. It might be thought that since text can only be visually resolved within the fovea, saccades in reading would proceed by moving from approximately one fovea-full of text to the next. In fact, Javal, listening to saccades through his stethoscope, noted that when viewing distance is changed over a large range, saccades modify their angular size so that about the same number of letters are crossed at each jump. This result, which has been confirmed many times (cf. Morrison and Rayner, 1981; O'Regan et al., 1983), is not consistent with the idea that the eye jumps one fovea-full at a time, since changing distance changes the number of letters falling in the fovea, and so should change saccade size measured in letters. An explanation for the fact that saccades actually cover the same number of letters independently of viewing distance will be given in section 7.1. Meanwhile, Javal's and subsequent results suggest that, rather than angular size, the number of characters is a more reasonable choice for measuring saccade size. However, alternative measures such as number of words or fractions of the line of print are also possibilities. A related question is whether 'average saccade size' should be an algebraic measure that takes account of the backwards regressive movements, or whether these should be considered separately.

It is clear that problems of what eye movement measures should be used in reading research cannot be resolved until we have a better theory. Until then, the choices we make for the discussion of existing experimental data will necessarily be arbitrary.

1.4. Brief history of eye movement research: 'local' and 'global' studies

Fig. 2 gives an idea of the variability of saccade sizes and fixation durations in reading. For each of several readers, the solid and the dotted histograms in the figure correspond to readings of a first and a second text. As has been found classically, mean progressive saccade sizes are about 7 letters long, with a standard deviation of 3 letters. Regressive saccades have a smaller mean size, about 3 or 4 letters. Fixation durations are about 250 ms (standard deviation 100 ms). It is interesting that distributions can be quite different from one reader to the next. But a given reader's distributions for first and second texts are similar when, as was the case here, the texts have identical word lengths and identical grammatical structure. Nevertheless, the precise positions that the same reader fixates in the first and in the second text will not necessarily be the same. This is also true of successive readings of the same text, as shown in Fig. 1B.

Parenthetically, it is worth noting that fixation duration distributions in reading are not normally distributed, but have a longer tail for long latencies. The same is true for the distribution of latencies for making a saccade to a suddenly appearing stimulus. It is of course obvious that fixation durations or latencies should not be normally distributed, because fixation durations can never be less than 0 ms, but can be infinitely long. In fact, as might be expected, fixation duration distributions resemble

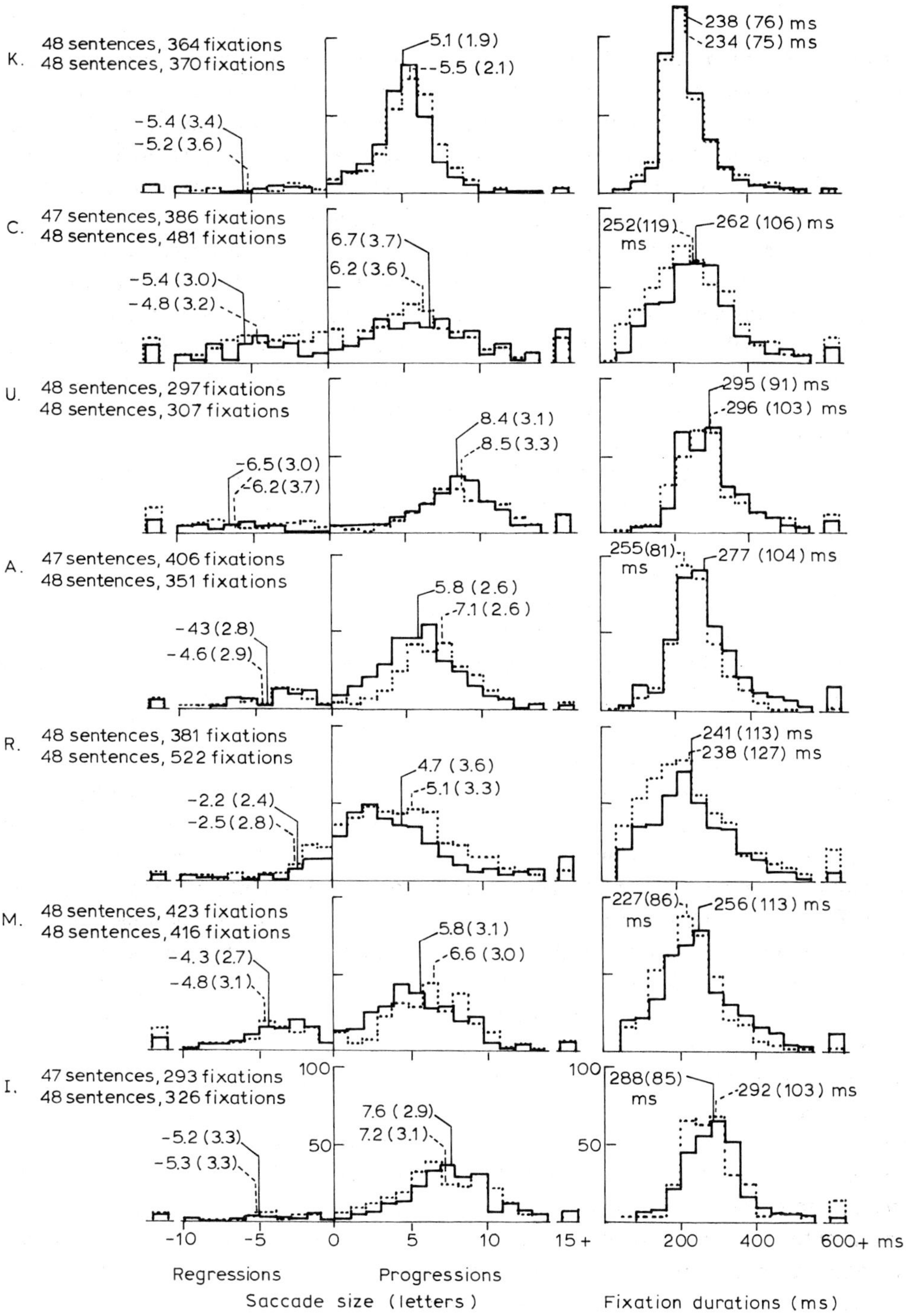

Fig. 2. Distributions of saccade size and fixation durations for seven subjects reading two blocks of 48 unrelated upper-case sentences. The sentences in the two blocks had identical word lengths and syntactic structures. The data for the first block are shown by solid lines, and for the second block by dotted lines. Note that on the second block saccade sizes are slightly larger and fixation durations slightly shorter. Means and standard deviations of the distribution of saccade sizes are indicated in letters and of the distribution of fixation durations in ms. (Adapted from O'Regan and Lévy-Schoen, 1978)

classic reaction time distributions. A rich literature exists to explain the shape of these, and aspects such as the fact that when the mean of a distribution changes, the standard deviation changes proportionately (see Ch. 10 of this volume).

Returning to Fig. 2, what is the source of the variability of fixation duration and saccade size? Undoubtedly there are several sources: inherent variability in oculomotor precision (this may possibly be affected by visual factors such as text layout, or by particular scanning strategies used by the reader), variability associated with perceptual processing, and variability associated with linguistic and cognitive processing. Up until recently, most research has been nourished by the hope that the variability does not reflect low-level visuo-motor processing, but mainly linguistic and cognitive, or at worst perceptual processing: for if this is true then eye movements can be used as a convenient online monitor of the reader's perceptual and thought processes.

The first step in making use of eye movements as a clue to cognitive and perceptual processes is to proceed backwards: manipulate processing in a known way, and try to understand the accompanying changes in eye movements. Later, when it is known how eye movements react to processing changes, one can use eye movements to understand the cognitive and perceptual processing that occurs in particular cases. But the first step, in which researchers try to understand how eye movements react to different cognitive or linguistic factors, has up to now given disappointing results. Systematic dependencies have been observed between eye movements and cognitive and linguistic processes. However, essentially all that can be said is that if things are hard to see or understand, the eye spends overall a longer time in the zone of difficulty: it may make more or longer fixations, it may make shorter saccades or more regressions. But which of these possibilities occurs, and exactly where in the difficult region, is not satisfactorily explained.

Early research on eye movements (up to about 1960) studied the effects of different factors on 'global' eye movement parameters, that is, the mean values of parameters such as fixation duration or saccade size, when measured not locally, but globally over a whole body of text. The goal was not to understand precisely where in the text eye movements were being modified, but it was hoped that particular patterns of eye movement effects would be associated with particular kinds of processing. However, in a review of this early work (O'Regan and Lévy-Schoen, 1978; Lévy-Schoen and O'Regan, 1978), we found that independently of whether the factors studied were the physical aspect of the text (e.g., type size, type font, spacing, color, contrast, viewing distance), the content of the text (type of text, difficulty) or aspects related to the reader (age, reading ability, familiarity with the material), no pattern emerged that enabled us to link particular factors to particular eye movement parameters.

Probably because, at the time, researchers were also aware of this unsatisfactory situation, a lull in interest occurred in the 1940s–60s (c.f. review by Tinker, 1958). Interest in eye movements built up again starting in about 1975. This rebirth was partly due to the impetus given by developments in psycholinguistics, which provided hypotheses about moment-to-moment processing in reading that could be tested using eye movements. An additional motivation has undoubtedly also been the technical fascination of building computer-aided measurement systems, and the possibility they give of changing what is displayed on a computer screen from moment to moment as a function of what part of the display the subject is looking at. (The first such systems were built by Reder, 1973, McConkie and Rayner, 1975, and O'Regan, 1975.) A large amount of work has been done using such computer-controlled eye-movement-contingent display change techniques.

A number of the modern studies, like the pre-1960 studies, were studies of global eye movement parameters and did not attempt to understand local behavior. The most successful of these have been studies of the 'perceptual span', that is, the zone around the instantaneous fixation point from which useful information is being extracted. These studies will be reviewed in section 2.1. They are the starting point for the line of argument to be presented in this chapter. The effects of viewing distance, of size and type, contrast, and spacing have also been looked at again, both in reading, and in the (probably) cognitively simpler task of scanning meaningless lines of letters in the search for a target letter. As was the case for the early studies, the rather obvious conclusion that emerges is that when things are difficult, reading slows down. But up to now no-one has been able to predict which eye movement parameters will be modified by which factors.

The real hope in modern computer-controlled eye movement measurement systems stems from their ability to pin down eye movement effects to fairly precise points in a text. Recent studies have attempted to measure local effects of perceptual and cognitive variables on eye movement parameters. Unfortunately, while a lot has been learned, if one is looking for a mechanistic explanation of why each saccade goes where it goes and why each fixation lasts the length of time it lasts, then the fruit is meagre.

Some success appeared to have been achieved by the influential work of Just and Carpenter (1980), whose production system model of reading correlated well with eye movement measures. However, the eye movement variable they showed to correlate with cognitive processing was 'gaze duration', defined as the total time spent by the eye on each word. This is not really a local measure, since the durations of several fixations occurring within a word are summed together. It tells us little about the moment-to-moment eye movement behavior, and so questions remain, such as: When will the eye skip the next word? What makes it fixate twice in a word? If it does, where will it refixate? Futher, Kliegl et al. (1982, 1983) have criticized Carpenter and Just's way of analysing the data, and claimed that the only strong correlation shown by Carpenter and Just's data was between word length and gaze duration: linguistic and semantic variables accounted for only a small part of the eye movement behavior (see Blanchard, 1985, for an excellent discussion). Analysis of a few of the more recent studies of linguistic variables will be done in section 7.4, after the strategy-tactics theory has been presented.

Studies looking at local variations in saccade sizes and fixation durations have not turned up any very strong dependencies with perceptual and cognitive processes. A number of studies show that if, by use of computer-controlled eye-movement-dependent display techniques, display changes are made to occur during reading, then these may immediately influence the fixation durations and the saccade sizes. But I will suggest in section 2.2 that these effects may be due not to changes in perceptual or cognitive processing, but to changes in visuomotor strategies caused by the display changes.

2. The perceptual span

One of the most obvious questions that might be asked when trying to understand eye movements in reading is: how much can be seen at each fixation pause of the eye? This question has been asked since the beginnings of psychology in the last century, and a number of the old studies were reviewed by Huey (1900, p. 296 ff) and in Woodworth's (1938) classic textbook.

While apparently innocent, the question has hidden depths. What do we mean by 'see'? It may be that at a fixation, information is 'seen' but not processed. It is known, for example, that in search and memory tasks a subject may directly look at the target and yet not notice or remember it (Mackworth et al., 1964; Mackworth and Mackworth, 1958). It happens to many people that when they get tired while they read, their eyes move over the lines, yet they are thinking of something quite different from the text. One might say they 'saw' the text, but 'perceived' nothing!

It is tempting to assume that the size of saccades in reading might be an indication of the span of perception in reading. But actually there is no guarantee that this should be the case. It is possible, for example, that at each fixation the material that can be seen comes from a wide region, but that the eye moves onwards only a fraction of that region so that semantic integration processes have time to occur.

It may also be the case that at each saccade, the eye moves further than the region from which information can be gathered. This might happen, for example, if the text is so easy to read that imperfectly viewed portions can easily be completed or guessed.

Most research has ignored these problems and has assumed that eye movement measures actually do indicate the extent of the perceptual span. Research has also been motivated by the converse hypothesis, namely that the edge of the perceptual span might be what is determining where the eyes go at each saccade: the eye might move forward in such a way that successive spans just touch each other. Temporarily setting aside the difficulties with the concept of perceptual span, I will now review a number of recent studies. However, it will become apparent that the notion is ill-defined. Section 2.4 will therefore define a new notion, that of 'visual span', and calculations and empirical data will be presented to show its dependence on viewing distance and character size. Section 2.5 will redefine 'perceptual span' in a precise way with respect to visual span, and section 2.6 will then show that in reading, eye movements are not directly linked to changes in perceptual span: an alternative theory to explain eye guidance in reading is needed.

2.1. Measuring perceptual span by perturbing the visual field in reading

Many of the early attempts to measure the span of perception during a fixation used tachistocopic presentations of text material (Cattel, 1885; Korte, 1923). However, as pointed out by Huey (1900, p. 298), tachistoscopic experiments must use presentation durations which are sufficiently short to prelude eye movements. This necessitates much shorter durations (< 100 ms) than the fixation durations commonly observed in reading (250 ms). This and other differences between reading and tachistoscopic experiments (cf. Rayner, 1975) led researchers to search for other techniques to measure perceptual span. Among these, Reder (1973), McConkie and Rayner (1975) and O'Regan (1975) pioneered the one that has recently generated the most attention, namely using a computer to create eye-movement-contingent perturbations in the text being read.

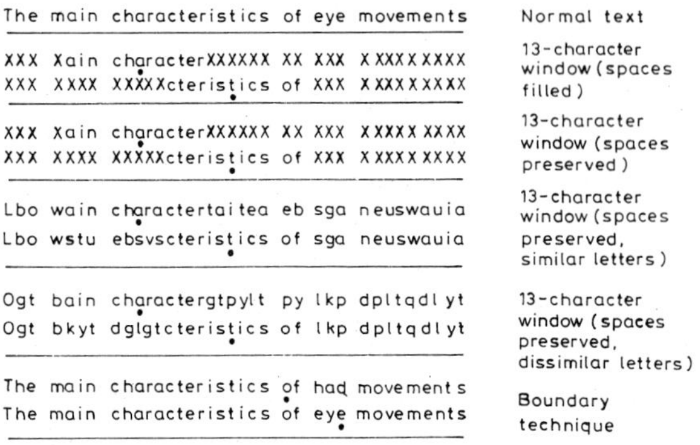

Fig. 3. Examples of techniques used to study the perceptual span. The top example shows a normal segment of text. The second to fifth examples show what is seen during two successive fixations in the moving-window paradigm. The eye's instantaneous position is indicated by the dot under the text line. The last example shows the boundary technique, where the word 'had' becomes the word 'eye' when the eye passes an invisible boundary after the word 'of'.

In one example of this technique, the 'moving window' method, a computer continuously monitors the eye's position during reading. The goal is to ensure that only the test material in a 'window' surrounding the instantaneous fixation point is visible to the reader at each moment. The letters of the text outside the window are replaced by other letters. The window of visible text may be of variable width, and the letters outside the window may be replaced by various other letters (see Fig. 3). In another example of the technique, the 'boundary' method, some portion of the text is replaced by an alternative portion, but only when the eye crosses a pre-defined, imaginary boundary placed at a particular position in the text (see Fig. 3, bottom).

These techniques are essentially 'perturbation' techniques: they perturb the information in parafoveal vision in various ways. The effect of these perturbations on eye movements (e.g., saccade size, fixation durations, gaze durations, total reading rate) are measured, and conclusions are reached concerning the kinds of information that are gathered by the eye at different eccentricities in parafoveal vision. For example, reading slows down when information about the length of words in parafoveal vision is removed by filling inter-word spaces outside the window by X's. Reading speed is not affected when the X's are further than 15 letters from the instantaneous fixation point. This suggests that word-length information is gathered up to 15 characters from the instantaneous fixation point: the perceptual span for word length is 15 characters. By doing other kinds of manipulations, such as replacing letters outside the window by letters that are more or less similar to the original letters, it is possible to deduce the size of the perceptual span for word shape or letter identity. A large number of studies have been done in this vein, and summaries of their results can be found in Rayner (1983) and Rayner and Pollatsek (1987). In the next paragraphs I will briefly sumarize the most important conclusions that were reached. But in the subsequent sections I will present some methodological and theoretical problems with these 'perturbation' techniques that have not been sufficiently considered.

One conclusion that has been reached about perceptual span is that there is not one perceptual span. Different spans are found, depending on the type of perturbation that is used. When gross features of the text, such as the position of the spaces that separate words, are perturbed, a large span will be found. When finer features such as individual letters are perturbed, a smaller span is found. This is coherent with the idea that different kinds of information can be extracted at different distances from the fixation point. Information about inter-word spaces can be obtained as far as 15 characters to the right of fixation (McConkie and Rayner, 1975; Rayner and Bertera, 1979; Rayner et al., 1981; Ikeda and Saida, 1978; Rayner, 1986). Word-shape information is no longer available beyond about 10 characters to the right of fixation (McConkie and Rayner, 1975; although see below for more on the problem of word shape), and information about specific letters is available no further than six to ten letters to the right of fixation (Underwood and McConkie, 1985; Pollatsek et al., 1986).

The size of perceptual span depends on the eye movement measure used. Fixation durations and saccade sizes are not affected when individual letters are perturbed beyond 8 letters to the right of fixation (Underwood and McConkie, 1985). Gaze duration is affected even when perturbations are 10 letters from fixation (Pollatsek et al., 1986). This kind of difference is reasonable when one considers that information takes time to be processed, and so the more subtle kinds of perturbations may affect more delayed eye movement measures such as gaze duration, which may include fixations occurring after the one in which the perturbation occurs.

The perceptual span appears to be asymmetrical, being greater on the right than on the left (the reverse is true for Hebrew; cf. Pollatsek et al., 1981). To the left of fixation, Rayner et al. (1980b) showed that the perceptual span extended to the beginning of the fixated word, or four letters leftwards, whichever was smaller. But to the right of fixation, Rayner et al. (1982) showed that perceptual span for individual letters went out to somewhere between 9 and 15 letters (also McConkie and Rayner, 1976; Rayner, 1986; although Underwood and McConkie, 1985, find a smaller value). Rayner et al. (1982) claim that to the right, perceptual span should be measured in letters, not in words. In addition, only the first three letters of the word to the right of fixation appear to facilitate the recognition of that word on the subsequent fixation (Rayner et al., 1980a, 1982).

A point related to perceptual span concerns whether the span can extend over word boundaries. Some controversy exists about this, since McConkie et al. (1982) present evidence that words in the parafovea are either completely identified or not identified at all, and that partial letter information can only be used if it enables the word to be completely identified. If not, processing must start anew on a subsequent fovealization of the word. However Balota et al. (1985), Inhoff and Rayner (1986) and Rayner and Pollatsek (1987) dispute the claim, citing various sources of evidence.

A further interesting point concerns the nature of

the information about individual letters which is integrated from one fixation to the next. Whereas older studies (but considered now to possibly contain artefacts related to display changes; see section 2.2) had suggested that word shape played a role in information extraction (Rayner, 1975; McConkie and Rayner, 1975; Rayner et al., 1978), recent results show no effect of word shape (Inhoff and Rayner, 1986). In fact several studies have now conclusively demonstrated that letter features such as line segments or global shape are not integrated across saccades. Rather, letter information is transformed into an abstract code, independent of the letter's physical appearance, typography or case, and only this code can be combined across successive fixations. This is shown by the fact that facilitation from parafoveal preview of a word is equally strong when the letters in the previewed word have a different case in parafovea than when they are subsequently directly fixated by the eye (McConkie and Zola, 1979; Rayner et al., 1980a). Two other studies also show that shape information as such cannot be integrated across the saccade (O'Regan and Lévy-Schoen, 1983; Rayner and Pollatsek, 1983).

2.2. Technical issues in the moving-window and the boundary techniques

The moving-window and boundary techniques have been extensively used to measure visual span in reading, and certain authors (e.g. Rayner, 1975; Pollatsek and Rayner, 1987) claim that they are preferable to tachistoscopic and other methods which do not involve normal reading. There is no doubt that a large amount of converging evidence and excellent research has been assembled using these techniques over the past decade. However, several problems sometimes make interpretation of results difficult, particularly with one of the two techniques, namely the moving-window technique. The first kind of problems are technical problems related to apparatus delays and persistence of displays on the screen. Because these problems have not been treated extensively, I shall list them in detail in this section. The second kind of problem is actually much more important and fundamental than the technical problems, and concerns the question of what is really meant by 'perceptual span'. It will be the subject of the next sections.

The basic assumption in the use of display changes is that they have their effect because of the kind of information they are perturbing (spaces, letter shapes, letter identities), and not as a result of the flicker or contrast changes associated with the display change. Thus, researchers have gone to great pains to ensure that display changes occur during saccades, and not during fixations, where flicker and contrast change would be readily noticed. However, in some of the earlier studies, delays in the eye movement recording apparatus or in the time taken by the computer to change the screen were long, with visible display disturbances lasting up to an estimated 20 ms (Rayner, 1975) or 40 ms (McConkie and Rayner, 1975; O'Regan, 1979) after the saccade ended, and this could have accounted for a portion of the observed effects.

Even in the more recent studies, delays in the recording apparatus or in the screen-change algorithms cannot be totally discounted. For example, in the experiments of Rayner et al. (1982) and Inhoff and Rayner (1986), possible delay before display changes were accomplished was estimated at 5 ms, and in Rayner et al. (1981) at 2–10 ms following saccade termination. If slight flicker is visible after the saccade, this may act as a warning stimulus which modifies saccadic latency. Changes in the display may also affect sensory information extraction and thereby fixation duration. Of course, masking and suppression phenomena associated with the saccade probably minimize the perceptual effects of these disturbances, and this may explain why in most cases display changes using modern techniques are invisible to the reader. Unfortunately however, there is evidence that even a subliminal flash occurring near the end of a saccade can modify the subsequent saccade endpoint (Deubel et al., 1984).

However, even if it could be proved that the delay in the recording apparatus or in the screen-change algorithms was too small to be of visual significance, there is still an inevitable delay associated with the persistence of the screen phosphor. Even for the fast P31 phosphor used in most reading research, where luminance drops to 1% after only 0.25 ms, after this, luminance remains fairly constant for many tens of milliseconds (cf. Hewlett Packard Application Note 115). Whether this 1% level will be visible or not depends on the initial luminance level from which the drop occurred, on what the background luminance is, and on what is superimposed on the decaying trace. If nothing is superimposed, the decaying trace may still be visible, particularly if the background is dark and the eye is adapted to dim conditions. Thus, when a letter is replaced by a new letter on the screen, then the parts of the old letter that lie in the gaps of the new letter may 'shine through' slightly, and diminish the contrast of the new letter. Again, metacontrast and masking may render screen changes subjectively invisible, and this may explain why subjects are usually unaware of the changes. But, objectively, the disturbance to the display may nevertheless have contributed to the observed effects on reading behavior. There are many examples in the eye movement literature where this problem may have occurred. My own work provides a case in point: In O'Regan (1980) I observed that when information about the upcoming word in parafovea was perturbed by writing the word backwards, then when the eye subsequently fixated that word, even though the word has returned to normal, the fixation on that word was longer than when no perturbation occurred. I claimed that the effect was evidence that when there was no parafoveal perturbation, parafoveally gathered lexical information about the word could be used to preprocess the word, thereby shortening the subsequent fixation. However an alternative interpretation is that in the case of the parafoveal perturbation, the contrast of the letters of the fixated word was poorer than in the unperturbed case, and so processing took longer.

Another point concerning the effect of screen persistence on contrast is important to note: the greater the difference in shape between the perturbing letters and the original letters, the larger the resulting 'smear' on the screen will be. In studies where similarity between perturbing parafoveal letters and original letters is manipulated, for example when experimenters attempt to determine the extent of the perceptual span for different kinds of information, there is thus a potential confounding factor. Effects assumed to be caused by differences in the type of information integrated across the saccade (word length, word shape, individual letters) may in fact be due to physical differences in contrast arising from the residual persistence of the screen.

Leaving aside the possible difficulties associated with display changes, other problems are associated with the visibility of the material outside the moving 'window'. Older studies (O'Regan, 1979; McConkie and Rayner, 1975) and some of the recent studies (Rayner et al., 1980a, 1982; Inhoff and Rayner, 1986) have employed sequences of X's or 'interlaced square wave gratings'. The edges of such spatially extended, repetitive patterns are detectable far from the fixation point even when the quickest display-change techniques are used, because they form blocks of uniform texture easily discriminable from the pattern formed by the letters they replace. Particularly when whole blocks of text are read with the masks present, as has been the case in the studies just cited, subjects may adopt specific strategies such as aiming saccades at the edge of the window or at least modifying their saccade aim (see the center of gravity effect, section 3.1). Effects observed using such masks may be specific to them, and may give no information about the zone normally used in reading to extract visual information. The situation is even worse when masks are used foveally rather than peripherally (Rayner and Bertera, 1979; Rayner et al., 1981).

Even when types of parafoveal mutilation other than gratings or X's are used as the stimuli outside the central window, strategy effects may appear when subjects read several sentences at a time in a given condition of parafoveal mutilation. For example, Rayner et al. (1982) suggested that, contrary to the usual claim that perceptual span extends only a small distance to the left of fixation, when span is artificially restricted to the right, more use of material to the left can be made. This may also have a strategic explanation, since the different window conditions were run in blocked rather than mixed groups. Underwood and McConkie (1985), aware of the possibility of strategic effects, did an experiment where mutilations occurred only 20% of the time at random text locations, and found a somewhat smaller perceptual span than had previous research.

2.3. The problem of defining the 'perceptual span'

As noted by McConkie (1983), Well (1983) and Hogaboam (1983), studies of the perceptual span using the moving-window technique fail to distinguish possible momentary changes in the region attended to during a single fixation, and the possible variations in the size of the span at different points in a text. McConkie et al. (1985b) have also pointed out that conclusions are often based on differences in the size of effects caused by different kinds of windows. Different-sized effects may occur because they occur with different frequencies, or because they occur with different amplitudes. Underlying these two possibilities may be two quite different mechanisms, with different implications for eye movement guidance.

But the most serious limitation of the work using window and boundary techniques is the problem of definition. This problem overshadows by far the technical problems discussed above. Researchers have generally assumed that the window and the boundary techniques measure the 'perceptual span'. This is taken as the region in which letters can be identified, or at least the region which contributes to recognition and language-processing. But the window and boundary studies did not measure the perceptual span in this sense. Instead they measured the region of the text whose contents can affect eye movement guidance and reading rate. As already noted briefly by McConkie (1983), this may not be the same. The reason is that in reading, eye movements may be determined not only by perceptual span (in the sense of region of perceptual information extraction), but also by a more or less independent eye movement guidance strategy that keeps the eye moving across the text. Whereas word recognition and language-processing require the extraction of certain kinds of information (e.g., letter identities) from the visual field, the eye guidance process may require other kinds. The perturbations in parafoveal vision created by the window and the boundary techniques may interfere either with the language-processing or with the eye guidance process, or both. For the effects of an experimental manipulation to be interpretable, these possibilities must be distinguished. Unfortunately, in the studies using display changes up to now, this has not been done.

In order to demonstrate that 'perceptual span' in the sense of 'what can be seen in a fixation' is not the only factor determining eye movement guidance, the following sections suggest first a way of calculating and estimating the perceptual span based on psychophysical rather than oculomotor measures, and then of testing how the eye movements react to changes in the span. It will appear that psychophysically measured changes of perceptual span do not produce the expected changes in eye movement parameters.

2.4. Visual span

Before discussing the estimation of the perceptual span by psychophysical means, it will be necessary to define a precursor to perceptual span, namely what I call 'visual span' (O'Regan, 1975, 1979; O'Regan et al., 1983). The difference between the two types of span is that 'visual span' refers to what can be seen without the help of linguistic knowledge or context, whereas perceptual span includes what can be seen with that help.

Fig. 4A shows a tangential cross-section of the human retina, with the center of the fovea indicated by the cross on the left. The circles are the cones, and the black dots that start to appear beyond an eccentricity of about 1 degree are the rods. Super-

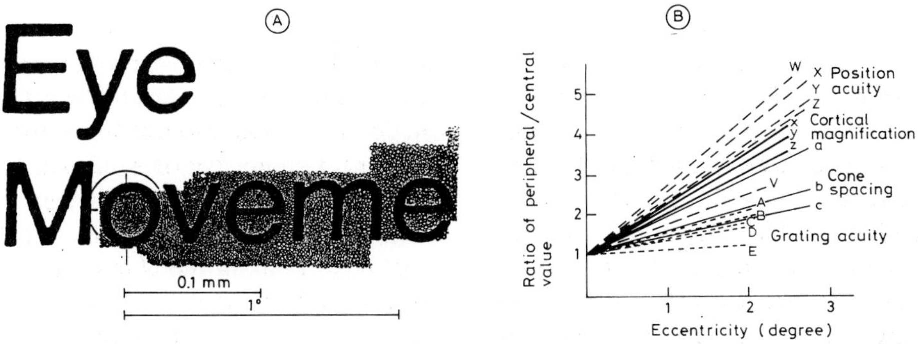

Fig. 4. A. A tangential cross-section of the human retina including the fovea, whose center (on the left) is indicated by cross-hairs. Small circles are cones; dots, appearing only beyond about 1 degree, are rods. The words 'Eye movement' are superimposed as they would appear on the retina when reading them in Vision Research at a distance of 30 cm (except they would appear upside down and in mirror image from). (Modified from O'Regan, 1989; Osterberg, 1935; Pirenne, 1967)
B. Ratio of eccentric to central values of various measures of resolution or cortical scale, as a function of eccentricity. Data compiled partially from tables given in Levi et al., 1985. Measures of grating acuity: A: Limb and Rubinstein, 1977; B and D: Levi et al., 1985; C: Westheimer, 1982; E. Wilson and Bergen, 1979, based on Hubel and Wiesel. Measures of position acuity: V: Jacobs, 1979, Landolt C without masking bars; W: Jacobs, 1979, Landolt C with masking bars; X and Z: Levi et al., 1985 (vernier); Y: Fendick and Westheimer, 1983 (stereoacuity); also Y: Klein and Tyler, 1981 (phase discrimination). Measures of cone spacing: a: Williams, 1988, using his moiré technique; also Williams' estimations from Osterberg, 1935; b: my estimation from the cross-section shown above, in A, also from Osterberg, 1935; c: Rolls and Cowey, 1970. Measures of cortical magnification: x: Dow et al., 1981; y: van Essen et al., 1984; z: Tootell et al., 1982.

imposed on the retinal mosaic is the image that would be formed by the words 'Eye movement' written in 8 point typography (as might be found in a journal article) viewed at 30 cm from the eye (each letter subtends about 10 minutes of arc), with the eye fixating the 'o'. If one defines the fovea as a zone of radius 1 degree around the optic axis, then the word 'movement' extends from the center to the edge of the fovea.

Although the letters shown are all within the fovea, they are being sampled by the retina in a dramatically different way. The 'o' being fixated centrally is sampled by a matrix of approximately 20×20 cones. The 'e', two letters from the 'o', is sampled by a matrix of approximately 15×15 cones, and the 'e' two letters further on is sampled by only 10×10 cones. Thus: four letters from the fixation point, but still well within the fovea, resolution has dropped to half its central value. The non-homogeneity of the retina is of course well-known physiologically and psychophysically, where an approximately linear increase in cone spacing or, equivalently, minimum angle of resolution, is observed up to eccentricities of about 10–14 degrees. However, the non-homogeneity exists even within the fovea. Some debate centers on the question of the actual rate of increase with eccentricity: in particular it appears that cortical receptive fields increase in size faster than cone spacing does. As suggested by Levi et al. (1985), this may explain why acuity measurements requiring position judgements, such as optotype or vernier acuity, give faster rates of drop-off than simple psychophysical tasks such as detecting gratings. Fig. 4B illustrates these ideas by plotting, for physiological and psychophysical measurements made at different eccentricities, the ratio of the eccentric value to the central value. The important point to be made from the figure is that, for all measures, the data fall on straight lines. Thus, sampling of the visual field at eccentricity Φ can be considered to take place at a sampling interval which is larger than sampling at the retinal center by a scale factor of $(1+m\Phi)$. Here, m is a constant between about 0.3 and 2, depending on which data you observe. If the scale factor for cortex and position acuity is used, which is reasonable for reading, then m is about 1.7 (when Φ measured in degrees; this gives $m = 100$ when Φ is measured in radians). Grating acuity and retinal cone spacing would give values around 0.5. The notion that parafoveal and eccentric vision can be considered a 'scaled-up' version of vision at the center of the fovea will be developed below.

In addition to the dramatic constraint on visibility imposed by the fall-off in retinal and cortical sampling rates, a further, very strong constraint is imposed by lateral interactions. As an illustration of this, consider the following example taken from Bouma (1978):

.	v
.	ovo
.	xvx
.	x v x
.	vs
.	sv

In the first line, if you fixate the central fixation point, it is fairly easy to identify the letter 'v' in the right parafovea. However, in the second line, when the 'v' is laterally flanked by other letters, identification becomes harder. Identification is even harder if the flanking letters have similar features to the target letter (third line). The phenomenon extends over fairly large retinal distances (about 0.4 Φ, where Φ is the target letter's eccentricity; cf. Bouma, 1970; Andriessen and Bouma, 1976), as shown by the fourth line. A further interesting fact is illustrated in the last two lines: it is easier to see a letter, here the 'v', when it is flanked by another letter on the foveal side than on the peripheral side (for studies of this curious asymmetry, see Chastain, 1985).

Most authors have argued that lateral interaction cannot be explained purely from the drop-off of resolution in parafovea, since it is hard to see how this would predict the large zone of interaction, the increased effects for similar letters, or the counter-intuitive fovea/periphery asymmetry. A higher-level explanation appears necessary. Krumhansl and Thomas (1977) suggested the existence of feature-specific interference, plus the idea that features tend to migrate towards the fovea. Detailed models have been proposed by Estes (1982), Wolford and Shum (1980) and others. However, it is also possible (O'Regan, 1989) that a contribution to the effects comes from the inhibitory part of the psychophysical point spread function (e.g., Blommaert and Roufs, 1985, or the N channel postulated by Wilson and Bergen, 1979). In any case, to get the effects over large retinal distances it must be assumed that in eccentric vision the cortical scale factor of about ($1+1.7\Phi$), rather than the smaller retinal scale factor, should be applied compared to central vision.

In order to permit simple modelling of the effects of acuity drop-off and lateral interactions on reading, it is convenient to lump them into a single measure, which might be called 'effective' resolution. Jacobs (1979) had compared acuity in peripheral vision for ordinary Landolt C's to acuity for Landolt C's flanked by bars. As expected from lateral interference, resolution was worse for the flanked targets than for the unflanked targets. Nevertheless the recognition of flanked targets still followed a linear function of the form:

$$r' = r_0'\,(1 + m\Phi)$$

where r' is the effective resolution at eccentricity Φ, r_0' is the effective resolution in the center of the field, and m is the scaling parameter; m is about 2 in Jacobs's data. Thus, in this case, a single simple expression sufficed to express the effects of both resolution and lateral interactions. Now, in general, when the flanking elements differ or are at different distances from the targets, the value of r_0' may differ. But, again, under the assumption that the properties of peripheral vision are simply a version of the properties of central vision scaled by the factor ($1 + m\Phi$), the function will remain linear.

With these assumptions it is possible to calculate how many letters should be visible on each side of the eye's fixation point in a text, that is, the 'visual span'. To make the calculation, it is necessary to make some assumption about the size of the smallest featural elements which allow the characters of a

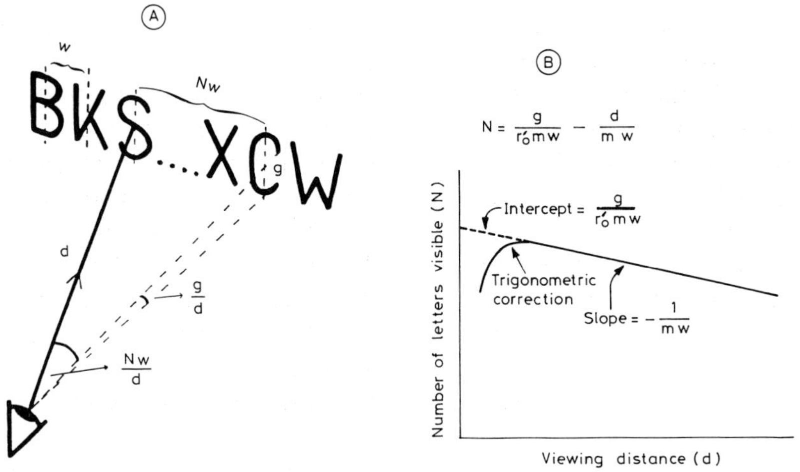

Fig. 5. A. Illustration showing how to calculate how far from the fixation point a letter can just be recognized. Assume the eye is looking directly at the letter S, from a distance *d*. Suppose the distance from letter to letter is *w*, and that, for them to be recognized, distinctive elements with characteristic size *g* (the 'grain size', measured in linear units, e.g., centimeters) must be resolved. Suppose the *N*th character can just be recognized. Then at the eye its distinctive features of size *g* subtend an angle of approximately g/d radians, and project on the retina at an eccentricity of approximately Nw/d radians. Effective resolution (which includes masking phenomona, see text) at this eccentricity is $r_0' \cdot (1 + m\Phi)$. If this is just sufficient to resolve the distinctive features of the letters, we must have: $g/d = r_0'(1 + m\Phi)$. This gives $N = g/(r_0'\, mw) - d/mw$, which is plotted in B. This relation applies only for small angles, and a trigonometric correction, necessary when *d* is small, is shown on the left-hand portion of the curve.

given typography to be distinguished from one another. Characters in a given typography differ, but one can define a parameter, *g*, which is the average resolution necessary to make all distinctions between the characters. I call *g* the 'grain size', in analogy with photographic grain. Factor *g* will depend on the particular typography, and, since it must include lateral interactions due to flanking letters, it will depend on the particular flanking letters and spacing. On average it will be of the order of some fraction of the character size. Note that grain might naturally be defined as an angular measure: that is, it would be related to the average angle subtended at the eye by the distinctive elements of the typography. However, this definition would have the disadvantage of making the grain change when the viewer changes his distance from the text. For this reason I prefer to use a definition in terms of the size, in *linear* units, for example centimeters, of the letters' distinctive features. This ensures that 'grain' is a characteristic only of the typography, and not of the viewer. Of course, the resolution needed to recognize letters viewed from a particular viewing distance, *d*, can be obtained by calculating the angle subtended by the grain, that is g/d radians (for *d* large compared to *g*).

Fig. 5 shows how to obtain theoretical predictions of the number of letters visible as a function of the eye's distance from the text. The calculation predicts that there should be an optimal value of the viewing distance, where the largest number of letters can be seen. When you move closer to the text than this optimum, the number of letters drops rapidly. However, when you move further away from the text, the number of letters also drops, but relatively slowly. The rate of drop-off should be $-1/mw$, where *w* is the character width and *m* is the parameter in the cortical scaling factor. Inserting the typical values $m = 100$ per radian and $w = 0.3$ cm, the prediction is that you should see one character less on either side of the fixation point for every 30 cm you move away from the text.

(Note that changing viewing distance is exactly equivalent, from the point of view of the retina, to

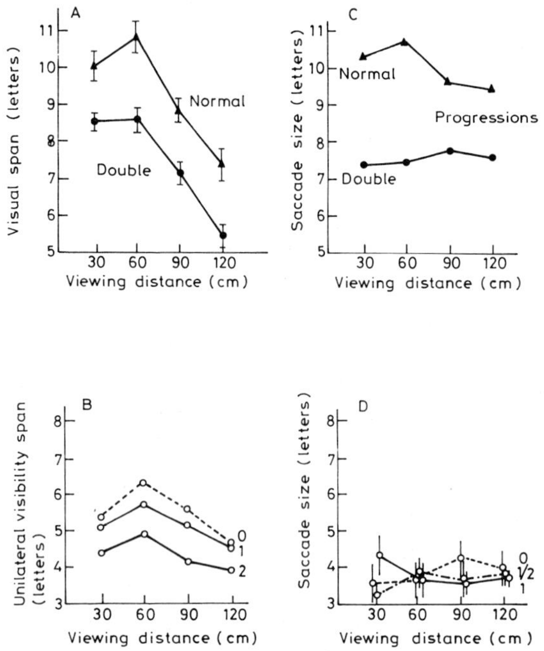

Fig. 6. A. Means and error bars (showing two standard errors on each side of the mean) over four subjects of empirically measured (unilateral) visual span, i.e., number of character spaces from the fixation point at which letters can be seen with 50% chance of being correctly reported, as a function of distance of the eye from the screen. The letters were lower case, and defined within an 8 × 8 matrix of pixels approximately 0.3 cm square. They were presented flanked on each side by a random numeral between 1 and 9. The letters were taken from a set of only ten possible letters. In the 'DOUBLE' condition, each letter (and numeral) contained additional white space on either side of it, so when words were written in the DOUBLE typography, they appeared doubly spaced as compared to the NORMAL condition. (From O'Regan et al., 1983)
B. The same as A, except a different letter set, upper-case letters, and different subjects, and using three degrees of spacing flanking each letter: 0 (equivalent to NORMAL in A), 1 (equivalent to DOUBLE) and 2 ('triple' spaced). (From Lévy-Schoen et al., 1984)
C. Mean progression saccade size made by the same four subjects as in A, reading texts printed in the same typographies as in A (but using all letters of the alphabet). Saccade size is measured in letter-spaces, so in the DOUBLE condition one 'letter-space' was twice as wide as in the NORMAL condition.
D. Mean progression saccade size made by the same subjects as in B, searching for the letter 'B' in lines of random letters taken from the set used in B. Three spacing conditions were used: 0 and 1, corresponding to 0 and 1 in B, and condition 1/2, with half as much spacing as 1.

changing character size. The same arguments above apply therefore.)

The small dependence on viewing distance (or character size) can be understood intuitively in the following way: suppose you move twice as far from the text. Characters now subtend an angle twice smaller, but they also move twice as close to the center of the visual field, where, because of the linear dependence with eccentricity, resolution is twice better. The characters therefore remain equally visible. (One can show that this argument would be exactly true if the minimum angle of resolution at the eye's center were zero. Since it is not, a slight drop-off with viewing distance is predicted. This corresponds to the right-hand sloping portion of the curve in Fig. 5B).

Fig. 6A,B shows some empirical data, which agree well with the predictions. An optimal viewing distance at about 60 cm is found, and a drop-off of about 1 character per 30 cm of viewing distance increase. The number of characters visible indicated in the data is the number of characters visible at a recognition criterion of 50%. The data show that, depending on the experiment and the conditions, about 3–11 characters were visible at this level of accuracy or better on each side of the fixation point. Several points should be noted about this number. First, had a 90% accuracy criterion been used instead of a 50% criterion, the estimate would have dropped considerably, to about 2–5 letters, depending on conditions. Second, in the experiments performed to obtain these data, only ten test letters rather than the whole alphabet were used. Third, the test letters were laterally masked by only a single flanking character on each side, rather than a whole string of flankers. For these reasons the present estimates are somewhat larger than the visual span in normal reading. Nevertheless, the dependence of the obtained values on viewing distance will not be influenced by these provisos, and I will use these curves in the next section as a basis for comparison with data on saccade size in reading and in visual search.

A more direct estimate of visual span, albeit without investigating the effect of changing viewing distance, can be found in the data of Townsend et al. (1971), who trained (with difficulty) three subjects to report letters in a letter string without moving their eyes. These authors found that the limit of 50% accuracy was attained at 5 letters from the fixation point using characters of size 1/3 degree, which is half-way between the angular size of our letters in the 30 cm and 60 cm conditions. This shows again that surprisingly few letters can be seen in normal reading conditions, where lateral masking is strong. I have recently confirmed this result using a method where, through an eye-contingent display technique, a string of letters is effectively stabilized at a given retinal location despite small eye movements. Work using brief displays also shows that only a few letters can be reported accurately around the fixation point (for an excellent review of studies on the recognition of letter sequences, see Estes, 1978).

2.5. Perceptual span as distinct from visual span

Visual span being so small, how is it then that when we look at a word, we have the impression of seeing the whole word, and not just the few letters being fixated directly? One factor is certainly the fact that eye movements can occur in the word. This will be considered later. Another factor is lexical knowledge. When characters form words, lexical constraints may help to disambiguate letters that cannot be properly seen, and the total span of perception may increase. The effect of lexical knowledge on word perception has been known since the work of Cattel (1885) and Erdman and Dodge (1898), who showed that while only a few letters could be reported in tachistoscopic presentations of random letter strings, whole words and sometimes groups of words could be reported. It is thought now that the effect of lexical knowledge is a truly perceptual effect, not just an effect of conscious guessing. Excellent reviews of recent theories can be found in Carr (1986) and Henderson (1982). The following example illustrates the effect: if you fixate at the arrow in the top sequence of letters you will only be able to report about 3 letters on either side. But in the same sequence of letters written in reverse order, you have the impression of seeing all the letters clearly!

YCNADNUDER
↑

REDUNDANCY
↑

The importance of knowledge and context in recognition creates the need to distinguish what can be seen without its help from what can be perceived with it. I will call what can be seen without making use of lexical knowledge and contextual constraints the ‘visual span’, and what can be perceived by additionally making use of them the ‘perceptual span’ (the idea is that ‘perception’ is ‘vision’ plus knowledge). The perceptual span will be larger than the visual span by an amount which will depend on the strength of the lexical constraints: for example, the internal statistical structure of the individual words, and, at a higher level, the predictability of the words within the surrounding text.

Exactly how much bigger will perceptual span be than visual span? For the purpose of the argument to be made below, I do not need to know the exact answer; rather, it will be sufficient to make the reasonable assumption that for a given reader, reading a given text, on average, the relation between visual span and perceptual span is a fixed monotonic function such that perceptual span is greater than visual span. The simplest such function would assume that perceptual span is a constant multiplicative factor k times visual span, where k is greater than 1. The exact function is unimportant; what is important is that the function is a measure of the disambiguation power of linguistic and knowledge constraints, and so depends only on the text being read (which may provide stronger or weaker constraints) and the reader (who may be better or worse at making use of these constraints), but which cannot depend on the physical characteristics of the text such as its typography, the letter spacing, or the reader’s distance from the page.

2.6. No simple relationship between perceptual span and saccade size in reading

In this section I return to the question of the relationship between perceptual span and saccade size. As implied in previous eye movement work, a tempting hypothesis to make about saccade size in reading is that the eye moves in such a way that (at least on average) the right edge of each perceptual span just coincides with the left edge of the next span (or overlaps with it by a constant amount). Under this 'perceptual span control' hypothesis about eye movement guidance in reading, manipulations in perceptual span should provide analogous changes in saccade size. Certainly in the literature on perceptual span (see sections 2.1, 2.2) changes in window size have always provoked approximately the expected changes in saccade size, with the smallest windows provoking the smallest saccades. But are the changes exactly those which would be expected under 'perceptual span control'? Given that we now have a way to estimate visual span and perceptual span, we can now test this more precisely by manipulating perceptual span in a known way, and seeing whether saccade sizes change in the expected manner.

The data in Fig. 6A estimate the visual span under conditions of different viewing distance, and for two different typographies, which I call 'normal' and 'double' spaced. If saccade size is proportional to perceptual span, and perceptual span is proportional to visual span, then saccade sizes should follow curves similar to the visual span curves. Fig. 6C shows saccade sizes for exactly the same subjects reading texts from the same viewing distances and with the same typographies. The curves for normal and double typographies are separated by 2–3 letters, which is consistent with the two-letter difference in visual span between these two conditions. However, the curves do not have the expected dependence on viewing distance: they are approximately flat, rather than changing by 4 letters over the range 60–120 cm as do the visual span curves.

It might be thought that the data could be explained if the relation between perceptual and visual span were a more complex function than simple proportionality. But this is not so. Any function relating visual span to perceptual span must be single-valued; that is, a given visual span must always give rise to the same perceptual span (if the reader and the text content is kept constant as was done here). Yet in the data there are cases where the same visual span provokes very different saccade sizes: for example, visual span is similar for the double-spaced typography at 60 cm and for the normal-spaced typography at 90 cm, yet the associated saccade sizes in reading are very different.

To account for the lack of correspondence between perceptual span and saccade size, we have previously suggested (O'Regan et al., 1983) that perhaps saccade size is determined partly also by linguistic factors. However, it is difficult to imagine how linguistic factors could have been the cause of the differences in saccade sizes that occurred when there were no visual span differences, since the subjects and texts (and therefore linguistic and context factors) were strictly the same.

Further experiments also discount linguistic factors as a sole explanation. In these experiments (Lévy-Schoen et al., 1984), we reasoned that if linguistic factors were the explanation for the incompatibility between visual span and saccade size changes, then, in tasks where linguistic factors were reduced to a strict minimum, visual span and saccade size should fall into step with each other. We used a task of searching for a target letter 'B' hidden in lines of random nontarget letters – assuredly a task requiring minimum linguistic processing. Fig. 6B shows the measured visibility span for letters in three spacing conditions (0, 1 and 2 blank characters between letters). Fig. 6D shows the saccade sizes observed in the similar conditions in the search task (note that only spacings 0 and 1 were common to both experiments). There is no correspondence between the two sets of graphs. The results seem again to show that something is wrong with the perceptual span control hypothesis, but we cannot be absolutely sure here, since the saccade sizes were not sensitive at all to the manipulations of spacing in this experiment: this time we cannot exclude the possibility that the relation between visual and perceptual span is more complicated than simple proportionality. However, in a third set of experiments, Jacobs (1986a,b) also directly adressed the question of the validity of the perceptual span control hypothesis in visual search. Although he concludes that overall there is a correspondence between perceptual span and saccade size, closer examination of his data shows exactly the same difficulties as in the earlier experiments we did: whereas changing visual span by one kind of manipulation (in his case by changing target-background similarity) creates a given change in saccade size, changing visual span by the same amount but through a different manipulation (e.g., by changing viewing distance or letter spacing) may give no change at all in saccade size. Similar observations apply to a study by Heller (1987), who varied letter size and spacing.

Since linguistic factors do not account for the incompatibility between saccade size and perceptual span, what other possibility exists to salvage the perceptual span control hypothesis? One possibility might be to take into account fixation durations: perhaps the amount of material that can be processed depends in a combined way both on the perceptual span and also on the time the eye stays at each fixation. For example, there might be an inverse relation between perceptual span and fixation duration: perceptual span might be smaller when fixation duration is short (see Jacobs, 1986, for other possibilities). It is certainly true in the studies discussed above that when changing the perceptual span produced no effect on saccades (e.g., for viewing distance changes), then fixation durations were affected (e.g., in Lévy-Schoen et al., 1984). However, as shown in a further study we did (Jacobs and O'Regan, 1987), this still leaves open the question of why under some circumstances saccade size reacts, under some circumstances fixation durations react, and under some circumstances both react to perceptual span changes. Also, in that study we found no evidence for an inverse relation between span and fixation duration. If there were such a trade-off on average in reading, one would expect that saccade size would be inversely correlated with preceding fixation duration. Neither we nor several other authors have found such correlations over large bodies of text (Andriessen and de Voogd, 1973; McConkie and Zola, 1984; Rayner and McConkie, 1976), although locally they may be found (Pollatsek et al., 1986).

The conclusion is that perceptual span does not determine saccades in reading and search in any simple way. So what does? In the strategy-tactics theory to be presented in section 6, the eyes are guided by a general scanning strategy, based mainly on gross visual characteristics of the text (not on perceptual span). To simplify: in reading, the eye moves from word to word, independently of how well words can be identified in parafoveal vision. Changing viewing distance thus changes nothing in this strategy, and no effect on saccade size is expected. Changing spacing, however, can have an effect on the visibility of the inter-word space, and thus may render inter-word aiming more or less difficult. This probably accounts for the fact that saccade sizes were smaller (measured in letters) in the double-spaced conditions of O'Regan et al. (1983).

2.7. Letters are the right units to measure saccades

One noteworthy point concerning all the experiments just discussed, as well as the results of Morrison and Rayner (1981), Javal (1878), Lamare (1893) and Huey (1908), is that viewing distance and letter size (cf. Heller, 1987; Tinker and Paterson, 1955) always has almost no effect on saccade size (when this is measured in letters). As explained above, this result is *approximately* predicted from perceptual span measurements and theoretical calculations. But unfortunately it is not *precisely* predicted, nor is it consistent with the results of other visual span manipulations. Nevertheless the result is a good reason for measuring saccades in letters rather than in degrees. It is amusing that ever since Javal, researchers have justifiably measured saccades in letters, but all the time without being aware of the underlying mystery.

3. Oculomotor constraints: spatial factors

Oculomotor constraints of different kinds may affect the way the eyes behave in reading. There may be spatial constraints, determining the accuracy with which the eye can attain a target, and temporal constraints, determining the latencies preceding saccades, and there may be interactions between the two. Temporal constraints in the oculo-motor system have received some attention in the reading literature (cf. Russo, 1978; McConkie, 1983) because there has been doubt about whether the apparently ponderous machinery necessary for saccade programming could actually leave any time for higher-level linguistic processing to influence the parameters of the immediately following saccade. Section 4 will consider the temporal constraints. However, recently, with the discovery of the 'center of gravity' effect to be described below, it has become apparent that spatial constraints can also be quite stringent in determining eye guidance in visually complex scenes.

3.1. The 'center of gravity' effect and a conceptual model of saccade programming

It is frequently said that saccades tend to undershoot a target, typically by about 10% of the target's eccentricity (Frost and Pöppel, 1976; Henson, 1978; Deubel et al., 1986). But this classical assertion applies to saccades made to an isolated target, that is, a target which can easily be seen within its surroundings. Recent work has shown that if a target is surrounded by other material in the visual field, then the eye's landing position will be deviated to a sort of 'center of gravity' of the the whole visual configuration around the target (Coren and Hoenig, 1972; Findlay, 1981, 1982, 1983; Ottes et al., 1984; Deubel et al., 1984, 1988; Coëffé, 1986; Coëffé and O'Regan, 1987). Thus, in Fig. 7A, the eye will have no trouble saccading to the target letter marked by crosses when it is present alone, but it will overshoot or undershoot it in the other examples because of the influence of the adjacent letters.

The phenomenon, which has also been called the 'Global Effect' (Findlay, 1983), can be conveniently explained by a model of saccade target selection which was proposed by Findlay (1983, 1987) and Deubel et al., (1984) and has been made most explicit by Coëffé (1987). There are two ideas behind these models. The first is that the visual processing which determines saccades must pass through the same stage of relatively slow spatio-temporal filtering that determines visual pattern recognition in general. The second is that two independent processes determine saccade generation: saccade triggering and saccade computation.

Saccade *triggering* is done by an external event which is independent of the saccade computation mechanism. At any moment, if a triggering signal occurs, the saccade will depart to the target location indicated by the current state of the ongoing saccade computation. Triggering can occur on the basis of visual information such as the visual transient produced by target onset, by visual recognition of some aspect of the target, but also on the basis of a non-visual event which is not related to the target onset, such as an auditory signal, the completion of some kind of cognitive processing of simply a voluntary decision. If (as for anticipatory saccades) the triggering signal occurs very early, before visual information has been properly analysed, the saccade will depart to an incorrect position or to a position determined by prior expectations.

Saccade *computation* is done continuously and automatically on the basis of the available visual information (Deubel et al., 1984), but is also modulated from moment to moment by attentional mechanisms (Coëffé, 1987). The saccade computation process is going on continuously without supervision, so that if a triggering signal occurs at any moment, the saccade will depart to the endpoint which is currently active. The visual information used in updating the saccade endpoint computation is assumed to come from low-level visual spatio-temporal filtering operations (possibly also involving texture-sensitive mechanisms; cf. Deubel et al., 1988), so its spatial extent and time course depend on the spatial and temporal characteristics of the

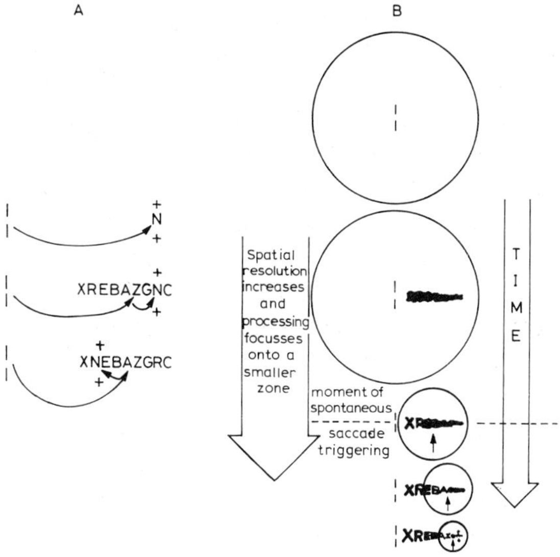

Fig. 7. A. Typical eye behavior observed by Coëffé and O'Regan (1987) on attempting to saccade to a target letter marked by crosses. If the letter is alone, the eye attains it after the primary saccade. If the letter is in a string of other, non-target, letters, the primary saccade will generally go to near the center of gravity of the whole string, and a correction movement will occur, bringing the eye on to the target.
B. Example of the course of excitation in a hypothetical sensory map of the visual field when saccading to a target as shown in A. The top circle is the zone of 'attention', which is initially large, and centered on the fixation mark. A moment later, a stimulus string appears on the right, but, because of spatio-temporal filtering in the early stages of the visual system, only a crude, low spatial frequency representation is at first available, so the letters cannot be distinguished. The representation is also distorted by cortical magnification, so the more peripheral parts of the stimulus are smaller and less clear. A moment later, the attentional circle has shifted and narrowed down to the general region of the stimulus. But since information as to the position of the crosses (indicating the target location) has not yet become available, the attentional circle can do no better than move to somewhere near the center of gravity of the whole configuration. With time, the crosses become visible, and the attentional circle can shift further rightwards and narrow down further to the region of the crosses, and the target letter becomes identifiable. As these processes occur, saccade coordinates are being continually calculated and updated. The endpoint being calculated at any moment is assumed to be the center of the attentional circle. If a signal to trigger a saccade happens to be given at the moment indicated by the horizontal dotted line, then the saccade will go to the place in the string shown by the small arrow. But if saccade triggering occurs later, the saccade will go further into the string, as shown by the arrows in the bottom two circles. The moment of saccade triggering is determined by independent processes, not shown on this diagram. They may depend on visual, but also cognitive processing, as well as on expectations, or even auditory or other stimuli. (From Coëffé, 1987)

filters. For example, immediately after target appearance, the information available about the target will be perturbed by transient phenomena, and accurate representation of the target will only appear after a certain integration period. Information of high spatial frequency will be available later than information of low spatial frequency. The temporal impulse response of the filters has been determined by Deubel et al. (1984), and shown to extend over a relatively long period of over 200 ms. The attentional mechanisms modify the way visual information is extracted, accelerating processing in the zone which the viewer is interested in. If the viewer has expectations about the target location, target extraction will be easier in the expected zone.

To illustrate how this conceptual framework explains the center of gravity effect, consider its operation in the situation of Coëffé and O'Regan (1987), where the eye starts at a central fixation point, and a string of letters appears in the left or right parafovea, at different eccentricities. The observer's task is to make a saccade to the letter in the string which is marked above and below by crosses, as shown in Fig. 7A.

Fig. 7B shows the sequence of events that will occur. The figure depicts successive states of excitation in a hypothesized sensory map in the brain. Before the stimulus appears, the sensory map is empty except for the fixation point, and the region being attended to, indicated by the large circle, is evenly distributed around it (top of figure). When the stimulus appears in parafoveal vision, activation builds up in the part of the map corresponding to the stimulated retinal location. The build-up of activation is represented by the increasing resolution of the image, with the idea that high spatial frequency information becomes available later than low spatial frequency information. In order to show the effect of reduced resolution in parafovea, the

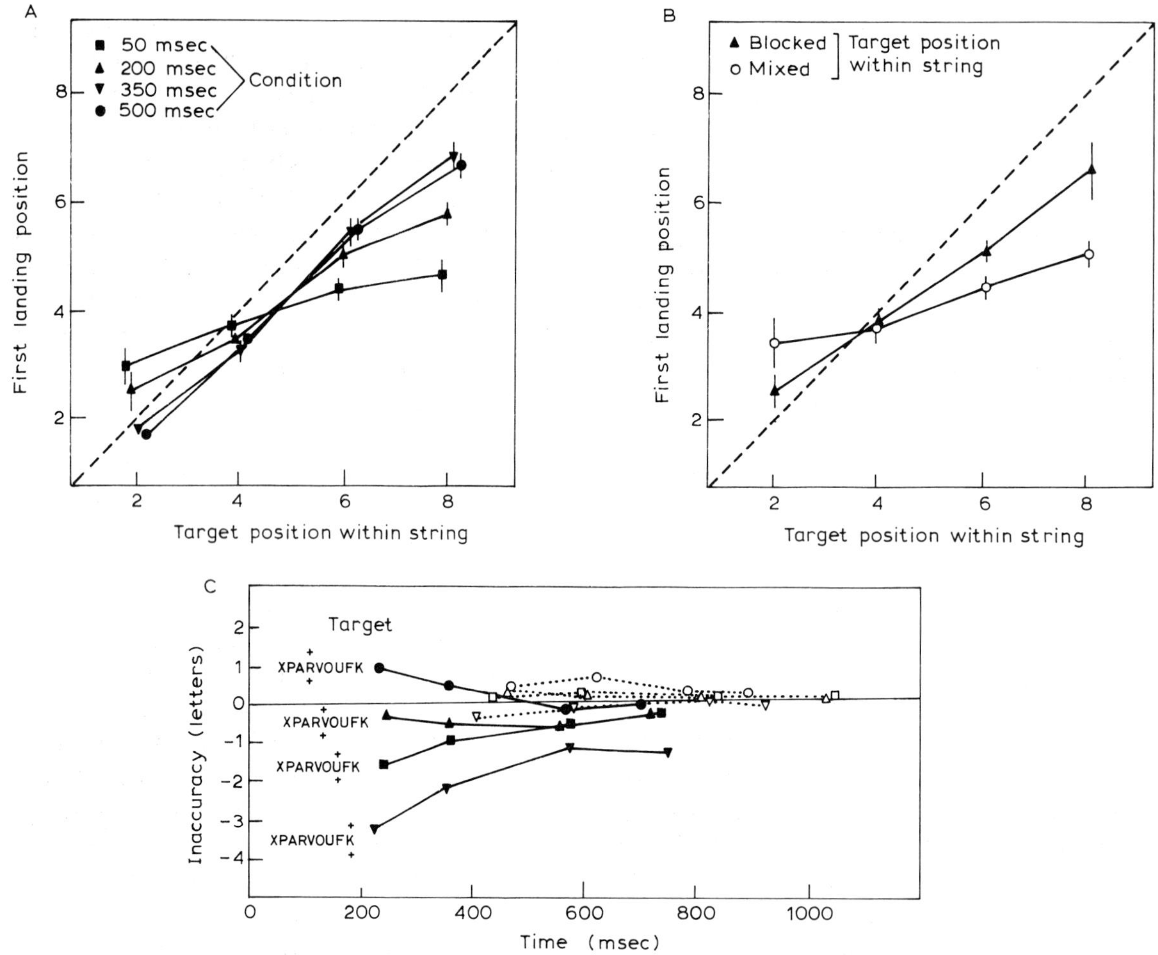

Fig. 8. A. Accuracy of primary saccades, meaned over 4 subjects, in attaining a target letter marked by crosses in a string of 9 letters, as shown in Fig. 7A, lower two examples. The task was to determine whether the target letter was a vowel or a consonant. The crosses appeared in random order at the 2nd, 4th, 6th or 8th letter position, the 8th being the most eccentric. The target string could occur in the left or the right visual field, with its least eccentric end starting at 8 or 16 letter spaces from the fixation mark. The ordinate gives the landing position in the string of the primary saccade, as a function of the target position on the abscissa. Data points with perfect accuracy would lie on the dotted diagonal line. The four curves correspond to four different latency conditions, in which the eye was detained at the intial fixation mark for varying amounts of time before being allowed to make the saccade. The eye was kept at the fixation position, despite the fact that the target string was already visible, by asking subjects not to make their saccade until the target mark disappeared. Disappearance occurred either 50, 200, 350 or 500 ms after the onset of the stimulus string. (From Coëffé and O'Regan, 1987)

B. The same as A, but comparing two conditions, one in which the crosses appeared randomly in one of the four positions in the string (mixed condition), and one in which the location of the crosses was always the same, so that at each trial, once the subject had located the side and eccentricity of the whole stimulus string, he knew where to look within it to find the target letter (blocked condition). (From Coëffé and O'Regan, 1987)

C. Solid curves: position that the eye has reached after a primary saccade at various moments following stimulus onset, on abscissa. Data points with perfect accuracy would lie on the horizontal line at ordinate 0. Dotted curves: position that the eye has reached after a primary and secondary saccade at different moments following stimulus onset. It can be seen that for target letters at positions 4, 6 and 8 within the stimulus string, after 400 ms the eye is closer to the target if it makes two saccades than if it makes only a primary saccade with 400 ms latency. (From Coëffé and O'Regan, 1987) stimulus is shown as deformed according to cortical magnification. As time progresses, higher- and higher-quality information becomes available in the sensory map, and the crosses become distinguishable: attention begins to direct itself onto this target region of the string. It is assumed that during this process of 'zooming in' and improving the resolution of information at the target location, potential saccade parameters are being continuously updated so that if the triggering command for a saccade is given, the saccade will go to the current center of attention, shown at the center of the circles in the figure. If triggering occurs early, accuracy will be poor, and the eye will go to the center of gravity of the whole visual configuration. If triggering occurs late, accuracy will be good, and the eye will go very near to the target.

The moment at which the saccade will be triggered will depend on processes independent of the 'zooming in' process. It may depend on cognitive processing of the visual information gathered, but it may also be determined by some other event necessitating little or no processing of the visual field, such as a tone that is heard or a rhythmic strategy adopted by the subject. It is seen from the figure that if the moment of saccade triggering occurs at the instant indicated by the dotted line, then the saccade will not attain the target accurately, but will go to the center of gravity of the (distorted) configuration. The center of gravity effect is explained.

It is important to stress two points about this model. The first point concerns the 'attentional' mechanism. Attention is a topic which has recently been accumulating an immense literature in experimental psychology. However, saccadic eye movements are rarely incorporated into this literature (though see Engel, 1971; also Groner, 1988, for a review, and Ch. 1 of this volume). The present rudimentary model has obvious similarities with 'zoom-lens' models (Eriksen and St. James, 1986) and 'spot-light' models (Norman, 1968; Posner, 1980; Shulman et al., 1979), but its details must be further developed before a comparison would be of interest. Meanwhile the model has constituted a sufficient framework from which to predict certain latency and expectancy effects that modulate the center of gravity phenomenon, as shown below.

The second point concerns the resemblance of the present scheme to the WHEN and WHERE mechanisms of Becker and Jürgens' (1979) often-cited model. However, the similarities are misleading, because Becker and Jürgens actually have two WHERE mechanisms: one that decides which side the target is on, left or right, and one which calculates the saccade amplitude. This latter mechanism is also not independent of the decision to move, since it is assumed to contain a temporal averaging window that only starts averaging after the decision to move has occurred. Further, the WHEN decision is determined purely by the retinal error signal, which is after all another kind of WHERE information. Thus, in Becker and Jürgens, WHEN and WHERE mechanisms are actually somewhat intertwined, whereas we suggest that they are completely independent. Another difference between the models is that in our case the spatial averaging that explains inaccurate saccades in the center of gravity effect (and also in double-step paradigms) comes not from a mechanism specific to the saccadic system, but simply from the early stages of the visual system, which is assumed to be continuously and automatically spatio-temporally filtering information as it falls on the retina. Finally, unlike Becker and Jürgens, in our model we assume that the WHEN decision is not triggered by the retinal error signal, but is based on a variety of kinds of information, including in particular non-visual information and voluntary decisions.

3.2. Latency and expectancy effects on the center of gravity phenomenon

The above model explains the data on the center of gravity effect, that is, the fact that the eye tends to be deviated towards the center of gravity of the visual configuration. In addition, two predictions can be made.

First, the deviation towards center of gravity should diminish when latency increases, since visual processing then has time to 'zoom in' closer to the true target position, and is less affected by the surrounding material. Indeed, Findlay (1981) has already shown that the center of gravity effect became less pronounced for longer-latency saccades, but the effects were weak owing to the fact that only a small range of latencies generally occur naturally. Coëffé and O'Regan (1987) and Jacobs (1987) therefore artificially increased the range of latencies by asking subjects to voluntarily delay their saccades until a central signal disappeared, or by giving subjects a simple perceptual task to do at the fixation point. We confirmed that saccade accuracy considerably improves at long latencies (see Fig. 8A).

It is also interesting to consider the literature on eye movement speed-accuracy trade-off in the light of the present model. Cohen and Ross (1978), Viviani and Swensson (1982), Findlay (1983), Kapoula (1984) and de Bie et al. (1986) have sometimes observed speed-accuracy trade-offs, but they have been weak for another reason. The reason is that the effect of latency on saccade accuracy will depend on the visual complexity of the target configuration. A single, isolated target has the same center of gravity when it is seen at low resolution in the early stages of processing as later, when higher resolution is available. This is not true of a target embedded in other material, since at early low-resolution stages of processing the target will not yet be isolated from its surroundings, and the center of gravity will include the whole configuration. Speed-accuracy trade-offs will thus only be strong for complex stimulus configurations.

A second prediction made by the present model is that the center of gravity effect should be weaker if visual processing can determine the target location rapidly: this would occur if the target is easy to isolate from the surroundings, but particularly also if its position is predictable in advance from coarse visual information, for example if it always occurs in the same place relative to some mark that can be localized using just coarse cues (e.g., the 'blob' constituted by a string of characters).

We have indeed confirmed that saccade accuracy improves in conditions where the subject knows in advance within the string where the target letter could occur (even if the string itself can occur at different places in the visual field) (Fig. 8B; Coëffé and O'Regan, 1987).

Apart from our study, evidence in the literature of the effect on saccade accuracy of prior knowledge about target position is scarce. Instead, work has concentrated on the effect of number of target alternatives or prior knowledge of target position on saccade latency, where no coherent picture emerges (cf. Heywood and Churcher, 1980). However, this is to be expected from the present theory, since we postulate that the time needed for target extraction will depend not just on the visual configuration, but also strongly on non-visual, task and strategy-specific factors.

3.3. Implications of the center of gravity phenomenon for saccade accuracy in reading

The importance of the center of gravity effect for reading will become apparent later in this chapter, after it is shown that each word has an 'optimal viewing position' where it is best to fixate. The question then arises of whether the eye will be able to accurately land on this optimal position: in particular do the surrounding words create a visual configuration that will deviate the eye from the desired position? How much time will be required before moving in order to get the eye accurately to the desired position?

With respect to the first point, note the following. In order to explain the Coëffé and O'Regan (1987) data, we found it necessary to assume that the sensory map is distorted in such a way as to give greater weight to stimuli that are near the center of the visual field. This is consistent with the concept of cortical magnification (Rovamo et al., 1978; Schwartz, 1980; Levi et al., 1985; Cavanagh, 1978), according to which the cortical area attributed to visual processing continuously diminishes as we move away from the center of the field. The implication of this for reading is that when the eye attempts to attain a target in the next word, the presence of words beyond that word will not strongly affect the saccade's accuracy (unless the current word is very short). I have confirmed this in my laboratory, by comparing saccades towards isolated words versus saccades towards pairs of words. I find that the presence of a word beyond the target word increases saccade size by at most half a letter, and only for the shortest (5-letter) words that I used. However, further work needs to be done on even shorter words, and also to explain some effects observed by McConkie et al. (1988) concerning the influence of the eye's starting position (see section 7.2).

With respect to the second question, namely of the time needed to accurately attain the 'optimal viewing position', an indication can be obtained from Fig. 8C, taken from Coëffé and O'Regan (1987), which concerns the accuracy of attaining a marked target letter in a string of non-target letters. The x-axis indicates time after stimulus onset. The solid curves give the deviations with respect to the target position of the endpoints of the saccades made to the target. The four curves correspond to four different target positions in the string of 9 letters. It can be seen that good accuracy is achieved only if the latency of the saccade is about 500–600 ms. Even then, targets which are far from the center of gravity of the string (target position 8) are not accurately attained (undershoot of 2 letters). The dotted curves in the figure give the position where the eye arrives after making a second, correction saccade, as a function of the arrival time after stimulus onset. A very interesting thing appears: at a moment 400 ms following stimulus onset, accuracy is better when two saccades have been made (dotted curves) than if only a single saccade with delayed latency has been made. It therefore seems that it is more efficient to make two saccades with short latency than to extend the latency of the primary saccade in order to increase its accuracy. Jacobs (1987) has reached a similar conclusion.

4. Oculomotor constraints: temporal factors

In the following sections I will review a number of factors that are known to influence saccade latency. These factors may presumably also act during reading, so they must be kept in mind when trying to understand eye movements in reading. In the discussion of these factors, I will pay particular attention to the question of whether some kind of incompressible motor latency period must precede each saccade. The question is important for reading, since if such a motor latency period exists, then only a portion of visual and linguistic processing done during a fixation can influence the following saccade, namely, the portion that occurs before the beginning of the latency period. This would limit the extent to which eye movements in reading could be under the direct control of the information extracted at each fixation. Note that McConkie (1983) has also considered this question in detail.

4.1. Minimum latency and oculomotor programming

It is generally said that saccades take a long time to program (cf. Carpenter, 1981). In simple tasks, saccade latencies are rather longer than the approximately 45–95 ms that would be expected from 35–60 ms afferent (Creutzfeldt and Kuhnt, 1974; Mohler and Wurtz, 1976; also Russo, 1978) and 10–35 ms efferent (Robinson, 1972) propagation delays (although these values, which are for animals, should probably be somewhat increased for humans). Saslow (1967b) says that the fastest latencies shown classically (Westheimer, 1954; Ginsborg, 1953) of 120–180 ms contain anticipatory saccades. When these are removed, fastest latencies of around 180 ms are found. The fastest values quoted by other authors are usually around 150 ms for latencies and about 180–220 ms for fixation durations in tasks where the fixation is preceded and followed by a saccade (Salthouse and Ellis, 1980; Rayner et al., 1983; Kapoula, 1983; although see later for 'express saccades' and the 'gap' condition).

These values represent the times necessary for saccades to be generated to a simple peripheral dot target. In addition to afference and efference, the processes involved are presumably as follows: building-up of visual information; recognition of the stimulus; selection of the saccade target; preparing the saccade characteristics; and triggering the saccade. Because making a saccade to a simple dot target seems to involve little in the way of recognition and target selection processes, it is often assumed that most of the time is taken in motor programming. It is thought that there is some kind of oculomotor programming delay which is necessary to get the motor apparatus ready to send the saccade onto target. Vaughan and Graefe (1977), Salthouse and Ellis (1980) and Rayner et al. (1983) estimate this oculomotor preparation to require 150–200 ms.

However, in fact, there is no firm evidence proving that the main portion of saccadic latency involves a preparation of the oculomotor apparatus. In the model I sketched above, all the latency comes from visual (stimulus localization) or decisional (saccade target selection) processes. This is not incompatible with current theories: in fact Young (1981), in his sampled data model, explicitly notes that the delay element may equally well be in the visual component. Becker and Jürgens (1979) explicitly refer to the delay of about 200 ms as being due to 'central decision and computation'. In the following brief overview of effects on saccade latency, while sometimes it may seem more natural to suppose that a factor acts via some motor mechanism, as far as I can see, alternative visual or attentional mechanisms are also feasible and have certainly not been empirically ruled out.

4.2. Factors affecting saccade latency

Factors affecting saccade latency and which are attributable to attentional effects include factors such as practice (Heywood and Churcher, 1980), warning signals (Saslow, 1967a; Becker, 1972), the number of stimulus alternatives or spatial uncertainty (Saslow, 1967b; for a review see Heywood and Churcher, 1980). Zingale and Kowler (1987) and Inhoff (1986) have also drawn attention to the extensive literature on the planning of sequences of limb movements, and compared this to planning sequences of saccades (see also Lévy-Schoen, 1977). It was found that the latencies of a pre-planned sequence of saccades depends on the number of saccades in the sequence.

Factors which may be visual in origin are target luminance (Wheeless et al., 1967; Prablanc and Jeannerod, 1974) and target-background similarity (Jacobs, 1987). An interesting, presumably visual or attentional effect, and which will be referred to later, is the 'gap' phenomenon, in which saccade latencies are significantly reduced when the central fixation point is extinguished before saccade occurrence (Saslow, 1967a; Deubel et al., 1982; Ross and Ross, 1983; Fischer and Ramsperger, 1984; Mayfrank et al., 1987; Kalesnykas and Hallett, 1987).

We shall see later that the effect of target eccentricity will be important in understanding within-word fixation durations in reading. Findlay (1983) cites a number of studies showing that for saccades larger than about 10–15 degrees, latency is often positively correlated with eccentricity. However, an interesting recent finding shows a strong effect on latency of the eye's final position in the orbit (Accardo et al., 1987). For large saccades this will often confound eccentricity measures, and so this renders most previous studies dubious.

For reading, we are more interested in saccades smaller than a few degrees. Wyman and Steinman (1973) found that for saccades of less than about 0.5–1 degree, latency was inversely correlated with amplitude, with very small saccades having longer latencies than larger saccades. More recently Kowler and Anton (1987) have observed a similar inverse correlation. The finding is also consistent with incidental observations on the latencies of corrective saccades, which are small and inversely correlated with saccade size (Becker and Fuchs, 1969; Prablanc et al., 1978; Robinson, 1964; Cohen and Ross, 1978; Viviani and Swensson, 1982; Deubel et al., 1982). There may be a relationship between this finding and the concept of saccadic dead-zone (cf. Rashbass, 1961; Wyman and Steinman, 1973; Young, 1981), or the idea that there are different modes of saccade programming depending on their size (Becker, 1976). The effect of eccentricity might naturally be considered a motor factor, but, since saccade size and target eccentricity are confounded in most experiments, it is impossible to rule out a visual explanation. In fact, I have found, in the conditions of an experiment to be mentioned in section 5.5, that the explanation must be perceptual not motor: it is not because small saccades are difficult to execute that their latencies are long.

A debate in the literature on saccade generation has concerned the question of whether there are separate mechanisms involved in deciding the amplitude and the direction of a saccade. This could be relevant to reading research, since it may determine how hard it is to make different kinds of modifications to a previously programmed saccade. Young (1981) has compiled data from various experiments concerning the latest moments before the saccade when certain types of modification of the target position can still just be taken into account. Young claims that inhibiting the saccade requires the least preparation and can be done almost up to the moment of occurrence of the saccade. Decreasing the saccade's magnitude can be done up to 50 ms before the saccade. Increasing the amplitude requires greater preparation and must be done at least 80 ms before the saccade. Reversing the saccade's direction must be done more than 100 ms before the saccade. Deubel et al. (1982) also find that correction saccades which change direction with respect to the primary saccade require about 30 ms more latency. However, there is some debate about the chronology suggested by Young, and about whether there exist separate amplitude and direction mechanisms (cf. Lévy-Schoen and Blanc-Garin, 1974; Becker and Jürgens, 1979; Hou and Fender, 1979; Findlay and Harris, 1984; Aslin and Shea, 1987; Deubel, 1987). But again it should be noted that all these effects may have either a visual or motor source.

The preceding discussion has shown that there is no need to postulate that the main portion of saccadic latency is an incompressible time delay needed for preparation of the oculomotor apparatus. But how can we then account for the fact that saccadic latencies to simple targets are so long?

Perhaps the visual, attentional and decisional mechanisms involved in attaining a simple target are not so simple after all. In fact the model outlined above suggests that even in the case of a simple target, before triggering saccade execution, the 'circle of attention' must have time to disengage from the region currently fixated (cf. Mayfrank et al., 1987), and move to the region where the target appears, otherwise gross undershoot will occur. Without prior knowledge of where to move attention, and particularly in cases where a central fixation point remains visible and thereby retains attention, an appreciable time may be necessary. Indeed, using a task where the central fixation point is extinguished before the saccade ('gap condition'), Kalesnykas and Hallett (1987) showed that accurate, visually guided (i.e. non-anticipatory) saccades can have latencies as low as 100–120 ms, a value which in humans is probably very close to the sum of the times for afference and efference.

4.3. Constraints on fixation durations in reading

Fixation durations in reading differ from saccadic latencies in simple step-tracking tasks in a number of ways. First, fixations are preceded and followed by saccades. There may be some basic oculomotor refractory period, perhaps needed for repotentiation of the muscles of their command centers, which prevents saccades occurring in rapid sequence. However, in fact this is not the case, as shown by the existence of 'back-to-back' saccades, that is, saccades with an effectively zero-duration fixation separating them, first observed by Lévy-Schoen and Blanc-Garin (1974) and now often found in the 'double-step' paradigm (Becker and Jürgens, 1979). Chapter 8 of this volume also shows examples of saccadic trajectories that slow down or stop briefly in the middle. In a task where subjects scanned sequences of crosses, and by investigating the effect on saccade latencies of delaying the onset of crosses with respect to the eye's arrival time upon them, Rayner et al. (1983) deduced that there was no oculomotor refractory period.

Another difference with saccadic latencies is the existence of the 'clearing-up period' suggested by

Dodge (1907). This period of poor vision after the saccade may be caused by forward masking following the smear created by the saccade, or by mechanical oscillation of the eye, dynamic overshoot (Kapoula et al., 1986), saccadic suppression (Volkmann et al., 1968) or vergence adjustments (Stromberg, 1938). Using computer-controlled, eye-contingent displays, the duration of the clearing-up period can be estimated by observing modifications in fixation durations when, at different moments following the end of the saccade, a mask is displayed which replaces the text being read. In evaluating such work it is important to bear in mind the possibility that if gross visual changes are involved, fixation durations may be determined not by visual processing, but simply by the warning signal created by the occurrence of the change itself (cf. Vaughan, 1983). Keeping this in mind, analysis of studies by Morrison (1984), Rayner et al. (1981) and Wolverton and Zola (1983) leads to 30 ms as the likely value for the clearing-up period – although its duration might also depend slightly on the size of the preceding saccade.

What conclusions can be reached about saccade control in reading? Even though, as shown above, there is actually no evidence for it, several previous authors had started from the (probably false) supposition that there is an irreducible oculomotor programming delay of about 150–200 ms preceding the saccade, to which must be added 30 ms of clearing-up period. Noting in addition that the average fixation in reading is 250 ms, they have argued that this leaves a time of only 20–70 ms at the beginning of each fixation during which saccade decisions must be made. In reading, these authors argue, saccades and fixation durations must therefore be predominantly governed by some simple pre-programmed strategy based on low-level visual information, and not on ongoing linguistic processing (Morton 1964; Bouma and de Voogd, 1974; Shebilske, 1975; Vaughan, 1978). Moreover, in an attempt to find some way of explaining how more time might be available for cognitive processing in reading, Salthouse and Ellis (1980) and Rayner et al. (1983) wondered whether the sequential, rhythmic, predictable nature of eye fixations in reading might reduce the difficulty of saccade programming in reading. But in a very elegant series of experiments they concluded that this was only minimally the case, and that even in reading there existed a 'minimal saccadic latency' of the order of 180–200 ms.

However, all these arguments are rendered unnecessary, given that the 150–200ms minimum saccadic latency may actually be part and parcel of the visual and attentional decision mechanisms that determine saccades. Nothing in the results of Salthouse and Ellis or Rayner et al., is incompatible with this idea. It is possible that in reading, visual and linguistic processes are at work, and require attention to be directed at various parts of the text. If a saccade is triggered at any moment, the eye will go to near the current focus of attention. The question is, when is the saccade triggered? Presumably different strategies may exist, depending on the reader, his attitude and abilities. McConkie (1983) and McConkie et al. (1985a) consider in detail the temporal characteristics of processing in reading, and suggest that it may be more efficient to trigger the eye before processing is complete; in that way additional visual information becomes available quickly, and processing need rely less on linguistic knowledge. This may be the case at some times. At other times it may be better to trigger saccades later, when processing has proceeded further.

4.4. Conclusion on visuo-motor constraints

An initial conclusion to be drawn from the above sections is that the visual or visuo-motor processing that determines saccade accuracy and latency is susceptible to a number of influences which will probably be present in normal reading, and which will contribute to variation in fixation durations and saccade lengths. We shall see later that some of these, in particular the center of gravity effect and the effect of eccentricity on the latency of small saccades, will be important in the strategy-tactics theory.

A second point concerns the time needed for

accurate saccades. Even in the case of an isolated target, but certainly in a complex field, the processes of extracting target location and disengaging attention from the preceding fixation point are time-consuming. It is quicker, instead of attempting to make a single, accurate saccade, to use a strategy of successive approximations: make a quick, approximate saccade, followed by a correction movement. This suggests an explanation for the findings in section 2.6, where it was shown that in reading, saccade size is not a simple function of perceptual span. For if at each saccade in reading the eye were to attempt to move to the edge of the zone of perceptibility, this would require a lot of processing: first using visual and linguistic information to process what can be processed around the fixation point, then determining the location where no further processing can be done, then disengaging attention from the current fixation point and making the saccade. Just as was the case for the isolated target, a more efficient strategy may actually be not to attempt to extract the location of the edge of the zone of perceptibility, but use crude, easily extractable visual cues such as the spaces between words, to move forward by some approximate amount that has a good chance of bringing the eye somewhere useful, and make local adjustments in the eye's position if necessary. If this were the strategy being used, then saccade size in reading would be mainly influenced, not by perceptual span, but by the crude cues being used in the eye guidance strategy. Perceptual span would only influence the probability and nature of the correction movements that occur when the general strategy fails to allow processing to continue.

A final point concerns the question of whether there is time for cognitive processing of information gathered at the fixation to influence its duration or the target of the next saccade. At present the question remains open. No firm evidence in the literature points to the existence of an incompressible motor programming period. In fact several models of oculomotor programming place most of the delay in initiating saccades at the visual and decisional levels. If this is true, then eye movements in reading may perfectly well reflect ongoing processing. However, reading strategies in which saccades are triggered before all processing is done at each point in the text may turn out to be more efficient. This may be the explanation, rather than oculomotor programming time, for the fact that many recent theorists suggest an appreciable lag between eye movements and cognitive or linguistic processing in reading.

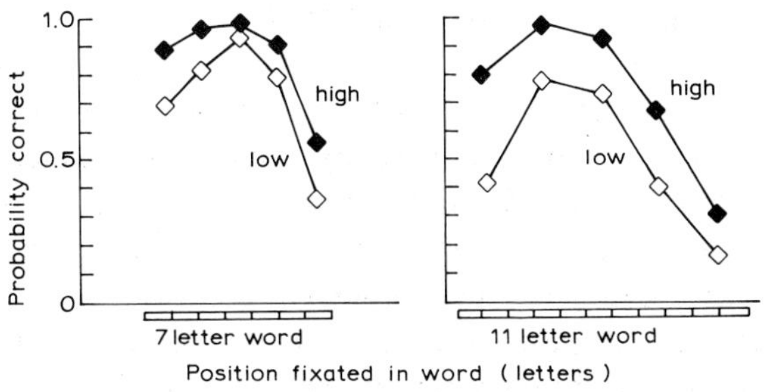

Fig. 9. Probability of correctly reporting words that appear at different positions with respect to the eye's fixation point. By use of a computer-controlled, eye-contingent display, the word was made to disappear if the eye attempted to move. The small rectangles on the abscissa represent the letters of the words where the eye could start fixating. 'high' and 'low' refer to words with high and low frequency of occurrence in French. Data points represent means over 10 words and 10 subjects. Fifty words contribute to each curve (latin square design).

5. The optimal viewing position phenomenon

Can words be recognized without eye movements? Psychologists using tachistoscopes have studied word recognition for almost a century now, and have never doubted that they can. But in their experiments the eye's fixation point is always placed near the middle of the word, where, even with visual resolution dropping off very rapidly, a maximum number of letters can be seen. Given the results in section 2.4 showing that visual span is very small, one can ask whether words can still be recognized when they are not fixated at their middles. It might be that word recognition depends critically on the position within a word that the eye fixates.

5.1. Optimal viewing position with the eye stationary

In an experiment I did to investigate this question, isolated words were presented displaced laterally by different amounts with respect to the eye's fixation point, so that on the appearance of a word the eye would be fixating one of five positions in the word. The subject's task was to read the word aloud. However, by the use of online eye-contingent control of the computer display, whenever the subject attempted to move his eye, the word being fixated disappeared and was replaced by x's. The subject was thus forced to attempt to identify the word from a single fixation point in the word, but he could keep his eye there as long as he liked.

Fig. 9 shows the probability of correctly reporting the words as a function of the position the eye was fixated. Note first that subjects cannot perfectly recognize the words. Especially in rare or long words, recognition can drop to 30–40% if the eye is fixated at an eccentric position in the word. Also interesting is the fact that frequent words were easier to report than rare words.

A second point is that there is an optimal viewing position where recognition is best. This was to be expected from the fact that visibility span is rather small, so fixating at the middle of the word would allow the most letters to be seen: the middle letters could be seen, but also the end letters, since they are not masked by flanking letters. However, contrary to expectations, the optimal viewing position is not at the middle of the words, but just left of the middle, especially for long words. We will see below that this shift is partially related to the internal informational structure of words, and partially to the mental processes responsible for word recognition.

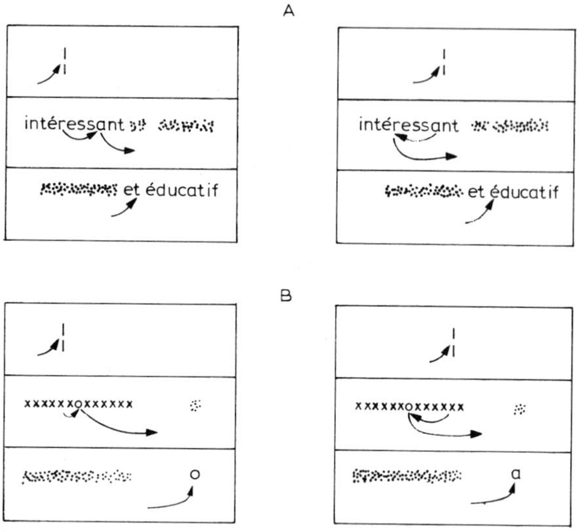

Fig. 10. A. Example of the technique used in experiments demonstrating the optimal viewing position effect. The eye fixates in the gap between two short, vertically aligned line segments. When the computer detects accurate fixation in the gap, it extinguishes the fixation marks and displays a short phrase in such a way that the eye initially fixates a certain position in the first word of the phrase, which is the word being tested. In the left hand example, this is the fourth letter, and in the right hand example it is the ninth letter. The words beyond the test word are initially masked off with random dots. The eye remains in the test word for a certain time (in the two examples it makes a second fixation in the test word, but it may make any number in the experiment), and then it makes a saccade to the next word. When the eye crosses the (imaginary) boundary between test word and remaining words, the dots are removed from the remaining words, and descend upon the test word so the eye cannot go back to re-examine it. The subject continues reading the phrase and then must make a decision as to whether it makes sense. In this case it does. An example of a phrase that does not would be: 'concombre de la solidité'.
B. The same technique as in A, but applied to a task in which the subject must fixate the middle letter of a string, and then move to a comparison letter on the right which may or may not be the same. His task is to respond 'same' or 'different'. The test string can be displayed in different positions with respect to the eye's initial position, so that on appearance the middle letter of the test string is at different distances from the fixation point.

5.2. Optimal viewing position when the eye is free to move

The finding that words cannot always be recognized from a single fixation raises the question of what happens in normal word recognition, when the eye is free to move. Obviously the word can now always be identified. But is there a penalty incurred when the eye must refixate the word because it started from a non-optimal place? A large number of experiments from my laboratory have addressed various aspects of this question, and they form the basis of the strategy-tactics theory to be described later. The main finding, which I call the 'optimal viewing position phenomenon', is that the total time the eye spends on a word before moving out of the word depends very strongly on the position where the eye starts fixating in the word.

The experiments use a method in which the eye's initial position in a word is varied, and the total time the eye spends on the word before moving on to other words is measured. The paradigm is the following (Fig. 10A). For each trial, the subject fixates a small fixation mark. When the computer detects an accurate fixation at the mark, it displays a word. The word can be displaced by varying amounts with respect to the eye, so that initially the eye may be fixating at one of several positions within the word. At the same time as the test word appears on the screen, an additional word or words is also displayed, starting at a position two letters to the right of the test word. The subject reads the test word, and then moves on, as in normal reading, to look at the remaining word or words. In one task a single non-test word is used, and the subject must decide whether it is identical to the test word. In a task more similar to normal reading, the test word plus several non-test words form a whole phrase, and the subject's task is to decide whether it is meaningful or not. In both tasks, in order to prevent processing of the non-test word or words while the eye is still on the test word, the non-test words are initially masked out by random dots so they are illegible. Only when the computer detects fixation upon them are the dots removed.

Typical data are shown in Fig. 11A. The graph shows the gaze duration on the test word, that is, the total time the eye stays on the test word before moving on to the remaining word or words. There is an optimal position, where the gaze duration on the test word is shortest. The position is at the middle or left of middle of the word, depending on its length, frequency and lexical structure, as we shall see later. The penalty for not starting to fixate at the optimal position is rather large: gaze duration increases by about 20 ms for each letter of deviation from the optimal position.

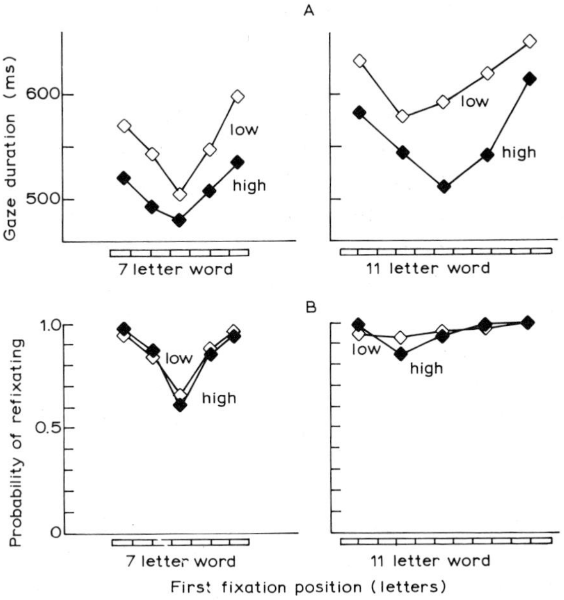

Fig. 11. A. The optimal viewing position phenomenon. The curves show the total time the eye spends on a word (gaze duration) before leaving it to read the remaining words displayed (see Fig. 10A), plotted as a function of the eye's initial fixation position in the test word (the small rectangles on the abscissa represent letters of the word). 'high' and 'low' refer to words of high and low frequency in French. Each data point represents a mean over 10 subjects reading 10 words, and 50 words contribute to each curve (latin square design).
B. For the same experiment as in A, the probability of making more than one fixation in the word as a function of the position initially fixated by the eye.

The optimal viewing position phenomenon has now been replicated in many different experiments. It is the main inspiration for the strategy-tactics theory to be presented later. I will now consider several aspects of it in detail.

5.3. Influence of lexical structure on optimal viewing position

What determines the optimal position in a word? If acuity and lateral masking were the only factors operating, it is clear that the most letters would be seen by fixating the middle of the word. However, the internal statistical structure of words may modify the situation: for example, consider a word like

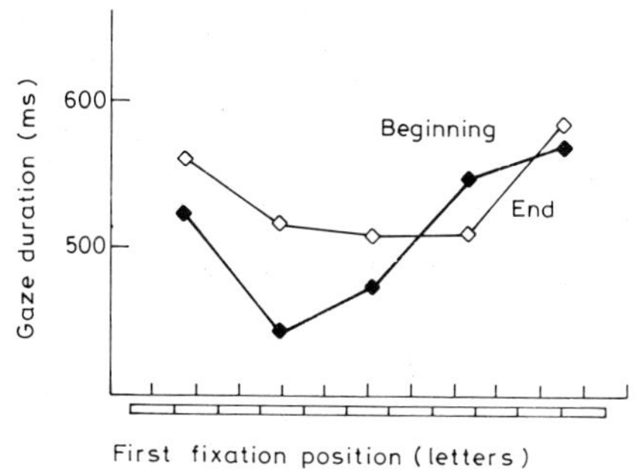

Fig. 12. Optimal viewing position curves for two types of word: words selected in the French dictionary in such a way that knowing their first six letters and approximate length allowed them to be uniquely determined ('beginning' words; examples: 'coccinelle', 'gladiateur'), and words such that knowing their last six letters and approximate length allowed the word to be uniquely determined ('end' words; examples: 'interview', 'transversal'). The words were matched for length and frequency. Each data point corresponds to 50 subjects and 2 words, with 10 words contributing to each curve in a latin square design. (From O'Regan and Lévy-Schoen, 1987)

'interview', where the first letters of the word are a commonly occurring prefix. These letters may provide less help in identifying the word than the last letters of the word. The optimal viewing position may therefore be located more to the right. The opposite might be true for words like 'elucubration', where most of the information is contained in the first half of the word. Here the optimal viewing position might be shifted towards the beginning of the word.

Fig. 12 shows the results of an experiment which attempted to verify this prediction. Whereas for words with information at the beginning, the optimal viewing position is near the beginning as expected, for words with information at the end, the optimal viewing position is not so clearly marked, and is certainly not located near the end of the words. The explanation for this asymmetry is undoubtedly related to how word-recognition processes operate. It seems that while information at the beginning of a word can be made use of efficiently, this is not true of information at the end of a word. If I give you the last few letters of a word, even if they uniquely determine the word's identity, the word may be hard to guess. It seems that the internal lexicon is organized in a left-to-right fashion, and that people cannot recognize words easily by their ends. Another point is apparent from the previous figure (Fig. 11A). Long words and rare words tend to have their optimal viewing position slightly left of the middle, whereas short words' and frequent words' optimal viewing position is closer to their middles (O'Regan and Lévy-Schoen, 1987). These differences could be related to differences in the distribution of information in words of different length and frequency, or to differences in lexical access processes. A review of the extensive psycholinguistic literature on lexical access can be found in Henderson (1982). Researchers are only now beginning to investigate the relationship between lexical structure, lexical access, and the optimal viewing position phenomenon (Holmes and O'Regan, 1987; O'Regan and Lévy-Schoen, 1987; Underwood et al., 1987, 1988).

The important point to note from all these results is that the optimal viewing position is not fixed: it is determined by the way visual constraints and internal word structure combine, and so may be different for each word. There is an unfortunate consequence for reading: the eye cannot know in advance, before landing in a word, where the optimal viewing position will be. I will come back to this problem in section 6.2.

5.4. Within-word eye movement tactics

Because it will turn out to be the 'tactics' in the strategy-tactics theory, I will now consider in detail the eye movement behavior that underlies the optimal viewing position phenomenon. For example, when the eye lands in a non-optimal position, where does the extra time needed to recognize the word come from? Presumably partly from extra fixations being made – but where and of what duration? How long does the eye stay in the non-optimal position before deciding to move? On what basis is the decision to move taken?

The natural hypothesis to make is that the eye's behavior is governed directly by the lexical processing occurring from moment to moment while the word is being recognized. At first sight all the evidence will appear to suggest that this is true. But it will turn out that in fact the situation is more complicated, with lexical processing only having an influence fairly late in the course of the scanning of a word.

Suppose that the eye lands at the optimal position. All lexical processing can be done from there, so the eye should saccade out of the word after making only a single fixation ('single-fixation tactic'). However, if the eye lands a little way from the optimal position, lexical processing will begin, but may not be able to terminate, since information about certain letters in the word is lacking. The eye would then have to refixate in the word to complete the recognition process. The probability of this 'two (or more) -fixation tactic' occurring should be higher if the initial fixation location is further from the optimal position. This indeed appears to be the pattern found (see Fig. 11B): (note by the way that even at the optimal position, the probability of refixating the word is quite high, especially for long words).

Where does the eye refixate in a word? Fig. 13 shows that when the eye is on one side of the word, it goes to the other. When it is near the middle, it goes to either one or other end. In other words, the eye is not attempting to get to the optimal viewing position. Rather, it is attempting to spread its fixations evenly over the word. This makes sense, given that once one fixation has occurred the best place to refixate will probably be on the other side of the word, where little information has as yet been gathered. This suggests that the eye's behavior is governed by lexical processing, but we shall question this later.

Things continue to look good for the hypothesis that the eye's behavior is governed by lexical processing when we examine the pattern of fixation durations in the two-fixation tactic. We expect the following: when the eye initially lands far from the optimal viewing position, very little processing can be done, and the fixation duration at this position should be very short. The eye then moves to another

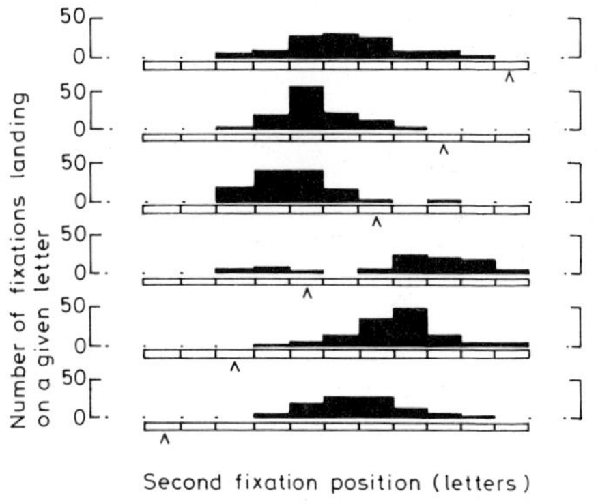

Fig. 13. Analysis of the subset of the data from O'Regan et al. (1984) when exactly two fixations were made in 11-letter words: histograms (unnormalized) showing the positions in the word where the second fixation occurred. A different histogram is plotted for each position where the first fixation could be (shown by arrows under each histogram). (Adapted from O'Regan and Lévy-Schoen, 1987)

position in the word, and there most of the processing can be done: fixation duration there should be long. On the other hand, if the eye lands near the optimal viewing position, more processing can be done on the first fixation, and less need be done on the second. There should be a trade-off between the durations of the first and second fixation in a word. Processing not done on the first fixation can be done on the second. This is also the pattern observed. To show this, Fig. 14A has been plotted in a special way. The solid curves represent first fixation durations as a function of the position where these fixations occurred. However, the dashed curves indicate the durations of the second fixations, NOT as a function of where they occurred, but as a function of where the preceding first fixations were. This was done in order to indicate for each abscissa position both the duration of the first fixation that occurred there, and the duration of the second fixation that followed that first fixation, even though it occurred somewhere else in the word. The expected trade-off between first and second fixation durations is found: when the first fixation is short because it occurs far from the optimal viewing position and little processing can be done, then the second fixation that occurs is long. Conversely, when the first

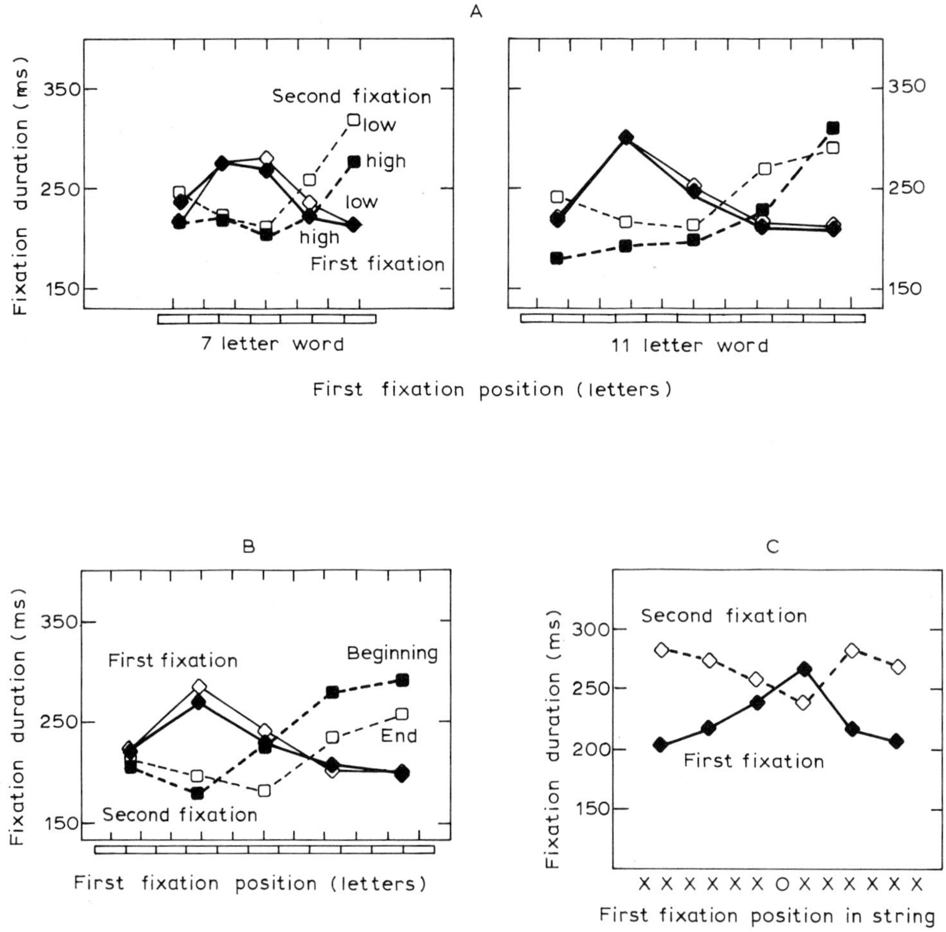

Fig. 14. A. Subset of the data of the experiment described in Fig. 12 when exactly two fixations were made: fixation duration as a function of the position of the first fixation, that is, the position of the eye at the moment the word appeared. The second fixation durations (dotted lines) are plotted at the abscissa positions where the corresponding first fixation (solid lines) occurred. In this way, the total time spent on the word as a function of the position that the eye initially fixated can be obtained by summing the data points aligned vertically at that position in the word. The thick lines (solid or dotted) correspond to high-frequency words, the thin lines (solid or dotted) to low-frequency words. (Adapted from O'Regan and Lévy-Schoen, 1987)
B. First and second fixation durations in the subset of the data of the 'beginning–end' experiment (Fig. 12) in which exactly two fixations occurred, plotted in the same way as in A. (From O'Regan and Lévy-Schoen, 1987)
C. Subset of the data of the string experiment (Fig. 10B) in which exactly two fixations occurred, plotted in the same way as in A.

fixation falls nearer the optimal viewing position, and its duration is long because more processing can be done, then second fixation duration is correspondingly shorter. In fact when the first and second durations are summed, the result is constant, independent of the position where the eye started fixating in the word. This suggests that the total amount of processing done is the same, wherever the eye starts fixating, it is just distributed differently over the word.

The above findings are again compatible with the idea that the eye's behavior is being governed by the moment to moment demands of lexical processing. But a problem appears when we consider the dif-

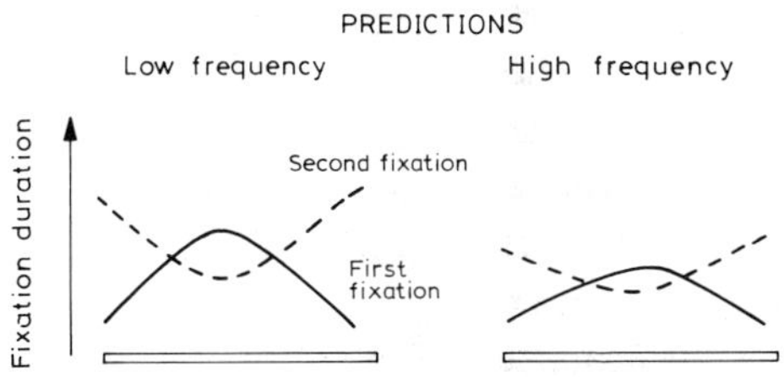

Fig. 15. Predictions that would be made for the subset of the data in which exactly two fixations occurred. For 'easy' words such as high-frequency words (a) the slopes of the first and second fixation curves should not be steep, and (b) the two curves should be fairly close together. This is because there is little processing to do, so (a) the advantage in fixating near the optimal position should not increase strongly as the eye's initial position approaches this position, and (b) the sum of the first and second fixation durations should not be great. The opposite should be true for 'hard' words like low-frequency words.

ference in behavior for words of different frequencies or different lexical structures. We would have expected that these differences would be reflected in the durations of first and second fixations. An easy word would require a smaller total time than a hard word. Fig. 15 shows the predictions: the trade-off between first and second fixation durations should continue to exist, but the curves would be flatter since their sum should be less. The thick solid or dotted lines in Fig. 14A correspond to high-frequency words, and the thin solid or dotted lines to low-frequency words. Curiously, for first fixation durations, the curves for high-frequency and low-frequency words are identical. The expected differences only appear for second fixation durations. Similar problems arise when considering words whose informational structure is manipulated. Again, virtually no difference appears on first fixation durations, only on second fixation durations (Fig. 14B).

5.5. Visuo-motor factors in the two-fixation tactic

An interesting experiment elucidates the mystery. I attempted to remove linguistic processing altogether, to see if the first/second fixation trade-off curves would become completely flat. To do this, I repeated the experiments above, but instead of having to recognize words, subjects had to simply look at a letter 'o' inserted in the middle of a string of 10 x's. Just as in the word experiments, the string appeared on the screen in a position that was displaced laterally with respect to the eye, so that subjects had to make a saccade to the 'o' at the center of the string before moving out of it. There was thus always a first fixation in some non-central string position, followed by a fixation in the middle of the string (cf. Fig. 10B). I observed that fixation durations followed exactly the same trade-off relation as for words, despite the fact that the processing involved in the task was virtually minimal, requiring only the (extremely easy) extraction of the central letter 'o' in the string of x's (Fig. 14C).

This result suggests that the hump in the first fixation duration curve, and the dip in the second fixation curve, may be caused by some mechanism other than perceptual or lexical processing. It may be that they are linked to purely visuo-motor phenomena.

One possibility to explain the hump in first fixation curves might be the eye's starting position. It is known that saccadic latency depends on the presence or absence of visual material at the fixation point (see the gap phenomenon of section 4.2). Perhaps latency also depends on how this material is arranged at the fixation point. The model presented in section 3.1 suggests that if the center of gravity of the material is at the fixation point, making a saccade to leave it might be harder than if the center of gravity is not there. We have done pilot experiments to check this hypothesis, but it appears not to be confirmed. The size and position with respect to the fixation point of a string of characters do not influence the latency of saccades made to leave the string.

Another possibility to explain the hump in the first fixation curve is the dependence of saccade latency on eccentricity: small saccades take longer to prepare than large saccades (for saccades less than about 1 degree, see section 4.2). However the simple suggestion that it is the angular size of saccades that influences their latency is not supported by an additional experiment we performed, similar to the experiment using strings of x's (Fig. 10B), but in which we doubled the subject's distance from the display. The saccades that occurred in this version of the experiment were all half as large, in angular terms, as those in the previous version. Yet their latencies did not increase in the expected way. In fact, when plotted using number of letters as abscissa, the curves for first and second versions of the experiment were exactly superposed. This shows that what is determining the latency is the number of letters the eye is moving over, irrespective of their angular size. A similar state of affairs was found in the study of perceptual span, above, where we showed that number of letters rather than angle determined perceptual span. It may be therefore that the hump in the first fixation duration curves has a perceptual and not a motor origin. In fact, more generally, the inverse correlation found for small saccades between saccade size and latency may also have a perceptual rather than a motor origin (cf. section 4.2).

One possibility might be that a target which is very easy to see does not serve as such a salient stimulus for a saccade as one which is hard to see. I have indeed confirmed that if a very visible target is used, the hump in first fixation duration curves is not so pronounced. In the case of words, where no particular visual target is present, the difficulty of judging where the eye is relative to the middle of the word may be less when the eye is near one end of the word than when it is already quite near the middle (it is easiest to tell that you are off-center when you are far off-center).

I now turn to the question of the dip in the second fixation curves. I will consider the case of the x-experiment first. Perhaps an explanation for these might be in terms of a kind of scanning rhythm in which the subject preprograms the moment at which he will make the large saccade out of the string of x's, irrespective of the moment when the first saccade in the string occurs. Preprogramming of spurts of saccades has been suggested before (Lévy-Schoen, 1981; Becker and Jürgens, 1979; Zingale and Kowler, 1987; cf. also Vaughan, 1983; Inhoff, 1986; Morrison, 1984). Another possibility might be that there is some oculomotor constraint that makes a short fixation more likely to be followed by a long one and vice versa. Yet another possibility is related to the size of the preceding saccade: when this is small, it might be easier (quicker) to make the next saccade than when the preceding saccade is larger.

We are only just beginning to study the visuomotor component, and have not yet looked at aspects such as the effect of word length, density of contours (though see Coëffé, 1985), character size and brightness, nor possible dependencies between the sizes, directions and durations of succeeding saccades or fixations. Nevertheless the finding that fixation duration trade-offs were found even in strings, where no lexical processing is involved, shows that the purely visuo-motor component in within-word tactics is important and must be further elucidated.

5.6. Conclusion on within-word eye movement tactics

Curves similar to those in Fig. 14A,B showing a trade-off between first and second fixation durations in the two-fixation tactic are very systematic and have now been observed in many different experiments performed in my laboratory. While initially we had thought that they reflected the way lexical processing is distributed over a word during recognition, closer examination showed that the fixation durations have an additional component related to visuo-motor phenomena. In fact, the lack of difference observed for words of different frequency in Fig. 14A suggests that the hump in the first fixation duration curves is probably related primarily to visuo-motor mechanisms. The dip in the second fixation duration curves also has a visuo-motor component, as suggested by the results of the experiment using strings of x's. However, in words, lexical effects are also apparent on the second fixation curves.

Similar conclusions can be reached from analysis of first and second fixation duration curves for words with different morphological or informational structure (Holmes and O'Regan, 1987; Lévy-Schoen and O'Regan, 1987): in the case of two-fixation tactics, first fixation curves are sensitive only to visuo-motor factors. Lexical processes become apparent only at the second of the two fixations that occur.

An obvious explanation for the fact that lexical processes act only on the second of the two fixations in the two-fixation tactic is that lexical processes take time, and so cannot determine the first stages of eye movement behavior. When the eye arrives in a word, its initial behavior must therefore be based on some tactic that requires no lexical knowledge. A reasonable tactic would be one that ensures that if the eye arrives in a place near one or other end of the word (from which the whole word is likely not to be visible), an additional fixation is programmed in the word. But if the eye lands near the position just left of center which is generally optimal for word recognition in French (and probably English), then no such additional fixation would be programmed. The eye would then remain in place until word recognition has been achieved. The length of time this takes would depend on the word's structure and frequency. In the case of very difficult words, a third fixation might be programmed. Their occurrence and durations could be under control of lexical processing. However, the duration of the first fixation (when several occur) would be determined purely by a visually based tactic depending only on the eye's position in the word.

This suggestion for eye movement control within words therefore consists of a superposition of two processes: a first, low-level visuo-motor process checks whether the eye is reasonably placed. It is driven by gross visual information and so can act rapidly. A second, linguistic analysis process slowly catches up on the visuo-motor process. Once it has, it can extend or shorten the currently occurring fixation.

There is an interesting consequence of the idea that, at first, only visuo-motor processes are driving the eye movement tactics within words. If this is true, then the decision as to whether or not to make a second fixation, as well as where to go, must also be based on a visuo-motor and not a lexical criterion. This is rather counter-intuitive for the following reason. One would have expected to find that the probability of making a second fixation should depend on how close the eye is to the optimal viewing location, with the likelihood of having to refixate being smallest at the optimal position. But the argument made here shows that this cannot be true, because the optimal location depends on the word's lexical structure. The decision whether to move can only be based on some purely visually definable cue, such as the closeness to the generally optimal position. That this may be true is suggested by the fact that even though high-frequency 11-letter words have their optimal viewing position near the middle (Fig. 11A), the probability of making more than one fixation in these words is actually lower near their third or fourth letters (Fig. 11B). Another prediction that must be made from the idea that lexical processing cannot influence the probability of refixating is that this probability should not be affected by a word's frequency or lexical structure. Fig. 11B shows that, as expected, there is little difference in the probabilities of refixating for high- and low-frequency words, although a small difference does appear in the middle of 7-letter words and near the 3rd or 4th letter of 11-letter words. This difference might arise because at this position, which is generally the optimal position, the eye will generally stay for a long time, so lexical processing may actually have a chance of being able to influence the probability of refixating after all.

5.7. Optimal viewing position versus 'preferred viewing position'

Up until now, studies on optimal viewing position have been done in conditions where a word appears at the eye's fixation point, and the subject must read the word and move on to a second word. This situation is different from normal reading in a number of respects, and we should ask whether in normal reading there still exists an optimal viewing position. Several studies in the past have looked at where the eye tends to land in words in normal reading, and

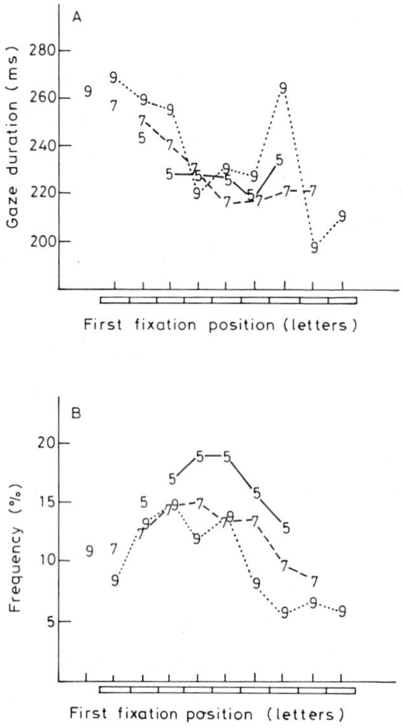

Fig. 16. Graphs plotted from data on continuous reading of texts, provided by Blanchard and McConkie (personal communication). The top graph gives the total gaze duration on words of length 5, 7 and 9 letters as a function of the first position the eye fixates in the word. The middle position on the abscissa corresponds to the middle of the words. The first point of the graph for each word length is not connected to the other points because it corresponds to a fixation occurring in the space preceding the word. For word lengths 5, 7 and 9, the data are derived from 2578, 1642 and 623 fixations, respectively. The last 3 data points for the 9-letter case are noisy because there were very few observations per data point. The lower graph gives histograms of the positions where the first fixations fell, expressed as a percentage of the total number falling on the word or in the preceding space. (From O'Regan and Lévy-Schoen, 1987)

have observed that this position is at the middle or left of middle of words (Rayner, 1979; Dunn-Rankin, 1978). But this position, where the eye 'prefers' to land (the 'preferred viewing position') need not logically be the same as the 'optimal' position, which is the position where recognition is most efficient. In fact, analysis of a large corpus of reading data I have obtained from Blanchard and McConkie shows that the position where the eye tends to land is in fact different from the generally optimal position, that is, the position where recognition was quickest, as measured from the same data. The generally optimal position is near the middle of words (Fig. 16A), while the 'preferred' landing position is nearer the third letter of words (Fig. 16B).

5.8. Optimal viewing position in normal reading

Research on the optimal viewing position in normal reading requires investigation of the total time taken to recognize a word as a function of where the eye happens to land in the word in reading. At present no published work exists on this question, but again the preliminary data from Blanchard and McConkie (see Fig. 16) show that the optimal viewing position continues to exist. However, two differences with my data on isolated words appear. First, the optimal viewing position is at the center of words, even for long words, whereas I have always found that for long, low-frequency words the optimal position is slightly left of middle (Fig. 11). This difference is not serious, because it is likely that in the (elementary) texts read by Blanchard and McConkie's subjects, mainly frequent words were used. A second difference is more serious: in Blanchard and McConkie's data, the penalty for not fixating at the optimal viewing position is about 10 ms per letter of deviation from the optimal position. This is half the value I have systematically found on the first words of short phrases, and some explanation for the difference is required.

Vitu and O'Regan (1988) tested two possibilities. The first explanation is that in normal reading, parafoveal information gathered during the fixation preceding the eye's arrival in each word allows processing of the word to begin. This might lessen the need to refixate the word when the eye lands in a non-optimal position. We found no evidence that this was happening. Preprocessing did in one experiment (but not in a more recent experiment) increase recognition speed, but it did not modify the penalty for not fixating the optimal viewing position (interestingly it also did not displace the optimal viewing position rightwards, as might have been expected).

A second possibility which might explain the lesser penalty in normal reading is the idea that in normal reading, a rhythmic fixation strategy which drives the eye onwards is used, suppressing many refixations in words. However, in another experiment where a reading rhythm was simulated by having subjects successively fixate two separated asterisks before fixating the target word, we found no evidence for this idea (Vitu and O'Regan, 1988).

It may be that the forward-going strategy suggested here could not be used in the simulated reading task. In normal reading, subjects can take the risk of now and then not successfully identifying a word, since context will generally help out. Adopting this risky tactic was perhaps not possible in our task, where no context was available. Context may also help in improving the ability to extract parafoveal visual cues (McClelland and O'Regan, 1981), thereby reducing the probability of refixation. Further work on the influence of context on the optimal viewing position phenomenon is needed.

More evidence in favor of the existence of the optimal viewing position in normal reading is provided by McConkie et al. (1989). These authors analysed the probability that a word will be refixated as a function of the position where the eye initially falls in the word. They found very clear evidence that the probability of refixating the word depends on the eye's landing position in the word, with an optimal position near the center of words.

6. A strategy-tactics theory of eye movements in reading

6.1. Summary up to now

I began this chapter by arguing that the perceptual span control hypothesis is false: sizes of saccades in reading do not correspond to estimates of the amount of material that can be seen at each fixation. An explanation for the discrepancy came from the findings in sections 3 and 4, showing how eye movements are restricted by visuo-motor constraints: aiming the eye accurately is a time-consuming process involving extraction of the target location and needing attention to be disengaged from the current fixation point. If the desired target location were defined as the edge of the perceptual span, determining its position would require not only visual, but also perceptual and perhaps preliminary lexical processing: saccadic latencies would have to be much longer than the 250-ms average fixation duration observed in reading. I therefore suggest that in reading a different strategy must be used in which eye movements and perceptual and linguistic processing are not so intimately yoked, but proceed autonomously. The proposal is that first, a global, preprogrammed scanning routine driven only by coarse visual cues guides the eye across the text; second, perceptual, lexical and linguistic analysis of the text is done continuously, and this can intermittently regulate the scanning routine by delaying the triggering of a saccade or by triggering it prematurely if the rate of information intake is too fast or too slow.

Similar proposals for eye movement guidance had been made by some early authors who also believed that saccade programming required long latencies. Thus, Buswell (1937), Morton (1964), Kolers and Lewis (1972), Andriessen and de Voogd (1973) and Bouma and de Voogd (1974), believed that the eye moved forward with a reading 'rhythm' which was adjusted in such a way that the rate of information intake kept approximately in step with the rate of linguistic processing. A minor difference between this old 'oculomotor' kind of theory and the theory I now wish to outline is that before, researchers thought that the necessity for long saccade programming delays came from an incompressible oculomotor programming delay, whereas it now seems more likely that the delay is due to the difficulty of extracting the target from its surroundings and disengaging attention from the present eye location. But the essential difference between the old 'reading rhythm' theory and the 'strategy-tactics' theory I will now present will be the fact that our greater knowledge about visuomotor constraints, and about the optimal viewing position phenomenon, allows much more precise predictions to be made about exactly where the eye goes in reading, and how long it stays where it does. Thus, although both the old oculomotor theories and the strategy-tactics theory postulate an autonomous scanning routine, in the strategy-tactics theory, because of visuo-motor constraints and the optimal viewing position phenomenon, this routine turns out not to be a rhythm, nor to have saccades of constant amplitude. The precise characteristics will be set out below.

6.2. A scanning routine for 'careful word-by-word' reading

In the proposal I wish to present, I will make the assumption that in reading the reader proceeds in a word-by-word fashion, completing recognition (or some stage of recognition) of each word before going on to the next word. I will call this 'careful word-by-word reading'. This kind of reading may not actually exist, but it will be a starting point which can be improved upon so as to correspond to more normal kinds of reading.

The existence of an optimal viewing position in words, and the large penalty in recognition time incurred when the eye fixates in a non-optimal position, suggests that in careful word-by-word reading it would be advantageous to aim the eye accurately to the optimal position in each word. In fact, if the penalty for not fixating the optimal position is the same in normal reading as for isolated words, then an error of only two or three letters in aiming precision would lead to a 40 or 60 ms increase in recognition time. Given that normal fixation durations in reading are 250 ms on average, this penalty would give rise to a 15–25% decrease in reading rate, which is considerable.

Of course there are probably differences between optimal viewing position in reading and optimal viewing position in isolated words. Parafoveal preprocessing or linguistic context might modify the phenomenon, perhaps by diminishing the penalty for not fixating the optimal viewing position, or by modifying its location in words (though see Vitu and O'Regan, 1988). Further, the notion of optimal viewing position in words should perhaps be generalized to groups of words: particularly groups of two or three very short words may be recognized in a single fixation if this fixation is appropriately placed. I will leave these issues for future work, and assume provisionally that in careful reading the optimal viewing position in each word is used, and that an efficient strategy for careful reading would be to move the eye from optimal viewing position to optimal viewing position.

But unfortunately, as we have seen in the preceding sections, the exact place where the optimal viewing position is located in each word depends on characteristics of the particular word (such as its informational or morphemic structure, frequency and length) and so cannot be known in advance. If the eye were to attempt to calculate, from poor-quality peripheral information, where this optimal viewing position might be, then we would be back to the situation of the perceptual span control hypothesis, where eye movements would be guided by the result of some time-consuming perceptual or linguistic calculation. If this were true, then we should have found a direct relationship between perceptual span and saccade size, which we didn't.

Instead of using the true optimal viewing position, an effective scanning routine must therefore somehow use coarse visual clues to take a bet on where in each successive word the optimal location generally is. Now, from the data available for French words of various length, frequency and structure, the 'generally optimal' position is at the middle or a little left of the middle of words. A reasonable bet for a scanning routine would therefore be to aim the eye to this 'generally optimal' position, i.e. to the middle or left of middle of each successive word (for French).

But can the eye attain this position accurately, and what happens when it misses? The section on visuo-motor constraints showed that even when the target position is defined in coarse visual terms, in the case of a complex visual field, as found in reading, accurate aim may still be quite time-consuming. In the 250 ms of an average fixation in reading, can the eye determine the location of the word's boundaries, estimate the middle of this region, and send the eye there? Evidence from studies with series of isolated crosses to fixate, which is presumably simpler than estimating the middle of a word, show that with fixation durations around 300 ms accuracy is far from perfect, and many correction saccades are made (Rayner et al., 1983; Kapoula, 1984). Thus, in reading, not only is it better not to wait for the edge of the perceptual span to be extracted, it may also not even be a good idea to wait for such an apparently easy-to-extract location as the generally optimal position to be located. It may be more efficient instead to program an approximate saccade quickly, and have a 'rescue tactic' ready when the eye arrives in the wrong place.

What exactly would the appropriate rescue tactic be? Presumably precisely the one I have observed in word recognition in the preceding sections, and which gives rise to the optimal viewing position phenomenon. That is, when the eye lands beyond a critical distance from the generally optimal viewing position, it rapidly makes a saccade bringing it to the other side of the word from where it is. (It might have been thought that an appropriate rescue tactic would be to make a correction movement bringing the eye accurately to the generally optimal viewing position. This would be analogous to the correction saccade that occurs when saccading to a target in a visual scene. However, the data (Fig. 13) for isolated words suggests that actually a more effective tactic is to move to the other side of the word – presumably even though the initial fixation was in a non-optimal place, some lexical processing would have started there, and it is better to move the eye somewhere where the most processing remains to be done.)

In summary: reading involves two fairly autonomous processes: a process of lexical and linguistic analysis which occurs on the basis of the available visual information; and a pre-programmed scanning routine which uses only coarse, easy-to-extract visual cues to guide the eye, but does so in such a way that (1) the eye quite frequently falls near the generally optimal viewing position of each word, but (2) when it does not, rescue tactics are engaged which allow the word still to be recognized. A suitable scanning routine would be the following (but see later for other possibilities).

Between-word strategy: When leaving a word, attempt (within the possibilities of visuo-motor constraints) to move to the 'generally optimal' viewing position (for French and probably English: middle or left of middle of the next word).

Within-word rescue tactics: If the landing error relative to the generally optimal position is greater than some critical value (to be defined), immediately make a saccade to the other side of the word from where you currently are. Then return to the between-word strategy.

6.3. Temporal aspects of the scanning routine, and cognitive intervention

As yet I have not discussed the temporal aspects of this scanning routine. What determines WHEN the between-word or within-word saccades occur? The hypothesis that can be made for 'careful word-by-word reading' is that the eye only moves to the next word when the word has been 'recognized' (i.e., some well-defined stage in the word recognition process has been attained – see later for other possibilities). Triggering the between-word saccades would thus be under the control of the ongoing lexical and linguistic processing. Triggering the within-word rescue saccades would be under the autonomous control of the scanning routine, and would occur automatically when the generally optimal position had been missed.

There is an interesting consequence of the idea that between-word saccades are triggered by word recognition. Consider the case when the fixated word is highly predictable or easy to recognize. Saccade triggering will occur very rapidly: in fact it may occur well before an accurate target can be determined for the saccade. The saccade may therefore be very inaccurate. This seems most likely to occur when the eye lands on a short, predictable word, or a word that was already partially processed in parafoveal vision before the eye landed on it. The consequence of this is that in reading easy text, it may often happen that the eye doesn't manage to land anywhere near the generally optimal viewing position of the next word, and may even land somewhere outside the next word. In particular, when the next word is a short word, because of the center of gravity effect, the word following the short word may exert an influence on the saccade, and the eye may tend to skip over the short word. But this is not a catastrophe, because if reading is easy, then there may be less need to land accurately at the generally optimum position.

An implication of this is also that despite the fact that I have called this kind of reading 'careful word-by-word' reading, the eye actually may not move from word to word. When the currently fixated word is easy to recognize, saccade size variability becomes greater.

6.4. Lexical influences on saccade size and fixation duration

A number of points about this proposition for eye movement guidance should be made. The first point concerns which kinds of information influence saccade size.

Saccade size is assumed to be determined only by coarse visual information concerning the inter-word spaces. The justification for this is the idea obtained from the section on visuomotor constraints that saccade size computation is difficult in a complex task such as reading. If the eye were to take account of perceptual cues such as letter or word identity, this would require even more time than taking account of coarse visual clues, and I concluded that doing this was difficult enough given the 250-ms fixation durations found in reading. Linguistic processing is, therefore, very unlikely to affect saccade sizes unless the prior fixation is unusually long.

The idea that saccade size generally does not depend on lexical or linguistic information implies that the eye cannot usually jump over a predictable word, or a word that is easy to recognize in parafoveal vision. In addition, when within-word tactics occur, the position the eye goes to when refixating a word cannot be determined by the identity of the word and, a fortiori, it cannot depend on where the true optimal viewing position of the word is, only on where the 'generally optimal' position is, since only this can be determined from coarse visual information about inter-word spaces.

Another point concerns what the present proposal predicts about fixation durations. Whereas saccade sizes are assumed to be exclusively determined by inter-word spaces, fixation durations are governed in two different ways, depending on whether they precede between-word saccades or within-word saccades. Between-word saccades are triggered by the completion of some stage of lexical processing. Fixation durations preceding them should be influenced by the difficulty of this processing, and therefore should reflect aspects of the word such as its frequency, length or morphemic structure. Within-word saccades, however, are governed by the autonomous scanning routine's detecting that fixation in the word is insufficiently near the generally optimal position. The visual processing necessary to detect that this has happened is probably in general more rapid than lexical processing. I therefore predict that when the eye lands far from the generally optimal viewing position and two fixations occur in a word, then the duration of the first of the two fixations will be determined purely by visuo-motor constraints. In particular, we have seen in the study of 2-fixation tactics in the case of isolated words that the duration of the first fixation of the two will depend on the position in the word where it occurs.

Another interesting aspect of the present model concerns the probability of making two fixations in a word. Again, the model supposes that a rescue tactic will be invoked when the eye misses the generally optimal viewing position. This is not dependent on the word's lexical structure and, in particular, it does not depend on where the optimal viewing position in the word really is, only on where the eye lands with respect to the 'generally optimal' position.

6.5. Alternative scanning routines for different occasions

The present proposition of 'careful, word-by-word' reading is only an idealized step towards more realistic models, and can be modified in various ways.

One possible modification concerns the moment at which between-word saccades are triggered. The suggestion made above that saccades leave a word after some phase of 'recognition' has occurred leaves open the question of exactly what phase of recognition is involved: is it the identification of the word's constituent letters, the generation of some preliminary access code, the completion of some phonological recoding process, access to knowledge of the word's presence in the internal lexicon, or the access to the word's meaning? These are open questions, but I suspect that the various intermediate stages of word recognition cannot normally generate 'signals' that can be used to trigger saccades, and attending to the covert stages of word recognition would require additional processes which are alien to normal reading. One candidate for a saccade-triggering signal might be the generation of an articulatory or 'pre-articulatory' response, as when one sub-vocalizes a word to oneself or 'hears' it while reading.

But this is only one of a range of other possibilities that might trigger between-word saccades. At the most 'motor' level, each saccade could serve as the warning stimulus to trigger the next saccade. This would lead to a very fast sequence of saccades, but they would be rather inaccurate, and frequently miss the generally optimal viewing position. In addition, there would be little time for the visual percept to clear up after each saccade. This kind of scanning can be experienced by moving the eyes in a very rapid series of saccades (not a smooth pursuit movement, which is impossible to make without a moving target) across the lines, so that the words seem to glide past the eye and appear blurred, and reading is impossible except at the ends of the lines where the eye stops for longer.

Another possibility for an event that might be used to trigger between-word saccades might be some visual event, such as detection of the retinal image becoming immobile or cleared up. Another possibility would be to trigger the saccade when the eye's position in the word can be ascertained (e.g. 'I am about in the middle of the word, I am on the left edge of the word, etc.').

These different possibilities would require varying amounts of time, and would therefore lead to latencies of different durations and saccades of varying degrees of accuracy, and so to different styles of reading. It would be the reader's choice which of such styles he or she wished to adopt, as a function of the amount of time he or she wished to assign to lexical processing and text-understanding, and of the risk he or she was willing to take of having to reread.

A further modification of the strategy-tactics model suggested here is certainly necessary to account for the way children or very slow readers read. For these readers, word recognition perhaps cannot usually be done in one or two fixations, and the simple, visually based within-word scanning tactics I proposed for normal reading would not apply. Instead, such readers may use some form of more extensive within-word scanning. Since, as seen in section 4.2, making small saccades is difficult, these within-word fixations will have to be long. This purely visuo-motor factor may be important in understanding children's eye movements. Other factors, such as an increased need to reread sentence portions, would of course also contribute.

Another place where the strategy-tactics model presented here might be modified is in its spatial characteristics. I have suggested that the eye should attempt to aim at the 'generally optimal' viewing positions in successive words. But an almost equally viable strategy might be to aim say three characters beyond the next space. It might equally be feasible simply to move forward a fixed number of letters. The reader might also adopt the riskier strategy of not fixating each word at all, and attempt to jump only to every other word. Different readers may have evolved different strategies. Certainly different strategies will have to be used in alphabetic languages where spaces between words are not marked, such as Thai, or in Chinese, where spaces between words and between within-word morphemes are not distinguished. In Japanese, function and content words can be distinguished on the basis of visual density (content words end in denser kanji symbols), and this may sometimes help to direct the eye. However, all these strategies will have to comply with the constraints of visuo-motor programming. In particular, inter-word strategies requiring precise aiming are probably unrealistic.

Another question concerns the within-word tactics. According to the suggestions made above, these were triggered by the eye's arriving 'too far' from the 'generally optimal' viewing position. Now different readers may use different definitions of the generally optimal position, and different definitions of 'too far', and in fact the adequacy of their definitions may explain part of the differences in their reading speeds. One factor contributing to the difference between fast and slow readers might be that fast readers have evolved an aiming strategy that tends to get their eyes more accurately on the generally optimal viewing position. A given reader could induce different reading styles by modulating the criterion used for refixation: for fast reading, a tactic of making no within-word refixations at all might be used.

7. Evidence for and against the strategy-tactics theory

Despite various modifications that might be made to the between-word strategy and within-word tactics to accommodate different reading styles, different readers, different languages and different tasks that the reader sets himself or herself, the main characteristics of the strategy-tactics proposal remain invariant and are amenable to testing. Since the theory is new, little work has as yet been done to test it directly. In the following sections I will review what already existing evidence is relevant.

7.1. Evidence on saccade size

An essential premise of the strategy-tactics theory is

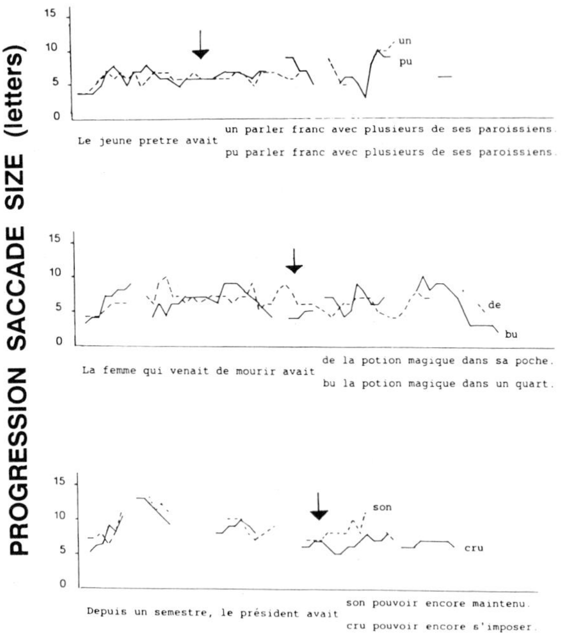

Fig. 17. Progression saccade size for saccades leaving each letter of the sentences shown on the abscissa. Each data point is a median over saccades made by 22 subjects leaving that letter and the two adjacent letters. The solid curves correspond to sentences containing the verb, the dashed curves to sentences containing the article. Gaps in the curves are places where there were fewer than six saccades contributing to the data. The arrows show the critical location where differences in saccade sizes should occur if the eye is making use of parafoveal information about word identity to aim saccades. The top sentence is an example where no differences appeared. Seven out of 10 of the sentences in this experiment gave data like this. The middle sentence is an example where a difference did appear in the critical region. However, this may have been noise, because similar differences appeared in other regions (see saccades leaving the word 'qui' at the beginning of the sentence). The third sentence is an example where the difference did appear to be significant. Further analysis showed the difference to occur only in those saccades which were preceded by long fixations.

the idea that saccades are hard to aim accurately, so neither between-word saccades nor within-word saccades should generally show influences of ongoing lexical processing. The only variables that should influence saccade sizes in reading should be variables related to crude visual information such as the lengths of words or the position of spaces in the text, and center of gravity effects should be strong. However, an exception to this principle might occur when the fixation duration before a saccade is particularly long (this might happen if the eye lands at the generally optimal position and the word is difficult to process). In that case, there would be time for the computation of the following saccade to take into account lexical factors.

Crude visual clues certainly influence saccade size: I have found that saccades leaving or going into long words are longer (O'Regan, 1979, 1980). More recent evidence comes from the careful study by McConkie et al. (1988), to be described in the next section. My interpretation of the experiments using moving windows of different sizes is also that crude visual clues influence saccade size (cf. section 2.2).

A more critical test of the strategy-tactics theory concerns the assertion that saccade sizes must generally not be affected by lexical factors. A potentially excellent test of this was my 'THE-skipping' experiment (O'Regan, 1979). In this experiment, I had constructed pairs of sentences which had a common beginning, but which could end in one of two ways, one with a segment beginning with the word THE and one with a segment beginning with a three-letter verb. Under the strategy-tactics theory, there should be no difference in behavior when saccading into the THE or the three-letter verb. The only exception to this would be cases when the fixation before the saccade was unusually long. This would allow parafoveal processing to be influenced by the frequency or the lexical category of the THE or three-letter verb, and a difference in saccade size might appear, presumably with the eye skipping over the THE more readily than over the three-letter verb.

At the time, I had found that saccades were longer when saccading towards the THE than towards the verb. The effect was weak, amounting to a difference of only 1–2 letters. Was the effect weak because in fact, as predicted by the strategy-tactics theory, THE-skipping was occurring only when the eye happened to make a long fixation in the previous word? Unfortunately at the time I did not test for this prediction, and the data are no longer available to check it. I have therefore repeated the experiment recently, using French readers, and sentences containing either the French definite and indefinite articles 'le', 'un', 'du', 'de' and 'des' (highly frequent), or the (less frequent) verbs 'bu', 'du', 'lu', 'vu', 'été', 'ri', 'cru', 'pu', 'va'. For seven out of the ten pairs of sentences, there was no difference between the saccade size approaching the article and the saccade size approaching the verb (an example is shown in the top graph of Fig. 17). For the remaining three sentence pairs, differences appeared (bottom two graphs in Fig. 17) similar to those found in my 1979 experiment. Analysis of the durations of the fixations preceding the saccades that are influenced by the article/verb distinction shows that differences only appear when preceding fixations are of particularly long duration. This is precisely as predicted by the strategy-tactics theory.

A number of other authors have also considered whether or not lexical or linguistic factors can influence the probability of skipping a target word. Some studies found no skipping (Zola, 1984; Ehrlich and Rayner, 1981, second experiment). Other studies found skipping (Pollatsek et al., 1986; Just and Carpenter, 1980; Ehrlich and Rayner, 1981, first experiment; Balota et al., 1985; Schustack et al., 1987). Of these, Pollatsek et al. (1986) analysed fixation durations prior to the word being skipped, and found, as predicted by the strategy-tactics theory, that these were longer than when no skipping occurred. Unfortunately the other studies did not check whether skipping occurred predominantly when prior fixation duration was long. Also, when skipping was found, it may have been caused by purely visual factors. This is because it is very difficult to design an experiment where visual factors are kept completely constant, and yet lexical factors change. For example, if you notice that function words tend to be skipped more often than content words, this may merely be because function words tend to be shorter (cf. Kliegl et al., 1982, 1983). As another example, suppose you want to manipulate the predictability of a word to see if this influences its probability of being skipped. To do this, you have to change the word itself, or the context in which the word appears. These changes will almost inevitably be accompanied by visual changes. In fact, even in my THE-skipping experiment mentioned above, the effects might be due to something about the overall shape of the word THE rather than on its lexical category.

Another test of the strategy-tactics theory was provided by experiments in which perceptual span was modified. According to the theory, since saccades from word to word are determined only by crude visual parameters, such as word length, so long as visibility is sufficient to see the block-shapes formed by words, word-to-word saccades in reading should be unaffected even in conditions of a small perceptual span. This is counter to the idea that saccade size might be approximately adjusted to perceptual span size. Evidence relevant to this issue has already been presented in section 2.6, where it was indeed noted that changes in perceptual span provoked by changing viewing distance did not affect saccade size in reading. A further study by Lévy-Schoen and O'Regan (1987), in which perceptual span was very strongly reduced by blurring the retinal image, also showed stability of saccade sizes, as predicted. However, in both this and the O'Regan et al. (1983) experiments, fixation durations did rise significantly when perceptual span decreased. This can be explained by invoking changes in the within-word tactics, which are sensitive to lexical processing and thus perceptual span.

7.2. Evidence on landing position

The strategy-tactics theory suggests that the eye in reading should ideally be aiming at the 'generally optimal' position in words, but that visuo-motor constraints, in particular the center of gravity effect, would prevent it from accurately attaining this position, particularly when preceding fixation durations are short.

Dunn-Rankin (1978) and Rayner (1978) had investigated the position in words where the eye tends to land, and found that this position, called the 'preferred landing position', is near the middle or left of middle of words. This certainly suggests that the eye is not moving randomly, and is aiming somewhere definite. But the result does not tell whether the position actually attained is the position being aimed at. In fact Blanchard and McConkie's data mentioned in sections 5.7 and 5.8 (Fig. 16) showed that the position the eye tends to attain is in fact different from the generally optimal position.

This is compatible with the pattern observed recently by McConkie et al. (1988), who examined landing positions in words of different length in reading as a function of the eye's launch site in the preceding word, and came to the conclusion that the eye was indeed attempting to aim for a particular location in words (which they called the 'functional target location'), but that it does not accurately attain it. When the eye starts very close to the next word it tends to overshoot this location, and when it starts very far from it it tends to undershoot the location. This kind of spread in landing positions is similar to the range effects observed by Kapoula (1985). It is compatible with the center of gravity effect, and is expected from the strategy-tactics theory when fixation durations are short.

7.3. Evidence on fixation durations

The predictions of the strategy-tactics theory concerning fixation durations are as follows.

A. (i) Gaze duration, that is, the sum of fixation durations on a word in reading, should be strongly dependent on the first location where the eye fixates in the word, and show an optimum viewing position curve as found in the experiments on individual words described in section 5. (ii) Gaze duration should also depend strongly on lexical processing.

B. (i) When a single fixation occurs in a word, its duration should not depend strongly on the eye's position. (ii) However, it should depend strongly on lexical processing.

C. When two fixations occur in a word, the duration of the first should depend strongly on its location in the word, but not strongly on lexical factors. The duration of the second should depend strongly both on the position of the first fixation and on lexical processing (with the trade-off curves as found in Fig. 14).

These predictions have never been tested in the literature, but in some cases partial evidence can be gleaned from existing work. Prediction A(i), the dependence of gaze duration in a word on the eye's initial fixation location in a word, is the cornerstone of the strategy-tactics theory. It has of course been confirmed for the first word of short phrases, since this is the optimum viewing position phenomenon described in section 5. In normal reading it has been confirmed in the unpublished data provided to me by Blanchard and McConkie (see Fig. 16, and discussion in section 5.8). However, further verification is necessary. In particular, it would be interesting to do a reading experiment in which words only become visible when the eye lands upon them. This would prevent parafoveal processing of upcoming words from modifying the optimum viewing position phenomenon, and similar optimal viewing positions should be found as in the experiments reported in section 5.

Prediction A(ii) that gaze duration should depend on lexical processes was confirmed in multiple regression analyses by Just and Carpenter (1980), although Kliegl et al. (1982, 1983) noted that most of the effects might not be lexical but merely related to word length. An explanation of the weakness of lexical effects on gaze duration may be the existence of a very strong effect of initial fixation location expected from the strategy-tactics theory, which might swamp lexical effects on gaze duration if first fixation location is not factored out. Further work must be done similar to Carpenter and Just's and Kliegl et al.'s, but in which initial fixation location is also used as a factor in the multiple regression.

An extremely interesting study by Hogaboam (1983) came very close to being a test for the strategy-tactics theory's predictions concerning the effect of initial fixation location on the duration of single, first of two, or second of two fixations (predictions B and C). Using a reading task, Hogaboam classified patterns of saccades into various classes, including within-word and between-word saccade sequences. He then applied multiple regression analysis to attempt to determine what factors influenced which fixation durations in the particular patterns. Of interest here is his analysis of the influence of lexical factors such as word frequency and length on fixation duration in the case where a single fixation on a word occurred, and in the case when two fixations occurred before the eye left the word. Hogaboam found that when a single fixation occurred, this fixation's duration was affected significantly by lexical factors. This is as predicted from the strategy-tactics theory. When two fixations occurred on the word, Hogaboam distinguished two patterns: a regressive one, where the second fixation was in the word, but to the left of the first fixation, and a progressive one, where the second fixation was in the word but to the right of the first. For the regressive pattern, lexical factors affected the second fixation duration, but not the first. This is expected from the strategy-tactics theory. However, for the progressive pattern, lexical factors affected the first fixation duration, but not the second. This result is not expected from the strategy-tactics theory. However, one of the stepwise regressions performed by Hogaboam in this case only showed a marginally significant contribution of lexical factors. It is possible that some of the progressive patterns were cases where the progressive saccade was aimed to the following word and undershot. The first fixation would have been at the generally optimum position and therefore reflected lexical processes. Further work must be done to check this. In addition, a better test of the strategy-tactics theory would have been possible if the initial fixation point in the word had been included as a factor in the multiple regression analysis.

Some other studies in addition to Hogaboam's are relevant to the question of the effects of lexical factors on the duration of fixations. But unfortunately these studies did not distinguish within-word tactics in which single fixations were made from tactics when two fixations were made. Authors have used the measures 'average fixation duration on a word', which may include contributions from first and further fixations, or 'first fixation duration', which means 'first' independently of whether there were one or more fixations in the word. Since both these measures include cases when a first and single fixation was made, I predict that both will reflect lexical processing somewhat. But because both of these measures are diluted by the presence of first fixations when there are two in a word, and these first fixations are not expected to depend on lexical factors, the composite measures will not be as sensitive as they could be to lexical factors. The eye's initial fixation location in a word will also influence these measures and increase their variability. Nevertheless, the strategy-tactics theory predicts that lexical processing should affect these measures, albeit weakly because of the confoundings.

Rayner (1977) studied eye behavior in sentences of the form 'The + subject + verb + the + object + prepositional phrase'. He found that 'average' fixation duration on the verb was longer by about 20–30 ms than on the subject or object. Ehrlich and Rayner (1981) tested the effect of context on fixation durations, and found that 'average' fixation duration on an unexpected word was longer than on an expected word. However, the authors did not use item statistics to verify that the effects were not due to one or two peculiar items in the experimental material. Zola (1984) showed that the 'first' fixation duration on a noun preceded by an adjective was 16 ms shorter if the noun was strongly rather than weakly constrained by the adjective (e.g., moviegoers desire 'buttered popcorn' vs. 'adequate popcorn'). First fixation duration was also longer if the noun was misspelled. However, again no item statistics were done. Underwood and McConkie (1985) did a study in which, during reading, the eye sometimes fell on a word in which several letters were replaced by dissimilar letters, so that the word could not be recognized. The authors observed that the duration of the affected fixation increased by 12 ms. Rayner and Duffy (1986) studied the effects of various lexical variables (frequency, lexical complexity and ambiguity) on eye movements. They found that 'first' fixation duration on a high-frequency word was shorter than on a low-frequency word by about 37 ms. Inhoff (1984) attempted to determine whether in word recognition during reading, lexical access and word interpretation are two separate processes or not. He studied the effect of word frequency and contextual constraint on first fixation and gaze duration in cases when there was or was not a small (1 or 3 letter) foveal mask that moved with the eye. Inhoff observed weak effects of frequency but stronger effects of predictability (contextual constraint) on 'first' fixation duration. On the other hand, Balota et al. (1985) observed that the 'first' fixation duration on a word was influenced by whether the parafoveal preview of that word was visually similar to it, but not by whether the word was predictable from its context.

All these findings, which generally show weak but consistent effects of lexical variables such as word frequency, contextual constraint, lexical category, are consistent with the strategy-tactics theory. But it is likely that stronger data would have been obtained if the effects on single and multiple fixations had been analysed separately, and if initial fixation location in words had been taken into account.

7.4. 'Immediacy'

The question of how tightly eye movements are yoked to perceptual and cognitive processing in reading has been called the 'immediacy' question, and has been a central issue in eye movement research over the last fifteen years. For an excellent treatment of some of the issues involved, see McConkie (1983). Ehrlich and Rayner (1983) also discussed the problem clearly, and distinguished between three groups of theorists: those who think that there is a cognitive or eye-mind delay between eye movements and processing (Kolers, 1976; Bouma and de Voogd, 1974; Morton, 1964), those who think eye movements reflect some but not all linguistic processing done on the fixated word or words ('process-monitoring hypothesis', Rayner, 1977, 1978), and those who think eye movements (at least gaze durations) reflect all the linguistic processing done at the point fixated, that is, the eye-mind delay is zero (Just and Carpenter, 1980).

The strategy-tactics theory has a compromise status with respect to these theories in the sense that it considers all of them to be right in some way. Thus, because of the difficulty of accurately extracting a saccade target, the strategy-tactics theory proposes that it is often more efficient for the eye to move on the basis of crude visual clues rather than on the basis of lexical or linguistic processing. There will thus appear to be an eye-mind delay between eye movements and processing. On the other hand, the idea that there should be a scanning routine which is modulated by ongoing processing is also comparable with the 'process-monitoring' view. Finally, since the strategy-tactics theory assumes that the eye moves on from one word to the next when some stage of lexical processing has been reached, the gaze durations on words should reflect that lexical processing. This is compatible with the idea that, for gaze durations, the eye-mind delay is zero.

The advantage of the strategy-tactics theory is that it makes precise predictions about which text factors should affect which eye movement variables and when. Crude visual clues should always act immediately on eye movements, since they determine where each between-word and within-word saccade goes. They also partially determine the duration of fixations when there are two fixations in a word. Lexical information, however, has a more subtle influence: it does not determine saccades (unless the prior fixation duration is long for some reason), and it determines fixation durations only sometimes: it determines the duration of single fixations in a word, and the duration of second fixations when there are two. Lexical information does determine gaze duration, but the influence is complicated by the simultaneous influence of the position of the first fixation in the word: when this is not at the optimal viewing position, a substantial penalty of 20 ms per letter of deviation from the optimal position is added to gaze duration.

Past studies concerned with immediacy have of course not been designed to test the predictions of the strategy-tactics theory, and so they do not make the distinctions the theory requires between single and multiple fixation tactics within words. What past studies have been concerned with is determining whether information gathered at the current fixation can immediately influence the next saccade or the current fixation duration. Unfortunately, however, the methodology that was used leaves open the possibility of alternative explanations.

For example, while there is no doubt that saccade sizes are affected by the length of the currently fixated word and that of the next word, (e.g., O'Regan, 1979, 1980), no one has up to now excluded the possibility that the word length effect occurs on the basis of word length clues extracted in peripheral vision *several fixations before* the eye gets to the current fixation. Another example concerns the effect of lexical processing of the currently fixated word on the current fixation duration. Several of the studies mentioned in the preceding section show effects of the currently fixated word's lexical properties on the 'first' fixation duration on the word, but in all but one of these studies parafoveal processing of the currently fixated word could have occurred on prior fixations, so there is no guarantee that lexical processing of the word was having a truly immediate effect on the current fixation duration. The study where no parafoveal processing of the word could have been done is that of Underwood and McConkie (1985), who looked at what happens when the eye falls on a misspelled word. In this study, by use of eye-contingent computer display, the misspelling appeared only when the eye landed on the word, so no prior parafoveal information was available about the error. Perhaps this is why the authors observed a much smaller lexical effect (12 ms) than the other studies (20–40 ms) cited above.

Another point concerns the use of the measure 'average fixation duration'. Three of the studies mentioned in the preceding section show lexical effects on average fixation duration. But since in some cases several fixations will have been made on a word, changes in average fixation duration may have come about because of changes not of the first fixation, but only of the second fixation in a word. These studies cannot be used as evidence for true immediacy of fixation durations.

Rayner and Pollatsek (1981) set out to give a definitive demonstration of the moment-to-moment influence on saccade size of the information gathered at the current fixation. The idea was to restrict parafoveal vision by means of a moving window whose size was changed from fixation to fixation. If saccade size adapts from moment to moment to the size of the window, this would be a good demonstration of moment-to-moment control of saccades as a function of locally gathered information. The authors did indeed demonstrate such immediate adaptation. However, the question arises of what information was driving the adaptation. If it was anything other than gross visual cues, then the strategy-tactics theory would be in trouble. But in fact the theory has no difficulty explaining the result, since the window used by the authors was a moving 'grating' that filled the spaces between words, and spaces are of course precisely the kind of gross visual cue that the theory proposes can be used to guide saccades on a moment-to-moment basis.

7.5. What eye movement measure for psycholinguistics?

Eye movements are being used increasingly often as an index of readers' cognitive processes during sentence comprehension. Excellent examples can be found in the reviews by Rayner and Pollatsek (1987) and Frazier (1987). In all this work, linguistic factors are generally manipulated, and the resulting changes in eye movements are used to make inferences about linguistic processing. The problem is that the changes in the text that must be made to manipulate linguistic structure are inevitably accompanied by changes which have visual correlates, such as changes in word length or number of words. Researchers have therefore attempted to use eye movement measures which are insensitive to these visual influences. Unfortunately no completely satisfactory measure has been developed as yet, and workers resort to using a range of measures: generally 'gaze duration', 'average fixation duration', 'time per letter', 'probability of fixation'. However, the strategy-tactics theory suggests that all these measures are strongly influenced by visuomotor factors related to the scanning routine. The following paragraphs give a few examples of how this can occur.

The use of gaze duration as a measure of processing has already been criticized in section 7.3: because of the optimal viewing position phenomenon, this measure will depend strongly on initial fixation location in the word. Gaze duration has also been criticized by Blanchard (1985), who pointed out that the principle underlying this measure is what he calls the 'trade-off' assumption, which is the idea that multiple short fixations are equivalent to one long one. This principle, he says, has not been proven. And indeed, evidence from my experiments shows (i) that when two fixations are made in a word, the sum of their durations is about 75–100 ms longer than when a single fixation is made (cf. O'Regan and Lévy-Schoen, 1987), and (ii) that two fixations occur for visuo-motor reasons, not for lexical processing reasons (when the eye fixates too far from the generally optimal position). Thus when two fixations occur, there will be a penalty of 75–100 ms linked to visuo-motor mechanisms, not to lexical processing. Coherent with this is Blanchard's (1985) finding, in a heirarchical regression analysis of eye fixations in text reading, that the number of fixations made in a word correlates only with word length, not with word frequency, whereas their durations correlate with word frequency, not with word length.

Frazier and Rayner's study (1982) is one example of a number of studies which use total time per letter as a measure of processing time. To test theories of sentence parsing, Frazier and Rayner considered sentences where an ambiguous noun phrase leads the reader's eye 'down the garden path' before it reaches a disambiguating region. An example is: "Wherever Alice walks her shaggy sheep dog will follow", compared with "Wherever Alice walks her shaggy sheep dog men follow". They observed differences in the total time per letter spent by the eye in critical regions of the sentences and used these differences as arguments to distinguish between possible theories of sentence parsing. They used the variable 'time per letter' in order to compensate for the fact that some of the sentence portions they wanted to compare were not of the same length. For example in the above case, what they called the 'disambiguating region' of the sentences was 'will follow' for the first and 'men follow' for the second sentence (one letter difference). More drastic differences in the length of the disambiguating region occurred in other sentences when they compared 'she laughed' to 'were laughing', or 'all the' to 'was running', or 'her history' to 'will be'.

Now it is not clear whether the variable 'time per letter' adequately compensates for the differences in length. By superimposing the high-frequency curves for words of 7 and 11 letters in Fig. 11 (and this is also true if 5- and 9-letter words are added: cf. O'Regan and Lévy-Schoen, 1987), it would be seen that the increment in gaze duration on these words when length is increased depends on where in the word the eye was fixated (there is virtually no increment if the eye fixates near the end of the word, whereas there is if the eye fixates near the beginning of the word). There is also an effect of the word's frequency (there is more increment for low-frequency words). These are confounding factors which will interact with the 'time per letter' measure. They will certainly have increased the variance of the data. Also, they may have appeared on particular sentence pairs and given rise to an apparent overall effect in the Frazier and Rayner experiment. (Unfortunately the authors did not verify this possibility by doing item statistics. This would have also allowed them to discount the possibility that the observed effects were due to other differences in the regions being compared, such as word frequency and semantic effects.)

Like many authors, Frazier and Rayner also used another measure of processing, namely average fixation duration over a given region. But this measure is also not wholly satisfactory. According to the strategy-tactics theory, when two fixations are made in a word both tend to be shorter than if a single fixation is made. Two fixations tend to be made for visuo-motor (not linguistic) reasons, when the eye's position is too far from the generally optimal position. This occurs primarily in long words. Thus, sentence portions with long words will tend to have shorter average fixation durations. Thus, as before, if average fixation duration is used to compare processing across sentence parts, these must contain words of identical length. Similarly, since word frequency may also affect fixation duration and the probability of making additional fixations, this factor should also be controlled when making comparisons. Ideally, sentence portions to be compared should be identical, and item statistics should be used.

As another example that suffers from similar problems, consider one experiment in a study by Ferreira and Clifton (1986). These authors attempted to verify the 'modularity' of syntactic processing by showing that prior contextual bias does not change the reader's low-level parsing strategy. One source of evidence for this view came from their finding that while prior context changed nothing in the 'reading time per letter' measure, a syntactic difference did change reading time per letter: in particular, when the syntactic ambiguity in: "Sam loaded the boxes on the cart..." was removed by reading the following sentence portion, 'onto the van', times were longer on this disambiguating region than on the purportedly easier 'before his coffee break' disambiguator. But this difference could have been caused by the fact that the 'before his coffee break' type disambiguators were always longer than the 'onto the van' type disambiguators. If (as is probably the case) the 'time per letter' measure does not actually compensate adequately for word length, then some of the effects observed in this experiment could be due to these systematic length differences.

What would be an appropriate measure of cognitive processing? O'Regan and Lévy-Schoen (1987) suggested a possibility in which gaze duration would be 'corrected' by subtracting an approximately 75–100 ms 'visuomotor penalty' for each additional fixation made after the first. But this suggestion is an extrapolation of data from studies on isolated words, and empirical justification in normal reading is still required. Also, other problems with this measure have still to be studied. For example, the penalty may not be the same going from the first to the second as going from the second to the third fixation in a word. There is also some suggestion that a better correction 'formula' should contain a small term depending on the eye's initial location in the word and on the word's length. Finally the 'formula' would probably be valid in what I have called 'word-by-word' reading, in which no parafoveal preprocessing of upcoming words is done, but it is unclear whether modifications must be made for normal reading. However, there is hope, if the strategy-tactics theory is right, that in future work a purer index of linguistic processing can be found than the measures that have been used up to now.

8. Conclusion

For the last fifteen years an impressive body of work has accumulated on the subject of eye movements in reading. Within this, one of the most intensively studied topics has been 'perceptual span', probably because of the underlying assumption that in reading the eye moves from span to span. This chapter started by reviewing a number of recent studies of perceptual span, and by showing that in fact something other than perceptual span must be determining where the eye goes at each saccade, and how long it stays at each fixation. This led to the conclusion that it might be necessary to give up the hope that instantaneous eye movement variability is purely caused by sensory or cognitive processing, and consider some of the low-level visuo-motor constraints that might also be active. It may be that eye movements have a life of their own that must be respected before they can be used as an indicator of cognitive processing.

An inventory of possible spatial and temporal visuo-motor constraints on eye movements then provided two important ideas which would help to understand eye movement behavior in reading. First, it appears that long latencies are necessary to aim the eye accurately, so it is usually better to program many quick, inaccurate saccades, based on crude visual cues, rather than few accurate ones based on fine cues. Second, visibility, even in the fovea, drops off catastrophically, and so even short words may need several fixations to be recognized.

The drastic drop-off of visibility even in the fovea led me to discover the optimal viewing position phenomenon: depending on its length, frequency and lexical structure, each word has a (possibly different) optimal viewing position, where the eye must first land in order to recognize the word most quickly. A study of the eye movement tactics underlying this very strong and reliable phenomenon provided the basis for a preliminary theory about eye movements in reading, the 'strategy-tactics' theory. In the final sections of the chapter I compared the predictions of the theory with the available evidence. Though the theory withstood the test successfully, more work needs to be done, since up to now its detailed predictions have not been tested.

A difference between the strategy-tactics theory and previous work on eye movements in reading is that the strategy-tactics theory is a 'mechanistic' model that attempts to describe as precisely as possible where the eye will go next and how long it will stay at each point in a text. In the past, workers have been concerned with studying the effects of various typographical or linguistic variables on eye movement parameters without trying (or at least without succeeding) to pin down the rules governing the behavior of individual saccades and fixations. I think the strategy-tactics theory is a breakthrough in this direction, because it sets out a preliminary testable set of rules, and thereby opens new lines of research, even if it turns out to need radical modifications. The breakthrough has come about, I believe, by giving greater respect to low-level constraints in the visuo-motor system.

Acknowledgements

I wish to particularly thank Arthur Jacobs, Françoise Vitu and Ariane Lévy-Schoen for their help, support, comments and suggestions. I also greatly appreciated the following people's comments on all or parts of the manuscript: Bruno Breitmeyer, Heiner Deubel, Danièle Dubois, John Findlay, Virginia Holmes, Albrecht Inhoff, George McConkie, Keith Rayner, Ronan Reilly, Liliane Sprenger-Charolles, Jonathan Vaughan.

References

Accardo, A.P., Inchingolo, P. and Pensiero, S. (1987) Gaze-position dependence of saccadic latency and accuracy. In: J.K. O'Regan and A. Lévy-Schoen (Eds.), Eye Movements: from Physiology to Cognition. North-Holland, Amsterdam, pp. 150–151.

Andriessen, J.J. and Bouma, H. (1976) Eccentric vision: adverse interactions between line segments. Vision Res. 16, 71–78.

Andriessen, J.J. and de Voogd, A.H. (1973) Analysis of eye movement patterns in silent reading. IPO Annu. Prog. Rep. 8, 30–35.

Arnold, D.C. and Tinker, M.A. (1939) The fixational pause of the eyes. J. Exp. Psychol. 25, 271–280.

Aslin, R.N. and Shea, S.L. (1987) The amplitude and angle of saccades to double-step target displacements. Vision Res. 11, 1925–1942.

Balota, D.A., Pollatsek, A. and Rayner, K. (1985) The interaction of contextual constraints and parafoveal visual information in reading. Cognitive Psychol. 17, 364–370.

Becker, W. (1972) The control of eye movements in the saccadic system. Bibl. Ophthalmol. 82, 233–243.

Becker, W. (1976) Do correction saccades depend exclusively on retinal feedback? A note on the possible role of non-retinal feedback. Vision Res. 16, 425–427.

Becker, W. and Fuchs, A.F. (1969) Further properties of the human saccadic system: eye movements and correction saccades with and without fixation point. Vision Res. 9, 1247–1258.

Becker, W. and Jürgens, R. (1979) An analysis of the saccadic system by means of double step stimuli. Vision Res. 19, 967–984.

de Bie, J., van den Brink, G. and van Sonderen, J.F. (1987) The systematic undershoot of saccades: a localization or an oculomotor phenomenon? In: J.K. O'Regan and A. Lévy-Schoen (Eds.), Eye Movements: from Physiology to Cognition. North-Holland, Amsterdam, pp. 85–94.

Blanchard, H.E. (1985) A comparison of some processing time measures based on eye movements. Acta Psychol. 58, 1–15.

Blommaert, F.J.J. and Roufs, J.A.J. (1981) The foveal point spread function as a determinant for detail vision. Vision Res. 21, 1223–1233.

Bouma, H. (1970) Interaction effects in parafoveal letter recognition. Nature 226, 177–178.

Bouma, H. (1978) Visual search and reading: Eye movements and functional visual field: a tutorial review. In: J. Requin (Ed.), Attention and Performance VII, Erlbaum, Hillsdale, NJ, pp. 115–146.

Bouma, H. and de Voogd, A.H. (1974) On the control of eye saccades in reading. Vision Res. 14, 273–284.

Buswell, G.T. (1937) How adults read. Supplementary Ed. Monogr. 45.

Boyce, P.R. (1967) Monocular fixation in human eye movement. Proc. R. Soc. B. 167, 293–315.

Carr, T.H. (1986) Perceiving visual language. In: K.R. Boff, L. Kaufman and J.P. Thomas (Eds.), Handbook of Perception and Human Performance, Vol II. Wiley, New York, pp. 29:1–29:92.

Carpenter, R.H.S. (1981) Oculomotor procrastination. In: D.F. Fisher, R.A. Monty and J.W. Senders (Eds.), Eye movements: Cognition and Visual perception. Erlbaum, Hillsdale, NJ, pp. 237–246.

Carpenter, P.A. and Just, M.A. (1983) What your eyes do while your mind is reading. In: K. Rayner (Ed.), Eye Movements in Reading. Perceptual and Language Processes. Academic Press, New York, pp. 275–307.

Cattell, J.M. (1885) Ueber die Zeit der Erkennung und Benennung von Schriftzeichen, Bildern und Farben. Philosoph. Stud. 2, 635–650.

Cavanagh, P. (1978) Size and position invariance in the visual system. Perception 7, 167–177.

Chastain, G. (1985) Positional differences in performance on members of confusable and nonconfusable letter pairs. J. Exp. Psychol. Hum. Percept. Performance 11, 752–764.

Coëffé, C. (1985) La visée du regard sur un mot isolé. Ann. Psychol. 85, 169–184.

Coëffé, C. (1987) Two ways of improving saccade accuracy. In: J.K. O'Regan and A. Lévy-Schoen (Eds.), Eye Movements: from Physiology to Cognition. North-Holland, Amsterdam, pp. 105–114.

Coëffé, C. and O'Regan, J.K. (1987) Reducing the influence of non-target stimuli on saccade accuracy: predictability and latency effects. Vision Res. 27, 227–240.

Cohen, M.E. and Ross, L.E. (1978) Latency and accuracy characteristics of saccades and corrective saccades in children and adults. J. Exp. Child Psychol. 26, 517–527.

Coren, S. and Hoenig, P. (1972) Effect of non-target stimuli upon length of voluntary saccades. Percept. Motor Skills 34, 499–508.

Cunitz, R.J. and Steinman, R.M. (1969) Comparison of saccadic eye movements during fixation and reading. Vision Res. 9, 683–693.

Creutzfeldt, O. and Kuhnt, U. (1974) Visually evoked potentials in animals. In: R. Jung (Ed.), Handbook of Sensory Physiology, Vo. VII/3. Springer, Heidelberg/New York, pp. 595–646.

Deubel, H. (1987) Adaptivity in gain and direction in oblique saccades. In: J.K. O'Regan and A. Lévy-Schoen (Eds.), Eye Movements: from Physiology to Cognition. North-Holland, Amsterdam, pp. 181–190.

Deubel, H., Wolf, W. and Hauske, G. (1982) Corrective saccades: effect of shifting the saccade goal. Vision Res. 22, 353–364.

Deubel, H., Wolf, W. and Hauske, G. (1984) The evaluation of the oculomotor error signal. In: A.G. Gale and F. Johnson (Eds.), Theoretical and Applied Aspects of Eye Movement Research. North-Holland, Amsterdam, pp. 55–62.

Deubel, H., Wolf, W. and Hauske, G. (1986) Adaptive gain control of saccadic eye movements. Hum. Neurobiol. 5, 245–253.

Deubel, H., Findlay, J., Jacobs, A.M. and Brogan, D. (1988) Saccadic eye movements to targets defined by structure differences. In: G. Lüer, U. Lass and J. Schallo-Hoffmann (Eds.), Eye Movement Research: Physiological and psychological aspects. C.J. Hogrefe, Inc., Toronto, pp. 107–145.

Ditchburn, R.W. (1973) Eye movements and visual perception. Clarendon Press, Oxford.

Dodge, R. (1907) An experimental study of visual fixation. The Psychological Review Monograph Supplements No. 35. The Review Publishing Co., Lancaster, PA.

Dow, B.M., Snyder, R.G., Vautin, R.G. and Bauer, R. (1981) Magnification factor and receptive field size in foveal striate cortex of the monkey. Exp. Brain Res. 44, 213–228.

Dunn-Rankin, P. (1978) The visual characteristics of words. Sci. Am. 238, 1, 122–130.

Ehrlich, K. (1983) Eye movements in pronoun assignment: a study of sentence integration. In: K. Rayner (Ed.), Eye Movements in Reading. Perceptual and Language Processes. Academic Press, New York, pp. 253–268.

Ehrlich, S.F. and Rayner, K. (1981) Contextual effects on word perception and eye movements during reading. J. Verbal Learn. Verbal Behav. 20, 641–655.

Ehrlich, K. and Rayner, K. (1983) Pronoun assignment and semantic integration during reading: eye movements and immediacy of processing. J. Verbal Learn. Verbal Behav. 22, 75–87.

Engel, F.L. (1971) Visual conspicuity, directed attention, and retinal locus. Vision Res. 11, 563–576.

Eriksen, C.W. and St. James, J.D. (1986) Visual attention within and around the field of focal attention: a zoom lens model. Percept. Psychophys. 40, 225–240.

Erdmann, B. and Dodge, R. (1898) Psychologische Untersuchungen ueber das Lesen auf experimenteller Grundlage. Niemeyer, Halle.

Estes, W.K. (1978) Perceptual processes in letter recognition and reading. In: E.C. Carterette and M.P. Friedman (Eds.), Handbook of Perception, Vol IX. Academic Press, New York, pp. 163–220.

Estes, W.K. (1982) Similarity-related channel interactions in visual processing. J. Exp. Psychol. Hum. Percept. Performance 8, 353–382.

Fendick, M. and Westheimer, G. (1983) Effects of practice and the separation of test targets on foveal and peripheral stereoacuity. Vision Res. 23, 145–150.

Ferreira, F. and Clifton, C. (1986) The independence of syntactic processing. J. Mem. Lang. 25, 348–368.

Findlay, J.M. (1981) Local and global influences on saccadic eye movements. In: D.F. Fisher, R.A. Monty and J.W. Senders (Eds.), Eye Movements: Cognition and Visual Perception. Erlbaum, Hillsdale, NJ.

Findlay, J.M. (1982) Global visual processing for saccadic eye movements. Vision Res. 21, 347–354.

Findlay, J.M. (1983) Visual information processing for saccadic eye movements. In: A. Hein and M. Jeannerod (Eds.), Spatially Co-ordinated Behaviour. Springer, Berlin.

Findlay, J.M. (1987) Visual computation and saccadic eye movements: a theoretical perspective. Spatial Vision 2, 175–189.

Findlay, J.M. and Harris, L.R. (1984) Small saccades to double-stepped targets moving in two dimensions. In: A.G. Gale and F. Johnson (Eds.), Theoretical and Applied Aspects of Eye Movement Research. North-Holland, Amsterdam, pp. 71–78.

Fischer, B. and Ramsperger, E. (1984) Human express-saccades: extremely short reaction times of goal-directed eye movements. Exp. Brain Res. 57, 191–195.

Frazier, L. (1987) Sentence processing: a tutorial review. In: M. Coltheart (Ed.), Attention and Performance XII: The Psychology of Reading. Erlbaum, Hillsdale, NJ, pp. 559–586.

Frazier, L. and Rayner, K. (1982) Making and correcting errors during sentence comprehension: eye movements in the analysis of structurally ambiguous sentences. Cognitive Psychol. 14, 178–210.

Frost, D. and Pöppel, E. (1976) Different programming modes of human saccadic eye movements as a function of stimulus eccentricity: indications of a functional subdivision of the visual field. Biol. Cybernet. 23, 39–48.

Groner, R. (1988) Eye movements, attention and visual information processing: Some experimental results and methodological considerations. In: G. Lüer, U. Lass and J. Shallo-Hoffmann (Eds.), Eye Movement Research: Physiological and Psychological Aspects. C.J. Hogrefe, Göttingen, pp. 295–319.

Ginsborg, B.L. (1953) Small involuntary movements of the eye. Br. J. Ophthalmol. 37, 746–754.

Haddad, G.M. and Steinman, R.M. (1973) The smallest voluntary saccade: implications for fixation. Vision Res. 13, 1075–1086.

Heller, D. (1987) Typographical characteristics and reading. In: J.K. O'Regan and A. Lévy-Schoen (Eds.), Eye Movements: from Physiology to Cognition. North-Holland, Amsterdam, pp. 487–498.

Henderson, L. (1982) Orthography and Word Recognition in Reading. Academic Press, New York.

Henson, D.B. (1978) Corrective saccades: effects of altering visual feedback. Vision Res. 18, 63–68.

Heywood, S. and Churcher, J. (1980) Structure of the visual array and saccadic latency: implications for oculomotor control. Q. J. Exp. Psychol. 32, 335–341.

Hogaboam, T.W. (1983) Reading patterns in eye movement data. In: K. Rayner (Ed.), Eye Movements in Reading. Perceptual and Language Processes. Academic Press, New York, pp. 309–332.

Holmes, V.M. and O'Regan, J.K. (1987) Decomposing French words. In: J.K. O'Regan and A. Lévy-Schoen (Eds.), Eye Movements: from Physiology to Cognition. North-Holland, Amsterdam, pp. 459–466.

Hou, R.L. and Fender, D.H. (1979) Processing of direction and magnitude by the saccadic eye movement system. Vision Res. 19, 1421–1426.

Huey, E.B. (1900) On the psychology and physiology of reading. I. Am. J. Psychol. XI, 3, 283–302.

Huey, E.B. (1908) The Psychology and Pedagogy of Reading. New York, Macmillan.

Ikeda, M. and Saida, S. (1978) Span of recognition in reading. Vision Res. 18, 83–88.

Inhoff, A.W. (1984) Two stages of word processing during eye fixations in the reading of prose. J. Verbal Learn. Verbal Behav. 23, 612–624.

Inhoff, A.W. (1985) The effect of factivity on lexical retrieval and postlexical processes during eye fixations in reading. J. Psycholing. Res. 14, 45–56.

Inhoff, A.W. (1986) Preparing sequences of saccades under choice reaction conditions: effects of sequence length and context. Acta Psychol. 61, 211–228.

Inhoff, A.W. and Rayner, K. (1986) Parafoveal word processing during fixations in reading: effects of word frequency. Percept. Psychophys. 40, 431–439.

Jacobs, A.M. (1986) Eye movement control in visual search: how direct is visual span control? Percept. Psychophys. 39, 47–58.

Jacobs, A.M. (1987) On localization and saccade programming. Vision Res. 27, 1953–1966.

Jacobs, A.M. and Lévy-Schoen, A. (1987) Le contrôle des mouvements des yeux dans la lecture: questions actuelles. Ann. Psychol. 65, 133–146.

Jacobs, A.M. and O'Regan, J.K. (1987) Spatial and/or temporal adjustments of scanning behavior to visibility changes. Acta Psycholog. 65, 133–146.

Jacobs, R.J. (1979) Visual resolution and contour interaction in the fovea and periphery. Vision Res. 19, 1187–1196.

Javal, E. (1878) Essai sur la physiologie de la lecture. Ann. Oculist. 79, 97–117; 240–274; and 80, 135–147.

Just, M.A. and Carpenter, P.A. (1980) A theory of reading: from eye fixations to comprehension. Psychol. Rev. 87, 329–354.

Kalesnykas, R.P. and Hallett, P.E. (1987) The differentiation of visually guided and anticipatory saccades in gap and overlap paradigms. Exp. Brain Res. 68, 115–121.

Kapoula, Z. (1983) The influence of peripheral preprocessing in a scanning task. In: R. Groner, C. Menz, D. Fisher and R. Monty (Eds.), Eye Movements and Psychological Functions: International Views. Erlbaum, Hillsdale, NJ, pp. 101–114.

Kapoula, Z. (1984) Aiming precision and characteristics of saccades. In: A.G. Gale and F. Johnson (Eds.), Theoretical and Applied Aspects of Eye Movement Research. North-Holland, Amsterdam, pp. 123–131.

Kapoula, Z. (1985) Evidence for a range effect in the saccadic system. Vision Res. 25, 1155–1157.

Kapoula, Z., Robinson, D.A. and Hain, T.C. (1986) Motion of the eye immediately after a saccade. Exp. Brain Res. 61, 386–394.

Klein, S.A. and Tyler, C.W. (1981) Phase discrimination using single and compound gratings. Invest. Ophthalmol. Vis. Sci. Suppl. 20, 124.

Kliegl, R., Olson, R.K. and Davidson, B.J. (1982) Regression analysis as a tool for studying reading processes: comments on Just and Carpenter's eye fixation theory. Mem. Cognition 10, 287–296.

Kliegl, R., Olson, R.K. and Davidson, B.J. (1983) On problems of unconfounding perceptual and language processes. In: K. Rayner (Ed.), Eye Movements in Reading. Perceptual and Language Processes. Academic Press, New York, pp. 333–343.

Kling, J.W. and Riggs, L.A. (1971) Experimental Psychology. Methuen, London.

Kolers, P.A. (1976) Buswell's discoveries. In: R.A. Monty and J.W. Senders (Eds.), Eye Movements and Psychological Processes. Erlbaum, Hillsdale, NJ, pp. 371–395.

Kolers, P.A. and Lewis, C.L. (1972) Bounding of letter sequences and the integration of visually presented words. Acta Psychol. 36, 112–124.

Korte, W. (1923) Ueber die Gestaltauffassung im Indirekten Sehen. Z. Psychol. 93, 17–82.

Kowler, E. and Anton, S. (1987) Reading twisted text: implications for the role of saccades. Vision Res. 27, 45–60.

Krumhansl, C.F. and Thomas, E.A.C. (1977) Effect of level of confusability on reporting letters from briefly presented visual arrays. Percep. Psychophys. 21, 269–279.

Lamare, M. (1893) Des mouvements des yeux pendant la lecture. C. R. Soc. Franç. Ophthalmol. 354–364.

Levi, D.M., Klein, S.A. and Aitsebaomo, A.P. (1985) Vernier acuity, crowding and cortical magnification. Vision Res. 25, 963–977.

Lévy-Schoen, A. (1977) Latence des réponses oculaires et manuelles àdes séquences de signaux visuels. In: G. Oléron (Ed.), Psychologie Expérimentale et Comparée, Hommage àPaul Fraisse. Presses Universitaires de France, Paris, pp. 123–135.

Lévy-Schoen, A. (1981) Flexible and/or rigid control of oculomotor scanning behavior. In: D.F. Fisher, R.A. Monty and J.W. Senders (Eds.), Eye Movements: Cognition and Visual Perception. Erlbaum, Hillsdale, NJ, pp. 299–314.

Lévy-Schoen, A. and Blanc-Garin, J. (1974) On oculomotor programming and perception. Brain Res. 71, 443–450.

Lévy-Schoen, A. and O'Regan, J.K. (1979) The control of eye movements in reading. In: P.A. Kolers, M.E. Wrolstad and H. Bouma (Eds.), Processing of Visible Language I. Plenum, New York, pp. 7–36.

Lévy-Schoen, A., O'Regan, J.K., Jacobs, A.M. and Coëffé, C. (1984) The relation between visibility span and eye movements in various scanning tasks. In: A.G. Gale and F. Johnson (Eds.), Theoretical and Applied Aspects of Eye Movement Research. North-Holland, Amsterdam, pp. 133–142.

Lévy-Schoen, A. and O'Regan, J.K. (1987) The effect of improper accommodation on the visual field and on eye movements in reading. In: L. Stark and G. Obrecht (Eds.), Presbyopia. Professional Press Books, Fairchild Publications, New York, pp. 178–184.

Limb, J.O. and Rubinstein, C.B. (1977) A model of threshold vision incorporating inhomogeneity of the visual field. Vision Res. 17, 571–584.

Mackworth, N.H. and Mackworth, J.F. (1958) Eye fixations recorded on changing visual scenes by the television eye marker. J. Opt. Soc. Am. 48, 438–445.

Mackworth, N.H., Kaplan, I.T. and Metlay, W. (1964) Eye movements during viglance. Percept. Motor Skills 18, 397–402.

Mayfrank, L., Kimmig, H. and Fischer, B. (1987) The role of attention in the preparation of visually guided saccadic eye movements in man. In: J.K. O'Regan and A. Lévy-Schoen (Eds.), Eye Movements: from Physiology to Cognition. North-Holland, Amsterdam, pp. 37–45.

McClelland, J.L. and O'Regan, J.K. (1981) Expectations increase the benefit derived from parafoveal visual information in reading words aloud. J. Exp. Psychol. Hum. Percept. Performance 7, 634–644.

McConkie, G.W. (1983) Eye movements and perception during reading. In: K. Rayner (Ed.), Eye Movements in Reading. Perceptual and Language Processes. Academic Press, New York, pp. 65–96.

McConkie, G.W. and Hogaboam, T.W. (1985) Eye position and word identification in reading. In: R. Groner, G.W. McConkie and C. Menz (Eds.), Eye Movements and Human Information Processing. North-Holland, Amsterdam, pp. 137–147.

McConkie, G.W. and Rayner, K. (1975) The span of the effective stimulus during a fixation in reading. Percept. Psychophys. 17, 578–586.

McConkie, G.W. and Rayner, K. (1976) Asymmetry of the perceptual span in reading. Bull. Psychonomic Soc. 8, 365–368.

McConkie, G.W. and Zola, D. (1979) is visual information integrated across successive fixations in reading? Percept. Psychophys. 25, 221–224.

McConkie, G.W. and Zola, D. (1984) Eye movement control during reading: the effect of word units. In: W. Prinz and A.F. Sanders (Eds.), Cognition and Motor Processes. Springer, Berlin, pp. 63–74.

McConkie, G.W., Zola, D., Blanchard, H.E. and Wolverton, G.S. (1982) Perceiving words during reading: lack of facilitation from prior peripheral exposure. Percept. Psychophys. 32, 271–281.

McConkie, G.W., Zola, D. and Wolverton, G.S. (1985b) Estimating frequency and size of effects due to experimental manipulations in eye movement research. In: R. Groner, G.W. McConkie and C. Menz (Eds.), Eye Movements and Human Information Processing. North-Holland, Amsterdam.

McConkie, G.W., Underwood, N.R., Zola, D. and Wolverton, G.S. (1985a) Some temporal characteristics of processing during reading. J. Exp. Psychol. Hum. Percept. Performance 11, 168–186.

McConkie, G.W., Kerr, P.W., Reddix, M.D. and Zola, D. (1988) Eye movement control during reading: I. The location of initial eye fixations on words. Vision Res. 28, 1107–1118.

McConkie, G.W., Kerr, P.W., Reddix, M.D., Zola, D. and Jacobs, A.M. (1989) Eye movement control during reading: II. Frequency of refixating a word. Percept. Psychophys. 46, 245–253.

Mohler, C.W. and Wurtz, R.H. (1976) Organization of monkey superior colliculus: intermediate layer cells discharging before eye movements. J. Neurophysiol. 39, 722–744.

Morrison, R.E. (1984) Manipulation of stimulus onset delay in reading: evidence for parallel programming of saccades. J. Exp. Psychol. Hum. Percept. Performance 10, 667–682.

Morrison, R.E. and Rayner, K. (1981) Saccade size in reading depends upon character spaces and not visual angle. Percept. Psychophys. 30, 395–396.

Morton, J. (1964) The effects of context upon speed of reading, eye movements and eye-voice span. Q. Exp. Psychol. 16, 340–354.

Norman, D.A. (1968) Towards a theory of memory and attention. Psychol. Rev. 75, 44–64.

O'Regan, J.K. (1975) Constraints on eye movements in reading. Unpublished doctoral dissertation, University of Cambridge, U.K.

O'Regan, J.K. (1979) Saccade size control in reading: evidence for the linguistic control hypothesis. Percept. Psychophys. 25, 501–509.

O'Regan, J.K. (1980) The control of saccade size and fixation duration in reading: the limits of linguistic control. Percept.

Psychophys. 28, 112–117.

O'Regan, J.K. (1989) Visual acuity, lexical structure, and eye movements in word recognition. In: B. Elsendoorn and H. Bouma (Eds.), Working Models of Human Perception. Academic Press, London, pp. 261–292.

O'Regan, J.K. and Lévy-Schoen, A. (1978) Les mouvements des yeux au cours de la lecture. Ann. Psychol. 78, 459–492.

O'Regan, J.K. and Lévy-Schoen, A. (1983) Integrating visual information from successive fixations: does trans-saccadic fusion exist? Vision Res. 23, 765–768.

O'Regan, J.K. and Lévy-Schoen, A. (1987) Eye movement strategy and tactics in word recognition and reading. In: M. Coltheart (Ed.), Attention and Performance XII: The Psychology of Reading. Erlbaum, Hillsdale, NJ, pp. 363–383.

O'Regan, J.K., Lévy-Schoen, A. and Jacobs, A.M. (1983) The effect of visibility on eye movement parameters in reading. Percept. Psychophys. 34, 457–464.

O'Regan, J.K., Lévy-Schoen, A., Pynte, J. and Brugaillère, B. (1984) Convenient fixation location within isolated words of different length and structure. J. Exp. Psychol. Hum. Percept. Performance 10, 250–257.

Osterberg, G. (1935) Topography of the layer of rods and cones in the human retina. Acta Ophthalmol. Kbh., Suppl. 65, 1–102.

Ottes, F.P., van Gisbergen, J.A.M. and Eggermont, J.J. (1984) Metrics of saccade responses to visual double stimuli: two different modes. Vision Res. 24, 1169–1179.

Pirenne, M.H. (1967) Vision and the Eye. Chapman and Hall, London.

Pollatsek, A., Bolozky, S., Well, A.D. and Rayner, K. (1981) Asymmetries in the perceptual span for Israeli readers. Brain Lang. 14, 174–180.

Pollatsek, A., Rayner, K. and Balota, D.A. (1986) Inferences about eye movement control from the perceptual span in reading. Percept. Psychophys. 40, 123–130.

Posner, M.I. (1980) Orienting of attention. Q. J. Exp. Psychol. 32, 3–25.

Prablanc, C. and Jeannerod, M. (1974) Latence et précision des saccades en fonction de l'intensité, de la durée, et de la position rétinienne d'un stimulus. Soc. EEG Neurophysiol. Clin. Lang. Franç. 1974, 6 mars, 484–488.

Prablanc, C., Massé, D. and Echallier, J.F. (1978) Error-correcting mechanisms in large saccades. Vision Res. 18, 551–560.

Rashbass, C. (1961) The relationship between saccadic and smooth tracking eye movements. J. Physiol. 159, 326–338.

Rayner, K. (1975) The perceptual span and peripheral cues in reading. Cognitive Psychol. 7, 65–81.

Rayner, K. (1977) Visual attention in reading: eye movements reflect cognitive processes. Mem. Cognition 4, 443–448.

Rayner, K. (1978) Eye movements in reading and information processing. Psychol. Bull. 85, 618–660.

Rayner, K. (1979) Eye guidance in reading: fixation locations within words. Perception 8, 21–30.

Rayner, K. (1983) The perceptual span and eye movement control during reading. In: K. Rayner (Ed.), Eye Movements in Reading. Perceptual and Language Processes. Academic Press, New York, pp. 97–120.

Rayner, K. (1986) Eye movements and the perceptual span in beginning and skilled readers. J. Exp. Child Psychol. 41, 211–236.

Rayner, K. and Bertera, J.H. (1979) Reading without a fovea. Science 206, 468–469.

Rayner, K. and Duffy, S.A. (1986) Lexical complexity and fixation times in reading: effects of word frequency, verb complexity, and lexical ambiguity. Mem. Cognition 14, 191–201.

Rayner, K. and Inhoff, A.W. (1981) Control of eye movements during reading. In: B.L. Zuber (Ed.), Models of Oculomotor Behavior and Control. CRC Press, Boca Raton, FL, pp. 210–231.

Rayner, K. and McConkie, G.W. (1976) What guides a reader's eye movements? Vision Res. 16, 829–837.

Rayner, K. and Pollatsek, A. (1981) Eye movement control during reading: evidence for direct control. Q. J. Exp. Psychol. 33A, 351–373.

Rayner, K. and Pollatsek, A. (1983) Is visual information integrated across saccades? Percept. Psychophys. 34, 39–48.

Rayner, K. and Pollatsek, A. (1987) Eye movements in reading: a tutorial review. In: K. Rayner (Ed.), Eye Movements in Reading. Perceptual and Language Processes. Academic Press, New York, pp. 327–362.

Rayner, K., McConkie, G.W. and Ehrlich, S.F. (1978) Eye movements and integrating information across fixations. J. Exp. Psychol. Hum. Percept. Performance 4, 529–544.

Rayner, K. and McConkie, G.W. and Zola, D. (1980a) Integrating information across eye movements. Cognitive Psychol. 12, 206–226.

Rayner, K., Well, A.D. and Pollatsek, A. (1980b) Asymmetry of the effective visual field in reading. Percept. Psychophys. 27, 537–544.

Rayner, K., Inhoff, A.W., Morrison, R., Slowiaczek, M.L. and Bertera, J.H. (1981) Masking of foveal and parafoveal vision during eye fixations in reading. J. Exp. Psychol. Hum. Percept. Performance 7, 167–179.

Rayner, K., Well, A.D., Pollatsek, A. and Bertera, J.H. (1982) The availability of useful information to the right of fixation in reading. Percept. Psychophys. 31, 537–550.

Rayner, K., Slowiaczek, M., Clifton, C. and Bertera, J.H. (1983) Latency of sequential eye movements: implications for reading. J. Exp. Psychol. Hum. Percept. Performance 9, 912–922.

Reder, S.M. (1973) On-line monitoring of eye-position signals in contingent and noncontingent paradigms. Behav. Res. Methods Instrum. 5, 218–227.

Robinson, D.A. (1972) Eye movements evoked by collicular stimulation in the alert monkey. Vision Res. 12, 1795–1808.

Rolls, E.T. and Cowey, A. (1970) Topography of the retina and striate cortex and its relationship to visual acuity in rhesus monkeys and squirrel monkeys. Exp. Brain Res. 10, 298–310.

Rovamo, J., Virsu, V. and Nasanen, R. (1978) Cortical magnification factor predicts the photopic contrast sensitivity of peripheral vision. Nature 271, 54–56.

Russo, J. (1978) Adaptation of cognitive processes to the eye movement system. In: J.W. Senders and R.A. Monty (Eds.), Eye Movements and the Higher Psychological Functions. Erlbaum, Hillsdale, NJ, 89–112.

Salthouse, T.A. and Ellis, C.L. (1980) Determinants of eye-fixation duration. Am. J. Psychol. 93, 207–234.

Saslow, M.G. (1967a) Effects of components of displacement-step stimuli upon latency for saccadic eye movements. J. Opt. Soc. Am. 57, 1024–1029.

Saslow, M.G. (1967b) Latency for saccadic eye movement. J. Opt. Soc. Am. 57, 8, 1030–1033.

Schustack, M.W., Ehrlich, S.F. and Rayner, K. (1987) Local and global sources of contextual facilitation in reading. J. Mem. Lang. 26, 322–340.

Schwartz, E.L. (1980) Computational anatomy and functional architecture of striate cortex: a spatial mapping approach to perceptual coding. Vision Res. 20, 645–669.

Shebilske, W. (1975) Reading eye movements from an information-processing point of view. In: D. Massaro (Ed.), Understanding Language. Academic Press, New York.

Shulman, G.L., Remington, R.W. and McLean, J.P. (1979) Moving attention through visual space. J. Exp. Psychol. Hum. Percept. Performance 5, 522–526.

Steinman, R.M., Cunitz, R.J., Timberlake, G.T. and Herman, M. (1967) Voluntary control of microsaccades during maintained monocular fixation. J. Opt. Soc. Am. 49, 901–908.

Stromberg, E.L. (1938) Binocular movements of the eyes in reading. J. Gen. Psychol. 18, 349–345.

Tinker, M.A. (1958) Recent studies of eye movements in reading. Psychol. Bull. 55, 215–231.

Tinker, M.A. and Paterson, D.G. (1955) The effect of typographical variations upon eye movement in reading. J. Educ. Res. 49, 171–184.

Tootell, R.B., Silverman, M.S., Switkes, E. and De Valois, R.L. (1982) Deoxyglucose analysis of retinotopic organization in primate striate cortex. Science 218, 902–904.

Townsend, J.T., Taylor, S.G. and Brown, D.R. (1971) Lateral masking for letters with unlimited viewing time. Percept. Psychophys. 10, 375–378.

Underwood, N.R. and McConkie, G.W. (1985) Perceptual span for letter distinctions during reading. Read. Res. Q. 20, 153–162.

Underwood, G., Hyona, J. and Niemi, P. (1987) Scanning patterns on individual words during the comprehension of sentences. In: J.K. O'Regan and A. Lévy-Schoen (Eds.), Eye Movements: from Physiology to Cognition. North-Holland, Amsterdam.

Underwood, G., Bloomfield, R. and Clews, S. (1988) Information influences the pattern of eye fixations during sentence comprehension. Perception 17, 267–278.

van Essen, D.C., Newsome, W.T. and Maunsell, J.H.R. (1984) The visual field representation in striate cortex of the macaque monkey: asymmetries, anisotropies and individual variability. Vision Res. 24, 429–448.

Vaughan, J. (1978) Control of visual fixation duration in search. In: J.W. Senders, D.W. Fisher and R.A. Monty (Eds.), Eye Movements and the Higher Psychological Functions. Erlbaum, Hillsdale, NJ.

Vaughan, J. (1983) Saccadic reaction time in visual search. In: K. Rayner (Ed.), Eye Movements in Reading. Perceptual and Language Processes. Academic Press, New York, pp. 397–411.

Vaughan, J. and Graefe, T. (1977) Delay of stimulus presentation after the saccade in visual search. Percept. Psychophys. 22, 201–205.

Viviani, P. and Swensson, R.G. (1982) Saccadic eye movements to peripherally discriminated visual targets. J. Exp. Psychol. Hum. Percept. Performance 8, 113–126.

Vitu, F. and O'Regan, J.K. (1988) Optimal landing position in words of different length and frequency. In: G. Lüer, U. Lass and J. Schallo-Hoffmann (Eds.), Eye Movement Research: Physiological and Psychological Aspects. C.J. Hogrefe, Inc., Toronto, pp. 286–294.

Volkmann, F.C., Schick, A.M.L. and Riggs, L.A. (1968) Time course of visual inhibition during voluntary saccades. J. Opt. Soc. Am. 58, 562–569.

Well, A.D. (1983) Perceptual factors in reading. In: K. Rayner (Ed.), Eye Movements in Reading. Perceptual and Language Processes. Academic Press, New York, pp. 141–150.

Westheimer, G. (1954) Eye movement responses to a horizontally moving visual stimulus. AMA Arch. Ophthalmol. 52, 932–941.

Westheimer, G. (1982) The spatial grain of the perifoveal visual field. Vision Res. 22, 157–162.

Wheeless, L. Jr., Cohen, G.H. and Boynton, R.E. (1967) Luminance as a parameter of the eye movement control system. J. Opt. Soc. Am. 57, 394–400.

Wilson, H.R. and Bergen, J.R. (1979) A four mechanism model for threshold spatial vision. Vision Res. 19, 19–32.

Williams, D.R. (1988) Topography of the foveal cone mosaic in the living human eye. Vision Res. 28, 433–454.

Wolford, G. and Shum, K.H. (1980) Evidence for feature perturbations. Percept. Psychophys. 27, 409–420.

Wolverton, G.S. and Zola, D. (1983) The temporal characteristics of visual information extraction during reading. In: K. Rayner (Ed.), Eye Movements in Reading: Perceptual and Language Processes. Academic Press, New York, pp. 41–51.

Woodworth, R.S. (1938) Experimental Psychology. Holt, Rinehart and Winston, New York.

Wyman, D. and Steinman, R.M. (1973) Latency characteristics of small saccades. Vision Res. 13, 2173–2175.

Young, L.R. (1981) The sampled data model and foveal dead

zone for saccades. In: B.L. Zuber (Ed.), Models of Oculomotor Behavior and Control. CRC Press, Boca Raton, FL, pp. 43–74.

Zingale, C.M. and Kowler, E. (1987) Planning sequences of saccades. Vision Res. 27, 1327–1341.

Zola, D. (1984) Redundancy and word perception during reading. Percept. Psychophys. 36, 277–284.

Eye movements and their role in visual and cognitive processes
E. Kowler, Editor

CHAPTER 10

Eye-movement models for arithmetic and reading performance

Patrick Suppes

Institute for Mathematical Studies in the Social Sciences, Stanford University, Stanford, CA 94305, U.S.A.

1. Introduction

In this chapter I propose various stochastic models of eye movement applicable to two important domains of cognition, namely, arithmetic and reading. I begin with the analysis of arithmetic because my own research has been concentrated there, but in the second half I consider the question of what changes have to be made in the axioms of the models proposed for arithmetic in order to deal with some well-known features of eye movements in reading. As might be expected and for reasons to be considered later, the changes are rather profound.

From the standpoint of fundamental science, it is somewhat disturbing that the axioms of different models for different cognitive tasks are changed so much depending upon the task. One would like to be able to isolate in clear and more definite form the fundamental assumptions that are invariant across different kinds of tasks, and then to impose various boundary and causal conditions to account for the changes. I do not think such an approach is hopeless, but it seems premature for the subject matter of this chapter.

On the other hand, the focus on examining the empirical adequacy of a small number of explicitly formulated models has necessarily led to simplifications of structure that do not accommodate all the many experimental findings. In the case of reading, for example, I begin with a minimal control model that probably no one would accept as correct. The purpose of this minimal model is to use it as a basis for examining, and then organizing in a more complex model, the most significant features of the reading process that are omitted. Deficiencies in the various models analysed highlight defects in current theories about arithmetic and reading performance.

Another methodological point of some importance concerns individual differences. The existence of individual differences does not count against the various models considered. It is assumed in their formulation, although not made explicit in the axioms, that parameters are estimated separately for each individual. What is required to reject a given model is not variation of such global parameters but the existence of individual distributions which violate the fundamental assumptions of the axioms, for example, distributions which are not convolutions of exponential distributions, or random-walk motions which are in violation of the basic assumptions. Global variables of text and task differences are especially present in reading, but also do not as such affect goodness of fit of a model, in contrast to local variables such as features of a particular arithmetic exercise or of a particular word in a reading text, which do affect fit.

2. Procedural theory for arithmetic

In previous publications a detailed procedural theory for the performance of standard algorithms of

TABLE 1

Example of one-column addition for sums ≤ 99

Pseudo machine-language program	English-addressable subroutines
Attend (1, 1)	Look at this number.
Readin	
Copy SS in NSS	Remember the number.
Attend (+1, +0)	Now look at this next number.
Readin	
Opr	
Attend (+1, +0)	Move down the column.
Readin	If there is another number, add as before and continue.
Jump (0–9)SS, Opr	
Attend (+1, +0)	If not, move down to the blank space.
Outright NSS	Write down the number of ones in the answer.
Deleteright NSS	
Attend (+0, +1)	Now look at the space to the left.
Outright NSS	Write down the number of tens in the answer (unless it is zero).
Deleteright NSS	
End	

arithmetic in column format was proposed (Suppes, 1972, 1980).

To give a concrete context for the later consideration of eye movements, I first describe the simple register machine and its language. To do so, I turn to a simple but natural example, children of seven or eight years of age being taught what it means to carry out the teacher's request "Add these numbers," where the numbers are written in a standard column form.

I first analyse the problem in terms of a pseudo-machine-language which has some psychological basis. Then I ask, how can we actually proceed with instruction, and so how do we communicate with the student? My answer is that we build up the complex procedure of adding – the meaning of *Add these numbers* – by using simpler commands whose meaning is already known to the student. We can thus say that our complex procedure of adding numbers is first synthesized for the student by calling up simpler subroutines that are the meaning of commands he already understands.

I now turn to the pseudo-machine-language used in the program at the left of Table 1.

For one-column addition, two registers suffice in our scheme of analysis. There is a stimulus-supported register [SS] which holds an encoded representation of a printed symbol to which the student is perceptually attending. In the present case the alphabet of such symbols consists of the 10 digits and the underline symbol '_'. As a new symbol is attended to, previously stored symbols are lost unless transferred to the second register, the non-stimulus-supported register [NSS], which provides longer-term storage for making computations.

I drastically simplify the perceptual situation by conceiving each exercise as being presented on a grid with at most one symbol in each square of the grid. For column addition we number the coordinates of the grid from the upper right-hand corner. Thus, in the exercise

$$\begin{array}{c} 5 \\ 4 \\ \underline{7} \end{array}$$

the coordinates of the digit 5 are (1,1), the coordinates of 4 are (2,1) and the coordinates of 7 are (3,1), with the first coordinate being the row number and the second being the column number (the column number is needed for the general case).

The restricted set of instructions we need for column addition is the following:

Attend (a, b):	Direct attention to grid position (a, b).
(±a, ±b):	Shift attention on the grid by (±a, ±b).
Readin [SS]:	Read into the stimulus-supported register the physical symbol in the grid position addressed by Attend.
Lookup [R1] + [R2]:	Lookup table of basic addition facts for adding contents of registers [R1] and [R2] and store the result in [R1].
Copy [R1] in [R2]:	Copy the content of register [R1] into register [R2].
Jump (val) R, L:	Jump to line labeled L if content of register [R] is val.
Outright [R]:	Write (output) the rightmost symbol of register [R] at grid position addressed by Attend.
Deleteright [R]:	Delete the rightmost symbol of register [R].
End:	Terminate processing of current exercise.

Of these instructions, only *Lookup* does not have an elementary character. In our complete analysis, it has the status of a subroutine built up from more primitive operations such as those of counting. It is, of course, more than a problem of constructing the table of basic addition facts from counting subroutines; it is also a matter of being able to add a single digit to any number stored in the non-stimulus-supported register [NSS], as, for example, in adding many rows of digits in a given column. I omit the details of building up this subroutine. It should also be obvious that the remaining instructions are not a minimal set.

The left-hand column of Table 1 shows a program for adding any single column of numbers such that the sum is equal to or less than 99. As would be expected, the program for multiple-column addition or subtraction is a good deal more complicated. A description of these programs may be found in Suppes (1972) or Suppes et al. (1983).

3. Axioms for eye movements in doing arithmetic

A detailed presentation of a mathematical model of eye movements in doing arithmetic is given in Suppes et al. (1982, 1983). The purpose here will be to review and comment on the basic axioms, with some modifications made, and then later to analyse the way in which the axioms must be changed as we move from arithmetic to reading. As would be expected, there are necessary simplifications of the theory of eye movements given here. We reach only a certain level of detail. For example, there is no treatment of the velocity or acceleration of the saccades, or of their angular length. We do emphasize the stochastic nature of eye movements, a point which is not always completely recognized in the literature. This leads to specific assumptions about the probabilistic distribution of the duration of fixations and also of the direction of movement. This stochastic aspect of eye movements has been well recognized in much of the literature, at least since Nachmias (1959).

The axioms fall naturally into two parts. The first part deals with the duration of fixation. An important point here is the underlying rationale of the axioms. Conceptualization is in terms of eye-control instructions being executed to control the duration of fixation. A fixation which executes only a single instruction is assumed to be exponentially distributed, and when n instructions are being executed internally as part of a single fixation then the duration of fixation is a convolution of n exponentials with the same parameter. The exponential is assumed for mathematical simplicity and is reasonably consistent with existing data. (For some recent data supporting the exponential distribution in infants and free-viewing adults, see Harris et al., 1988.) This assumption, which was used in Suppes et al. (1983) for arithmetic, applies in a very natural way, as we shall see, to the case of reading. It should be emphasized that the internal instructions are not ones that I am attempting to identify in the present context. They do not, for example, correspond directly to the instructions shown in the left-hand column of Table 1. I think of these eye-control instructions as the fine-grained instructions needed for performing a cognitive task, such as executing an algorithm of arithmetic or reading a passage of text. The coarser instructions of Table 1, for example, are best thought of as subroutines, constructed from these fine-grained instructions.

3.1. Axioms on duration of fixation

AXIOM F1. *The execution time of each eye-control instruction is independent of past processing and the present stimulus context.*

AXIOM F2. *Each fixation lasts for the execution of* n *internal instructions, for* n = *1,2,. . ..*

AXIOM F3. *The execution times for the* n *instructions executed during a given fixation are identically distributed.*

The first axiom by itself implies that each eye-control instruction is executed in exponentially distributed time, undoubtedly a simplification but a reasonable approximation for present purposes. The second axiom, together with the first, implies that the duration of each fixation is distributed as a convolution of exponential distributions. The third axiom implies that the instructions executed during a given fixation are identically distributed, that is, have the same exponential parameter. The axioms are stated in a general form, because without knowing the number of instructions occurring during a fixation, a direct parametric test of the distribution of fixation durations is not possible. However, results were not too bad when the following special axiom was assumed.

AXIOM F4. *In processing arithmetic algorithms,* n = *1 or* n = *2.*

On the basis of this axiom it is possible to compare histograms of fixation durations to the combination of two distributions, one of which is an exponential distribution and the other a convolution of two exponential distributions with the same parameter. This distribution of fixations has the form:

$$f(t) = \frac{\alpha}{\lambda_1} e^{-t/\lambda_1} + \frac{(1-\alpha)t}{\lambda^2_2} e^{-t/\lambda_2} \qquad (1)$$

Direction of saccades. The next set of axioms is concerned with the direction of saccadic movement. This is conceptualized as a random walk, and some data on the Markovian character of this random walk are presented below. Note that the direction of saccades, not their temporal duration, nor the direction of fixations, is assumed to be a random walk in discrete trials. The full process is continuous in time. This discrete part is abstracted for purposes of data analysis. For the grid display described earlier, there are seven kinds of motion in the random-walk model. The first motion is simply the *stay put*, which means that the *region of regard* stays within a given square of the grid display. It is important to note that several saccades can occur within the same region of regard. The stay put motion is such a saccade. Here the region of regard is taken to be a square of the grid. The region of regard is similar to the concept of gaze in Just and Carpenter's reading studies (1980). They define *gaze* as the aggregate of fixations on a single displayed word.

The second type of movement is the *forward* step, which represents progress in the standard normative formulation of the algorithmic sequence. In general, this means moving down in the column or, when the column is completed, moving to the top of the next column on the left. The third, fourth and fifth movements correspond to three forms of backtracking. *Backtrack1* is the motion from the second row to the top row. The step *backtrack2* is the motion back to the top of the column but with two or more steps, and *backtrack3* is the motion from a row to the preceding row if the preceding row is not the top row. In the axioms we do not formulate each type of backtrack motion explicitly, but these three are the actual cases used in order to break up the analysis in the most significant way.

The sixth step is that of *skipping* over a square on the grid. There is good evidence in the arithmetic data that for a certain percentage of the time a square on the grid is not fixated even though the stimulus there is cognitively, and therefore visually, comprehended. This implies that skipping was due to the use of extrafoveal vision to recognize the numbers displayed. The important point is that stimuli at some distance from the fixation point may be recognized, a phenomenon that needs to be accounted for by any theoretical model. The seventh motion is the catchall *other*, which includes all the cases of motion that do not satisfy the standard algorithm and that do not have a clear cognitive interpretation. Given the stochastic character of eye movements, it is important to report and analyse this seventh class of movement in order to give a sense of how faithfully the algorithm of the register-machine model is being followed.

These assumptions about the random motion are made explicit in the following axioms:

3.2. Axioms on saccades in arithmetic

AXIOM D1. *If processing is complete in a given region of regard, then jump to the next grid square in the register-machine model, i.e., the normative model of the algorithm.*

AXIOM D2. *If processing in a given region of regard is not complete and non-stimulus-supported memory has not decayed, stay put on present grid square.*

AXIOM D3. *If processing in the present region of regard is not complete and non-stimulus-supported memory has decayed, backtrack to the immediately preceding row in the same column or to the beginning of the column.*

AXIOM D4. *If the present region of regard also provides a perceptual image of the next grid square and processing it is complete, then skip over the next square to the following one.*

AXIOM D5. *A saccade is independent of past motion and earlier stimuli.*

It should be noted that these axioms do say something, of course, about the length of a saccade but only in terms of the random walk on the grid. Axiom D5 is an informal statement of the independence-of-path assumption needed to imply the Markovian character of the random walk. For the purposes of studying the algorithms of arithmetic, this level of generality can be accepted although it would still be useful to have a more detailed study of the actual angular length of saccades, and to relate these angular lengths to the random walk. This, however, will have to be a subject for future study in which stimuli and tasks are chosen to encourage variation in saccade length.

4. Survey of the data analysis on arithmetic performance

I will present here a summary of the data analysis. The experimental methodology and methods of analysis are presented in detail in Suppes et al. (1982, 1983). The subjects were two adult male college students, one eighth-grade girl, and two fifth-grade boys. The subjects were selected from a pool on the basis of the capacity of the eye-tracking device to properly generate eye-tracking data for them. The computer-based eye-tracking system known as PERSEUS (Anliker, Floyd, Morf, Kailath)* incorporated as a peripheral hardware device a two-dimensional double-Purkinje-image eye-tracker (Cornsweet and Crane, 1973; revised by Crane and Steele, 1978). The system determines eye position with an accuracy estimated to have less than five minutes of arc error over a field of 20 × 20 degrees in good subjects.

4.1. Distributions of fixations

First we present data on two subjects, comparing the histogram of fixations to the mixture distribu-

* Anliker, J., Floyd, R., Morf, M. and Kailath, T. Biocybernetic Factors in Human Perception and Memory. Final report for the Advanced Research Projects Agency of the Department of Defense. ARPA Order Number 3177, July 1977. Stanford University, Center for Systems Research.

tion given by Eqn. 1, with parameters α, λ_1 and λ_2 to be estimated from the data. The scale on the abscissa is measured in seconds, and the frequency of fixations is shown on the ordinate. The threshold for a recorded fixation was 25 ms, so each histogram is for fixations of more than 25 ms. This amount should be added to each column of the histogram to get the total duration of a fixation. Eqn. 1 was fitted to the 'delayed' histograms, i.e., those shown below without the added 25 ms. (This methodological point is being made explicit to make clear how an approximately exponential distribution was fitted to each histogram.) Since saccades of about 5′ of arc or more were detected and recorded, the histograms contain a number of fixations of short duration, which were interrupted by what are called microsaccades, those of less than 12 or so minutes of arc (McConkie, 1983).

Fig. 1 shows the histogram and fitted distribution for one adult subject. The data are combined for both addition and subtraction exercises, with slightly more than 108,000 fixations. This adult subject had 12 sessions on addition exercises and 9 sessions on subtraction. The three parameters in this distribution (see Eqn. 1) are $\alpha = 0.75$, that is, the weighting of the exponential distribution, $\lambda_1 = 0.272$, which is the mean of the exponential distribution, and $\lambda_2 = 0.121$, which is one-half the mean for the convolution of the two exponentials. The histogram of Fig. 1 is consistent with reading data on fixation durations: means of 200–300 ms and large standard deviations (Kliegl et al., 1983).

Fig. 2 shows the histogram and fitted distribution of fixation durations for a 14-year-old child subject with over 16,000 fixations in 12 sessions of mixed exercises on addition and subtraction. The most interesting feature of this distribution is its nonmonotonic character. The estimated parameters of the mixture distribution express this feature of the data but are not able to fit it completely satisfactorily. The values of the parameters are $\alpha = 0.04$, $\lambda_1 = 0.009$ and $\lambda_2 = 0.130$.

In the case of both subjects the fits of the distributions are reasonably good, but, given the very large number of observations, there are clearly significant deviations. For present theoretical purposes, it is probably not wise to try to improve the fit of these distributions by more complicated theoretical assumptions, although this should be a point of concentration in the future.

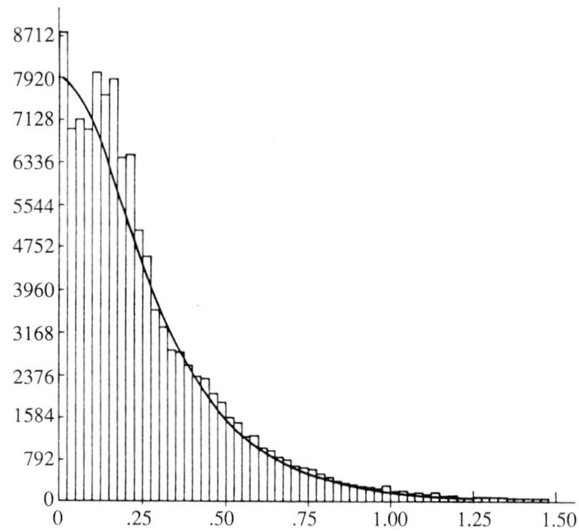

Fig. 1. Histogram and fitted distribution of fixation durations for one adult subject.

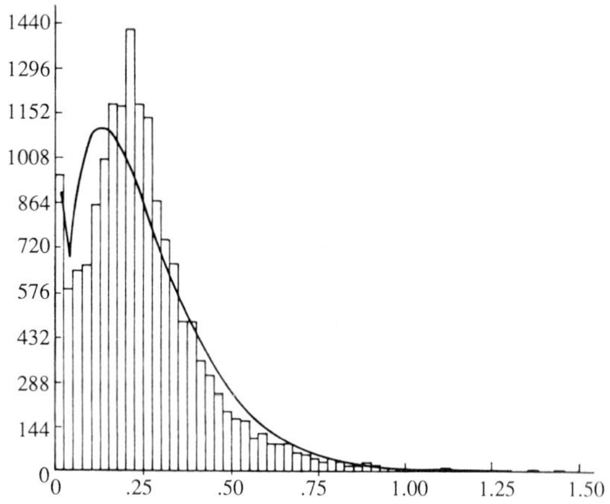

Fig. 2. Histogram and fitted distribution of fixation durations for one child subject.

An immediate point of theoretical concern is the *rate* of microsaccades and fixations of short duration. It was consistent with that reported in the literature for various experimental conditions. For example, in a well-known study of microsaccades in reading (Cunitz and Steinman, 1969) one subject reading 30 paragraphs made 82 microsaccades dur-

TABLE 2

Means of relative frequency data for the random-walk model with seven possible movements

Subject	Stay put	Forward	bktrck1	bktrck2	bktrck3	Skip	Other
1A	.585	.214	.027	.008	.024	.057	.085
1S	.487	.187	.034	.014	.019	.099	.161
2A	.668	.172	.017	.005	.011	.036	.091
2S	.608	.119	.035	.005	.014	.067	.152
3	.340	.108	.067	.022	.073	.030	.361
4	.622	.094	.051	.008	.029	.025	.170
5	.609	.048	.034	.007	.046	.010	.247

ing 1712 fixations with a mean fixation of 473 ms. Assume now, as a simplification of Eqn. 1, that fixation durations are exponentially distributed. Then the probability of a microsaccade in the initial duration segment of a fixation can be equated to the probability of a fixation duration of not more than 50 ms. Using the mean of 473 ms as the mean of the exponential distribution, the probability of a microsaccade in the initial duration segment of 50 ms is approximately 0.05, and the rate observed, assuming independence and stationarity, was 0.048. (This comparison is only a qualitative one to show that the rate is comparable to that observed in arithmetic. A more detailed analysis is not appropriate here.) The point is that this use of the exponential distribution, or for a more detailed analysis, Eqn. 1, supports Cunitz and Steinman's conclusion that a single process governs both microsaccades (together with very short fixations) and larger saccades (with longer intersaccadic fixations). Such a single process is implied by the axioms given above for eye movements in arithmetic. The properties of approximately exponential distributions have not as yet been widely used in the theoretical analysis of fixations.

4.2. Direction of saccades

Table 2, taken from Suppes et al. (1983), shows the means averaged over sessions of relative-frequency data for the random-walk model with seven possible movements. The first two lines of the table show the data for the first adult subject. The *A* refers to the results on addition exercises and the *S* to subtraction. Lines 3 and 4 of the table are defined similarly for the second adult subject. The three young subjects received mixed exercises. They are shown respectively as lines 5, 6 and 7 in the table. The S.D.s for all subjects and movement types are relatively small, the largest being 0.060. Over 70% of the S.D.s are less than 0.02.

The data of Table 2 are quite stable across subjects, in many respects to a surprising degree. For example, *stay put* is the dominant motion for all subjects with the exception of subject 3, and in the case of this subject the higher probability of the catchall movement *other* is only slightly higher. This unusually high percentage for *other* in the case of subject 3 indicates very poor following of the standard algorithms of addition and subtraction. The step *backtrack2* has the minimum mean frequency for all subjects. When that step is removed, *backtrack3* for the adults and *skip* for the children are minimal.

In contrast to the kinds of differences that have been observed for different regions of regard in reading, presumably corresponding primarily to cognitive characteristics of different words, in the case of arithmetic no striking quantitative differences for means of average fixations were found to be associated with the seven different steps of the random walk. These data are presented in Table 3.

TABLE 3

Means of average fixation durations for different steps in the random-walk model

Subject	Stay put	Forward	bktrck1	bktrck2	bktrck3	Skip	Other
1A	.288	.256	.253	.129	.257	.275	.212
1S	.318	.238	.289	.149	.302	.275	.247
2A	.288	.350	.177	.341	.181	.321	.158
2S	.253	.232	.234	.152	.166	.294	.169
3	.246	.248	.304	.240	.295	.226	.252
4	.148	.147	.197	.142	.153	.096	.128
5	.145	.186	.156	.127	.200	.178	.160

TABLE 4

Mean correlations of successive fixation durations

Subject	Number of sessions	Number of fixation durations: Mean	Number of fixation durations: S.D.	Mean correlation of successive fixations
1A	11	4542	655.9	−.0006
1S	10	2398	143.5	−.0193
2A	12	6470	882.7	.0326
2S	9	3371	647.8	.0180
3	12	1309	171.2	.0472
4	7	4075	728.3	.1171
5	10	3119	272.0	.0871

It is also to be noted that the range of mean average fixations to be found in Table 3 falls very much within the range ordinarily observed in fixations in reading. Here the range is from 127 ms to 350 ms: I emphasize again these are the ranges of means, not of individual observations. It can be seen from the histograms of Fig. 1 and 2 that there were individual fixations with much longer durations, as would be expected under any reasonable probabilistic theory of fixation durations.

4.3. Immediacy and eye-mind assumptions

In a number of publications on eye movements in reading, Carpenter and Just (for a good summary see 1983) have emphasized the importance of two assumptions. The first is the immediacy assumption, which is that a reader tries to interpret each word of a text immediately rather than waiting to interpret or process it after a number of words have been perceived. This assumption is reflected directly in the axioms F1–F3 on duration of fixations. One way to test the immediacy assumption, which is common to their analysis and to that given here for arithmetic, is to examine the correlation of successive fixation durations. The examination of the data in this fashion does not settle all aspects of testing the immediacy assumption, but it is a test that should pick up any strong effects of violation of immediacy. Data on this question from Suppes et al. (1983) are shown in Table 4, which shows the means and standard deviations of a number of fixation durations for individual subjects averaged across sessions. For each subject there are a very large number of fixation durations in each session and therefore substantial data to analyse for the correlations of successive fixation durations. The mean autocorrelations of lag one are shown in the fourth column of Table 4. The autocorrelation statistic can be written as follows, where d_i represents the ith fixation duration, and $\bar{d}$ their average:

$$\sum_{i=1}^{n} (d_i - \bar{d})(d_{i-1} - \bar{d}) / \mathrm{sqrt} \left[\left(\sum_{i=1}^{n} (d_i - \bar{d})^2 \right) \left(\sum_{i=2}^{n} (d_{i-1} - \bar{d})^2 \right) \right]$$

The striking thing about the data in Table 4 is that the correlations are all quite small. There is really no evidence of the duration of one fixation affecting that of the next fixation. In this respect, the data strongly support the immediacy assumption for arithmetic, for, given the very low autocorrelations of lag one, it is unlikely that there are other forms of temporal dependence in the data.

Carpenter and Just's eye-mind assumption, the second one mentioned above, is that the reader continues to fixate a word until all the cognitive processes initiated by receiving that word have been completed. In terms of the axioms stated above, the eye-mind assumption would be reflected for arithmetic in Axiom F2, which asserts that a fixation lasts for the time required to execute some number of internal instructions. Assuming that different regions of regard in executing an algorithm should lead to different control instructions being executed, fixation duration should vary with the region of regard. This seems unlikely, because, as is already evident from the analysis given, we got reasonably good fits to the histograms of fixation durations by assuming that the number of control instructions is no more than two (see Fig. 1 and 2). However, it is quite possible that certain structural features of the arithmetic problems, such as the region of regard where a carry is required in addition or a borrow in subtraction, would lead to a structurally determined variation in fixation duration. Such variation would be very much in the spirit of Carpenter and Just's eye-mind assumption for reading. Data and analysis bearing on such structural variations are taken from Suppes et al. (1983). The fixation durations were regressed on the following variables, which are local variables in the terminology introduced at the beginning of the chapter:

ROW, the row the fixation is in,
COL, the column the fixation is in,
LENGTH, the number of digits in the top row,
ONOFF, an indicator in subtraction of whether a borrow was needed from the next column, and in addition of whether a carry was given to that column from the previous one.

The regression equation was therefore

$$y_i = a_0 + a_1 \,\mathrm{LENGTH}_i = a_2\mathrm{ROW}_i + a_3\mathrm{COLUMN}_i + a_4\mathrm{ONOFF}_i$$

The results of these regressions are shown in Table 5 in the form of means of estimated regression coefficients. As can be seen from the size of the various coefficients, the regression on the structural variables accounts for only a relatively small part of the variation in fixation durations: the range of the square of multiple correlation is 0.0003 to 0.0912. So, significant effects of structural characteristics on fixation durations are not found, contrary to the results for reading. Unlike the immediacy assumption, the eye-mind assumption does not contribute to our understanding of the processes involved in doing arithmetic.

TABLE 5

Means of estimated regression coefficients

Subject	Row	Column	Length	Onoff
1A	.0296	.0133	−.0185	−.0350
1S	.0326	.0148	−.0214	.0300
2A	.0164	−.0188	.0162	.0316
2S	.0161	−.0152	.0177	.0437
3	−.0090	.0150	−.0238	.0352
4	−.0022	−.0046	−.0170	.0155
5	.0168	−.0090	−.0160	.0220

4.4. Scanpath fit

In the normative register-machine model the random-walk motion in addition and subtraction should reduce to just two motions, namely, *forward* and *stay put*. Backtracking is evidence of memory decay which is excluded in the normative model, and *other* is indication of wandering attention. What is to be said about goodness of fit, of course, could easily include backtracking as well, but that is not the issue.

For the normative models of addition and subtraction, three distinct measures of fit were tested for the random-walk model with just the two motions of *forward* and *stay put* (Suppes et al., 1983). The first measure, designated fit-1, is constructed as follows. A perfect scanpath was defined to be moving top to bottom in each column, with a fixation at the bottom of a column being immediately succeeded by a fixation in the first row of the column immediately to the left. The sequence begins in the upper right-hand grid position. In accordance with the register-machine model, we denote the duration of the fixation at time t as *conforming* to the model when the position p_t of a fixation at time t is either p_{t-1} or $p_{t-1} + 1$. In other words, fixation is conforming if it is either staying put in the same grid or advancing one square. When this is not the case, we denote the fixation time as nonconforming. The analysis given here is for addition. It is only slightly different for subtraction. The statistic is then simply the ratio of the conforming time to the overall time. Note of course that this measure, as can be seen from Table 6, is somewhat optimistic because so much of the time is spent in the *stay put* movement.

The second fit errs on the side of being too pessimistic. In this case the *stay put* durations, i.e., all the durations that constituted a repeated fixation on the same grid square, were deleted. Therefore, the ratio of forward motions to all other motions constituted fit-2.

The third measure of fit is probably the best and is, as a fit, a genuine correlation. To compute this measure for each arithmetic exercise we first determined how many fixation positions, say n, actually occurred in a particular exercise. Then two sequences are defined. First, the sequence $1,\ldots,n$, i.e., the actual sequence, and second, the sequence of grid positions predicted by the register-machine model, without any staying-put motion. The correlation of these two sequences is fit-3. These correlations are then averaged across the exercises for a given subject, and, in the case of the adult subjects, for a given type of exercise, addition or subtraction. Note that fit-3 is somewhat pessimistic. It would be natural to make a monotonic transformation on the sequence to naturally allow for repetitions, which were not included in the normative register-machine model.

TABLE 6

Means of measures of fit of the scanpaths to the register-machine model

Subject	Fit-1	Fit-2	Fit-3
1A	.819	.518	.874
1S	.703	.284	.772
2A	.878	.619	.833
2S	.759	.301	.728
3	.462	.171	.708
4	.721	.299	.701
5	.627	.165	.583

The data for these three measures of fit of the scanpaths to the register-machine model are shown in Table 6. The data are means from averaging over sessions for each subject. As suggested above, fit-1 is too optimistic and fit-2 is probably too pessimistic. The discrepancy between the two is especially strong for subtraction. Fit-3, which is the correlation of the actual and the normative sequence of grid positions, is perhaps the most appropriate of the three measures, and the fit is reasonably good for all subjects. I do not want to suggest that these three measures of fit are necessarily the best. They are certainly not the only ones. They do tackle the problem of relating our normative ideas of arithmetic to actual behavior.

5. Minimal control model of reading

It does not take much reflection to realize that, in principle, models of reading must inevitably be more complicated than models for performing arithmetic algorithms. In arithmetic the algorithms are, in one obvious sense, self-contained, which means that the interpretation of perception beyond the recognition of symbols is minimal. Reading is quite the opposite. The meaning of lexical items and the way syntax and semantics are interlocked to put together the meaning of phrases, entire sentences and passages of discourse introduce direct complications that do not exist in arithmetic. From a formal standpoint, the student can learn to do the algorithms of arithmetic, and his eye movements can be trained to perform accordingly, without any understanding of the concept of number being required. This is not at all the case for reading. Of course, as an experimental matter and perhaps occasionally for applications in some highly specialized domains, individuals can be taught to read aloud the written text of a language they do not understand at all. But in ordinary reading, perceptual and cognitive aspects of the task are inextricably intertwined, and I shall not attempt to deal with each separately. In particular, there is no review here of the general literature on eye movements in perception.

There is very considerable controversy as to the relation between eye movements and reading. Even direct phenomenological questions do not seem to be finally and decisively settled. In order to address some of the most important considerations, I begin by constructing a minimal control model which lets the process of reading influence eye movements in only a minimal way. Probably no one would be willing to accept this model as correct, but it constitutes an interesting model from which to examine the way in which the context of reading text forces deviations from this minimal control model. The model is called one of minimal control because the control of eye movements introduced as part of the cognitive process of reading is minimal in character. It is assumed that most of the process is an automatic low-level process, little disturbed by cognitive and linguistic aspects of reading. The two basic assumptions of the minimal control model are, first, that durations of fixations are not affected by stimulus context, that is, by the content of the reading text, and, second, the length of saccades is not influenced by text content, but only by the physical layout of the page.

5.1. Axioms on duration of fixation

AXIOMS F1–F4. *As stated for arithmetic.*

The important point of the axioms is that little variation in the distribution of durations is permitted, only that based upon the number of internal instructions $n = 1$ or $n = 2$, which leads to the mean distribution (1). It is not clear that the mixture distribution as represented in Eqn. 1 will fit the distribution of fixation durations in reading as well as it did for arithmetic, where even there, as already noted, it can certainly be improved upon. One of the difficulties is the lack of studies of fits of theoretical distributions to durations of fixation in reading. Lacking such evidence, the present assumptions provide an appropriate mathematically simple start.

Some histograms shown in the literature, such as in Lévy-Schoen and O'Regan (1979, p. 13), suggest that Eqn. 1 would not fit very well because the unimodal histogram at about 180 ms falls away rapidly for shorter fixation durations, contrary to the ones shown in Fig. 1 and 2 in this chapter. Some of this variation, however, may be an artifact of the way in which fixations are calibrated for short time intervals, and without a much more technical analysis than is appropriate here will not be examined with any care. (See the earlier remarks on microsaccades in connection with Fig. 1.) Other aspects of the distribution given by Lévy-Schoen and O'Regan would fit fairly well, although the right-hand tail seems somewhat short. On the other hand, the distribution is based on a relatively small number of fixations, namely 3,499, whereas those given in Fig. 1 and 2 are based on a much larger number of observations.

The implications of the minimal control model for the theory of fixation duration need some further emphasis. The model is stated in such a way that variations in duration are not due to variation in stimulus conditions, that is, variations in reading text, but are due simply to the probabilistic nature of the process. Assumptions of this kind have not been discussed very extensively in the eye movement literature, but to assume an exponential, or convolution of two exponentials, as the distribution of duration is to make the process highly probabilistic. Much of the reading literature appears to be based on the assumption that durations should not have this much probabilistic 'slack' in their variation, i.e., the process should not be as random as required by an exponential or convolution of exponential distributions. But such distribution questions are not discussed at all in the many excellent and detailed articles in the volumes on eye movements in reading edited by Rayner (1983) or by Gale and Johnson (1984). Most commonly, only mean data rather than distributional data are presented.

I now turn to the axioms on saccades. With appropriate rewording for the case of reading they have really the same content as axioms D1–D5 for arithmetic. One of the things that will not be made explicit in the axioms is the movement back to the left at the beginning of each new line: this will be left as part of the forward movement of the motion as characterized abstractly for arithmetic as well. There is a very similar phenomenon in arithmetic as one moves from the bottom of one column to the top of the next column on the left. Obviously, in a detailed physical account of the saccadic movements, specific recording and analysis of this special movement would be carried out.

5.2. Axioms on saccades in reading

AXIOM D1. *If processing is complete in a given region of regard, then move to the next word of text.*

AXIOM D2. *If processing in a given region of regard is not complete, stay put on the same word.*

AXIOM D3. *If processing in the present region of regard is not complete and non-stimulus-supported memory has decayed, backtrack to the immediately preceding word or phrase.*

AXIOM D4. *If the present region of regard also provides a perceptual image of the next word and the processing of it has been completed, then skip over the next word to the following one.*

AXIOM D5. *Independence-of-path assumption the same as for arithmetic.*

These axioms then give us something very similar to what was examined in arithmetic, namely, a random walk consisting of four movements: forward, stay put, backtrack, and skip. It will also be obvious in any real data that the catchall motion *other* needs to be added for a fifth possibility. The division of backtrack into several kinds can also be done here by examining whether the backtracking is to the immediately preceding word or two words preceding, etc. Data from various sources, for example, Hogaboam (1983), support the hypothesis that regression or backtracking beyond the two preceding words rarely occurs.

Direction and size of saccade are under cognitive control in this minimal model. It is to be noted, therefore, that this is not in any true sense a minimal model. A strong minimal model would put a probability distribution on the four types of saccadic movement formulated in the axioms and then limit cognitive control to the choice of movement. Given the overwhelming data showing that saccadic movements do move from word to word and very seldom, for example, focus on the empty spaces between words, it seems reasonable to reject a strongly minimal model for the weaker one formulated here. For evidence of the essential role of blank spaces in search procedures which do not involve reading, see Jacobs (1987). Almost any salient stimulus pattern irregularity probably has an effect on size of saccade. Notice that Just and Carpenter's concept of gaze is easily accommodated within the minimal control model because of its essential equivalence to the concept of region of regard used earlier and in the above axioms.

6. Data support for minimal control model of reading

6.1. Independence

The axioms of the minimal control model embody, as in the case of arithmetic, some very strong assumptions about independence and stationarity. First, consider independence. It is natural to ask whether the low correlations of successive fixation durations observed in arithmetic and reported in Table 4 are also found in reading. The bulk of the data seems to support this assumption of independence of fixation duration from previous fixation durations. Correlations reported in the literature seem to be quite small. Good examples are Andriessen and Devoogd (1973), Rayner and McConkie (1976) and Hogaboam (1983).

6.2. Stationarity

The evidence for stationarity of process seems to be quite positive, in the sense that, once adulthood is reached, reading behavior remains quite stable, but there are two riders to this conclusion. First, there is a developmental process which is not meant in any way to be covered by the axioms stated for the minimal model. Second, there is the issue, not to be addressed at this point, of whether the type of text influences the parameters of the distributions and random walk assumed as part of the minimal model. The basic assumption of stationarity excludes such contextural effects, which are addressed below.

6.3. Robustness

There is one conclusion which seems to be generally agreed upon and which supports the robustness of the axioms of the minimal model. This is the conclusion that direct training of ocular activity does not have very much effect, in fact no more or perhaps less than well-motivated reading practice alone (Tinker, 1958; Morton, 1966).

6.4. Random walk

The basic axioms of the minimal control model concerned with the random walk incorporate effects of the reading context on the probability of forward, stay put, backtrack or skipping motions. The model is not compatible with probabilistic sequential dependencies. An example of such a sequential dependency would be that the probability that a forward motion is followed by a forward motion is greater than that a stay put motion is followed by a forward motion. It is to be noted that the nonexistence of such dependencies in the random motion itself does not, of course, prove that the reading context itself will not have significant effects on the random walk, a matter already postulated in the basic axioms.

What I have not been able to find in the literature on reading is a summary of data for the random-walk motion corresponding to Table 2 given above for arithmetic. For example, I have not been able to determine any estimate of the miscellaneous category *other* for competent adult readers. Hogaboam's (1983) data do show that backtracking or regression beyond two words apparently occurs with quite low probability.

6.5. Other tests needed

The current literature on eye movements in reading has not been oriented toward the testing of overall models of the reading process. To evaluate the minimal control model we need, in addition to the random-walk analysis mentioned above, tests of independence of successive fixation durations of the sort shown in Table 4 for arithmetic, and tests of scanpath as shown in Table 6 for arithmetic. The point is that the thing I have found especially difficult to obtain from the literature on eye movements in reading is some idea of how good the fit is to various normative models. In particular, it has been especially difficult to get a sense of how many of the fixations and thus saccadic movements are to be classified as *other* in the terminology used for arithmetic. What would be especially interesting would be the data on wandering fixations on the part of good readers. Notice that the lowest percentage of *other* movements in the case of arithmetic was something of the order of 9% for the two adults doing addition exercises. In the case of subtraction, a notably more difficult task for everyone, the category of *other* movements rose to above 15%. For the child subjects these percentages were higher. One might conjecture that reading is a more disciplined activity for most people than arithmetic, one that is certainly engaged in more regularly as adults, and therefore we might expect that the category *other* should, for good readers with text of normal difficulty, be below 5%. But it would be most desirable to have extensive data on this question.

6.6. Status of global variables

In evaluating the fit of the minimal control model, it is necessary to distinguish global variables from local ones. Local variables such as features of individual words are considered in the next section. Only local variables affect the evaluation of fit. Global variables are determined by individual differences in readers, individual differences in entire texts, and individual differences in approach to the task, which can vary with a given subject from one occasion to another. Broadly speaking, it is these three different kinds of global variables – those of reader, text and task – which do not affect the validity of the minimal control model for the following reason. We expect the parameters of the minimal control model to vary for each of these global variations. Typically, the length of fixation durations and, even more, length of saccades will vary directly with the skill of the reader. Early studies of eye movements tended primarily to look in fact at variations caused by global variables (Woodworth, 1938). More recently, good examples of dependence of length of saccade on type of text are to be found in Heller (1982). The differences in mean number of fixations per line, as a function of text, are not large but are completely systematic in the mean. He also obtained (see his Table 1) variation in the number of fixations, depending upon the task instruction: silent reading for comprehension, internal speaking, reading in a low voice for comprehension, and oral reading. Similar results have, for example, been found by Lévy-Schoen (1980). The Lévy-Schoen results and also those of Heller show that instructions to adjust reading speed have systematic effects in the intended direction. Another interesting effect of task instruction reported by Heller (1982) is that when subjects are instructed to look for typing errors a significantly greater number of corrective saccades followed the return sweep. A radically different sort of global variable is the language being read. Eye movements in reading English and Chinese are in many ways surprisingly similar (Sun et al., 1985), but as yet only eye movements in reading English, French or German have been studied in real detail. The changes in the minimal model discussed below are probably in the right direction, even if not correct in detail, for reading many different languages.

A quite different kind of global variable is generated by tasks such as solving word problems in mathematics or science. At least in the case of arithmetic word problems, the data and analysis in de Corte and Verschaffel (1987) indicate the feasibility of beginning with the minimal control model, even though the evidence of incomplete reading is much more extensive than in standard reading experiments. As could be expected, incomplete reading of the problems was a main cause of failure to find a correct solution. Greater deviations from eye movements in standard reading are to be found in the studies by Groner and his associates of eye movement behavior in multi-term series problems (Groner and Groner, 1982, 1983).

This is only a sample of the many different studies showing the effects of global variables on reading. In qualitative terms, none of the effects is enormously surprising. It is important to establish them and also to have a sense of their quantitative magnitude. The existence of so many different significant global variables in no way directly invalidates the minimal control model because it is assumed in this model that changes in the global variables simply mean different parameter values in the model. In this sense, the model makes fundamental assumptions about the qualitative character of eye movements in reading. It is left to specification of the global variables to fix the numerical values of the various parameters. Of course, an important task for the investigation of global variables which I have not considered here is actually that of determining what is a sufficient list of global variables beyond which very little additional improvement in fit will be found. Although this is an important and significant problem, I have set it aside in order to turn to the more critical one of examining ways in which the minimal model fails owing to local variables that cannot in principle be taken account of in the model as formulated.

7. Evidence against minimal control model of reading

First, a demurrer about what is to come as evidence against the model needs to be made. Details of oculomotor characteristics that go beyond the specification of the model will be ignored. This does not mean that such characteristics are not important. For example, determination of the latency time for a saccadic movement is an important consideration in determining the correctness of the immediacy assumption of Just and Carpenter and others. The minimal control model is not sufficiently refined to take account of this latency period. Ballistic characteristics of the saccadic eye movement are also ignored, as is variation in saccadic size smaller than the length of a word. Such variables are ignored because my primary goal is to describe and test a normative model of saccadic eye movement that looks at the most important features of the cognitive task. Thus, for example, in the conception of a random walk I have ignored the difference between forward movement along a line and the return sweep with a possible corrective saccade movement, just as was also done in the case of arithmetic. This simplification helps to concentrate the analysis of the kinds of saccadic patterns that should characterize good reading.

The number of local variables relevant to testing the minimal control model of reading is still enormous. McConkie (1983) gives a table of more than thirty such local influences, as he calls them. Most of them would fall within what I have termed cognitive variables. In spite of the large number of references to experimental studies McConkie gives to document his list, it is still only a small sample of the many relevant experiments. For the model-theoretic orientation I have adopted here, I want to cluster local variables into certain main categories which raise various cognitive questions that are of importance in trying to improve on the minimal control model. I do not mean to suggest that the categories I consider here are necessarily the best ones, and certainly not the only ones, but they are ones that naturally arise in any discussion of reading as a cognitive activity.

As a preliminary step, it is natural to divide the consideration of local variables into two classes, those which affect duration of fixations and those which affect saccadic movements.

7.1. Fixations

I have divided the local variables affecting fixations into three broad classes, which I have identified as line, word, and grammatical variables, with it understood that the grammatical variables refer to grammatical features of a word in the context of its grammatical role or to a more global structure of a grammatical kind, for example, the end of clauses, end of sentences, distinctions between adverbs and verbs, etc.

(i) Line variables. That there are variations in fixation durations, with a special feature being that the first fixation on a line tends to be longer, has been known for some time and has also been recently confirmed (Woodworth, 1938; Rayner, 1977). A more recent study is that of Heller and Müller (1980), cited in Heller (1982). Heller and Müller give a histogram of the variation in fixation times across the line. The greater length of fixation at the beginning of the line is striking. What is also interesting about their data is that when subjects were

asked to scan a random-order arrangement of the same words, thereby generating meaningless text, the variation in fixation time along the line was very much less.

(ii) Word variables. The evidence on the influence of word features is overwhelming in terms of the number of significant studies. But the exact assessment of these effects in terms of their magnitude is more difficult. There is no doubt that there are effects which can easily be demonstrated. For example, fixation durations are longer on shorter words (O'Regan, 1981). It is understood of course that there is usually more than one fixation on longer words.

A more complicated controversy surrounds some variables which are relatively highly correlated. These are the effects of number of letters in a word, number of syllables, and relative frequency of the word. In various publications, Carpenter, Just, and their collegues (for example, Dee-Lucas et al., 1982) show regression on gaze duration which indicates effects of number of syllables and frequency. Their concept of gaze, as discussed earlier, is very similar to that of region of regard. But it is to be noted that gaze duration is not necessarily positively correlated with fixation duration. In fact, according to the O'Regan results just mentioned, the correlation between gaze duration and fixation duration should be negative in the sense that words requiring a longer gaze, and therefore more than one fixation, have individual fixations that are shorter. Fortunately the untangling of these various variables has been done in some detail by Kriegl et al. (1982, 1983). They show that the fits of eye fixation data are better when not just number of syllables and frequency are considered but also number of letters. Moreover, once the number of letters is introduced in a stepwise regression, for example, the additional effect of syllable length is nonexistent and the contribution of word frequency is "decreased from 12 to 3%". They make the point that this dominance of number of letters over the other two variables makes a case for the reduction of cognitive variables to perceptual ones.

(iii) Grammatical variables. One of the relatively clear results concerning the impact of grammatical function on fixations is that short function words are often skipped. One of the better experiments in this area is certainly that of O'Regan (1979), in which the effect of the impact of *the* is separated from the impact of high-frequency three-letter verbs (*are*, *had* and *was*) and also lower-frequency verbs (*ate*, *met* and *ran*). The relative rate of skipping was significant at the 0.001 level, but, as might be expected, the effect was stronger in comparison with the low-frequency verbs. (It should be mentioned that the O'Regan experiment was really concerned with control of saccadic movement rather than fixation but the skipping data are also pertinent for discussion of fixation.) The result concerning skipping of function words opposed to correspondingly short content words has also been duplicated by Carpenter and Just (1983).

At a more general level the conviction is widespread, and surely grounded in some respects, that grammatical structure has an influence on fixation durations. For example, a common hypothesis would be that the fixation duration on less frequent passive forms of verbs would be different from that on active forms. More generally, another kind of hypothesis is that major breaks in grammatical structure will have an effect on fixations. For example, using their measure of gaze, Dee-Lucas et al. (1982), summarizing earlier work, report on the significance of an increase in gaze for the last word in a sentence and the last word in a paragraph. As usual, the fact that the gaze duration increases does not itself directly mean that fixation duration increases.

A natural hypothesis is that when anaphoric reference is appropriate and unambiguous, fixation time will be less than when it is ambiguous or incongruous. Kerr and Underwood (1984) found that this was true, but the results are not at all strong. For example, the duration of first fixations for congruous pronouns was at a mean value of 231 ms, for ambiguous pronouns 232 ms, and for incongruous ones 261 ms. The small differences in these numerical results indicate the difficulties of identifying, in a highly significant form, grammatical effects on fixation durations. As will be shown below, the evidence is better for the impact of grammatical structure on saccadic movements than it is for its impact on fixation duration.

7.2. Saccadic movements

I have grouped local effects on saccadic length under the same three categories of line, word and grammatical variables.

(i) Line variables. The obvious effect of position on the line on saccadic movement is the return sweep. I have ignored that in the minimal control model and will also in the revised model stated in the next section, but I emphasize that in any more complete model it must be taken into account. What is also important is to take particular account of small corrective movements following the return sweep. The rather complicated character of the data is well illustrated by Heller (1982), who found that the number of corrective saccades associated with easy, average and difficult text did not have a simple monotonic relation, that is, with more corrective saccades when the text was more difficult, but depended on the physical length of the line, ranging from 7 cm through 11 cm to 15 cm. Again I emphasize that it is not my purpose here to take account of corrective saccades in the models being considered.

(ii) Word variables. O'Regan (1979) reports two effects on length of word. The saccadic movement is longer when a longer word lies to the right of the fixated word, that is, when enough information about the word to the right is given in peripheral vision to control the central tendency of the movement to that word. A second related effect is that a longer movement occurs following a fixation on a longer word. The purpose of O'Regan's experiment was to reject the rhythmical scan hypothesis, that is, the hypothesis that saccadic movements follow a rhythm of movement independent of the character of text being read. O'Regan's results are significant but, as in the case of many local effects, it is not easy to assess with precision their quantitative magnitude. For example, when the word fixated is short rather than long and the word in peripheral vision to the right is short, mean saccadic movement goes from slightly less than eight to slightly less than twelve letters, an increase of nearly 50%, but the significance level is only 0.05 because, presumably, of the variance in response, which is not reported. A stronger effect occurred when the word to the right in peripheral vision was long. In this case the median saccadic movement size in going from short to long fixated words was from about four letters to about nine, and the significance level is 0.001.

Experimental variations of these effects have been studied by a number of investigators. For example, saccade length decreases when, in the peripheral vision on the right, erroneous letters replace correct letters in words. A similar effect is observed when letters in peripheral vision are replaced by a grating. Relevant studies include those of McConkie and Rayner (1975), McConkie and Underwood (1981), O'Regan (1980), Rayner and Bertera (1979), Rayner et al. (1981) and Rayner and Pollatsek (1981).

(iii) Grammatical variables. The expected difference between active and passive verb forms has already been alluded to. Wanat (1976) showed that the number of regressive eye movements differed between active and passive sentences. The effects were stronger in oral than in silent reading but present in both cases. A well-known study is that of Mehler et al. (1967), who tried to relate both movement and fixation to surface syntactic structure, but general results, including theirs, have not been successfully replicated or clearly established. For example, in an attempted replication, O'Regan (1975) obtained quite different results. In addition, Communale (1973) and Rayner (1975b) found no differences in eye-movement behavior in the immediate neighborhood of the main verb of a sentence, perhaps the most significant grammatical element of a sentence.

The O'Regan (1979) results on the skipping of *the* must also be regarded as showing a grammatical influence on saccadic length, for when a word is skipped the saccadic movement is, in general, longer than when it is not. Rayner (1975a) and O'Regan (1980) show that the degree of linguistic control on saccadic movement does not extend in any significant way beyond six or seven letters to the right of a given fixation point.

Without providing a detailed structural theory, Frazier (1983) shows that eye movement is affected by complex structural features, for example, the number of regressions, as would be expected, is greater for garden-path sentences, that is, sentences in which the reader is led down a certain path of analysis but then finds he is mistaken and must retreat and begin again. Garden-path sentences represent a particularly strong form of local ambiguity. Frazier makes the excellent point that purely lexical considerations cannot account for these kinds of difficulties, and consequently any theory that attempts to reduce structural grammatical features to lexical features alone is bound not to be successful.

8. Revised control model of reading

The evidence reviewed against the minimal control model provides a systematic basis for formulating a better one. This revised model, for reasons which will become apparent, I call the *text-dependent probabilistic control* model of reading or, for short, the TDPC model. The model is called *text-dependent* because characteristics of saccades, excluding those properties such as velocity which are not likely to be under cognitive control, depend in specific ways on the characteristics of stimulus context, that is, the reading text. On the other hand, by taking account of these context dependencies the TDPC model definitely differs from the minimal control model of reading, or the arithmetic model presented earlier, in being dependent on the characteristics of stimulus context, that is, the reading text. Processing varies from moment to moment depending on immediate features of the text. Second, the model is called a *probabilistic control* model to emphasize the importance of probabilistic considerations. Much of the research on eye movements in reading is written as if at bottom there is no probabilistic element: we just have to pursue a research program with sufficient vigor and compulsion to reach a point at which we will not have probabilistic distributions but will deterministically account for essentially a hundred percent of the variance in fixations and saccadic movements. In my own view this is a piece of fantasy. The phenomena are too complicated, and the movements involved are too unstable ever to hope to have anything like a complete deterministic account. Not only now but a hundred years from now, probability distributions will be an important part of the best fundamental account of eye movements in reading. Consequently, not only in the title but, of course, in the revised axioms, probabilistic aspects enter in a fundamental way into the TDPC model – a property shared with the minimal control model.

A probabilistic model is also supported by evidence not stressed earlier about reading but already exhibited in the case of artihmetic (e.g., Table 4); namely, that correlations between and within eye-movement parameters are essentially zero. Rayner and McConkie (1976) showed that saccade size and fixation duration are not correlated. In fact, they found an absence of correlation between successive fixation durations, between successive saccade movements, and between the size of the saccade and the preceding and following fixation time. Similarly, very weak correlations have been reported by Andriessen and Devoogd (1973), and Just and Carpenter (1980) also did not find significant autocorrelations. The absence of such dependencies strongly points to probabilistic elements. Of course, the argument for probabilistic elements at a fundamental level is not conclusively established by nonsignificant correlations, because in principle the introduction of textual, neurophysiological and ballistic variables could still render the process deterministic, but my skepticism that we shall ever be successful in incorporating enough factors to account for all sources of variation has already been expressed.

The revised model takes into account the local variables that have the largest effects on eye movements. Variables with little or no effect are ignored. For example, it is my assessment that almost no studies show a significant text effect on fixation durations. Most of the variables that affect fixations, summarized in the previous section, have only relatively small effects. The only substantial effect is that of the monotonic decrease of fixation duration as the eye moves from left to right along the line of reading text. This effect is taken account of in revision of the axioms. The relationship that Just and Carpenter (1980) show to number of letters or number of syllables or frequency, which is pretty much reduced by Kliegl et al. (1983) to number of letters, is not really an effect on fixation duration but on the random-walk movement. With an increase in number of letters there is an increase in the probability of a *stay put* motion on a given word. Similarly, the fact of often skipping function words (O'Regan, 1979) and, therefore, having zero fixations, is really again a matter of saccadic movement. It is therefore the saccadic movements that are more dependent on text than fixations.

It seems to me that the summary given in the previous section leads to five features that need to be taken account of in the revised model. (i) The probability of a *stay put* motion increases with the number of letters in a word; (ii) a saccadic movement is longer when a longer word is to the right; (iii) a saccadic movement is longer when the current fixation is on a longer word; (iv) high-frequency function words have the highest probability of being skipped; (v) ambiguous or difficult grammatical structures increase the number of regressive movements.

8.1. Revised axioms on fixation duration

AXIOM F1. *The execution time of each eye-control instruction monotonically decreases along the line of text, but is independent of task processing and the present word context.*

AXIOM F2. *Each fixation lasts for the execution of* n *internal instructions, for* n = *1,2,. . ..*

AXIOM F3. *The execution times for the* n *instructions executed during a given fixation are identically distributed.*

AXIOM F4. *In processing reading text,* n = *1 or* n = *2.*

Note that the only change in the axioms for fixation from those for the minimal control model is in axiom F1, which takes account of the change in duration of fixation as the eye moves along the line of text. On the basis of the change in this axiom the distribution of fixations as given in Eqn. 1 in section 2 is replaced now by the following equation:

$$f_x(t) = \frac{\alpha}{g_1(x)}\, e^{-t/g_1(x)} + \frac{(1-\alpha)t}{g_2^2(x)}\, e^{-t/g_2(x)} \qquad (2)$$

where $g_1(x)$ and $g_2(x)$ are both monotonically increasing functions of x, which measures position in the line of text. Note that the functions $g_i(x)$ are monotonically increasing because we want the mean of the distribution to be monotonically decreasing as the eye moves to the right in reading a line of text. It would, of course, be desirable in formulating the new axioms to give a specific parametric form to $g_i(x)$ and similarly for the other probabilistic axioms on saccadic movement to be considered below, but this seems unrealistic in view of the fact that the text context will vary too much to be able to pin down to specific parametric forms the various functions. Still, it would be useful to do this in some restricted cases. It is also obvious that Eqn. 2 needs to be tested more directly by detailed fits of distributions of fixation durations in the reading literature.

I turn now to the revised axioms on saccadic movement, which change a good deal more than the axioms on fixation, as would be anticipated from the remarks at the beginning of this section.

8.2. Revised axioms on saccades in reading

AXIOM D1. *If processing of a given word is complete, then move to the approximate center of the next word of text.*

AXIOM D2. *If processing in a given region of regard is not complete, stay put on the same word.*

AXIOM D3. *The probability of processing a word*

in a single fixation monotonically decreases with increasing number of letters in the word.

AXIOM D4. *If processing of the word in the region of regard cannot be completed, backtrack to the immediately preceding word or phrase.*

AXIOM D5. *The probability of having to backtrack monotonically increases with increasing ambiguity or difficulty of the grammatical structure in which the word in the present region of regard is embedded.*

AXIOM D6. *If the present region of regard also provides a perceptual image of the next word and the processing of it has been completed, then skip over the next word to the following one.*

AXIOM D7. *The probability of skipping over a word monotonically decreases with increasing length and, for words of the same length, is highest for frequently occurring function words.*

AXIOM D8. *The various probabilities mentioned are independent of the path by which the current region of regard has been reached, and the length of the next saccade is independent of the current fixation duration or the previous length of saccade.*

It is worth reviewing where the various features mentioned at the beginning of this section are taken into account in the axioms. For example, Axiom D3 takes into account the effect of the number of letters in a word on the number of fixations (Kliegl et al., 1983). The effect of word length on the length of the saccadic movement (O'Regan, 1979) is expressed in Axiom D1. The greater distance is taken care of by the reference to the approximate center of the next word. It should be noted, however, that O'Regan et al. (1984) have shown that the saccadic movement is actually on average slightly to the left of the center of words having more than five letters. O'Regan calls this the *convenient viewing position*, justified in the case of English and French by the fact that the first letters of a word carry more information than its last letters (Boerse and Zwaan, 1966; Eriksen and Eriksen, 1974). The effect is not large, so it has not been explicitly included in the axioms. The relatively higher probability of skipping function words (O'Regan, 1979) is covered in Axiom D7, and the effects of grammatical structure (e.g., Frazier, 1983) are covered in Axiom D5.

It seems to me that Axiom D5 is to be regarded as the most defective because it does not spell out the various kinds of ambiguous or difficult grammatical structures. It would be desirable to replace Axiom D5 by a set of more specific axioms as greater agreement is reached on the effects of grammatical structure. I should also mention that backtracking beyond the immediately preceding word or phrase is not covered in the axioms, because the data of Hogaboam (1983) and others show that almost all backtracking is for a short distance only.

The monotonicity assumptions expressed in the various axioms are not surprising. Their presence is meant to reflect the fact that a significant effect of variables such as word length has been found. That the probabilities of different types of movement and length of movements satisfy strong independence of path assumptions as represented in Axiom D8 is supported by experimental studies cited earlier, e.g., Rayner and McConkie (1976), although still further tests would be desirable.

It is quite obvious that the axioms can be improved by reducing the level of abstraction and by introducing additional variables that affect saccades. How much these additional variables will improve the account of reading is on present evidence not clear. One issue that would be clarified by the introduction of additional variables is the issue of whether saccades are programmed only on the basis of present processing of a word, or whether they are preprogrammed. Saccades during performance of simple tasks, e.g., fixating a sequence of dots, may be preprogrammed (Zingale and Kowler, 1987). A better understanding of saccadic programming during reading is needed to settle this rather important cognitive issue, which at the present is still open.

The TDPC model is also defective as a general model of reading, because it does not provide an explicit parsing mechanism and semantic analysis of the meaning of words, phrases and sentences, i.e., the model provides neither syntactic nor semantic parsing. In that sense a model which concentrates on eye movement as the TDPC model does is quite insufficient as a complete model of reading. The real scientific question, however, is whether the introduction of detailed mechanisms of syntactic and semantic parsing can be shown to be at all closely related to eye movements in reading. It is at least a reasonable conjecture that the relationship is rather weak. For example, it may not be possible at the level of different eye-movement data to distinguish possible parsing mechanisms, which reflect different current theories of syntactic and semantic parsing. It does seem possible that by examining eye movements for readers of texts in different languages some insights into grammatical parsing might be obtained. Although most of the main current varieties of grammars put forth by linguists are not really formulated with psychological processing as a central concern, it would still be of interest to see whether eye movements in reading could shed light on the internal parsing that takes place, and the same is possibly even more true for semantic parsing and representation. For this purpose, more psychologically and computationally realistic parsing mechanisms will need to be developed.

9. Summary

Three stochastic eye-movement models for arithmetic and reading performance have been proposed, one for arithmetic and two for reading. Each model characterizes a real-time stochastic process in terms of fixation durations and saccadic movement, but only direction and length of saccades are considered, not acceleration or velocity. Aspects of the models that are emphasized, partly because of their general neglect in the literature, are the probability distribution of fixation durations and the random walk of saccade directions.

The distributions of fixation duration are approximately exponential, but systematic deviations can be accounted for in the models, even though the fit to data is not perfect. In the case of the arithmetic algorithms of addition and subtraction, the random walk of the normative model has only two possible moves. Data are also presented on backtracking, skipping and wandering eye movements, each of which has a significant relative frequency.

The first reading model is called a minimal control model, because it does not take account of the effects of many local variables, e.g., word length, that have been extensively studied. The axioms on fixation duration for the minimal control model are the same as for the arithmetic model. Abstracting from the different arrangement of stimuli in arithmetic algorithms and in linear text, the axioms on saccadic motion for the two models are also essentially identical.

The stochastic nature of both models is strongly supported by data on the independence of fixation durations from previous fixation durations. Additional detailed evidence is presented for the arithmetic model.

To better account for a great variety of experimental results concerning significant effects on eye movements in reading, a text-dependent probabilistic model of reading is introduced. Significant local effects fall into three classes, identified as line, word and grammatical variables. The revised axioms embody five features of text known to be significant: (i) fixation duration depends on the number of letters in a word; (ii) a saccade is longer when a longer word is to the right; (iii) a saccade is longer when the current fixation is on a longer word; (iv) high-frequency fixation words have the highest probability of being skipped; (v) ambiguous or difficult grammatical structures increase backtracking.

References

Andriessen, J.J. and Devoogd, A.H. (1973) Analysis of eye movement patterns in silent reading. IPO Annu. Prog. Rep. 8, 30–35.

Boerse, A.C. and Zwaan, E.J. (1966) The information value of initial letters in the identification of words. J. Verbal Learn. Verbal Behav. 5, 441–446.

Carpenter, P.A. and Just, M.A. (1983) What your eyes do while your mind is reading. In: K. Rayner (Ed.), Eye Movements in Reading: Perceptual and Language Processes, Academic Press, New York, pp. 275–307.

Communale, A.S. (1973) Visual selectivity in reading: a study of the relationship between eye movements and linguistic structure. Diss. Abstr. Int. 34, 1692–1693.

Cornsweet, T.N. and Crane, H.D. (1973) Accurate two-dimensional eyetracker using first and fourth Purkinje images. J. Opt. Soc. Am. 63, 921–928.

Crane, H.D. and Steele, C.S. (1978) An accurate three-dimensional eyetracker. Appl. Opt. 17, 691–705.

Cunitz, R.J. and Steinman, R.M. (1969) Comparison of saccadic eye movements during fixation and reading. Vision Res. 9, 683–693.

De Corte, E. and Verschaffel, L. (1987) Oogbewegingen van eersteklassers tijdens het oplossen van redactie-opgaven. (Eye movements of first graders during word problem solving.) Pedagog. Stud. 64, 137–149.

Dee-Lucas, D., Just, M.A., Carpenter, P.A. and Daneman, M. (1982) What eye fixations tell us about the time course of text integration. In: R. Groner and P. Fraisse (Eds.), Cognition and Eye Movements, North-Holland, Amsterdam, pp. 155–168.

Eriksen, B.A. and Eriksen, C.W. (1974) The importance of being first: a tachistoscopic study of the contribution of each letter to the recognition of four-letter words. Percept. Psychophys. 15, 66–72.

Frazier, L. (1983) Processing sentence structure. In: K. Rayner (Ed.), Eye Movements in Reading: Perceptual and Language Processes. Academic Press, New York, pp. 215–236.

Gale, A.G. and Johnson, F. (Eds.) (1984) Theoretical and Applied Aspects of Eye Movement Research, North-Holland, Amsterdam.

Groner, R. and Groner, M. (1982) Towards a hypothetico-deductive theory of cognitive activity. In: R. Groner and P. Fraisse (Eds.), Cognition and Eye Movements. North-Holland, Amsterdam, pp. 100–121.

Groner, R. and Groner, M. (1983) A stochastic hypothesis testing model for multi-term series problems, based on eye fixations. In: R. Groner, C. Menz, D.F. Fisher and R.A. Monty (Eds.), Eye Movements and Psychological Functions. International Views, Hillsdale, NJ, pp. 257–274.

Harris, C.M., Hainline, L., Abramov, I., Lemerise, E. and Camenzuli, C. (1988) The distribution of fixation durations in infants and naive adults. Vision Res. 28, 419–432.

Heller, D. (1982) Eye movements in reading. In: R. Groner and P. Fraisse (Eds.), Cognition and Eye Movements. North-Holland, Amsterdam, pp. 139–154.

Heller, D. and Müller, H. (1980) Augenbewegungen beim Lesen von Sprachapproximationen. Forschungsbericht 1979 des Psychologischen Instituts der Universität Würzburg, Würzburg, pp. 63–81.

Hogaboam, T.W. (1983) Reading patterns in eye movement data. In: K. Rayner (Ed.), Eye Movements in Reading: Perceptual and Language Processes. Academic Press, New York, pp. 309–332.

Jacobs, A.M. (1987) On the role of blank spaces for eye-movement control in visual search. Percept. Psychophys. 41, 473–479.

Just, M.A. and Carpenter, P.A. (1980) A theory of reading: from eye fixations to comprehension. Psychol. Rev. 87, 329–354.

Kerr, J.S. and Underwood, G. (1984) Fixation time on anaphoric pronouns decreases with congruity of reference. In: A.G. Gale and F. Johnson (Eds.), Theoretical and Applied Aspects of Eye Movement Research. North-Holland, Amsterdam, pp. 195–202.

Kliegl, R., Olson, R.K. and Davidson, B.J. (1982) Regression analysis as a tool for studying reading processes: comment on Just and Carpenter's eye fixation theory. Memory Cognition 10, 287–295.

Kliegl, R., Olson, R.K. and Davidson, B.J. (1983) On problems of unconfounding perceptual and language processes. In: K. Rayner (Ed.), Eye Movements in Reading: Perceptual and Language Processes. Academic Press, New York, pp. 333–343.

Lévy-Schoen, A. (1980) La flexibilité des saccades et des fixations au cours de la lecture. Ann. Psychol. 80, 121–136.

Lévy-Schoen, A. and O'Regan, K. (1979) The control of eye movements in reading. In: O.A. Kolers, M.W. Wrolstad and H. Bouma (Eds.) Processing of Visible Language. Plenum Press, New York, pp. 7–36.

McConkie, G.E. (1983) Eye movements and perception during reading. In: K. Rayner (Ed.) Eye Movements in Reading: Perceptual and Language Processes. Academic Press, New York, pp. 65–96.

McConkie, G.E. and Rayner, K. (1975) The span of the effective stimulus during a fixation in reading. Percept. Psychophys. 17, 578–586.

McConkie, G.E. and Underwood, N.R. (1981) Some temporal characteristics of perception during a fixation in reading. An unpublished manuscript. (Available from George W. McConkie, Center for the Study of Reading, 51 Gentry Dr., Champaign, IL 61820.)

Mehler, J., Bever, T.G. and Carey, P. (1967) What we look at when we read. Percept. Psychophys. 2, 213–218.

Nachmias, J. (1959) Two dimensional motions of the retinal image during monocular fixation. J. Opt. Soc. Am. 49, 901–908.

Morton, J. (1966) A two hours reading course. Nature 211, 323–324.

O'Regan, K. (1975) Structural and contextural constraints on eye movements in reading. Unpublished doctoral thesis, University of Cambridge.

O'Regan, K. (1979) Saccade size control in reading: evidence for the linguistic control hypothesis. Percept. Psychophys. 25, 501–509.

O'Regan, K. (1980) The control of saccade size and fixation duration during reading: the limits of linguistic control. Percept. Psychophys. 28, 112–117.

O'Regan, K. (1981) The "Convenient Viewing Position" hypothesis. In: D.F. Fisher, R.A. Monty and J.W. Senders (Eds.) Eye Movements: Cognition and Visual Perception, Erlbaum, Hillsdale, NJ, pp. 289–298.

O'Regan, J.K., Lévy-Schoen, A., Pynte, J. and Brugaillère, B.

(1984) Convenient fixation location within isolated words of different length and structure. J. Exp. Psychol. Hum. Percept. Performance 10, 250–257.

Rayner, K. (1975a) The perceptual span and peripheral cues in reading. Cognitive Psychol. 7, 65–81.

Rayner, K. (1975b) Parafoveal identification during a fixation in reading. Acta Psychol. 39, 271–282.

Rayner, K. (1977) Visual attention in reading: Eye movements reflect cognitive processing. Memory Cognition 4, 443–448.

Rayner, K. (1983) The perceptual span and eye movement control during reading. In: K. Rayner (Ed.), Eye Movements in Reading: Perceptual and Language Processes. Academic Press, New York, pp. 97–120.

Rayner, K. and Bertera, J.H. (1979) Reading without a fovea. Science 206, 468–469.

Rayner, K., Inhoff, A.W., Morrison, R.E., Slowiaczek, M.L. and Bertera, J.H. (1981) Masking of foveal and parafoveal vision during eye fixations in reading. J. Exp. Psychol. Hum. Percept. Performance 7, 167–179.

Rayner, K. and McConkie, G.W. (1976) What guides a reader's eye movements? Vision Res. 16, 829–837.

Rayner, K. and Pollatsek, A. (1981) Eye movement control during reading: evidence for direct control. Q. J. Exp. Psychol. 33A, 351–373.

Sun, F., Morita, M. and Stark, L.W. (1985) Comparative patterns of reading eye movement in Chinese and English. Percept. Psychophys. 37, 502–506.

Suppes, P. (1972) Facts and fantasies of education, Phi Delta Kappa Monograph. Reprinted in M.C. Wittrock (Ed.), Changing Education: Alternatives from Educational Research. Prentice-Hall, Englewood Cliffs, NJ, 1973, pp. 6–45.

Suppes, P. (1980) Procedural semantics. In: R. Haller and W. Grassl (Eds.), Language, Logic and Philosophy (Proceedings of the 4th International Wittgenstein Symposium, Kirchberg/Wechel, Austria, 1979). Hölder-Pichler-Tempsky, Vienna, pp. 27–34.

Suppes, P., Cohen, M., Laddaga, R., Anliker J. and Floyd, H. (1982) Research on eye movements in arithmetic performance. In: R. Groner and P. Fraisse (Eds.), Cognition and Eye Movements. North-Holland, Amsterdam, pp. 57–73.

Suppes, P., Cohen, M., Laddaga, R., Anliker, J. and Floyd, R. (1983) A procedural theory of eye movements in doing arithmetic. J. Math. Psychol. 27, 341–369.

Tinker, M.A. (1958) Recent studies of eye movements in reading. Psychol. Bull. 55, 215–231.

Wanat, S.F. (1976) Language behind the eyes: some findings, speculations and research strategies. In: R.A. Monty and J.W. Senders (Eds.), Eye Movements and Psychological Processes. Erlbaum, Hillsdale, NJ.

Woodworth, R.S. (1938) Experimental Psychology. Henry Holt, New York.

Zingale, C.M. and Kowler, E. (1987) Planning sequences of saccades. Vision Res. 27, 1327–1341.

Subject index